TWELFTH EDITION

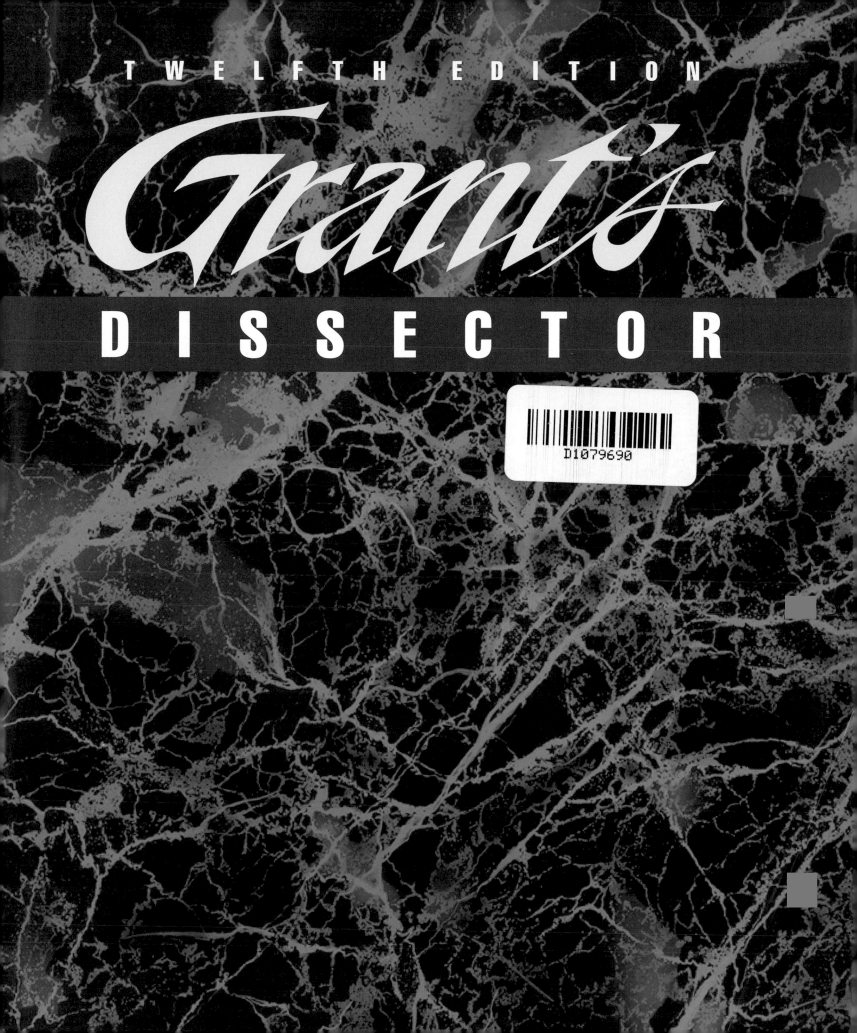

Grant's

DISSECTOR

Eberhardt (Ebo) K. Sauerland has a diversified and multifarious background. With doctoral degrees in medicine and neurophysiology, he started his career as a researcher in aerospace medicine. He joined the faculty at UCLA where he taught gross anatomy and met Dr. Grant, a visiting professor at the time. Later, he taught anatomy as a professor in the University of Texas System. In addition, he served as a major in the military, coordinating medical research in the US Air Force. With residency training in radiology and psychiatry, Dr Sauerland is an accomplished clinician with a passion for teaching. More recently he has been instrumental in improving mental health care in the forensic setting. However, anatomy continues to play a major part in Dr. Sauerland's life, and he enjoys teaching as a visiting professor at various institutions.

Wanda S. Sauerland's background and interests range from journalism to applied computer science. Wanda has been working for nearly a decade with various advanced *Adobe* software, and she is in the process of obtaining certified teaching credentials in this specialized computer field. For the 12th Edition of the Dissector, she created images and artwork in *Adobe Photoshop*, using special techniques for layering and composition. She composed the general layout for the *Dissector* in *Adobe PageMaker*. Wanda enjoys teaching computer basics to beginners. She is particularly interested in information technology and in the future of the Internet.

TWELFTH EDITION

Grant's

DISSECTOR

EBERHARDT K. SAUERLAND, M.D.

Adjunct Professor of Anatomy

Department of Cellular and Structural Biology
The University of Texas Health Science Center
San Antonio, Texas

WANDA S. SAUERLAND

Adjunct Professor of Anatomy

LIPPINCOTT WILLIAMS & WILKINS
A Wolters Kluwer Company
Philadelphia • Baltimore • New York • London
Buenos Aires • Hong Kong • Sydney • Tokyo

Editor: Paul J. Kelly
Managing Editor: Kathleen Scogna
Marketing Manager: Christine Kushner
Production Manager: Susan Rockwell
Digital Art and Composition: Wanda S. Sauerland

351 West Camden Street
Baltimore, Maryland 21201-2436 USA

530 Walnut Street
Philadelphia, Pennsylvania 19106-3621 USA

Printed in the United States of America

By J.C.B. Grant and H.A. Cates:
First Edition, 1940
Second Edition, 1945
Third Edition, 1948
Fourth Edition, 1953

By J.C.B. Grant:
Fifth Edition, 1959
Sixth Edition, 1967

By E.K. Sauerland:
Seventh Edition, 1974
Eighth Edition, 1978
Ninth Edition, 1984
Tenth Edition, 1991
Eleventh Edition, 1994

Sauerland, Eberhardt K., 1933-
Grant's dissector.--12th ed. / Eberhardt K. Sauerland; digital arrangements of text and illustrations by Wanda S. Sauerland.
p. cm.
Includes index.
ISBN 0-683-30739-8
1. Human dissection Laboratory manuals. I. Grant, J.C. Boileau (John Charles Boileau), 1886-1973. II. Title. III. Title: Dissector
[DNLM: 1. Dissection Laboratory Manuals. QS 130 S255g 1999]
QM34.G75 1999
611--dc21
DNLM/DLC
for Library of Congress 99-25214
CIP

To purchase additional copies of this book, call our customer service department at **(800) 638-3030** or fax orders to **(301) 824-7390**. For other book services, including chapter reprints and large quantity sales, ask for the Special Sales department. International customers should call **(301)714-2324.**

Visit Lippincott Williams & Wilkins on the Internet: **http://www.lww.com**. Lippincott Williams & Wilkins customer service representatives are available from 8:30 am to 6:00 pm, EST.

00 01 02 03
3 4 5 6 7 8 9 10

140 Ohs

PREFACE

THE BUSY PROFESSOR, who is accustomed to quickly come to the point, might comment:
"So, you have a new edition here. Tell me in a few words what has and what has not changed."

What HAS NOT changed:
The method of dissection; the sequence of dissections; the sequence of chapters.
All are identical to what was presented in the previous 11th edition.

What HAS changed:
There are 25% more illustrations, and they are in full color to increase clarity.
The text is now referenced to five major atlases and a video atlas.
Human anatomical dissections can now be more time-efficient than ever.

* * * * *

The first edition of *GRANT'S DISSECTOR* appeared over half a century ago in 1940. During the following six editions in three decades, this manual became an almost indispensable item for American and Canadian students engaged in human anatomical dissections. In 1972, Professor J. C. Boileau Grant asked me to prepare the seventh and subsequent editions of the *DISSECTOR* and to adapt this manual to the ever-changing needs of medical school and/or health sciences curricula. This mandate is particularly applicable at the present time.

We live in an age of information explosion. Nowhere is this more evident than in the medical sciences. The modern medical student is accustomed to utilizing rapid changes in information technology; and as technology changes, so does the student's approach and *modus operandi* of learning. A keen academician recently noted that "students are changing significantly from year to year now."

This realization presents an enormous challenge to medical educators, particularly in the field of anatomy. Health sciences curricula tend to allocate fewer and fewer hours to anatomy. Yet, experienced educators and clinicians recognize the fact that the gross structural substrate of the human body, including three-dimensional conceptualization, *must* be mastered before dealing with it in the diagnostic setting, the emergency room, or the operating suite; this is only fair to those we want to serve, our patients.

The dichotomy between available and actually needed time for adequate teaching, learning, and reinforcement, presents a dilemma for the teaching faculty. A partial remedy is to increase time efficiency in the laboratory. Therefore, every effort has been made in the current 12th edition to save time or to use a more time-efficient approach. This was done by offering speedy referencing to atlas illustrations, color coding between text and figures, and increasing the clarity of anatomical structures shown in illustrations.

The 12th edition of *GRANT'S DISSECTOR* offers detailed instructions for students who perform dissections. Yet, at the same time, it is an informative guide for students who review gross anatomy. Thus, this manual is intended to serve two purposes: (1) to guide human anatomical dissections and (2) to facilitate the study and review of gross anatomy, preferably in the context of clinical significance. The *DISSECTOR* is **not** a replacement for a textbook. Although amply illustrated, it is **not** an atlas.

Well-informed, contemporary students have more choices now than in the past; for example, it is not uncommon that students select an anatomical atlas of their personal choice. Furthermore, the teaching faculty and individual professors have their own preferences concerning anatomical atlases. Atlas references save our students an enormous amount of time, particularly when it is of the essence in the dissecting lab. We have recognized that need when, in 1974, we first referenced exclusively to the 6th edition of *GRANT'S ATLAS*. Now, we have vastly expanded our reference system. We have created an unobtrusive middle reference column that allows us to refer to the right and left page halves without cluttering the text. The new 12th edition of *GRANT'S DISSECTOR* offers more than 6,500 citations of illustrations in five major atlases: ***Grant's Atlas of Anatomy***, 10th ed., Anne M. R. Agur, Ph.D., Ming J. Lee, M.D.; ***Color Atlas of Anatomy: A Photographic Study of the Human Body***, 4th ed., Prof. Johannes W. Rohen. M.D., Prof. Chihiro Yokochi, M.D., Prof. Lütjen-Drecoll, M.D.; ***A.D.A.M. Student Atlas of Anatomy***, Todd R. Olson, Ph.D.; ***Atlas of Human Anatomy***, 2nd ed., Frank H. Netter, M.D.; ***Anatomy: A Regional Atlas of the Human Body,*** 4th ed., Carmine D. Clemente, Ph.D.

In addition, the middle reference columns provide nearly 700 references to ***The Video Atlas of Human Anatomy*** by Dr. Robert D. Acland. These high-quality videotapes show clear three-dimensional views of real, unembalmed cadaver dissections. They provide an invaluable teaching and learning resource for understanding human anatomical structure. All four videotapes have built-in visible timers that help the user to precisely locate the stated reference.

The importance of pertinent and clear illustrations is obvious because they guide the student in time-efficient dissection and recognition of significant structures. In comparison with the previous edition, we have increased the overall number of illustrations by 25%; and 35% of all illustrations have been newly created. Most importantly, we are now showing all illustrations in full color, thus increasing clarity and faster recognition of key structures.

Each chapter of the *DISSECTOR* stands alone as an independent unit. Thus, anatomical dissections may be carried out in any sequence desired and as specified by the instructor. The teaching staff may choose to delete certain parts of this manual from the class assignment. This is often necessary because many gross anatomy courses across the nation are under severe time constraints. On the other hand, additional dissection projects may be desirable, particularly for students on special assignments or on elective rotations. These projects have been grouped together in the *APPENDICES* and include such topics as the lumbar approach to the kidney, dissection of smaller joints, dissection of the bull's eye, and the dissection of fetus and placenta. The dissection procedures for fetus and placenta was last offered in the 9th edition. However, in response to numerous requests, we are reintroducing this clinically relevant and important section into the current 12th edition.

The new format of the *DISSECTOR* allows the student to quickly cover anatomy point by point, stressing the clinical significance of anatomical structures. It is our objective to save time whenever possible without loss of quality education. Consequently:

- The text is concise. Often a step by step approach is used, highlighting each topic with a highly visible bullet.
- Dissection instructions are clearly identifiable because they stand out on a bright yellow background in slightly larger print.
- New and improved illustrations and diagrams in full color quickly convey information and concepts.
- Thousands of references to appropriate illustrations of five major atlases ensure the most time-efficient and complete use of an accompanying atlas during anatomical dissections or review.
- Since rapid and competent dissections (as well as clinical examinations) often depend on a thorough knowledge of pertinent bony reference points, a brief discussion of relevant bony landmarks of each anatomical region is included.
- At the end of each chapter, the *DISSECTOR* offers one or more self-tests for the student's achieved competence in three-dimensional anatomical concepts. These tests are called GAPP, an acronym standing for **G**ROSS **A**NATOMY **P**RACTICAL **P**RIMER. It is intended to help the student build confidence and prepare for modern diagnostic modalities such as CT and MRI.
- Studies in gross anatomy are more meaningful to students if they are aware of the *clinical significance* of various structures. Clinically relevant comments complement the regular text. These clinical correlations are set in smaller type and boxed for special attention and quick referral.

IN SUMMARY, the present 12th edition of *GRANT'S DISSECTOR* has been carefully designed to offer a solid and useful core of anatomical knowledge in an educational environment where time is of the essence.

E. K. SAUERLAND, M.D.

ACKNOWLEDGMENTS

Personal Considerations

Most authors, when involved in a major undertaking, have to apologize to their extended family for their seeming detachment and lack of time. Not only do I fall into this category, but I also had to ask my wife Wanda, a medical writer and expert in computer graphics, to live and breathe "The Dissector" day in and day out for well over a full year. I wish to thank her for her conceptual contributions, the interviews she conducted with students in the dissecting lab, and the resulting practical suggestions. Her greatest contribution was the difficult artwork that demanded full color rendition of over 400 illustrations, many of them newly designed. And then there were the countless hours during which she put all text, illustrations, labels and captions into digital format and generally managed and edited a vast amount of digital data. In addition, my daughter Laura Burnett, an Executive Coordinator in her own right, spent considerable time proofreading for the 3rd printing of this edition. Her valuable services are much appreciated.

Student Input

The composition of this edition of the Dissector has benefitted from the many suggestions made by students either through Internet communications or in actual interviews. In this regard, we especially thank the Medical Class of 2001 of the University of California at San Diego and Dr. Mark C. Whitehead, who made this valuable access possible. We invite our students, past and future, to send continued input and suggestions to acerland@hotmail.com.

Esteemed Colleagues

I am grateful to my friend and mentor, the late Professor J.C.B. Grant, as well as to a number of colleagues who have provided excellent ideas and suggestions for the improvement of various past editions of this manual. Their names are cited here in *alphabetical order*: Doctores Susan Abbondanzo, Erle Adrian, Anne Agur, J. Collins, R.V. Gregg, Craig Hammes, R.M. Harper, Linda Johnson, R.D. Laurenson, G.F. Lewis, D.I. Lewis-Jones, R.G. MacKenzie, Roger Marchand, Keith Moore, R.R. Peterson, Tracey Sauerland, C.H. Sawyer, M.F. Teaford, K. Thibodeau, J.S. Thompson, and Robert Trelease. The time and thought of the following recent reviewers is gratefully acknowledged: Doctores Nancey Bookstein, Andrew Evan, Gary Mattingly, and N. Anthony Moore. Many other anatomists and reviewers have contributed anonymously by providing comments to the Editorial Staff at Williams & Wilkins; their constructive ideas are greatly appreciated. We also acknowledge with thanks the contributions of Dr. Robert DePhilip and his staff at Ohio State University for pointing out inaccuracies that were corrected in the second and third printing of this edition. The constructive comments by Dr. Micheal Iwanik, University of Virginia School of Medicine, were most helpful. The Author expresses special appreciation to Dr. Ernest W. April, College of Physicians and Surgeons at Columbia University, N.Y., for his detailed and exhaustive review of the text and illustrations.

Illustrations

The production of over 400 color images for this 12th edition of ***Grant's Dissector*** required a monumental effort on part of the Sauerland Team. Fortunately, we had at our disposal numerous black and white line drawings previously published by Williams & Wilkins in ***Grant's Dissector*** (6th through 11th editions), in ***Grant's Method*** (7th and 8th editions), and in ***Grant's Atlas*** (5th and 8th editions). Most of these original line drawing were the work of two of Dr. Grant's favorite artists: Dorothy Chubb and Nancy Joy; one illustration was drawn by A. Porter.

Some of our new illustrations were inspired by classic atlas illustrations. For example, Figure 3.40 is a modified drawing of Figure 419 in Clemente, *A Regional Atlas of the Human Body*, 4th edition. Figures 2.28 and 2.51 are modifications and adaptations from Netter's *Atlas of Human Anatomy*, 2nd edition, Plate 253. Netter's classic illustrations in the *CIBA Collection* also inspired the drawings of our Figures 2.7 and 3.11. One classic art illustration by Richter, *Anatomie Artistique*, Paris (1890), served as the background for our surface anatomy depictions, Figures 4.1, 6.1, and 6.12. The radiographic material shown in this edition (Figures 1.44, 7.11, and 7.86) belong to the author's personal collection of radiographic images. Several of the new illustrations in this edition were borrowed, with permission, from the *Well-Informed Patient Series* (WIPS), which is also authored and produced by the Sauerland Team.

The Team at Lippincott Williams & Wilkins

At Lippincott Williams and Wilkins, the cast of dedicated contributors to every aspect of the book publishing business is most impressive. Their efforts under the leadership of *Tim Satterfield, Executive Vice President, Education and Reference Publishing*, are gratefully acknowledged. In particular, I appreciate the professional dedication and foresight of *Paul Kelly, Acquisition Editor*, who embraced our efforts to include full color illustrations and multiple atlas references into this edition. *Crystal Taylor,* the accomplished and proficient *Managing Editor*, exerted persistent pressure on various parties to get the necessary work done in a timely fashion; yet she did so with understanding, compassion, and in a very professional manner. The concerted efforts of the following members of the team have been truly outstanding: *Susan Rockwell, Production Manager, Copyediting; Christine Kushner, Marketing Manager;* and *Mike Standen, Editorial Assistant.* In addition, *Kathleen Scogna*, *Senior Development Editor*, coordinated the important aspects for the 3rd printing of this edition.

In general, the staff at this publishing house deserves greatest praise; I should know because it has been my pleasure to work with Williams & Wilkins, now Lippincott Williams & Wilkins for more than 25 years.

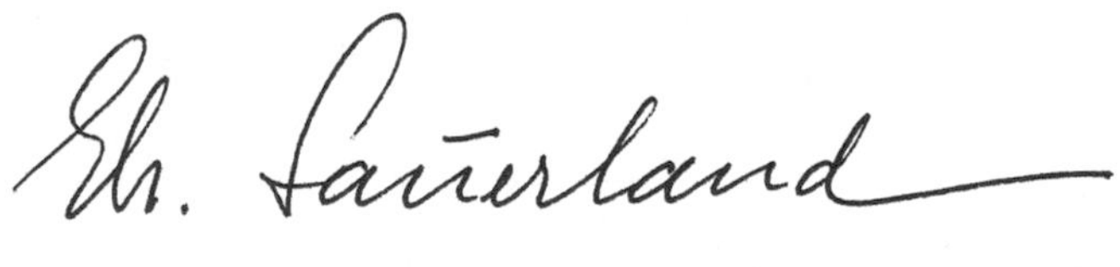

CONTENTS

3 The Pelvis And Perineum

4 The Back

5 The Lower Limb

6 The Upper Limb

7 The Head and Neck

The Appendices

Before You Begin

How To Use This Manual

The 12th edition of *Grant's Dissector* has been designed to aid the student in performing comprehensive and yet time-efficient dissections. This concept is reflected in a number of special features:

- General informative text that is preparatory to dissection is printed in black on a white background.

The text for dissection procedures is in black on a yellow background. Therefore, it is easily identified. The font size is slightly larger. As a result, the text stands out clearly.

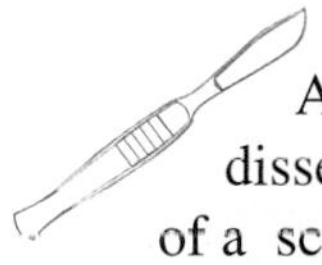

At the beginning of each anatomical region, the dissection instructions are also indicated by the icon of a scalpel.

- Individual dissection steps are highlighted by round bullets.

- The names of *important structures* are shown in **bold print.**
- *Important anatomical terms* that are **bolded** in the **text** for emphasis are also labeled with **bold type** in the accompanyiing **illustrations**.

Clinical Correlations and *Dissection Notes* are set in black text boxed by blue lines.

- Figure **references** in the text are color coded to figure legends; the figure call-outs are set in red. In that manner, the student is prompted to instantly establish a link between illustration and text. He/she is easily referred back from the illustration to the original text location to continue with reading or dissection.
- Atlas references to five major atlases (*atlantes*) are unobtrusively placed in a special middle column. These references are positioned next to the text under discussion. Small arrows point to either the left or the right text column.
- In the beginning of each chapter, there is a reminder concerning the referenced atlases, their editions, and the use of either plate numbers, figure numbers, or page numbers.

Grant's Dissector is referenced to the following five atlases and the Video Atlas of Human Anatomy as follows:

⇦
GRANT'S 6.20
ROHEN 390
A.D.A.M. 6.22
NETTER 400, 401
CLEMENTE 26-28
A.V.A. 1: 0.17.07

- **Grant's Atlas of Anatomy, 10th ed.**
  Anne M. R. Agur, Ph.D.
  Ming J. Lee, M.D.
  Lippincott Williams & Wilkins, 1999, Philadelphia

- **Color Atlas of Anatomy:**
  A Photographic Study of the Human Body, 4th ed.
  Prof. Johannes W. Rohen. M.D.
  Prof. Chihiro Yokochi, M.D.
  Prof. Lütjen-Drecoll, M.D.
  Williams & Wilkins, 1998, Baltimore

- **A.D.A.M. Student Atlas of Anatomy**
  Todd R. Olson, Ph.D.
  Williams & Wilkins, 1996, Baltimore

- **Atlas of Human Anatomy, 2nd ed.**
  Frank H. Netter, M.D.
  Arthur F. Dalley II, Ph.D., Consulting Editor
  Novartis, 1997, East Hanover, NJ

- **Anatomy:**
  A Regional Atlas of the Human Body, 4th ed.
  Carmine D. Clemente, Ph.D.
  Williams & Wilkins, 1997, Baltimore

- **The Video Atlas of Human Anatomy**
  Four Video Tapes by Robert D. Acland, FRCS
  Williams and Wilkins, 1998, Baltimore

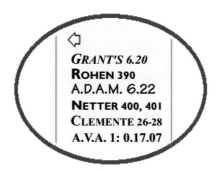

About Dissection

The Purpose of Dissection

There is no substitute for dissection, i.e., a three-dimensional approach to the structures of the human body. In the dissection lab, the student will:

- Observe and palpate the topographic relations of various structures to each other;
- Feel the texture of blood vessels, nerves, and various tissues;
- Test the rigidity of bones and the strength of ligaments;
- Explore and appreciate the three dimensions of anatomical structures;
- Prepare for an intelligent approach to physical examination and surgery.

About The Cadaver

What will the student find when assigned to a cadaver?

- The body is already preserved or embalmed.
- The whole body has been kept moist by adequate wrappings or by submersion into suitable preservative fluid.
- The veins are sometimes full of clotted blood, and sometimes empty.
- Occasionally, the arteries are injected with a (red) coloring matter.

What is the proper care for the cadaver?

- Uncover only those parts of the body to be dissected.
- Inspect every part periodically, and renew and moisten wrappings as the occasion demands.
- No part must ever be left exposed to the air needlessly.
- Special attention must be given to the face, hands, feet, and external genitalia.

Once a part is allowed to become dry and hard, it can never be fully restored, and its proper dissection is impossible. Plastic bags are particularly useful to prevent drying.

The student must always remember that former living persons have donated their bodies for medical studies benevolently and in good faith. Therefore, the cadaver must be treated with respect and dignity. Improper behavior in the dissecting laboratory (such as eating, drinking, making crude jokes, playing entertaining music, taking photographs without permission, illegally removing body parts from the laboratory, mutilations, or grave robbery, for example, by enriching oneself with the gold teeth of the deceased) cannot be tolerated.

Working Conditions in the Lab

Be sure that the light falls on the part under investigation. Adequate light is essential for efficient dissection. Work in a position that is comfortable and not tiring. Make use of blocks to stabilize parts of the cadaver and to maintain its most suitable posture. Protect clothing by wearing a long laboratory coat or apron. Wearing protective gloves has become common practice for anyone handling human material (dead or alive). You may be required to wear disposable latex gloves. When cutting bony structures, protect your eyes with glasses or goggles against flying chips.

Instruments Used for Dissection

Usually, the student will be provided with a list of dissecting instruments preferred by the faculty or individual instructors. If in doubt, procure the following instruments:

A seeker or probe (Fig. I.1) consisting of rigid steel with a bent, blunt tip. In addition, a flexible blunt probe is useful for insertion into vessels or ducts (e.g., during exploration of such structures as coronary arteries, uterine tubes, urethra, etc.). Pointed needle-like seekers, as well as abruptly hooked instruments are dangerous and should not be used.

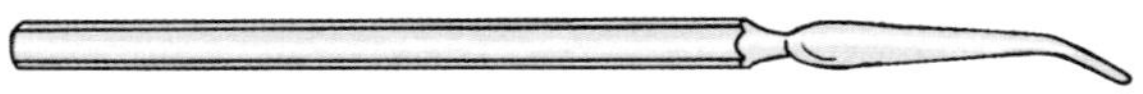

Figure I.1. A seeker.

Two pairs of forceps (Fig. I.2) with transversely ridged handles to prevent slipping. The ends should be blunt and rounded and the gripping surfaces should be corrugated. The second pair is needed for distracting the tissue. Many students find it advantageous to use one big and one small pair of forceps. The small one, mouth-toothed or sharp-pointed, is used to hold on to delicate structures.

Hemostats may be used in place of forceps. The firm clamping action of a hemostat offers many advantages.

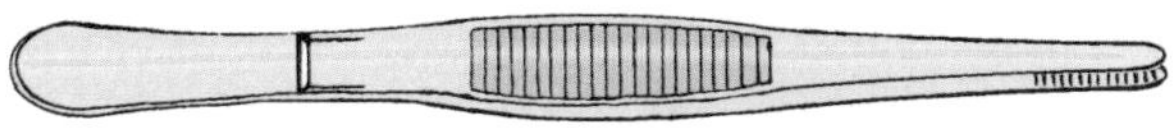

Figure I.2. A forcep.

A scalpel (Fig. I.3) designed for detachable knife blades. The scalpel handle should be made of metal (not plastic). The blade should be about 3.5 to 4 cm long. The cutting edge must have some convexity near the point. The blade must be sharp at all times. No one can do good work with a dull knife. Therefore, a sufficient supply of blades will be needed. The rounded end of the handle can be conveniently used to separate soft tissues.

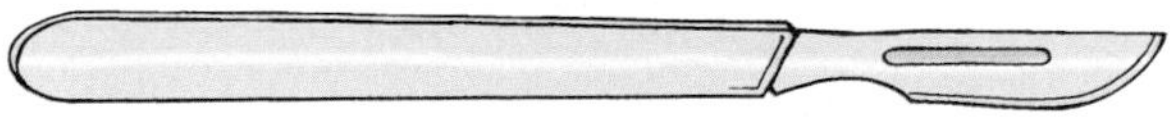

Figure I.3. A scalpel.

Two pairs of scissors (Fig. I.4): a larger, heavy dissecting scissors about 15 cm in length, and a fine pair of scissors with two sharp points for the dissection of delicate structures. Consult your instructor.

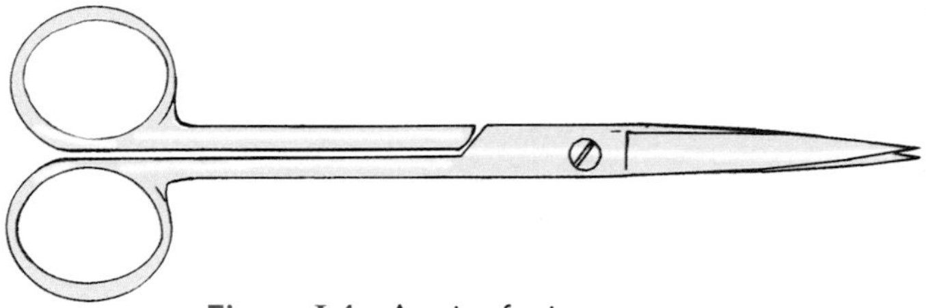

Figure I.4. A pair of scissors.

Dissecting Techniques

Keep in mind that a variable amount of subcutaneous fat lies immediately deep to the skin. That fat contains superficial nerves and vessels, particularly veins. Therefore, in removing skin, all fat should be left behind (unless instructed otherwise). In those subjects nearly devoid of fat, one needs to exercise special care; deeper structures can be easily damaged.

The thickness of skin varies from region to region. For example, the skin is relatively thin in the anterior region of the forearm; in contrast, it is considerably thicker in the area of the back. Generally, incisions should be made cautiously and not exceeding the thickness of the skin. If, during removal of skin, you see brownish muscular fibers shining through the filmy deep fascia, your cut is too deep.

Always remember to put *traction on the skin* as it is being removed (Fig. I.5), to keep the sharp knife directed against it (Fig. I.6), and to leave the fat in place (unless specified otherwise). In this manner, you will work faster and encounter fewer difficulties.

The unnecessary destruction of many soft structures can be avoided and a great deal of time can be saved by employing the method of *blunt dissection*, utilizing one's fingers or the blunt handle of the scalpel to separate various structures gently from each other. Delicate structures (e.g., fine blood vessels and nerves adhering to each other) can be efficiently separated by utilizing the *scissor technique*. As illustrated in Figure I.7, use a fine pair of scissors of the sharp-sharp type and gently force the blades apart in a direction parallel to the structures of interest.

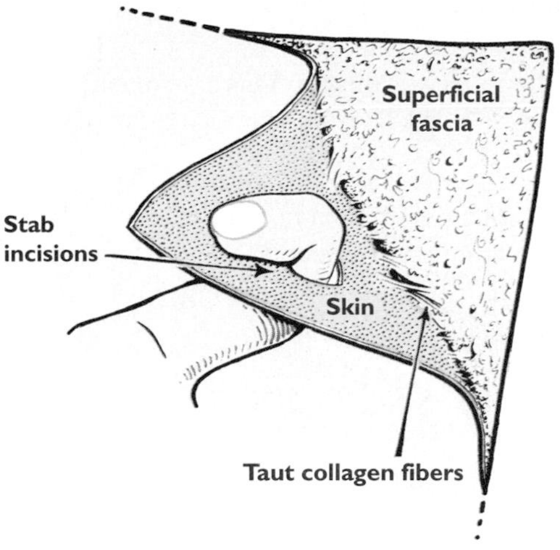

Figure I.5. When removing skin, apply traction.

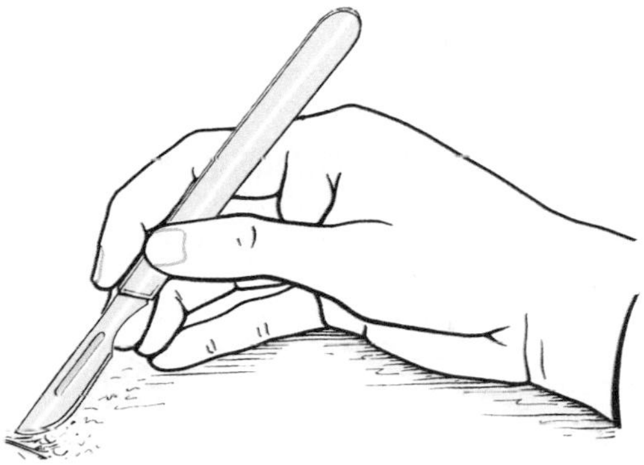

Figure I.6. When dissecting, rest the hand. Eliminate unsteady movements.

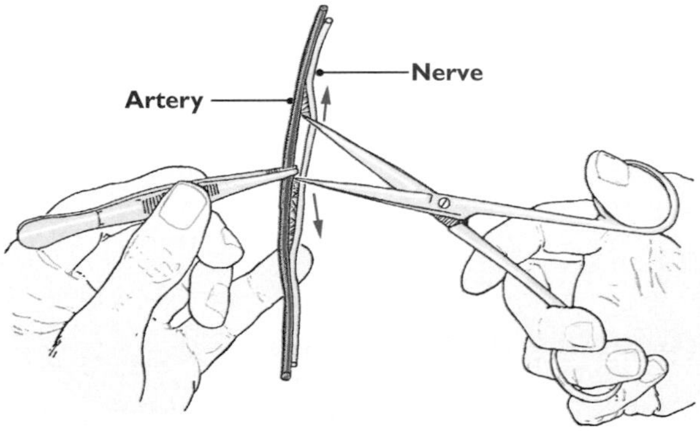

Figure I.7. Scissors technique: separating delicate structures.

Efficiency

Time is immensely valuable. Learn as much as possible in the shortest possible time. The following suggestions will help to increase efficiency.

- Acquire a *theoretical concept* of the area under investigation *before* attempting to dissect it. Do not "dig around" and happen to find "something interesting." You must deliberately search for certain structures.
- Make full use of a good *atlas* of your choice. Refer to the reference middle column to find appropriate illustrations or video demonstrations speedily and without loss of valuable time.

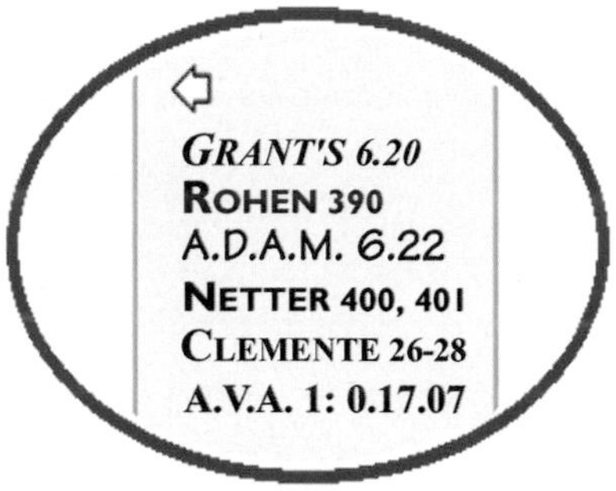

- Always palpate *bony landmarks* because they are keys in the search for related soft structures. It is mandatory to have a skull available when dissecting the head.
- *Use your time wisely*. To spend an hour tracing the terminal twigs of a cutaneous nerve when the general skin area supplied by the nerve is obvious is spending an hour for little gain. To spend 3 minutes to define the exact fiber direction of a ligament is to spend 3 minutes for great gain; you will understand why and how that ligament restrains or prevents certain movements of bony structures.
- Demonstrate the *essential features* of a given anatomical region with *clarity*. Remove fat, connective tissue, and smaller veins. If a clear-cut display of arteries is obtained, the general arrangement of the companion veins will be obvious.

Finally, we must be aware that no doctor or anatomist can please all. Instructors and professors, like students, have their own individual preferences concerning dissection methods, clinical approaches, instruments, and safety precautions. In most instances, individual variations or requirements are based on experience and good reason. Therefore, modifications of procedures are sometimes advisable.

Terminology

Anatomical Position

Anatomists have agreed to relate everything they describe to a universally approved and accepted position of the body

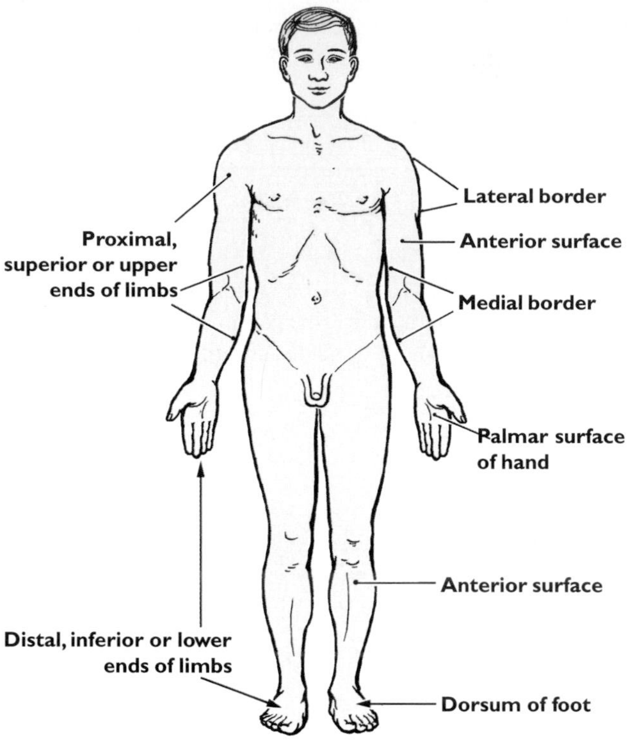

Figure I.8. Anatomical position.

(Fig.1.8). It is that position in which the body stands erect with the feet together, arms by the side and the palms facing forward. That the dissector is (on most occasions) working with the cadaver lying on its back makes not the slightest difference. The statement that a given structure is inferior to another one is clearly understood by anatomists and surgeons: it means that this given structure is nearer to the feet. Figure I.9 illustrates such essential terms as ***superior (cranial), inferior (caudal), anterior (ventral)***, and ***posterior (dorsal)***.

Anatomical Planes and Sections of the Body

The terms ***coronal, sagittal***, and ***transverse*** *(horizontal)* are explained in Figure I.10.

From a clinical point of view, the most important sections (slices) are the *cross sections or transverse sections*. These are slices of the body or of body parts that are cut at right angles to the longitudinal axis of the body. Such sectioning techniques are widely used for diagnostic purposes in *computerized tomography (CT)* and *magnetic resonance imaging (MRI)*. By established convention, slices of diagnostic images are viewed "from below"; i.e., the examiner views the sections as if looking from the feet toward the

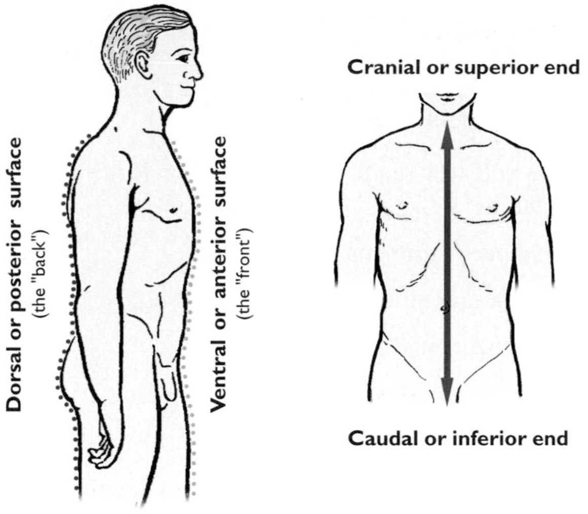

Figure I.9. Essential terms for orientation.

head. In such a view, the liver appears on the left side of an abdominal transverse section; the left lung is displayed on the right side of a section through the chest. It is very important to become familiar with this convention. Therefore, most cross-sectional images in this manual are presented in the same manner as CT or MR images.

Descriptions

Anatomical structures can be precisely described. Learn and practice to give an *accurate account* of each important structure in an *orderly* and *logical fashion.* Always project yourself into a future professional situation: Remember, you must give orderly and logical accounts when reporting on radiological findings, on performed surgery or autopsies, etc. When encountering a *muscle* during dissection or review, be aware of its size and shape, its origin and insertion, its function and its nerve supply.

Usually, muscles act on *joints*. You should be able to describe the type of joint and the extent of its movements. When studying *blood vessels*, be cognizant of their proximal and distal connections. In any region under consideration, you should know the origin and destination of encountered *nerves* as well as their functional composition (motor, sensory, mixed, autonomic).

Variations

No cadaver will conform in all details of its anatomical construction to the patterns outlined in the pages of this book. This manual describes the most *common patterns* encountered in the adult. Minor and even major

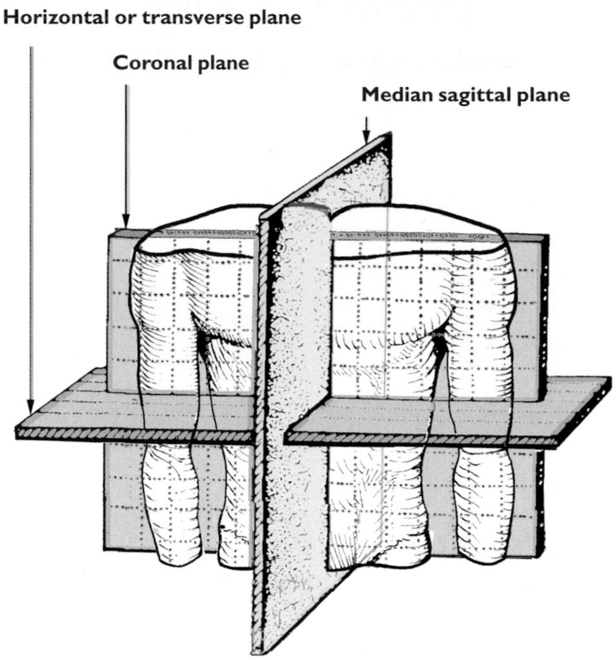

Figure I.10. Fundamental planes in the body: sagittal, coronal, and transverse.

variants frequently occur. Arteries may arise from sources other than those indicated or may pursue different courses. Muscles may have extra heads of origin or be absent entirely. Organs may vary from their usual shape and/or be found in other than "normal" positions. There may be accessory organs. The usual anatomical relations may be distorted by disease processes (e.g., cancer) or by prior surgical intervention. This is particularly true for the abdomen and thorax.

Regard the cadaver you are working on as a "typical example." In a sense, you are studying *generic anatomy*, and you will retain generally applicable information of a generic heart, generic mandible, generic foot, etc. In clinical practice, you will appreciate the individual overlay or embellishment that makes the generic principle unique. By all means, examine as many different subjects as possible. Only in this manner will you be able to familiarize yourself with the accepted "normal" and with variations and anomalies. Variations, particularly in arteries and nerves, will be mentioned in this manual whenever indicated.

Prior to dissection, the student is encouraged to make careful observations concerning the assigned cadaver and to enter these data into the provided ***Observation Box***. This information is valuable and particularly useful if clinically relevant questions arise during later dissection.

OBSERVATION BOX

CONCERNING THE ASSIGNED BODY - (CADAVER):

DATE OF ENTRY OF THIS LOG:

BODY NUMBER (TANK OR TABLE NUMBER):

BODY SEX:

GIVEN OR ESTIMATED AGE OF BODY:

BODY HEIGHT:

ESTIMATED BODY WEIGHT:

GENERAL CONDITION OF THE BODY:
(WELL NOURISHED; EMACIATED OR CACHECTIC; OBESE):

PHYSICAL CHARACTERISTICS
(SKIN COLOR; FORM OF HAIR; IS HEAD SHAVEN?):

DEFORMITIES, IF ANY:

IF BODY IS PARTIALLY DISMEMBERED?
STATE WHICH BODY PARTS ARE MISSING (E.G., LEFT LOWER LIMB):

ARE THERE CERTAIN BODY PARTS THAT HAVE BEEN PREVIOUSLY DISSECTED?

ARE THE EYEBALLS ABSENT?
(IN CASE OF DONATION OF CORNEA):

SPECIAL BODY MARKS?
TATTOOS; INDICATE AREA OF MARKED WINDOWS FOR IRRADIATION; OLD (HEALED) SCARS; FRESH (UNHEALED) INCISIONS INDICATING:

(1) ORGAN DONATION:

(2) RECENT SURGERY:

(3) PARTIAL AUTOPSY:

(4) SITES OF EMBALMMENT:

PRESERVATION:

IS THE CADAVER WELL EMBALMED?

ARE THERE GREENISH MOLD SPOTS INDICATING BODY AREAS NOT SUFFICIENTLY INFILTRATED WITH PRESERVATIVE FLUID?

CAUSE OF DEATH (IF KNOWN):

GAPP TESTS

GAPP is an acronym for Gross Anatomy Practical Primer. GAPP was conceived with several pedagogic concepts in mind. In summary, it:

- Is a self-test requiring a solid knowledge in gross anatomy;
- Enhances 3-dimensional concepts;
- Encourages students to study thoroughly;
- Boost students' self-confidence;
- Requires intelligent deductive reasoning;
- Increases professional competence;
- Prepares the student well for modern diagnostic modalities, such as CT and MRI;
- Offers a comprehensive review of each major anatomical
  region;
- Is a teaching tool.

One or more **GAPP** tests will be offered at the end of each chapter. Each GAPP test contains several anatomical images: some are conventional, others are transverse sections similar to CT or MR images. Unidentified structures are labeled with a letter or are numbered. It is the student's challenge to match the correct number/letter combination. The key for each GAPP test is printed upside down at the bottom of the page. If a student passes the GAPP self-test, she or he can be proud and confident of newly gained knowledge.

Illustrations

This book contains over 400 illustrations that are intended to orient the dissector and to facilitate the approach to a given anatomical region. They are designed to offer explanations, increase comprehension, and attract attention to a useful point of reference. The additional use of a good atlas is desirable.

CHAPTER 1
THE THORAX

GRANT'S ATLAS OF ANATOMY, 10TH ED.:	*GRANT'S FIG. #*
ROHEN, COLOR ATLAS OF ANATOMY, 4TH ED.:	ROHEN PAGE #
A.D.A.M. STUDENT ATLAS OF ANATOMY:	A.D.A.M. PLATE #
NETTER, ATLAS OF HUMAN ANATOMY, 2ND ED.:	NETTER PLATE #
CLEMENTE, ANATOMY, 4TH ED.:	CLEMENTE FIG. #
ACLAND'S VIDEO ATLAS OF HUMAN ANATOMY	A.V.A. Vol: hr.min.sec

Thoracic Wall

General Remarks

The main function of the thorax is to house and protect the vital heart and lungs. The thoracic wall is mobile to accommodate volume changes of the thorax during respiration. The main components of the thoracic wall are vertebrae, ribs, sternum, and muscles. The deep fascia covers the muscles of the thoracic wall. The superficial fascia is of variable thickness. It is located between skin and deep fascia. It contains blood vessels, lymph vessels, superficial nerves, and sweat glands. In addition, the superficial fascia of the anterior thoracic wall contains the mammary glands.

GRANT'S 1.23
A.D.A.M. 2.3, 2.6
NETTER 184
CLEMENTE 160

Bony Landmarks and Surface Anatomy

Vertebra. Examine individual bones or an articulated skeleton. Refer to a **thoracic vertebra** and note the following (Fig. 1.1):

GRANT'S 4.7, 4.8
ROHEN 184
A.D.A.M. 1.11, 1.12
NETTER 143
CLEMENTE 658-661
A.V.A. 3: 0.03.30

- Identify the weight-bearing **body** and a protective vertebral arch, which is made up of two rounded pedicles (roots) and two flat plates or laminae.
- At the junction of the **pedicle** and **lamina**, a **transverse process** projects laterally, and **articular processes** project superiorly and inferiorly.
- At the junction of the two laminae, a **spinous process** projects posteriorly in the median plane. The bodies and transverse processes of the thoracic vertebrae have facets for the ribs.

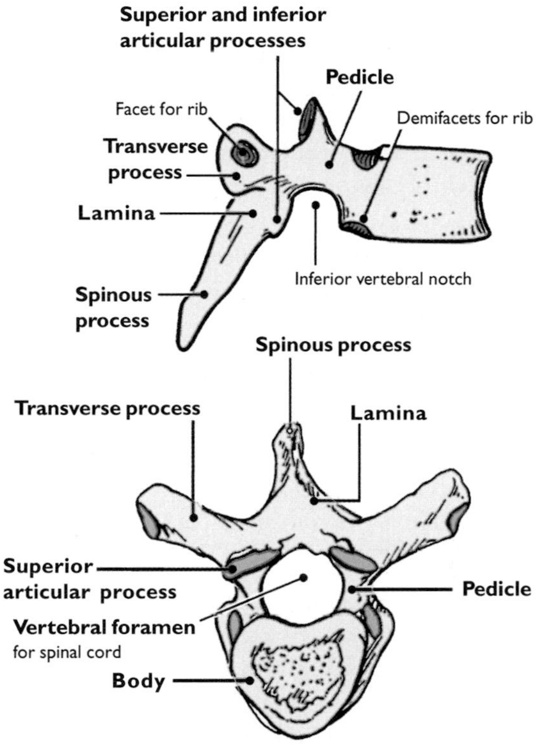

Figure 1.1. Typical thoracic vertebra in lateral and superior view.

- Place your index finger in the **vertebral foramen** of a vertebra. Observe that the size and shape of the vertebral foramina differ from vertebra to vertebra. In the articulated vertebral column, the vertebral foramina collectively form a bony tube, the **vertebral canal**. This canal encloses and protects the spinal cord.

> ***Clinical Correlation:*** Abnormal curvatures of the spine (kyphosis, with convexity backward; scoliosis, lateral curvature or deformity) may be seen in the dissecting laboratory. These clinical conditions may produce alterations of the shape and volume capacity of the thoracic cavity.

Ribs. Refer to one or more **ribs** and note the following features (Fig. 1.2):

- Identify **head, neck, tubercle,** and **body**.
- On the external surface, observe the angle where the body takes a bend and also a twist; therefore, a rib will not lie flat on a table.
- The lower border of a typical rib is sharp with an internal flange-like **costal groove** to shelter the intercostal nerve and vessels.
- Note the distinctly different shape of the **first rib** (Fig. 1.4). It is the highest, shortest, broadest, and most curved. On occasion, there may be a cervical rib, which is usually due to an enlarged costal element of the 7th cervical vertebra. A bicipital rib occurs when there is partial fusion of two adjacent ribs.

◁
GRANT'S 1.9, 1.10
ROHEN 188
A.D.A.M. 1.16
NETTER 171
CLEMENTE 155
A.V.A. 3: 0.39.54

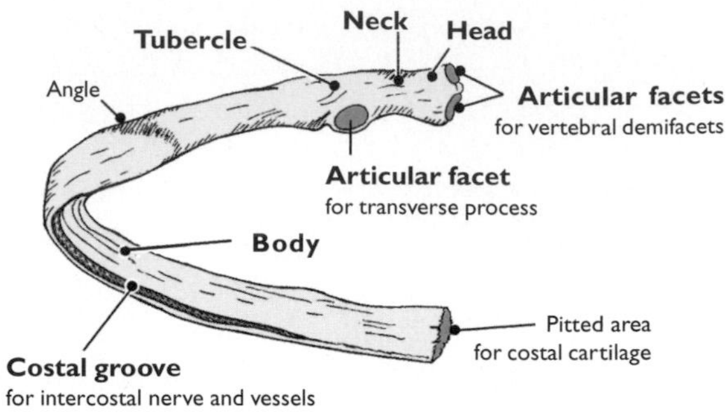

Figure 1.2. Typical left rib, posterior view.

Articulated Vertebral Column. Refer to an **articulated vertebral column** and note the following (Fig. 1.3):

- Two adjacent vertebral bodies are united by a fibrocartilaginous **intervertebral disc**. This is a joint of the symphysis variety.
- Two adjacent vertebral arches are united by their articular processes.
- An **intervertebral foramen** is completed between the pedicles of two adjacent vertebrae. It transmits the spinal nerve of the corresponding segment and associated spinal blood vessels.
- The **head** of a rib articulates typically with two vertebral bodies and the intervening disc. The **tubercle** of a rib articulates with the transverse process of the vertebra with the same segmental number. Example (Fig. 1.3): The head of rib 5 articulates with vertebral bodies T4 and T5. The tubercle of rib 5 articulates with the transverse process of T5.

◁
GRANT'S 1.13, 1.14
ROHEN 186, 189
A.D.A.M. 1.11
NETTER 172
CLEMENTE 657, 670
A.V.A. 3: 0.41.02

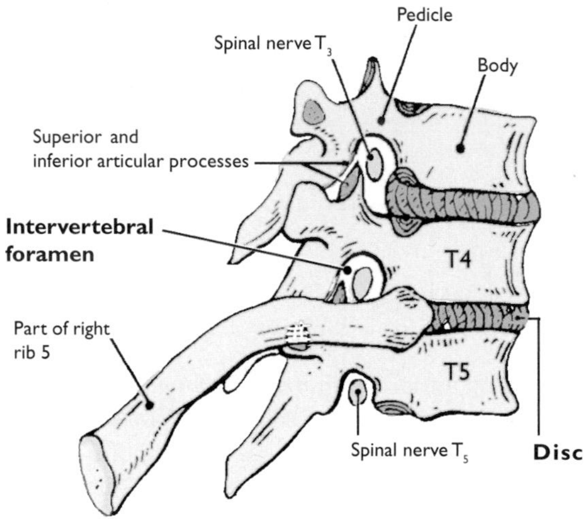

Figure 1.3. Part of vertebral column, thoracic region, intervertebral disc; intervertebral foramen with spinal nerve; rib.

Sternum and Other Landmarks.
Examine the **sternum** (Fig. 1.4):

- Identify its wide upper segment, the **manubrium**.
- The **body** of the sternum is made up of four distinguishable bony segments.
- The pointed lower extremity of the sternum is the **xiphoid process** (Gr. *xiphos*, sword). It is cartilaginous in youth, but ossified in the middle-aged and older person. Occasionally, the body of the sternum may be perforated. This hole may be mistaken as a bullet wound when, in fact, it is the result of a relatively common defect in the ossification process of the sternum.

◁
GRANT'S 1.11
ROHEN 186
A.D.A.M. 1.3
NETTER 171
CLEMENTE 153
A.V.A. 3: 0.37.23

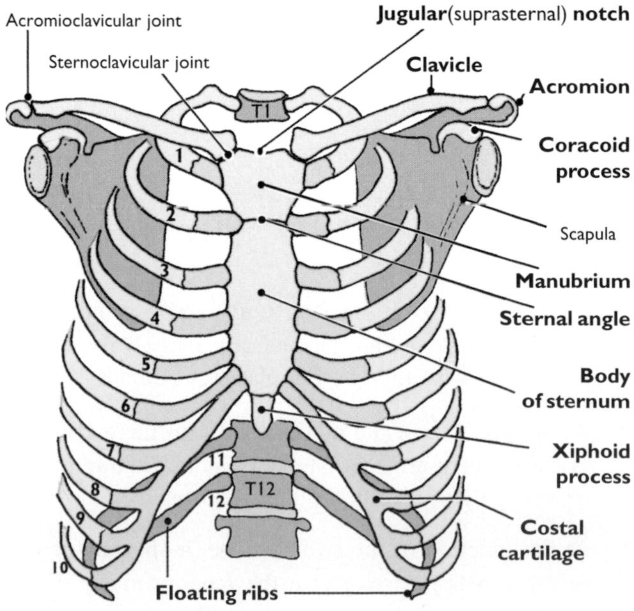

Figure 1.4. Bony landmarks of thoracic region.

- The anterior extremity of each rib is connected to the sternum by means of a bar of hyaline cartilage. These **costal cartilages** become progressively longer from 1st to 7th rib. Costal cartilages 8, 9, and 10 reach only as far as the cartilage next superior.
- Ribs 11 and 12 have free pointed ends; therefore, they are also known as "**floating ribs**."
- **Jugular notch** (suprasternal notch).
- **Sternal angle** marking the junction of manubrium with body of sternum. At this level, the 2nd rib can be palpated.
- Medial end of **clavicle** marking the **sternoclavicular joint**.
- Lateral end of clavicle marking the acromioclavicular joint.
- **Acromion** of scapula forming the point of the shoulder.
- **Coracoid process** of scapula.

Clinical Correlation: As a useful practical exercise for the student's future activities in **physical diagnosis**, the following study is recommended (Fig. 1.5):

With a grease pencil, mark the subject's sternum, clavicle, and ribs 2 through 6. Identify and number the intercostal spaces (ICS). The 2nd ICS is located between ribs 2 and 3. The mammary papilla (nipple) lies at the level of ICS 4 in the male, more inferiorly in the female.

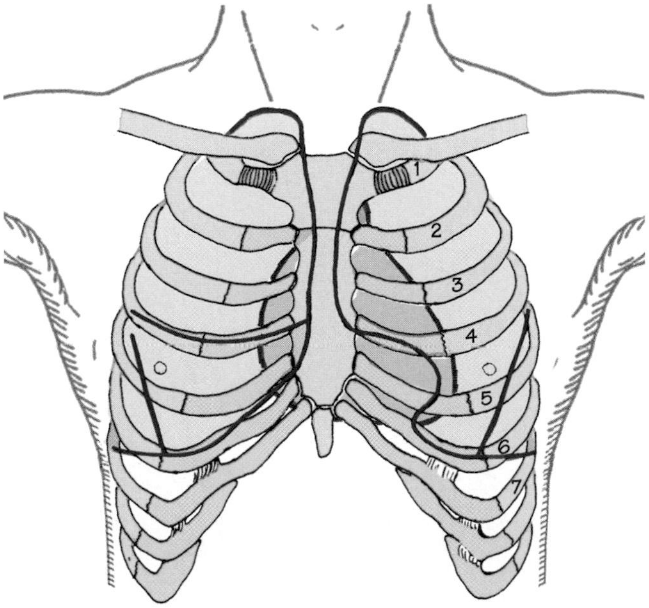

Figure 1.5. Projections of heart (red lines) and lungs (blue lines) on anterior chest wall.

GRANT'S 1.8B
ROHEN 186
A.D.A.M. 1.3, 1.17
NETTER 170
CLEMENTE 1.49
A.V.A. 3: 0.36.38

GRANT'S 1.11
ROHEN 347
A.D.A.M. 1.3, 1.17
NETTER 170, 171
CLEMENTE 148
A.V.A. 3: 0.37.46

GRANT'S 1.23, 1.24
ROHEN 232, 236
A.D.A.M. 2.3, 2.6
NETTER 184
CLEMENTE 159, 160

Outline the **borders of a normal heart** : The apex lies in ICS 5 and about 8 to 10 cm to the left of the midsternal line. Mark the right border by a vertical line 2.5 cm (1 inch) lateral to the right sternal margin. The inferior border crosses the junction between the xiphoid process and the body of sternum. The left border curves superiorly from the apex to ICS 2, about 2.5 cm from the left sternal margin. Part of the aortic arch projects on ICS 1, just to the left of the manubrium. In the living person, in erect posture, these borders will shift.

Outline the **borders of the lungs:** The apex of each lung extends up into the neck for about 2.5 cm (cupula). The anterior borders of both lungs approach the midsternal line. The left lung deviates laterally at the level of ribs 4 and 5 to form the cardiac notch. Mark the approximate position of the horizontal fissure that begins near the right midaxillary line and extends forward along the right 4th costal cartilage. The oblique fissures of both lungs extend inferiorly and end near the 6th costochondral junction.

Review the projections of the heart and lungs on the thoracic wall. Correlate your observations with a posterior-anterior (PA) radiograph of the chest. *Note:* The complex lateral radiographic view of the chest will be discussed at the end of this chapter.

Clinical Observations. Inspect, observe, and note. Examine the anterior and lateral chest wall for evidence of trauma or apparent abnormalities. Palpate the clavicles. Are they smooth or is there an irregular thickening suggesting a previous fracture? Always compare the right and left side for symmetry. Are the breasts present, absent, or asymmetrical? Is there a bulge in the pectoral region that may indicate the presence of an implanted pacemaker? Look for surgical scars. A scar in the midsternal region may have resulted from a coronary bypass operation. In that case, the sternum had been split vertically in the midline. Be prepared for sharp stainless steel wires that were used to hold the sternum together. A scar along an intercostal space would suggest a previous lateral approach to structures within the thorax. Scars near a breast could have resulted from a mastectomy.

Removal of Skin

Before you begin ...

Skin and Superficial Fascia. Collectively, the **skin** is an enormous protective organ that is responsible for nearly 20% of the body weight. The skin consists of two layers, the external **epidermis** and the deeper **dermis** (or corium). The dermis contains hair follicles, sebaceous glands, sweat glands, small blood vessels, and the terminal branches of cutaneous nerves. Deep to the skin is the **subcutaneous tissue or superficial fascia**, which contains various amounts of fat, blood vessels, and superficial nerves. Deep to the superficial fascia lies the **deep fascia**, which envelops muscles. Fibrous bands of connective tissue, the **retinacula cutis**, pass from the skin through the fat of the superficial fascia to the deep fascia, thus attaching the skin to deeper parts of the body but allowing considerable mobility. During dissection, the skin is reflected first, leaving the superficial fascia (subcutaneous tissue) behind. After identifying superficial blood vessels and nerves in the superficial fascia, the deep fascia with its underlying musculature can be approached.

Do *not* dissect at this time. Understand the **objectives** of the contemplated dissection. First, consideration must be given to the superficially positioned mammary gland. Subsequently, the muscles of the chest wall will be dissected. The thoracic wall is covered anteriorly with muscles that belong to the upper limb. If you have already covered CHAPTER 6, UPPER LIMB, these muscles (pectoralis major and minor; subclavius) have already been dissected. If you are beginning your cadaver dissection with this first chapter (thorax), these muscles must be dissected and reflected before the intercostal spaces and their contents can be approached. Subsequently, the anterior thoracic wall will be removed to provide access to the thoracic cavity. It is essential that, despite the dissection process, all major anatomical structures can be repositioned into their original 3-dimensional configuration; e.g., a muscle with adjacent nerves and vessels can be reflected or repositioned; or the removed anterior chest plate can be placed back into its original position.

Skin Incisions. With the cadaver in the supine position (face up), commence with the skin incisions. Do not cut too deep. You may inadvertently damage superficially positioned nerves. Disregard the following instructions for skin incisions if you have already dissected CHAPTER 6, UPPER LIMB. If you are beginning your cadaver dissection with the THORAX, make the following skin incisions now (Fig. 1.6):

- From jugular notch *A* along the clavicle and across the acromion *B* to point *E*, about 10 cm distal to the acromion.
- From *A* to the xiphoid process *C*.
- From *C* horizontally and laterally until stopped by the table *D*.
- From *C* superiorly and laterally and along the anterior axillary fold to point *E*. Avoid the nipple.
- From *E* halfway around the medial side of the arm to point *F*.
- Reflect the outlined flaps and discard them.

> ***Dissection Note:*** If you have already dissected the mammary gland, platysma, pectoralis major, pectoralis minor, and subclavius as part of a previous assignment of CHAPTER 6, UPPER LIMB, skip these sections and continue with the INTERCOSTAL MUSCLES. Otherwise, proceed with the dissection of the mammary glands.

The Breasts

GRANT'S 1.3, 1.6
ROHEN 245
A.D.A.M. 1.41, 1.42
NETTER 167
CLEMENTE 6, 9
A.V.A. 3: 1.21.36

Mammary Glands (Fig. 1.7). The two mammary glands are modified sweat glands. Therefore and by definition, they lie in the superficial fascia. Each gland is positioned anterior to the deep fascia of the pectoralis muscle. Between gland and deep fascia, there is a loose connective tissue plane, the **retromammary space**, which allows the breast to move freely; i.e., there is no firm attachment of the gland to the deep fascia of the pectoralis major muscle. In contrast, the gland is firmly attached to its overlying skin by means of fibrous bands, the **suspensory ligaments** (Cooper's ligaments) that pass from the deep fascia to the deep layer of the skin. The connective tissue network of the breast can be readily demonstrated in a mammogram. The rounded contour of the female breast is due to fat lying in compartments bounded by these areolar septa. The **nipple** (or mammary papilla) is often found at ICS 4; however, it varies considerably in position. It rises from the center of the pigmented **areola**. The surface of the areola is rough due to small subcutaneous glands that produce lubrication for the nipple. Each mammary gland contains approximately 15 to 20 **lactiferous ducts** that drain corresponding glandular lobules and then converge and open on the nipple. The extent of the lactiferous duct system can be demonstrated radiologically by means of a galactogram.

GRANT'S 1.7B
A.V.A. 3: 1.22.09

ROHEN 245
A.V.A. 3: 1.22.44

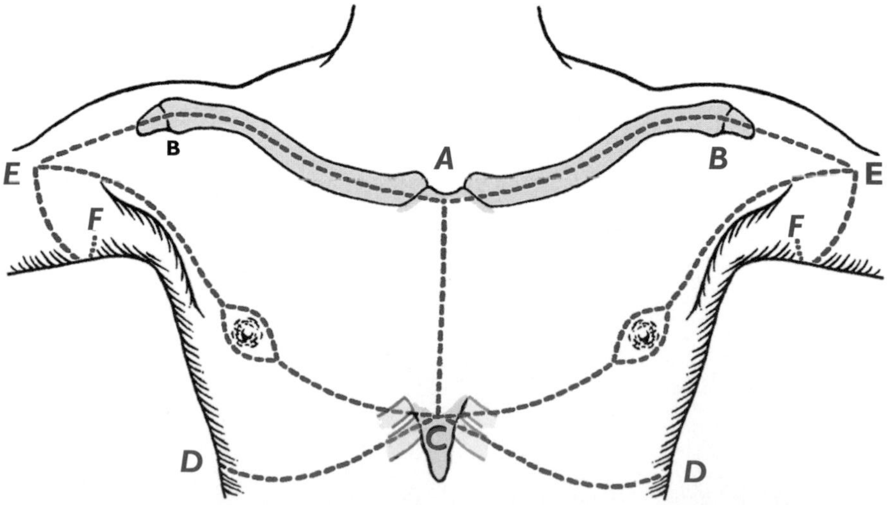

Figure 1.6. Skin incisions for dissection of thoracic wall.

Dissect the mammary gland in female specimens only (Fig. 1.7). *Note*: Old age of the cadaver and the process of preservation may make it difficult to dissect and identify all the structures listed.

GRANT'S 1.3, 1.6
ROHEN 245
A.D.A.M. 1.41, 1.42
NETTER 167
CLEMENTE 6-10
A.V.A. 3: 1.22.18

- Identify the gland in the superficial fascia just anterior to the pectoralis major muscle.
- Pull the area of the **nipple** and **areola** anteriorly and thus render taut the **suspensory ligaments** (of Cooper). These ligaments or septa form the boundaries of compartments that contain fat.
- With the rounded handle of a scalpel, scoop collections of fat out of several compartments. Next, probe through the fat deep to the nipple.
- Find and clean several of the 15 to 20 **lactiferous ducts** that converge on the nipple.
- Trace a duct proximally to its corresponding lobe of glandular tissue that is embedded in dense fibro-areolar stroma. Trace the duct distally to the nipple, identify its **orifice** at the nipple, and mark this opening with a bristle or fine wire.

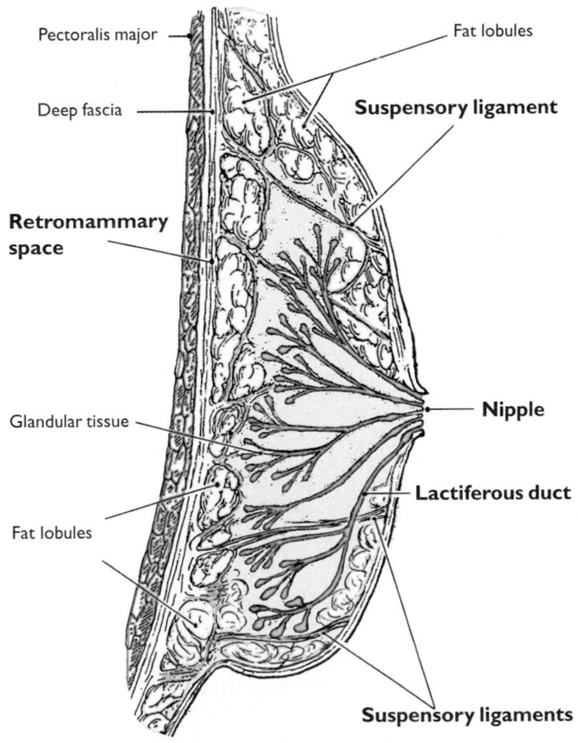

Figure 1.7. Schematic drawing of female breast in sagittal section.

- Make a parasagittal cut through the nipple. Note its circularly arranged smooth musculature which is responsible for nipple erection and compression of lactiferous ducts.
- Insert your fingers into the **retromammary space**. Note that, within this space, the normal mammary gland can be easily separated from the deep fascia of the pectoralis major muscle.
- For future examination and review, store the removed breasts in a plastic bag.

Clinical Correlation: The size of glandular tissue varies greatly and is subject to hormonal regulation. In older females, the glandular parenchyma is diminished.

For descriptive purposes, clinicians often divide the female breast into four quadrants. Of particular clinical interest is the superolateral (upper outer) quadrant. It contains a large amount of glandular tissue; the majority of breast cancers develop here. From this quadrant, an "axillary tail" often extends into the axilla.

GRANT'S 1.3
A.D.A.M. 1.37

In advanced carcinoma of the breast, the tumor may grow through the retromammary space and subsequently invade the underlying pectoralis major muscle and its fascia. Understand that this condition leads to a fixation of the malignant breast lesion to the chest wall.

Advanced cancer of the breast (and its accompanying fibrosis) also has a tendency to shorten the suspensory ligaments of Cooper. Understand that the resulting traction of the suspensory ligaments on the skin leads to a characteristic, irregular dimpling of the skin overlying the lesion.

GRANT'S 1.5
A.D.A.M. 1.41
NETTER 169
CLEMENTE 11

Although the **lymphatic drainage** of the breast is difficult to demonstrate during routine dissection, it must nevertheless be thoroughly understood by any physician. Familiarize yourself with the arrangement of lymph channels and lymph nodes draining the breast tissue. Cancer has a tendency to spread along these lymph passages, particularly into the axillary lymph nodes. Occasionally, cancer will block the lymphatic system on the side of the malignant lesion. In that case, lymph drainage (including transportation of cancer cells) may go to the opposite breast and its lymphatic drainage. Usually, some breast pathology can be seen in the dissecting room. Find out and examine!

GRANT'S 1.7A
CLEMENTE 12

GRANT'S 1.7B

Study a **lymphogram** of the nodes involved in the lymphatic drainage of the breast. Pay particular attention to the important axillary nodes. Also, study a lateral **mammogram** and observe the characteristic connective tissue network of the female breast anterior to the shadow of the pectoralis major muscle.

On occasion, the mammary tissue in males may be hypertrophied, a condition known as gynecomastia. In most cases, this is due to an abnormally high level of circulating estrogens. Carcinoma of the male breast is rare; however, it does occur.

Muscles, Nerves, and Vessels

GRANT'S 8.1
ROHEN 60, 61, 77
A.D.A.M. 1.41
NETTER 21
CLEMENTE 696
A.V.A. 5: 0.05.20

Platysma. The platysma muscle is a wide, thin sheet of striated musculature that belongs to the muscle group of facial expression. It tenses the skin of the neck and widens the mouth. Superiorly, its fibers blend with those of the oral facial musculature. Therefore, it is logical that the platysma and other facial muscles share a common motor nerve supply, the facial nerve (CN VII); specifically, the platysma is innervated by the cervical branch of the facial nerve. The inferior portion of the platysma passes anterior to the clavicle into the pectoral region. This part of the muscle may be encountered at this stage of dissection.

GRANT'S 1.2
ROHEN 193
A.D.A.M. 1.32, 6.17
NETTER 175
CLEMENTE 17-19

Dissect the inferior portion of the platysma. Since it lies in the superficial fascia, it may have been inadvertently removed with the skin.

GRANT'S 1.2
CLEMENTE 16
A.V.A. 3: 0.05.30

- Look for its brownish-red muscle fibers as they cross the clavicle. The platysma is no thicker than a sheet of paper. Do not attempt to search for the platysma in the neck region superior to the clavicle.
- Turn the platysma superiorly.

Cutaneous Branches of Spinal Nerves. It is essential to be familiar with the distribution of a typical spinal nerve. Study a suitable diagram (Fig. 1.8).

GRANT'S 1.20
ROHEN 214
A.D.A.M. 1.35
NETTER 166, 179
CLEMENTE 13

The thin anterior cutaneous twigs emerge from the intercostal spaces just lateral to the sternal margin. The **lateral cutaneous branches** are substantially larger, and one representative (thoracic segments 4, 5, or 6) should be dissected. The lateral cutaneous branch of T2 is also known as the **intercostobrachial nerve.** This nerve supplies the skin and subcutaneous tissue on the back and medial side of the arm. The lateral cutaneous branches course in the superficial fascia; they may be surrounded by substantial amounts of fat.

GRANT'S 1.2
NETTER 175
CLEMENTE 19

Dissect one representative lateral cutaneous branch of either segments T4, T5, or T6 (i.e., in ICS 4, 5, or 6):

GRANT'S 1.2
ROHEN 202
A.D.A.M. 1.34, 1.35
NETTER 174, 175
CLEMENTE 19

- Make a vertical cut through the superficial fascia just lateral to the sternum.
- Make a horizontal cut corresponding to the lower horizontal skin incision. Reflect the flap of superficial fascia laterally.
- Identify an intercostal space by fingertip palpation between two ribs. Search for the **lateral cutaneous branch** where it leaves its intercostal space and passes between the digitations of the **serratus anterior** (Fig. 1.9). Follow the nerve through the fat of the superficial fascia.
- Trace its **anterior and posterior branches** for a short distance.
- Next, identify the lateral cutaneous branch of T2, the **intercostobrachial nerve**. If you have already dissected CHAPTER 6, UPPER LIMB, establish the continuity of the intercostobrachial nerve. If you are beginning with the THORAX, follow the nerve into the subcutaneous tissue of the posterior axillary fold.

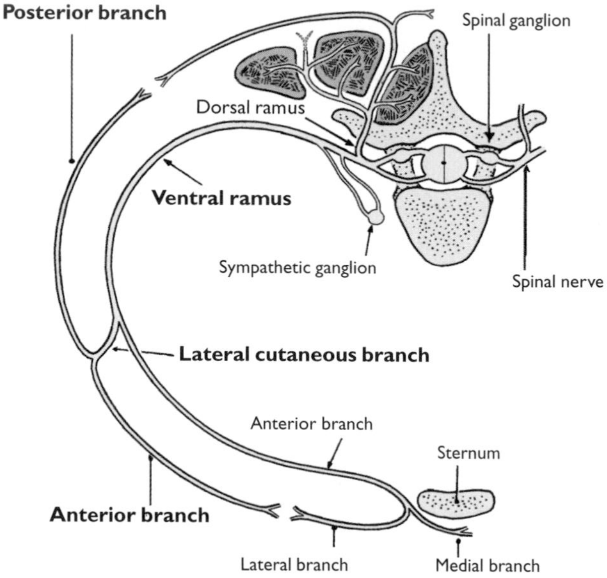

Figure 1.8. Distribution of typical spinal nerve.

Clinical Correlation: The **intercostobrachial nerve** is often involved in the phenomenon of "referred pain" in cases of angina pectoris. Referred pain is perceived in an area other than its actual origin. In cases of angina pectoris, the actual problem resides in the insufficiently perfused heart, but the resulting visceral pain is also referred to upper thoracic nerve segments, i.e., to an area of the anterior chest wall, often extending to the left arm. Understand that sympathetic nerves supplying the heart also carry afferent cardiac pain fibers back to the upper thoracic (T) segments of the spinal cord. Thus, the intercostobrachial nerve (T2) becomes involved in the phenomenon of referred cardiac pain.

Pectoralis Major. This substantial, fan-shaped muscle consists of two heads: a large **sternocostal head** originating mainly from the sternum and ribs, and a smaller **clavicular head** originating from the medial half of the clavicle. Observe that the two muscle heads meet at the sternoclavicular joint. Distally, the muscle converges, and its tendon attaches to the lateral lip of the intertubercular groove of the humerus. The pectoralis major constitutes the most important part of the anterior wall of the axilla. Palpate your own anterior axillary fold, and activate its muscular components. One of its functions is adduction of the humerus. Study a transverse section through the axilla. Note that lateral pectoral nerve arises from the lateral cord of the brachial plexus and then enters the deep surface of the pectoralis major muscle. The medial pectoral nerve, arising from the medial cord, supplies the pectoralis minor muscle and part of the pectoralis major.

GRANT'S 1.2
ROHEN 195
NETTER 174
CLEMENTE 18
A.V.A. 1: 0.18.26

GRANT'S 6.13
A.V.A. 1: 0.33.43

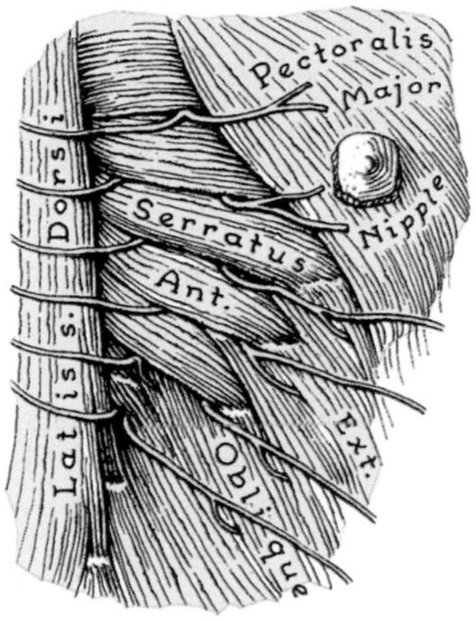

Figure 1.9. Anterior and posterior branches of lateral cutaneous nerves passing between digitations of the serratus anterior muscle.

Dissect the pectoralis major muscle.

GRANT'S 1.2
ROHEN 195
A.D.A.M. 1.37
NETTER 174
CLEMENTE 18
A.V.A. 1: 0.18.26

- Clean its entire anterior surface. Identify its **clavicular head** and **sternocostal head** (on rare occasions absent). With blunt dissection (handle of knife), separate the clavicular and sternocostal parts. Observe their meeting point at the sternoclavicular joint.
- Trace the tendon of the muscle to its insertion in the humerus. Observe: The anterior lamina of the tendon belongs to the clavicular head; the posterior lamina is folded on itself and belongs to the sternal head.

GRANT'S 6.14
ROHEN 385
A.D.A.M. 1.37, 1.38
CLEMENTE 20
A.V.A. 1: 0.24.55

- Superior to the clavicular head, and between it and the adjacent deltoid muscle, define and clean the **deltopectoral triangle** and the contained **cephalic vein**.

- Using a scalpel and cutting close to the clavicle, carefully detach the clavicular head from the clavicle.

ROHEN 196
CLEMENTE 24
A.V.A. 1: 0.29.52

- Gently reflect the muscle head laterally toward the arm until the reflection is stopped by strands of tissue entering the deep surface of the clavicular head. Probe and clean these tissue strands. They are the **lateral pectoral nerve** and muscular branches of the thoracoacromial artery.

The next objective is to reflect the **sternal head of the pectoralis major** without disturbing the underlying pectoralis minor.

GRANT'S 6.13
A.V.A. 1: 0.27.58

- Relax the sternal head of the pectoralis major by flexing and adducting the arm of the cadaver. Gently insinuate your fingers posterior to the sternal head. Your fingers are now in the space between the posterior surface of the pectoralis major and the **clavipectoral fascia**, which envelops the pectoralis minor. The firm strands of tissue you can palpate with your fingers are the vessels and nerves entering the deep surface of the pectoralis major.

GRANT'S 6.19B, 6.22
NETTER 404

- Reflect the **pectoralis major** in the following manner: Using a scalpel, detach the sternal head from its sternal and costal origins, and reflect it toward the arm. Note that the **medial pectoral nerve** pierces the **pectoralis minor** before it enters the sternal head of the pectoralis major.
- Cut a representative piece (or "button") out of the pectoralis major and leave it attached to the nerves and blood vessels for subsequent identification.
- Reflect the remainder of the pectoralis major laterally, thus exposing the clavipectoral fascia.

GRANT'S 6.14-6.16
ROHEN 385
A.D.A.M. 1.38
NETTER 403
CLEMENTE 20
A.V.A. 1: 0.17.07

Clavipectoral Fascia, Pectoralis Minor, and Subclavius. After reflection of the pectoralis major, the **clavipectoral fascia** is exposed. It encloses the **subclavius**, a slender muscle immediately inferior to the clavicle, and the **pectoralis minor**. The pectoralis minor attaches proximally to the costal cartilages of ribs 2 through 5; distally it is inserted into the coracoid process of the scapula, an important landmark for surgeons. Two major blood vessels pierce the clavipectoral fascia: the cephalic vein and the thoracoacromial artery. The **cephalic vein** crosses the pectoralis minor tendon anteriorly and then joins the **axillary vein**. The **thoracoacromial artery** is a branch of the axillary artery (Fig. 1.10). Expect to find variations.

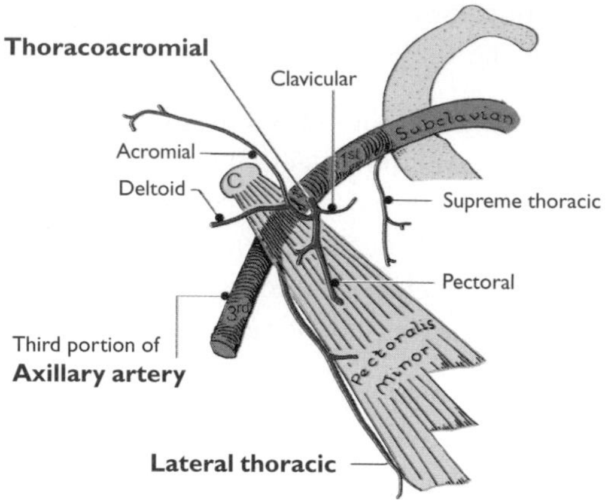

Figure 1.10. Axillary artery and its branches.

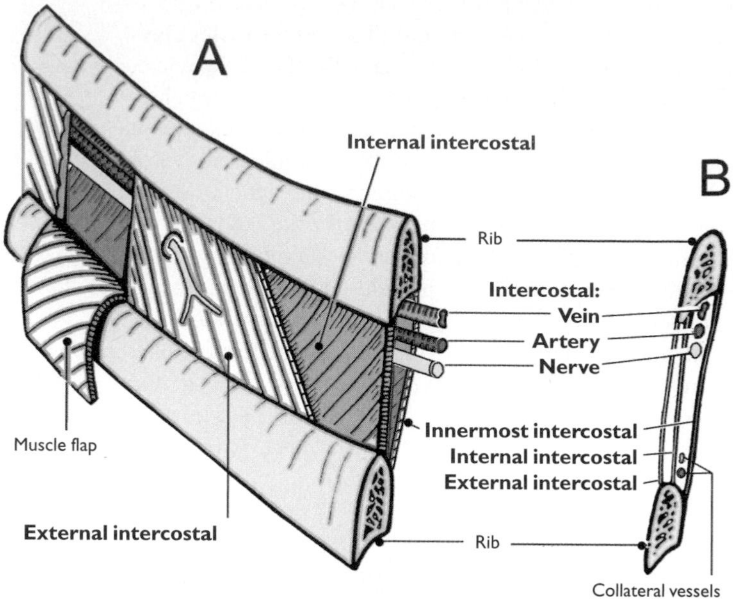

Figure 1.11. ***A.*** Intercostal space and related structures; ***B.*** Intercostal space on coronal section.

Dissect the structures related to the clavipectoral fascia.

- Clean and trace the **cephalic vein** as it crosses the pectoralis minor tendon anteriorly and pierces the clavipectoral fascia medial to the pectoralis minor and together with the **thoracoacromial artery** and the **lateral pectoral nerve**. Clean these structures and maintain them.
- Next, detach the **pectoralis minor** from its costal origin and reflect it superiorly. Leave the muscle attached to its insertion in the coracoid process of the scapula.
- Remove the remains of the clavipectoral fascia and any fat between the pectoralis minor and the rib cage.
- The remainder of the **thoracoacromial artery** can now be traced to its origin from the **axillary artery**.
- Medial to the pectoralis minor, clean and define several branches of the thoracoacromial artery: a pectoral branch to the pectoralis major and minor, a deltoid, a clavicular, and an acromial branch (Fig. 1.10).
- Lateral to the pectoralis minor, demonstrate the **lateral thoracic artery**.
- Trace the cephalic vein to the axillary vein. Do *not* disturb or destroy the contents of the axilla.

⇦
GRANT'S 6.22
ROHEN 385
A.D.A.M. 1.23, 1.24
NETTER 402
CLEMENTE 23
A.V.A. 1: 0.25.12

Intercostal Spaces and Intercostal Muscles. Three layers of muscles are located in the intercostal spaces. From superficial to deep, these muscle layers are: **external intercostal, internal intercostal, and innermost intercostal.** These muscles are supplied by the corresponding **intercostal nerve and intercostal vessels** that are strategically located between the muscle layers (Fig. 1.11). The intercostals are inspiratory muscles; they elevate the ribs and keep the rib spaces rigid. The **internal thoracic vessels** run vertically across the intercostal spaces, just lateral to the sternum. These vessels communicate with the intercostal vessels. Note that the **internal thoracic (internal mammary) arteries** are branches of the corresponding subclavian arteries (see Figures 1.12, 1.13).

⇨
GRANT'S 1.15, 1.18
ROHEN 193, 194
A.D.A.M. 1.38, 1.39
NETTER 175-177
CLEMENTE 146, 147
A.V.A. 3: 0.55.58

Dissect at least one intercostal space and its contents.

- Observe and palpate **ribs** and **intercostal spaces.**
- Note the oblique course of the **external intercostal muscles**. Anteriorly, these muscles are replaced by tough connective tissue, the external intercostal membrane.
- Incise this membrane at the 4th intercostal space (ICS 4), i.e., the space between ribs 4 and 5. Insert the flat handle of the scalpel or forceps deep to the membrane. Push the handle along ICS 4 into the areolar tissue deep to the external intercostal muscle.

- With the handle as a guide, cut the muscle from the rib above and turn it inferiorly (Fig. 1.11**A**). Follow the external intercostal muscle laterally until you reach the digitations of the serratus anterior.
- Focus your attention on the next deeper layer of the intercostal musculature, the **internal intercostal muscles** that run at right angles to the external intercostal fibers.
- In ICS 4, carefully detach the internal intercostal muscle from the inferior margin of rib 5 and reflect it superiorly.
- With the aid of a probe, and starting laterally, locate the 4th **intercostal nerve** and the **intercostal artery and vein** just inferior to rib 4. Verify that the intercostal nerve and vessels run in the space between **internal intercostal** and **innermost intercostal muscles** (Figs. 1.11 and 1.12).

GRANT'S 1.20
ROHEN 214
NETTER 179
A.V.A. 3: 1.09.20

Display portions of the internal thoracic vessels.

GRANT'S 1.15
ROHEN 197
A.D.A.M. 1.40
NETTER 175
CLEMENTE 146
A.V.A. 3: 1.07.46

- Create a window in ICS 2 or 3 by removing all intercostal structures just lateral to the sternum.
- Identify the vertically orientated **internal thoracic artery and vein.**
- Deep to these vessels observe the gray and glistening **parietal pleura.**

> ***Clinical Correlation:*** If a needle must be inserted through an intercostal space (e.g., during a pleural tap), painful puncture of the intercostal nerve should be avoided. Refer to Figure 1.11. The needle should be passed close to the superior border of a rib to circumvent nerve injury.

Anterior Thoracic Wall

To open the thoracic cavity, the anterior thoracic wall or breastplate must be removed. This procedure is similar to the one used by pathologists during autopsy. Removal of the anterior chest wall should be accomplished without significantly damaging the underlying parietal pleural membrane. The area to be removed includes the anterior and lateral portions of **ribs 2 through 6** with the contents of their intercostal spaces, and most of the **sternum.** The first ribs, the most superior part of the manubrium and the most inferior part of the body of the sternum, will remain attached to the trunk. Study "a view from inside"; i.e., a posterior view of the anterior thoracic wall. The **internal thoracic vessels** are firmly attached to the anterior thoracic wall by several muscle slips of the **transversus thoracis** as

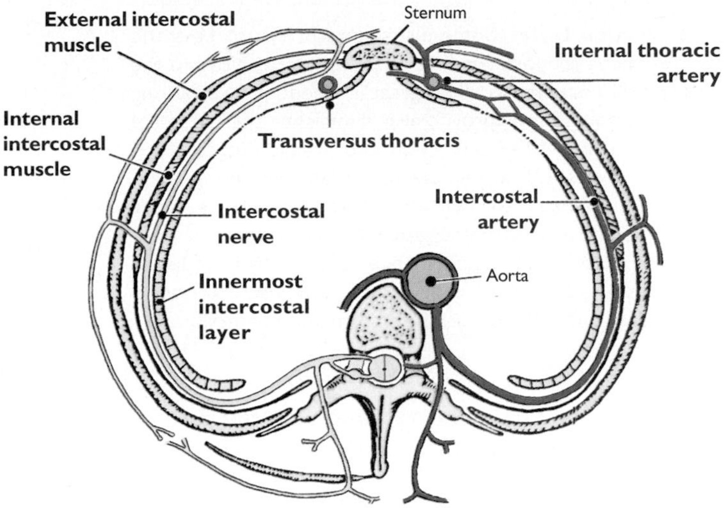

Figure 1.12. Schematic transverse section through thorax. The intercostal nerve and vessels run in the space between internal intercostal and innermost intercostal muscles.

well as by segmental arterial branches and venous tributaries. Therefore, it is most time efficient to sever these vessels on both sides just superior and inferior to the breastplate and to remove these vascular segments together with the anterior chest wall.

Removal of the anterior thoracic wall (Fig. 1.13). Secure a hand saw. Proceed as follows:

- Identify the digitations of the serratus anterior and cut ribs 2 through 6 just anterior to these digitations and on both sides.
- Cut the ribs only. Leave the underlying parietal pleura intact (see *Dissection Note*, page 10).
- Next, envision a line from right to left in ICS 1 just inferior to the first ribs. Saw along this line (*Saw Cut 1*) through the manubrium of the sternum.
- In a similar manner, saw across the inferior part of the sternum at ICS 6 (*Saw Cut 2*).
- Gently elevate the inferior part of the sternum together with the attached portions of severed ribs. Cut remaining soft tissue connections. Reflect the anterior chest wall superiorly.
- Note the **right and left internal thoracic vessels.** Sever them just inferior to the first ribs. Now remove the isolated anterior rib cage.

GRANT'S 1.16
ROHEN 194
NETTER 176
CLEMENTE 162
A.V.A. 3: 1.08.01

Dissection Note: Some instructors prefer to have the ribs cut as far posteriorly as possible (i.e., as close to the table as possible) to allow greater freedom in exploring the thorax. This approach also diminishes the hazard of injury to the dissector's hands and fingers due to sharp edges of ribs. Use a hand saw to prevent splintering of the bones. An instructor may assist with an electric autopsy saw. Some instructors suggest that cloths or paper towels be placed on the jagged edges of the ribs in order to protect students from injury. Ask your instructor as to the preferred method of rib removal and protection.

Examine the **removed** and **isolated anterior thoracic wall**.

GRANT'S 1.16
ROHEN 194
A.D.A.M. 1.43, 1.44
NETTER 176
CLEMENTE 162
A.V.A. 3: 1.08.01

- On its posterior surface, clean the **internal thoracic vessels.**
- Identify the **internal thoracic artery** and demonstrate at least one of the **anterior intercostal branches**, marking the area with a piece of paper slipped between the vessel and the inferior margin of the corresponding rib.
- Identify and clean the **transversus thoracis.**
- Examine and dissect one of the **sternocostal joints**. Cut through fine ligaments and the joint capsule, and open the **synovial cavity.** Understand that slight gliding movements occur in the sternocostal joints during (respiratory) movements of the ribs.

GRANT'S 1.12
A.D.A.M. 1.17
NETTER 171
CLEMENTE 148, 156

- Place the isolated thoracic wall in anterior view. With a scalpel, slit the perichondrium of costal cartilage 3 or 4 by making H-shaped cuts as shown in Fig. 1.13. Peel the membrane superiorly and inferiorly off the costal cartilage; shell out a segment of cartilage; leave the membrane intact. Similarly, a surgeon may shell a segment of a bony rib out of its surrounding periosteum; later, a new bony rib regenerates from the remaining membrane.

GRANT'S 1.15

- Finally, with bone pliers or a fine saw, remove some of the cortex of the sternum and of one of the bony ribs (Fig. 1.13). Expose the spongy bone that, in the living, contains red bone marrow.

You have now finished the dissection of the anterior thoracic wall. Restore all body parts into their original anatomical configuration. In doing this correctly, you will once again appreciate the anatomical topography. This exercise is also necessary so that other students may begin their studies and review of the region.

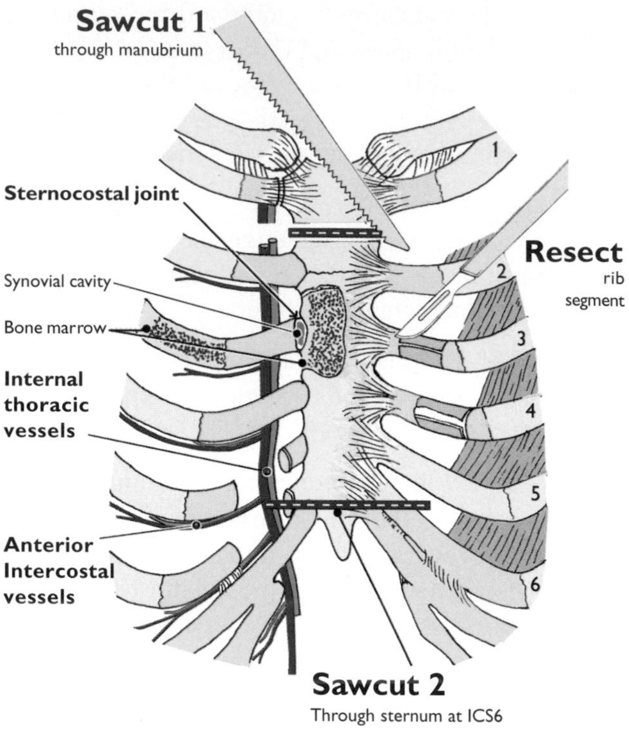

Figure 1.13. Removal of anterior thoracic wall, examination of sternocoastal joints; resection of rib segment.

- First, place the anterior chest plate into its original anatomical position.
- Next, reposition the pectoralis minor, making sure that its slips of origin touch ribs 3, 4, and 5. Arrange associated blood vessels and nerves.
- Restore the two heads of the pectoralis major to their original anatomical positions on the chest wall.
- Finally, place the dissected mammary gland anterior to the pectoralis major, positioning the nipples approximately over the 4th or 5th intercostal space. Moisten the entire region well with preservative fluid and cover the properly prepared prosection specimen.

Clinical Correlation: There are two main surgical approaches to the contents of the thorax. (1) The anterior route is accomplished by splitting the sternum vertically in the midline and spreading it apart with retractors. This approach allows good access to major blood vessels and to the heart. It is commonly used for coronary bypass surgery. At the conclusion of this vascular operation, the sternum is held together with stainless steel wires that can be readily detected later on chest radiographs. (2) The lateral route uses an opening along an intercostal space to access the lungs or structures posterior to the heart. Often, the operating field must be widened by surgical rib resection.

You may be interested in the principle of surgical rib resection. Note the demonstration of this procedure in the prosected anterior thoracic wall. When a surgeon needs wide access to thoracic structures, parts of one or more ribs may have to be removed. The surgeon will slit the periosteum along the external surface of the targeted rib portion, peel the membrane off the bone superiorly and inferiorly, and remove the desired portion of the bony rib. The periosteum itself remains intact. With retractors, it can be sufficiently displaced to offer a suitable operating field within the thorax. Following surgery and in time, some replacement bony substance is generated from the periosteum.

The marrow cavity of the sternum is readily accessible for the aspiration of red marrow through a large bore needle (sternal puncture). The bone marrow is used for diagnostic purposes and for treatment in patients who need healthy bone marrow transplants.

Pleural Cavities

General Remarks and Definitions

The thorax has two openings or apertures (Fig. 1.4). The **superior thoracic aperture** is relatively small and bounded by the manubrium of the sternum, the paired first ribs, and the first thoracic vertebra. Through this aperture, also known as the **thoracic inlet**, pass structures between the thorax and the neck (e.g., trachea, esophagus, vagus, major vessels) and between the thorax and the upper limbs (e.g., major blood vessels). At the level of the **inferior thoracic aperture** or **thoracic outlet**, the musculotendinous thoracic diaphragm separates the thoracic cavity from the abdominal cavity. Several structures (e.g., aorta, inferior vena cava, esophagus) pass between thorax and abdomen through special openings in the diaphragm.

GRANT'S 1.21
ROHEN 231
A.V.A. 3: 0.47.52

The space within the thorax contains two **pleural cavities**, a right and a left one, and the **mediastinum** (Fig. 1.14). The mediastinum (L. *quod per medium stat*, what stands in the middle) is the median space between the two pleural cavities. It contains the heart and many other structures such as the aorta, trachea, and esophagus. The two pleural cavities occupy the lateral parts of the thoracic cavity. Under normal circumstances, each inflated lung fills most of its respective pleural cavity. When a lung is collapsed, however, the extent of its corresponding pleural cavity becomes particularly obvious (Fig. 1.15). Each **lung** is completely covered with a smooth glistening membrane, the **pulmonary or visceral pleura**. Each lung is attached to the mediastinum by an isthmus through which the airways and blood vessels enter or leave the organ. This area of attachment to the mediastinum is known as the **root of the lung**. Here, the visceral pleura is continuous with the parietal pleura that lines the walls of the pleural cavity.

GRANT'S 1.21
ROHEN 232
A.D.A.M. 2.7
NETTER 184, 185
CLEMENTE 164, 165
A.V.A. 3: 0.48.01

The **parietal pleura** (Fig. 1.15) can be subdivided into the following portions: **costal** pleura (lining the rib cage); **mediastinal** pleura (lining the mediastinum); **diaphragmatic** pleura (lining the diaphragm); and **cupula or cervical pleura** (extending into the neck).

The lines along which costal pleura becomes diaphragmatic and mediastinal are known as **pleural reflections** (see Fig. 1.16). At *three sites*, these reflections are so acute that the two portions of the parietal pleura are not only continuous but also *in actual contact with one another* by their inner or serous surfaces. No lung tissue with its visceral pleura intervenes between the apposing pleural layers. These sites of reflections of parietal pleura are known as **pleural recesses**. The **costomediastinal recess** is part of the left pleural cavity. It is defined as the parietal pleural reflection from the anterior portion of the thoracic wall to the mediastinum. Both pleural cavities have a **costodiaphragmatic re-**

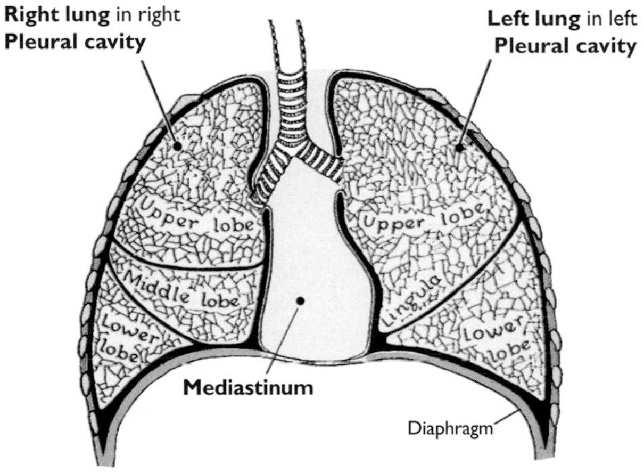

Figure 1.14. Diagram of the respiratory system.

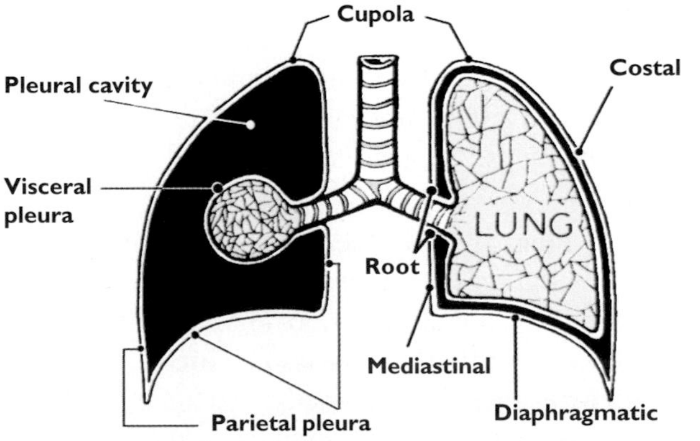

Figure 1.15. Schema of pleural membranes (pleurae) and pleural cavity. Named portions of the parietal pleura are shown to the right.

cess that is located at the most inferior limits of the parietal pleura (Fig. 1.16). Here the diaphragm lies so close to the costal wall as to bring costal and diaphragmatic surfaces of the parietal pleura into apposition. During ordinary inspiration, the thin inferior margin of the lung does not extend into the costodiaphragmatic recess. Rib cage and parietal pleura are separated from each other by a small amount of loose connective tissue, which provides a cleavage plane for surgical (and other manipulative) separation of the pleura from the thoracic wall. This tissue plane is known as the **endothoracic fascia**.

⇦ A.D.A.M. 1.43
CLEMENTE 239, 370

Clinical Correlation: The two pleural cavities are two separate and closed spaces. Normally, they contain only a small amount of serous lubricating fluid. This substance reduces friction between parietal and visceral pleura during respiratory movements.

The costodiaphragmatic recesses are potential spaces into which the lungs extend during deep inspiration. Under pathological conditions, the *potential space* of the pleural cavity may become a real one. Considerable amounts of fluid (up to several liters in extreme cases) can accumulate in the costdiaphragmatic recess and extend from there into other parts of the pleural cavity. This excess fluid, clinically known as effusion, can compress the corresponding lung and thus produce breathing difficulties. Pleural effusions can be visualized on a chest film. In advanced cases, the effusion may totally obscure the radiographic picture of the lung.

If air enters a pleural cavity, the lung within that cavity collapses due to its own elasticity (Fig. 1.15) and, therefore, cannot function properly. This condition is known as pneumothorax. If blood is accumulated in the pleural cavity, we speak of "hemothorax."

Pleurisy is an inflammation of the pleurae. It usually leads to the formation of pleural adhesions between parietal and visceral pleura. You may encounter such adhesions in the cadaver. These adhesions must be broken down before the lung can be completely mobilized.

The parietal pleura, particularly the costal pleura, is exquisitely pain sensitive. In contrast, the visceral pleura is not sensitive to pain. This fact has obvious clinical implications.

⇦ *GRANT'S 1.25*
NETTER 184
CLEMENTE 163
A.V.A. 3: 0.50.20

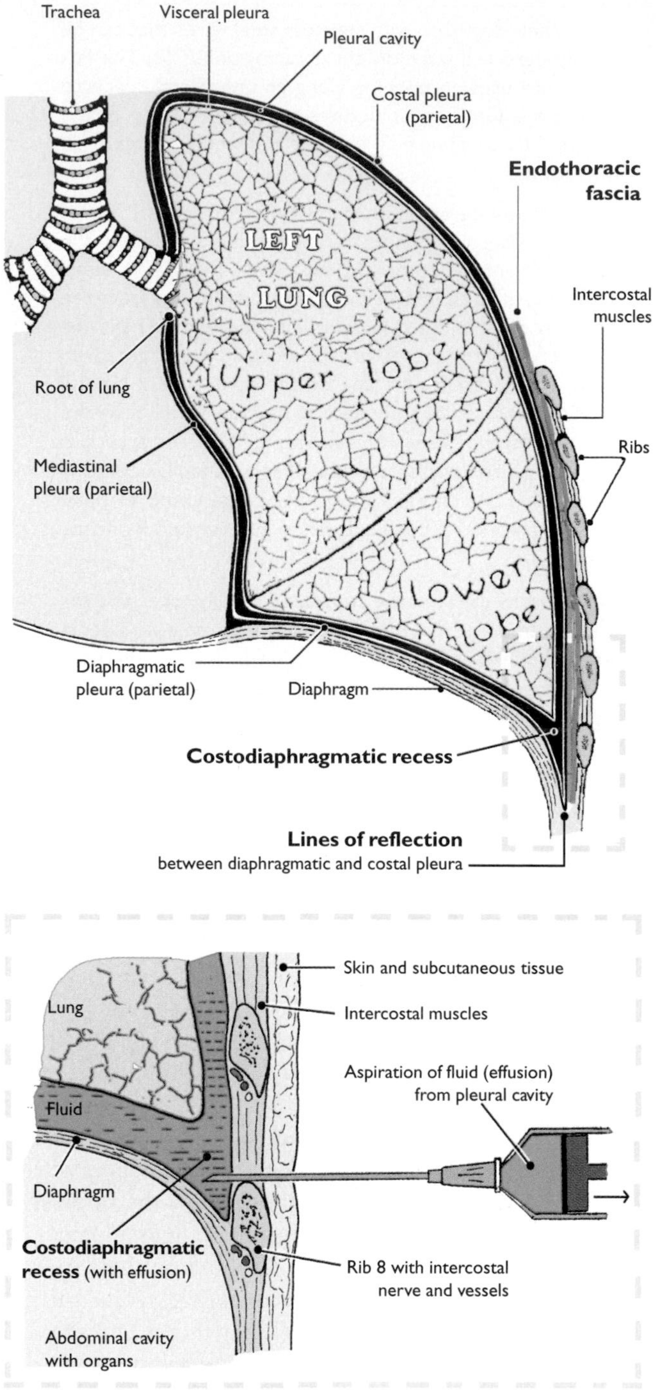

Figure 1.16. Schema of parietal pleura, line of pleural reflection, recess and pleural cavity. At the root of the lung, the parietal pleura is continuous with the visceral pleura. The costal parietal pleura is separated from the thoracic wall by endothoracic fascia. The *INSET* shows anatomical relation pertaining to a pleural tap.

Exploration of Pleural Cavities

If possible, all students should explore the right and left pleural cavities before removal of the lungs.

Pleural Sacs. Identify the right and left pleural sacs. The parietal pleura may have been damaged during removal of the anterior thoracic wall. Using scissors, **incise both pleural sacs** longitudinally. To gain wide access to the pleural cavities, remove the anterior portion of the pleural sacs. Note the lungs in their respective **pleural cavities.**

⇦ *GRANT'S 1.25*
ROHEN 249, 250
A.D.A.M. 1.40
NETTER 186
CLEMENTE 163
A.V.A. 3: 0.50.03

- Place your hand into the right or left **pleural cavity**.
- Palpate the root of the lung. Verify that it is attached to the mediastinum.

- All other portions of the lung are free within the pleural cavity. However, you may encounter pleural adhesions in various places as a result of old pleurisy. Sever these adhesions with your fingers.
- Explore with your hand the various parts of the parietal pleura: **parietal pleura: costal, diaphragmatic, mediastinal,** and **cupula**.
- On the left side, place your fingers into the **costomediastinal recess**. Find it in the region of the cardiac notch where the costal and mediastinal parts of the parietal pleura come into contact with each other.

GRANT'S 1.23
CLEMENTE 169
A.V.A. 3: 0.48.20

- In both pleural cavities, palpate the extensive and deep **costodiaphragmatic recesses**.
- Appreciate the extent of the right and left costodiaphragmatic recesses in a suitable transverse section.

GRANT'S 1.40
ROHEN 265
A.D.A.M. 2.39, 2.40
NETTER 180
CLEMENTE 245

Clinical Correlation: **Pleural Tap (Thoracentesis).** The aspiration of pathological material (serous fluid, fluid mixed with tumor cells, blood, pus, etc.) from the pleural cavity is of important diagnostic value. Another reason for a pleural tap is the drainage of excess fluid (effusion) to allow better pulmonary function. The pleural tap is performed in the midaxillary line or slightly posterior to it. Usually, ICS 6, 7 or 8 is selected for the puncture.

As shown in Figure 1.16 (*Inset*), a large-bore needle is passed close to the superior border of the lower rib in the intercostal space to avoid injury to the intercostal nerve and vessels. The presence of fluid is confirmed by aspiration into a syringe. Subsequently, a small flexible catheter is passed through the needle (cannula) into the tapped pleural cavity and then fed inferiorly into the costodiaphragmatic recess. The external end of the catheter is connected to a vacuum source for controlled removal of excess fluid. If the needle is passed through ICS 8 or 9 and pushed too deep, it will penetrate the diaphragm and enter the abdominal cavity with its contents. After traversing the diaphragm, the needle would reach the spleen on the left side or the liver on the right side.

Chest Tube Insertion. Large amounts of pleural fluid (pleural effusions), blood (hemothorax), or air (pneumothorax) can cause considerable respiratory distress and require removal through a flexible chest tube with an inner diameter much larger than that of a needle. When indicated, the insertion of one or more chest tubes into the pleural cavity is an important and often life-saving clinical procedure in the emergency department.

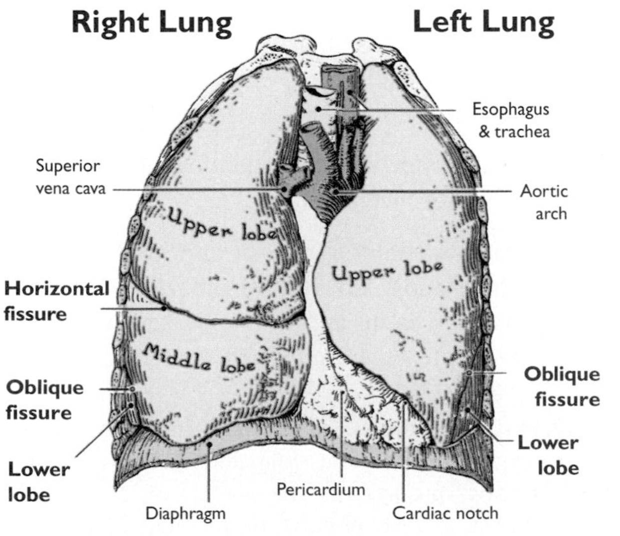

Figure 1.17. The lungs *in situ*.

GRANT'S 1.26
ROHEN 249-252
A.D.A.M. 2.7, 2.8
NETTER 186
CLEMENTE 163

Study the lungs *in situ* (Fig. 1.17).

- Interlobar **fissures** divide the lungs into lobes. Observe the long and deep **oblique fissure** of both lungs.
- Identify the **horizontal fissure** of the right lung.
- Note that the right lung has three **lobes** (*superior or upper, middle, and inferior or lower*).
- The left lung has only two lobes (*superior and inferior*).
- Identify the pericardial sac that contains the heart.

Clinical Correlation: Clinicians often refer to the **oblique fissure** as **major fissure**. The **horizontal fissure** is also known as **minor fissure** or transverse fissure. Occasionally an extra fissure may be present or a fissure may be absent.

GRANT'S 1.28, 1.29
ROHEN 233
A.D.A.M. 2.9, 2.10
NETTER 187
CLEMENTE 176, 177
A.V.A. 3: 0.50.35

Root of Lung. The mediastinal pleura becomes visceral pleura at the root of the lung. The connecting portion between parietal and visceral pleurae is a tube or sleeve of pleura. In its upper half lie all the structures that pass from and to the lung. This is the actual **root** of the lung. The lower half of the sleeve is empty, except for a few lymph vessels. It is collapsed and known as the **pulmonary ligament**. This ligament reaches caudally nearly to the diaphragm. It is difficult to see or to palpate at this time.

Removal of Lungs

The right and left phrenic nerves pass anterior to the roots of the lungs; the vagus nerves course posteriorly. These nerves must **not** be damaged during removal of the lungs.

Proceed with the removal of both lungs as follows:

GRANT'S 1.44
ROHEN 251
NETTER 200, 201
CLEMENTE 190
A.V.A. 3: 1.16.43

- Identify the **phrenic nerves**. They are closely applied to the sides of the pericardial sac. Note that they course about 1.5 cm anterior to the root of each lung (Fig. 1.44.). Preserve the nerves.

- Place your hand into the pleural cavity between lung and mediastinum. With one hand push the lung laterally, thereby stretching and exposing the **root of the lung.**
- With a scalpel in the other hand, carefully transect the root in the middle between lung and mediastinum. Take care *not* to cut into the mediastinum.
- Remove both lungs and store them for future studies, using the storage method required by your instructor. A plastic bag is convenient for this purpose.

Pleurae

Mediastinal Pleura. Explore the **mediastinal pleura**.

- Note that you can palpate through the mediastinal pleura certain mediastinal structures, such as the esophagus on the right and the descending aorta on the left.
- Follow the right and left layers of the **mediastinal pleura** dorsally.
- Posterior to the pericardial sac, they pass to the sides of the **esophagus.**
- Posterior to the esophagus, the two layers come together (to form a "mesoesophagus"). Place one hand in each pleural cavity and bring the fingertips together between esophagus and aorta (*Arrows* in Fig. 1.18).
- Follow the pleura further dorsally to the **descending aorta** where the two layers separate to reach the sides of the vertebral bodies.
- Subsequently, each layer becomes **costal pleura.** Verify these facts.
- Note that certain structures are conspicuous through the pleura. To examine these structures in detail, the pleural membranes must be removed.

Removal of Pleura. Remove the **costal and mediastinal pleura**. Proceed as follows:

- Peel off the **parietal pleura** from the rib cage, starting at the level of the cut ribs 2 to 6.
- The **endothoracic fascia** (Fig. 1.16) provides a natural cleavage plane for manipulative separation of pleura from the adjacent thoracic wall.
- Gently remove the pleura where it covers the vertebral column, aorta, esophagus, and pericardium (Fig. 1.18).

Grant's 1.37, 1.38
Rohen 262, 263
A.D.A.M. 2.29-2.32
Netter 218, 219
Clemente 186-189
A.V.A. 3: 0.48.17

Grant's 1.37, 1.38
Rohen 262, 263
A.D.A.M. 2.29-2.32
Netter 218, 219
Clemente 186-189
A.V.A. 3: 0.48.17

Grant's 1.37
Rohen 262
A.D.A.M. 2.31, 2.32
Netter 218
Clemente 187
A.V.A. 3: 1.09.20

Grant's 1.37, 1.38
Rohen 262, 263
Netter 218, 219
Clemente 187, 189
A.V.A. 3: 1.19.05

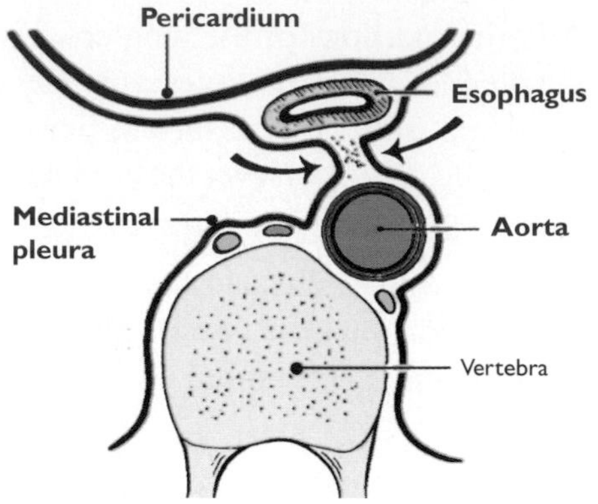

Figure 1.18. Mediastinal layers of pleura.

- Be careful not to injure the **phrenic nerves.** These nerves are positioned between the mediastinal pleura and pericardium about 1.5 cm anterior to the root of the lung.

Intercostal Structures. With the costal pleura removed, you have access to intercostal structures and the bilateral sympathetic trunks (Fig. 1.12). Proceed as follows:

- On the left side of the thorax , note the aortic arch and the **descending aorta.**
- Verify that the **intercostal arteries** arise from the aorta. Clean one artery and follow it into the intercostal space.
- On the right side of the thorax, identify and clean at least one **intercostal artery.** Follow it distally into the intercostal space. Follow it proximally and note that it disappears in the space between esophagus and vertebral column. The right intercostal arteries are also derived from the aorta.
- On both sides, identify and clean at least one of the **intercostal veins** that accompany the intercostal arteries.
- On both sides, identify and clean at least one of the **intercostal nerves**.
- Follow it distally until it disappears dorsal to the **innermost intercostal muscle.** Follow it proximally as far as possible. Note fine nerve connections to the **sympathetic trunk.**

Sympathetic Trunk. The right and left chains of sympathetic ganglia are part of the sympathetic component of the autonomic nervous system. The chains have cervical, thoracic, lumbar, and sacral parts. In the thorax, you will be able to see and examine the **thoracic part of the sympa-**

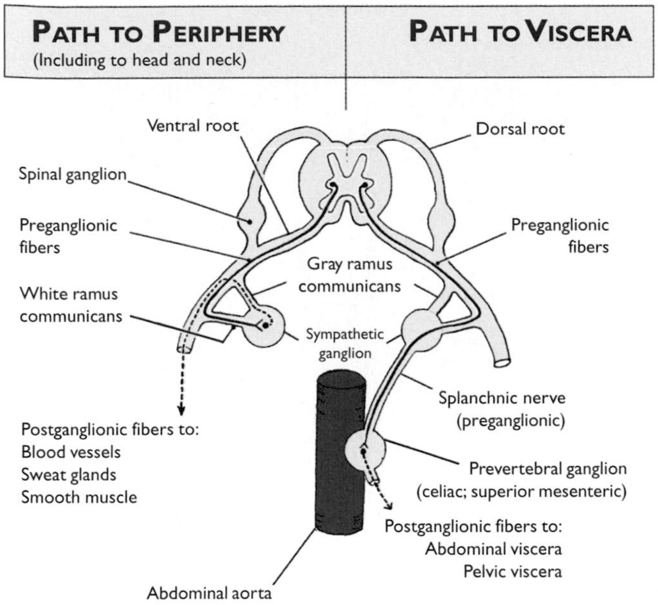

Figure 1.19. General plan of sympathetic nerve distribution.

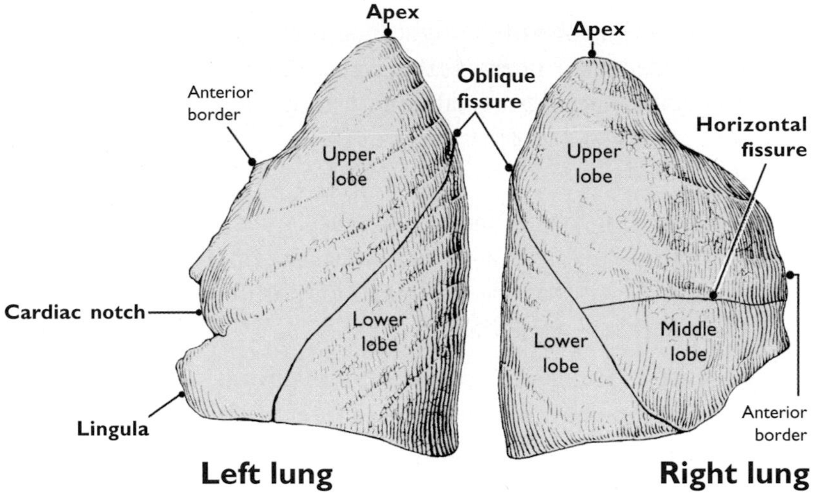

Figure 1.20. Lateral views of left and right lungs.

thetic trunks (chains). Familiarize yourself with a general schema or plan of sympathetic nerve distribution (Fig. 1.19). Preganglionic sympathetic fibers are efferent fibers that pass from the spinal cord through the ventral roots to the spinal nerves. The preganglionic fibers (relatively thick and whitish) then pass through white rami communicantes to the ganglia of the sympathetic chain. From that point on, the fibers may take one of the following two pathways:

(1) Without interruption, they may continue on as preganglionic fibers, pass through the thoracic splanchnic nerves, and terminate in the prevertebral ganglia (celiac; superior mesenteric). These ganglia contain the cell bodies of secondary neurons. The preganglionic fibers synapse in these ganglia. Postganglionic fibers of the secondary neurons then reach the abdominal and pelvic viscera.

(2) Preganglionic fibers may synapse in these sympathetic ganglia. Postganglionic fibers (relatively thin and grayish) pass through the gray rami communicantes to the peripheral nerves. These postganglionic fibers supply blood vessels, sweat glands, and smooth muscle fibers of hair follicles. The vertical connections between the individual ganglia of the sympathetic chain contain fibers that run between various segments. The sympathetic chains also contain afferent fibers that carry sensory information from viscera and blood vessels to the central nervous system.

Demonstrate the **sympathetic trunk** and some of its branches in the cadaver.

- On both sides, identify and clean the **sympathetic trunk.**
- Starting as high as possible in the thorax, follow it inferiorly as it crosses successively the heads of ribs 2 to 9. Subsequently, it lies on the sides of the lower thoracic vertebrae.
- Note that the sympathetic trunk has a series of swellings, the **sympathetic ganglia**, one for each segment.

GRANT'S 1.19, 1.71
ROHEN 262, 263
A.D.A.M. 2.31, 2.32
NETTER 2.18, 2.19
CLEMENTE 239
A.V.A. 3: 1.19.18

- Demonstrate the fact that *two rami communicate* with each **intercostal nerve** and its corresponding **sympathetic ganglion.** These are the **rami communicantes**. It may be difficult to distinguish white and gray rami.
- Identify the largest of the three splanchnic nerves, the thoracic **greater splanchnic nerve**.
- Verify that it receives contributions from several sympathetic ganglia of the trunk.

The Lungs

Examination of Lungs. Refer to the two isolated lungs and examine them. Note the following (Fig. 1.20.):

GRANT'S 1.27-1.29
ROHEN 233
A.D.A.M. 2.9-2.12
NETTER 186, 187
CLEMENTE 172-177

- The right lung is shorter but more voluminous than the left.
- The **apex** of the lung rises as high as the neck of the 1st rib, but not higher.
- Each lung is divided into a **superior** (upper) and an **inferior lobe** (lower lobe) by an **oblique fissure**. Identify these lobes.
- Observe that most of the inferior lobe occupies the posterior part of the thoracic cavity.
- Most of the superior lobe occupies the anterior part of the thoracic cavity.

- The superior lobe of the right lung is further subdivided by a **horizontal fissure**, thereby producing anteriorly a small **middle lobe**. This lobe reaches laterally only as far as the midaxillary line.
- The superior lobe of the left lung has a wide **cardiac notch** on its anterior border. The **lingula** is the most inferior and anterior portion of the left superior lobe.
- Identify the lung **surfaces**. These are: **costal**, **medial** (having a mediastinal and vertebral part), and **basal or diaphragmatic.**
- The **borders** are anterior and inferior. They are thin and sharp.

Contact Impressions. In the well-embalmed and hardened lung, contact impressions from topographically related structures can be observed.

- On the mediastinal surface of the right lung, identify the **cardiac impression** and the **groove for the esophagus**.
- On the mediastinal surface of the left lung, identify the **cardiac impression** and the continuous **groove for aortic arch and descending aorta.**

GRANT'S 1.28, 1.29
ROHEN 233
A.D.A.M. 2.9, 2.10
NETTER 187
CLEMENTE 176, 177

Hilus and Related Structures (Fig. 1.21). At the hilus, various structure enter or leave the lung. Note the following:

- At the **hilus**, observe the relative positions of **bronchus, pulmonary artery, and pulmonary veins**. Generally, the bronchus lies posterior, the artery superior, and the veins lie inferior.
- Force apart the fat-free lung tissue with the blunt ends of two pairs of forceps.
- Identify the **main bronchus**. If the root of the lung was cut close to the lung tissue, the main bronchus was left behind in the mediastinum. In this case, only the subsidiary bronchi can be seen at the hilus.
- In the *left* lung, identify the **superior (upper) and inferior (lower) lobar bronchi** (Fig. 1.22).
- In the *right* lung, identify the **superior, middle, and inferior bronchi.**
- Note that the **right superior bronchus** has a special location. It is more superior (higher) than any other bronchus, and even higher than the pulmonary artery (Fig. 1.22). Therefore, this bronchus has also been named "eparterial bronchus."

GRANT'S 1.30
ROHEN 230, 231
A.D.A.M. 2.11
NETTER 190
CLEMENTE 180, 181

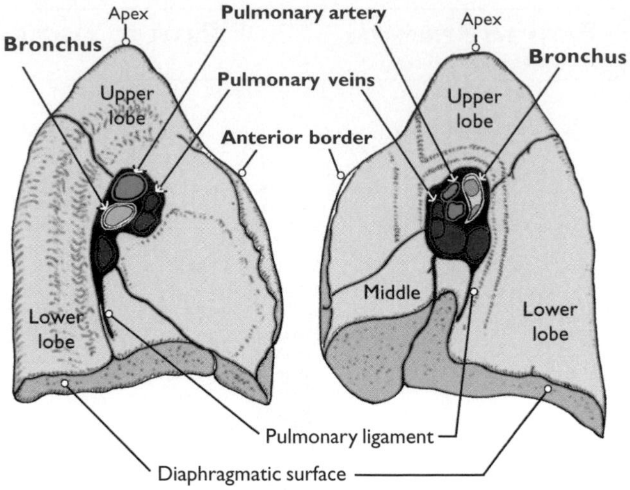

Figure 1.21. Mediastinal surfaces of left and right lungs. Hilus and related structures.

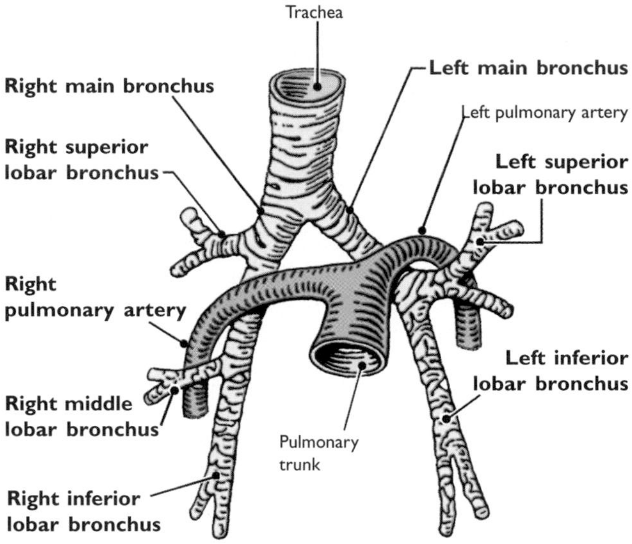

Figure 1.22. Topographic relations of pulmonary arteries and bronchi.

Segmental Bronchi. Next, identify the **segmental bronchi**.

- Verify by palpation that they contain pieces of cartilage.
- Pass a probe into each segmental bronchus. Follow each structure for 2 to 3 cm into the lung tissue.
- Remove intervening (black) lymph nodes. Cut away some lung tissue near the hilus.

- Select one segmental bronchus. Open it with a pair of scissors, and follow it and its ramifications far into the lung tissue.
- Identify the **pulmonary artery** and its branches, which carry deoxygenated blood. Look for blood clots. These vessels are distributed together with the bronchial tree. Bronchioles and arterioles are intrasegmental.
- In contrast, the tributaries to the pulmonary veins lie at the periphery of any pulmonary unit, e.g., at the periphery of a segment; they are intersegmental. The pulmonary veins carry oxygenated blood.

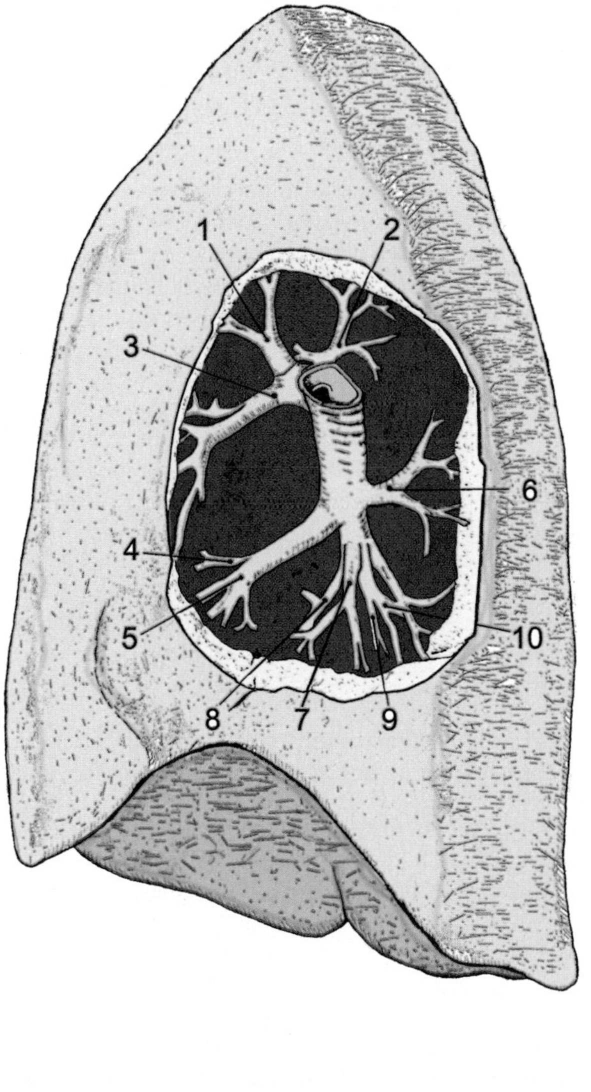

Figure 1.23. Right bronchial tree. The segmental bronchi are labeled as follows: *1*, apical; *2*, posterior; *3*, anterior; *4*, lateral; *5*, medial; *6*, superior; *7*, medial basal; *8*, anterior basal; *9*, lateral basal; *10*, posterior basal.

GRANT'S 1.33, 1.34
ROHEN 231
A.D.A.M. 2.9, 2.10
NETTER 194, 195
CLEMENTE 176, 177

GRANT'S 1.30-1.32
ROHEN 235
A.D.A.M. 2.11, 2.12
NETTER 188-191
CLEMENTE 174-179

- There are additional structures at the hilus: bronchial arteries that are nutrient vessels for the lung tissue, lymph nodes and lymph vessels, and autonomic nerve fibers. Be aware of their existence.

Dissection Notes: **Specific Segmental Bronchi and Bronchopulmonary Segments.** Each lung has 10 bronchopulmonary segments. These segments are of considerable clinical importance. A bronchopulmonary segment is that part of lung tissue aerated by a tertiary bronchus and supplied by a single branch of the pulmonary artery. Students may or may not be required to identify all segmental bronchi and their corresponding bronchopulmonary segments. Check with your instructor. If you are required to be specific, identify all segmental bronchi in the right and left lung.

Right Lung (Fig. 1.23):

- Superior lobe
  1. apical
  2. posterior
  3. anterior
- Middle lobe
  4. lateral
  5. medial
- Inferior lobe
  6. superior
  7. medial basal
  8. anterior basal
  9. lateral basal
  10. posterior basal

Left Lung:

- Superior lobe
  1. + 2. apical-posterior
  3. anterior
  4. superior lingular
  5. inferior lingular
- Inferior lobe
  6. superior
  7. + 8. anterior-medial basal
  9. lateral basal
  10. posterior basal

You have now finished the dissection of the pleural cavity and lungs. Prepare the specimen for review by yourself and others.

- Place the isolated, dissected lungs either back into their respective pleural cavities (or into a plastic bag, if so specified by your instructor).
- Moisten the entire region well with preservative fluid and cover the properly prepared prosected specimen.

Clinical Correlation: Knowledge of the **segmental bronchial distribution** is a necessary prerequisite for pulmonary radiology, surgery, and medicine. Frequently, a specific diseased segment is identified and surgically removed. Obstruction of a bronchus prevents proper ventilation to the lung peripheral to the obstruction. The air trapped peripherally is absorbed slowly with time, resulting in volume loss of the concerned lung tissue (atelectasis; collapse).

The trachea and bronchi (tracheobronchial tree) can be visualized by endoscopic examination using a flexible bronchofiberscope. Thus, endobronchial inflammatory processes, tumors, or aspirated foreign bodies can be visualized and photographed. In the management of pulmonary diseases, fiberoptic bronchoscopy may be combined with lavage of individual bronchi. The concerned bronchus is irrigated with saline. Subsequently, thick mucus plugs or inspissated bronchial secretions can be suctioned and removed. As a result, the corresponding pulmonary segment receives better ventilation. The **bronchial tree** can also be demonstrated radiographically by injecting contrast material into the various parts of the air passages.

The vascular **pulmonary trunk** and its branches can be demonstrated radiographically in the living person by injecting contrast material into the right side of the heart. In this manner, radiographically visible branches of the pulmonary arteries can be followed into individual pulmonary segments.

Realize that the lungs have a rich nerve supply via the anterior and posterior pulmonary plexuses. Sympathetic contributions are received from the right and left sympathetic trunks, while parasympathetic contributions are received from the right and left vagus.

Clinical Observations, Lungs: Describe the nature of fluids (if any) in the right and left pleural cavities. Were you able to remove the lungs easily, or were there adhesions that had to be broken down? Are both lungs complete, or is there evidence of surgical removal of lobes or pulmonary segments? Remember, embalmed cadaver lungs are hard and discolored. The dark, mottled surface markings are most likely due to a life-long accumulation of carbon particles. Are there any surface bullae? These emphysematous cysts may rupture and cause pneumothorax. Are there any whitish nodules on the lung surface or inside the lung? These lesions may represent cancer. If you see such nodules in close association with bronchi, a bronchogenic carcinoma may be suspected. Cavities in the lung may be associated with pulmonary tuberculosis. Did you find blood clots in the pulmonary artery or its branches? In the clinical setting, such blood clots could be the result of a dangerous pulmonary embolism, a real emergency and a major cause of death in hospitalized patients.

Mediastinum

Definitions and Subdivisions

The median region between the two pleural sacs is the mediastinum (Fig. 1.14). It extends from the superior aperture of the thorax to the diaphragm, and from the sternum anteriorly to the bodies of the 12 thoracic vertebrae posteriorly. Purely for descriptive purposes, this extensive region is arbitrarily subdivided into subsidiary parts (Fig. 1.24).

Grant's 1.31

Grant's 1.22
A.D.A.M. 2.28
Clemente 191
A.V.A. 3: 1.03.55

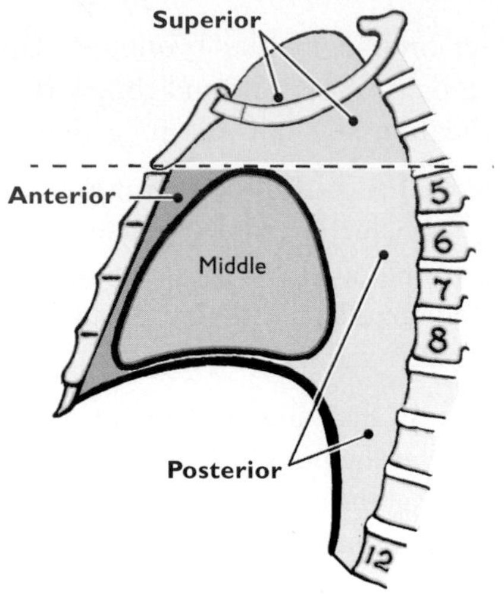

Figure 1.24. The four classic anatomical subdivisions of the mediastinum.

At the level of the sternal angle (i.e., between body and manubrium of sternum), a horizontal plane passes through the intervertebral disc between thoracic vertebrae 4 and 5. Superior to this imaginary plane lies the **superior mediastinum.** This plane is especially important since it indicates the level of the superior border of the fibrous pericardium and the level of the bifurcation of the trachea, i.e., the superior border of the root of the lung.

Grant's 1.41
Netter 198, 199
Clemente 236

The remaining portion of the mediastinum (inferior to the superior mediastinum) is divided into three parts (Fig. 1.24):

1. **Anterior mediastinum**, the small and relatively unimportant portion between sternum and pericardium; in children and adolescents, the thymus gland may reach inferiorly into the anterior mediastinum;

2. **Middle mediastinum**, containing the pericardium with the enclosed heart and the roots of the great vessels;

3. **Posterior mediastinum**, the portion posterior to the pericardium and anterior to the bodies of the lower 8 thoracic vertebrae. Certain structures traversing the length of the mediastinum (e.g., esophagus, vagus nerve, phrenic nerve, thoracic duct) lie, of course, in more than one mediastinal subdivision.

Clinical Correlation: The foregoing definition of the divisions of the **mediastinum** is the **classic anatomical description**. However, clinicians often use a more simple and pragmatic description in an attempt to aid in differential diagnosis. For example, the noted radiologist Benjamin Felson finds the divisions of the mediastinum, as defined by anatomists, not suitable for roentgen diagnosis of mediastinal lesions. Therefore, he uses radiographic subdivisions as follows: The "anterior" and "middle" mediastinum are divided by the line extending along the posterior aspect of the heart and anterior to the trachea. The "middle" and "posterior" mediastinal compartments are separated by the line connecting a point on each thoracic vertebra about a centimeter behind its anterior margin. With these pragmatic subdivisions, the "anterior" mediastinum contains the classic anterior and middle mediastinal compartments. The "posterior" mediastinum delineates the thoracic paravertebral space with its characteristic neurogenic lesions. The "middle" mediastinum is the area between the "anterior" and "posterior" mediastinum. It includes all the longitudinal structures with their characteristic pathological lesions. The classic anatomical term "superior mediastinum" becomes superfluous. Unfortunately, the medical profession does not use a consistent definition for subdivisions of the mediastinum. The student should be aware of these circumstances and be ready to adapt to different definitions later in the clinical years. At this time and during this gross anatomy course, the student will use and be responsible for the **classic anatomical descriptions of the mediastinum.**

It must be stressed that, in the living person, the mediastinum is a highly mobile region. Observe the loose fat and areolar tissue of the mediastinum. It is perfectly suited to accommodate movements and volume changes in the thoracic cavity (e.g., movements of trachea during respiration, pulsations of great vessels, volume changes of esophagus).

Radiologists and clinicians are often confronted with a so-called "widening of the mediastinum" seen on a chest film. Conceptually, any structure located in the mediastinum can contribute to this pathological widening. Often it is seen after trauma resulting in hemorrhage into the mediastinum from one or more lacerated great vessels (e.g., aorta or superior vena cava). Commonly, lymphoma leads to vast enlargement of lymph nodes in the mediastinum with resulting widening. Tumors of the esophagus or of the thymus as well as inflammatory processes in the mediastinum can lead to a widening of the mediastinum. A thorough knowledge of the mediastinum and its contents is a prerequisite for a logical diagnostic approach.

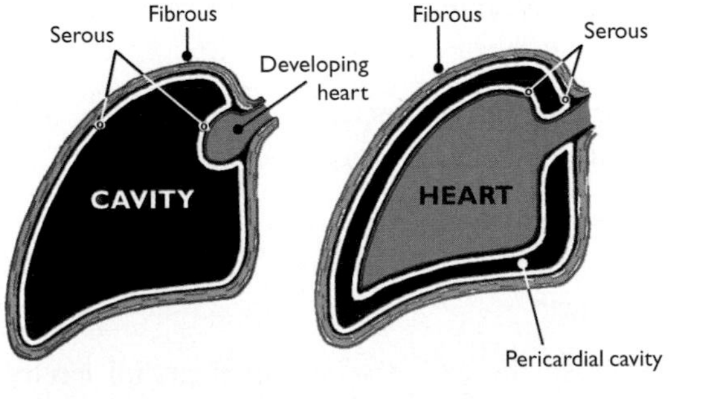

Figure 1.25. Invagination of developing heart into layers of pericardium.

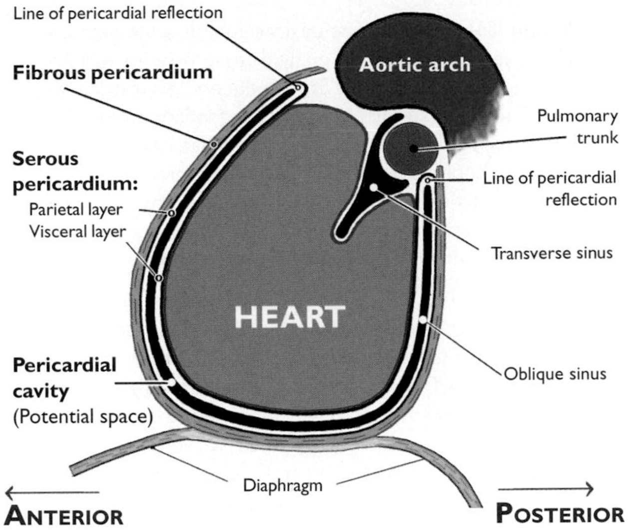

Figure 1.26. Schema of pericardium and heart in sagittal section. Pulmonary trunk with subsequent bifurcation into right and left pulmonary arteries.

Middle Mediastinum and Heart

Pericardium

GRANT'S 1.26, 1.44
ROHEN 249, 250
A.D.A.M. 2.16
NETTER 200
CLEMENTE 190
A.V.A. 3: 1.04.34

The **middle mediastinum** contains the pericardium (with adjacent phrenic nerves), the **heart**, and the roots of the great vessels passing to and from the heart. The **pericardium** is a sac enclosing the heart and pierced by the roots of eight vessels (two arteries, two caval veins, four pulmonary veins). The outer surface of the pericardium is fibrous and tough. Its inner surface is serous and smooth. Envision that, during development, the growing heart invaginates into the pericardial sac, taking the serous layer with it (Fig. 1.25). With these facts in mind, consider the following (Fig. 1.26):

- The inner surface of the fibrous pericardium is covered with the *parietal layer* of smooth, **serous pericardium.**
- The serous pericardium is reflected onto the heart as the *visceral layer* of **serous pericardium.** This smooth visceral layer is also known as **epicardium.**
- Between the opposing surfaces of parietal and visceral layers of serous pericardium is a potential space, the **pericardial cavity.**
- Posteriorly, the oblique sinus is a blind recess of the pericardial cavity between pulmonary veins and inferior vena cava.
- The transverse sinus is a transversely running passageway between venous and arterial poles of the heart.
- The inferior part of the tough, fibrous pericardium is densely attached to the tendinous part of the diaphragm. Thus, the function of the heart is influenced by diaphragmatic movements during respiration.

> ***Clinical Correlation:*** The pericardium and the pericardial sac can be involved in many disease processes. Certain inflammatory diseases can produce a "pericardial effusion" in which significant amounts of inflammatory fluids are accumulated in the pericardial sac. As a result, the heart becomes compressed and ineffective. A chronically inflamed and thickened pericardium may actually calcify and seriously hamper cardiac efficiency. Non-inflammatory pericardial effusions commonly occur in congestive heart failure.
>
> Bleeding into the pericardial sac or "hemopericardium" is commonly associated with penetrating heart wounds or perforation of a weakened heart muscle following myocardial infarction. Arterial bleeding into the tough, fibrous and nonextensible pericardial sac leads to compression of the encased heart and the roots of the great vessels associated with the heart. This potentially lethal condition is known as "cardiac tamponade."
>
> In patients with pneumothorax, air under pressure may dissect along connective tissue lines into the pericardial sac, producing a "pneumopericardium." This condition is particularly serious in newborns. Pneumopericardium can be demonstrated radiographically.
>
> On a congenital basis, the pericardium may be partially or totally absent.

Before opening the pericardial sac and removing the heart, identify the following structures:

- **Superior vena cava**
- **Ascending aorta** and **arch of aorta**
- **Pulmonary trunk or artery**
- Gently probe in the interval between aortic arch and pulmonary trunk and identify the **ligamentum arteriosum**. This structure passes from the root of the left pulmonary artery to the arch of the aorta.
- With a probe, identify the **left vagus** nerve as it passes over the lateral aspect of the aortic arch.
- Inferior to the aortic arch and just lateral and posterior to the ligamentum arteriosum, identify the initial portion of an important branch of the left vagus nerve, the **recurrent laryngeal nerve.**

⇦
GRANT'S 1.45
ROHEN 251, 252
A.D.A.M. 2.16
NETTER 200, 201
CLEMENTE 190, 192
A.V.A. 3: 1.12.17

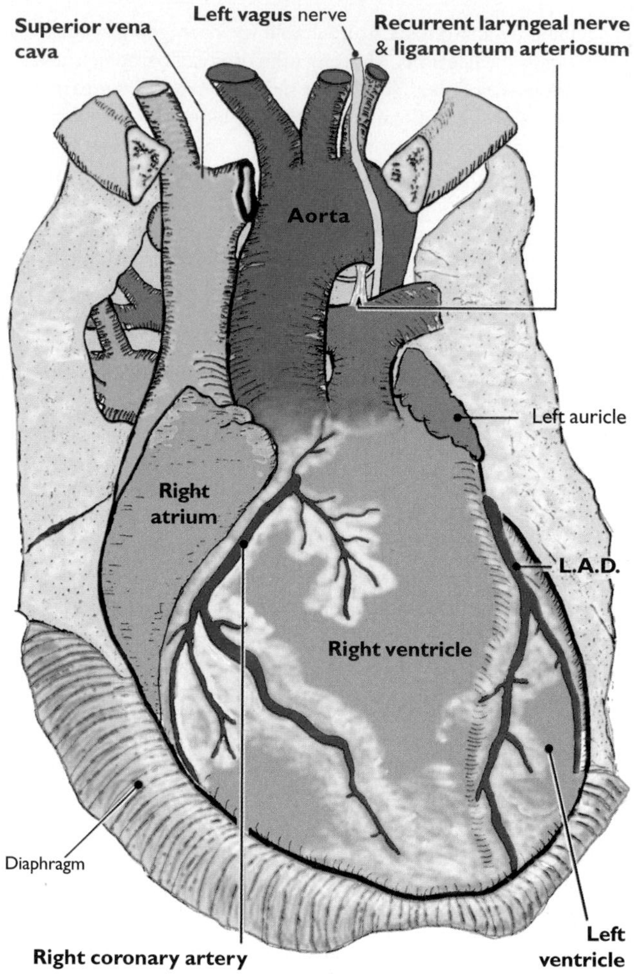

Figure 1.27. Sternocostal surface of heart and great vessels *in situ*. *L.A.D.*, left anterior descending branch of left coronary artery.

Before you begin ...

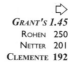

The pericardial sac must be opened to provide access to the heart (Fig. 1.27). After manual exploration of the pericardial cavity and its two sinuses, the heart must be detached from its eight great vessels. Subsequently, the isolated heart will be dissected.

Pericardial Sac. Open the pericardial sac in the following manner:

- With a pair of forceps, pinch up a fold of the pericardial sac where it overlies the right atrium.
- With scissors, nick the fold and enter the pericardial cavity. Open the pericardial sac widely.
- Remove the entire anterior portion of the pericardial sac to ensure sufficient access to the heart. Do not remove the posterior portion.
- Sponge the interior of the pericardial sac with water.

⇨
GRANT'S 1.45
ROHEN 250
NETTER 201
CLEMENTE 192

Pericardial Reflections. Demonstrate the pericardial reflections as follows:

- Observe that the smooth *visceral layer* of pericardium, the **epicardium**, intimately invests the heart.
- Establish the extent of the **pericardial cavity.** Push a probe anterior to the ascending aorta to the superior limit of the cavity.

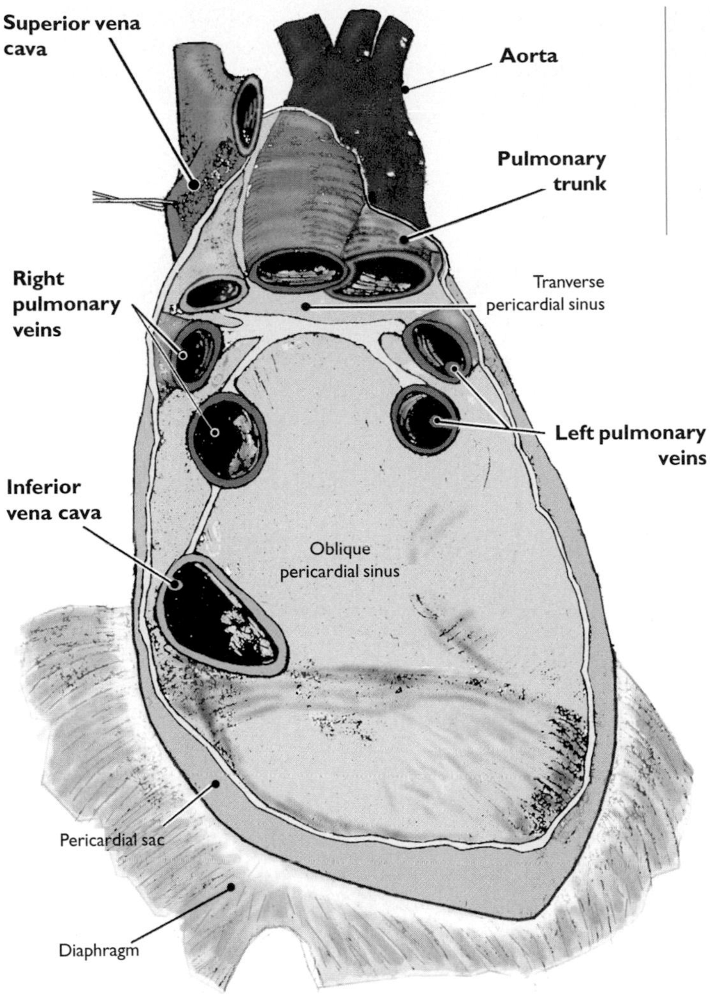

Figure 1.28. Interior of pericardial sac.

- Insinuate a finger between the superior vena cava and ascending aorta. Then, push the finger posterior to the pulmonary artery. Now your finger lies in a serous-lined tunnel known as the **transverse pericardial sinus**. Mark the sinus by placing a probe through it.
- Push two fingers posterior to the heart into the **oblique pericardial sinus**. It is a serous-lined cul-de-sac bounded by the inferior vena cava and the four pulmonary veins.
- With your fingers, explore the lines of reflection from the visceral to the parietal pericardium at the entry and exit points of the eight major vessels (compare Fig. 1.28, which illustrates these lines of reflection).
- The heart will eventually be detached along these lines of reflection. First, however, examine the heart and the great vessels *in situ*.

Heart and Great Vessels in Situ

GRANT'S 1.45
ROHEN 252
A.D.A.M. 2.16
NETTER 201
CLEMENTE 193

Heart *in situ*. Note the following (Fig. 1.27):

- Identify the surfaces of the **right atrium** and **right ventricle.**
- Observe the **right coronary artery** and the **anterior interventricular branch** (LAD, left anterior descending) **of the left coronary artery.**
- Superior to the heart, identify the **superior vena cava, ascending aorta, the left vagus nerve,** and the **recurrent laryngeal nerve** in relationship to the **ligamentum arteriosum.**

Removal of Heart

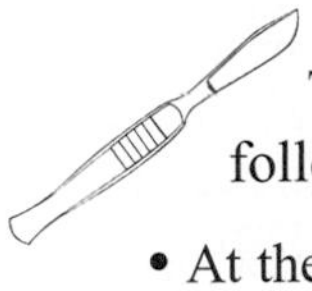

To remove the heart, proceed as follows:

- At the level of the marked transverse sinus, cut across the **ascending aorta** and the **pulmonary trunk.**
- Next, cut the **inferior vena cava** as inferior as possible within the pericardial sac.
- Transect the **superior vena cava** about 1 cm superior to its junction with the right atrium.
- Lift the heart anteriorly and superiorly by its apex. Cut across the **four pulmonary veins** where they bound the oblique sinus. Careful! Cut the pulmonary veins very close to the pericardial sac, or you will injure the left atrium.
- Now, the heart is held in place posteriorly by merely two layers of pericardium. (These layers separate the oblique from the transverse sinus. However, they cannot be discerned at this time). Cut through this posterior attachment. Remove the heart.
- Next, examine the posterior aspect of the pericardial sac. The field of dissection should compare with that of Figure 1.28 or a similar atlas illustration.

GRANT'S 1.53B
ROHEN 254
NETTER 203
CLEMENTE 194

Inspection of Heart

GRANT'S 1.43
ROHEN 255
A.D.A.M. 2.17, 2.18
NETTER 202
CLEMENTE 199, 200

Inspection. In the isolated heart, note the following:

- Identify the **coronary or atrioventricular groove (sulcus)** that runs obliquely around the heart, separating atria from ventricles.
- At right angles to the coronary sulcus are the **anterior and posterior interventricular grooves.** These grooves separate the ventricles from one another and, therefore, denote the position of the interventricular septum.

- Note that the grooves or sulci contain blood vessels. The coronary grooves are typically filled with fat. If the fat is not removed, both grooves and blood vessels are difficult to locate.

- Study the surfaces of the heart (Fig. 1.27). The **right ventricle** makes up the largest part of the anterior surface of the heart. The **right border** consists of the **right atrium**. The **left border** is formed by the **left ventricle**, which is responsible for the **apex** of the heart. At the superior end of the left border, the **auricle of the left atrium** can be seen. The **inferior border** belongs to the **right ventricle**, except for a small portion on the extreme left that belongs to the left ventricle.

⇦
GRANT'S 1.45, 1.60
ROHEN 236
A.D.A.M. 2.17, 218
NETTER 202
CLEMENTE 199, 200

- Examine the heart in superior view. Identify the **aorta and its valve**, the **pulmonary trunk and its valve**, and the **superior vena cava.**

⇦
GRANT'S 1.58
ROHEN 241
A.D.A.M. 2.19
NETTER 210
CLEMENTE 196

> ***Anatomical Position:*** It is clinically important to orientate the heart in its correct anatomical position. Proceed as follows:
>
> • Remove the dissected heart from the cadaver. Hold the isolated heart in its correct anatomical position in front of your own chest.
>
> • How sure are you that you are holding the heart correctly?
>
> • *Solution:* Use the roots of the pulmonary veins and of the venae cavae as reference structures. Pass two pencils or rods through the openings of the pulmonary veins in the left atrium, as indicated in Figure 1.29. Pass one probe from the superior vena cava through the right atrium into the inferior vena cava. In the anatomical position, the probes through the venae cavae are in a vertical position, whereas the probes through the pulmonary veins are horizontally oriented.
>
> *Note*: For instructive purposes, the heart can be conveniently placed back into the pericardial sac. This should be done whenever clarification of anatomical orientation and position is required (e.g., *anterior or posterior* papillary muscle, *plane* of base of heart, or *plane* of interventricular septum).

⇦
GRANT'S 1.43
ROHEN 236
A.D.A.M. 2.19
NETTER 202
CLEMENTE 200

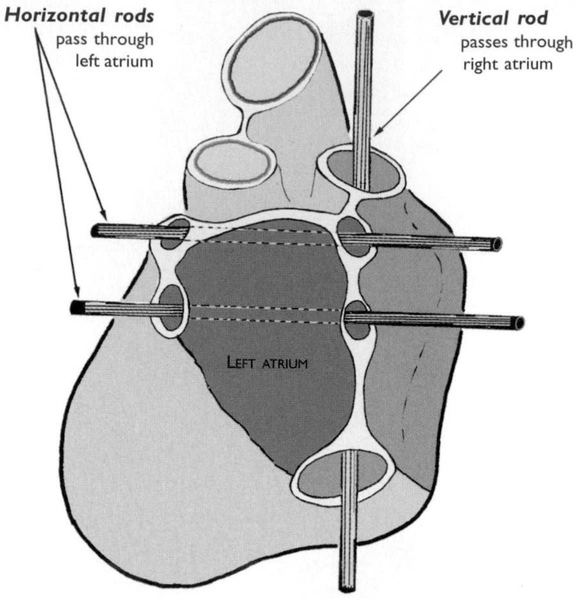

Figure 1.29. Posterior aspect of heart in anatomical position.

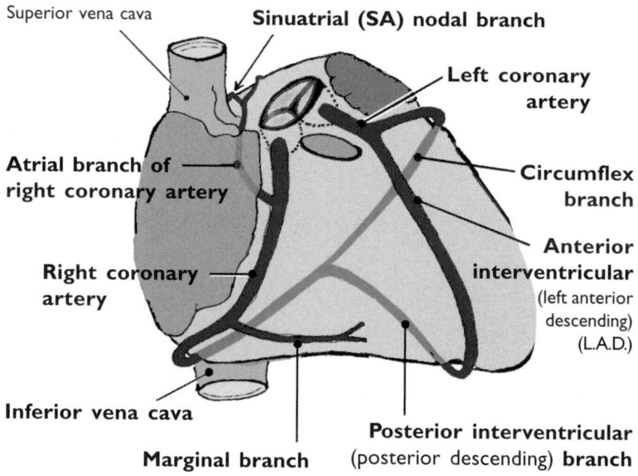

Figure 1.30. Coronary arteries. Locations of anastomoses between named coronary arteries are variable and, therefore, indicated as continuations.

Dissection of Heart

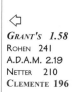

Cardiac Vessels. When dissecting these vessels, it will be necessary to remove piecemeal the epicardium and fat. Using blunt forceps, remove only enough fat and connective tissue to visualize the course of the vessels. The arteries are accompanied by veins, which will be identified subsequently. Begin with the two **coronary arteries** that originate from the **ascending aorta**.

⇦
GRANT'S 1.46
ROHEN 244
A.D.A.M. 2.19, 2.21
NETTER 204
CLEMENTE 201-204

Left Coronary Artery. Identify this vessel and proceed as follows (Fig. 1.30):

- First, identify the opening of this artery as it arises from the **ascending aorta** within the excised heart.

- Look into the remaining stump of ascending aorta and identify the **three aortic valvules** or cusps. Identify the left coronary cusp.

- Find the origin and **orifice of the left coronary artery** just superior to the left aortic cusp. Insert a probe into the coronary orifice.
- Palpate the tip of the probe between the left auricle and the cut pulmonary trunk. You have now positively identified the initial portion of the left coronary artery.
- Using blunt dissection, trace the short stem of the left coronary artery, which divides into the **anterior interventricular branch** and the **circumflex branch**.
- Follow the **anterior interventricular branch** as it travels in the anterior interventricular sulcus to the apex (clinicians refer to this vessel as the left anterior descending artery or LAD; Fig. 1.30).
- Follow the **circumflex branch** along the coronary sulcus and around the left border of the heart to the posterior aspect of the left ventricle.
- Expect to find variations of the left coronary artery and its branching patterns.

Right Coronary Artery. Identify this vessel and proceed as follows (Fig. 1.30):

- Identify the opening of the right coronary artery just superior to the right aortic valvule. Insert a probe. Palpate the tip of the probe to the left (anatomical position) of the right auricle.
- Follow the artery along the coronary sulcus to the right border of the heart, where it usually gives off the prominent **marginal branch**.
- Trace the artery along the posterior interventricular sulcus in which it descends toward the apex as the **posterior interventricular branch.**
- If time permits, identify the small but functionally important **anterior right atrial branch** (Fig. 1.30). This branch arises close to the origin of the right coronary artery and ascends along the anteromedial wall of the right atrium.
- Expect to find variations of the right coronary artery and its branching patterns.

Clinical Correlations: The **anterior right atrial artery** gives off a branch, the **superior vena caval branch**, also known as **nodal artery or sinus node artery** (Fig. 1.30). It supplies the sinuatrial (S-A) node, which is the "pacemaker" of the heart and determines the heart rate. Occlusion of the nodal artery will lead to failure of the sinus node (sinus arrest, sinus block, cardiac arrhythmia). The nodal artery can be demonstrated radiographically with selective coronary arteriography.

Expect to find variations of the coronary arteries and their branching patterns. These are common. In about 75% of the cases, the right coronary artery is dominant, i.e., posteriorly it crosses to the left side to supply the left ventricular wall and posterior portion of the interventricular septum. In about 10% of the cases, the circumflex branch of the left coronary artery, in addition to supplying all of the left ventricle, may send branches to the posterior portion of the interventricular septum and the right ventricular wall. In the remaining 15%, the posterior portion of the interventricular septum is supplied by both. The fields of distribution of the coronary arteries can be demonstrated radiographically with selective coronary arteriography. The ascending aorta and its related structures (cusps of aortic valve; coronary arteries; aortic arch) can be visualized radiographically by injecting contrast material into the root of the ascending aorta (aortic root angiogram).

GRANT'S 1.58
A.D.A.M. 2.19
NETTER 210, 211
CLEMENTE 196

GRANT'S 1.48
NETTER 205
CLEMENTE 203, 204

GRANT'S 1.47
A.D.A.M. 2.20
NETTER 206, 207
CLEMENTE 205

GRANT'S 1.48B

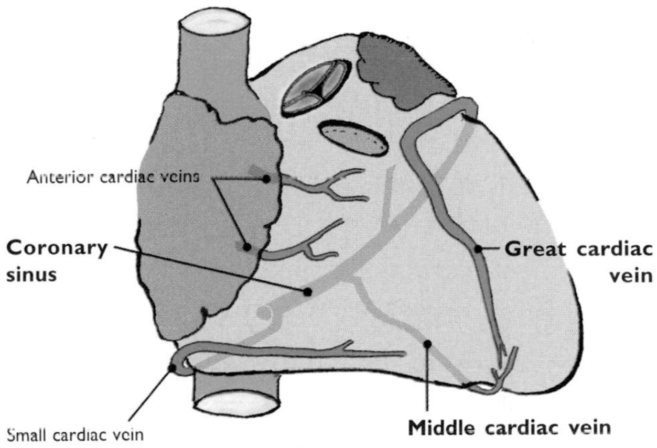

Figure 1.31. Cardiac veins.

Cardiac Veins. Observe the following (Fig. 1.31):

- Note that most veins of the heart are tributaries to the **coronary sinus**.
- Identify and clean this sizable venous channel that lies in the posterior part of the coronary sulcus. The coronary sinus is about 2 to 2.5 cm in length. Its opening into the right atrium will be seen later.
- Realize that it empties into the right atrium.
- It has **numerous tributaries.** Identify and clean the two most important ones, the **great cardiac vein** and the **middle cardiac vein.**

GRANT'S 1.49
ROHEN 240
A.D.A.M. 2.22
NETTER 204
CLEMENTE 197, 198

GRANT'S 1.46
NETTER 204
CLEMENTE 203, 204

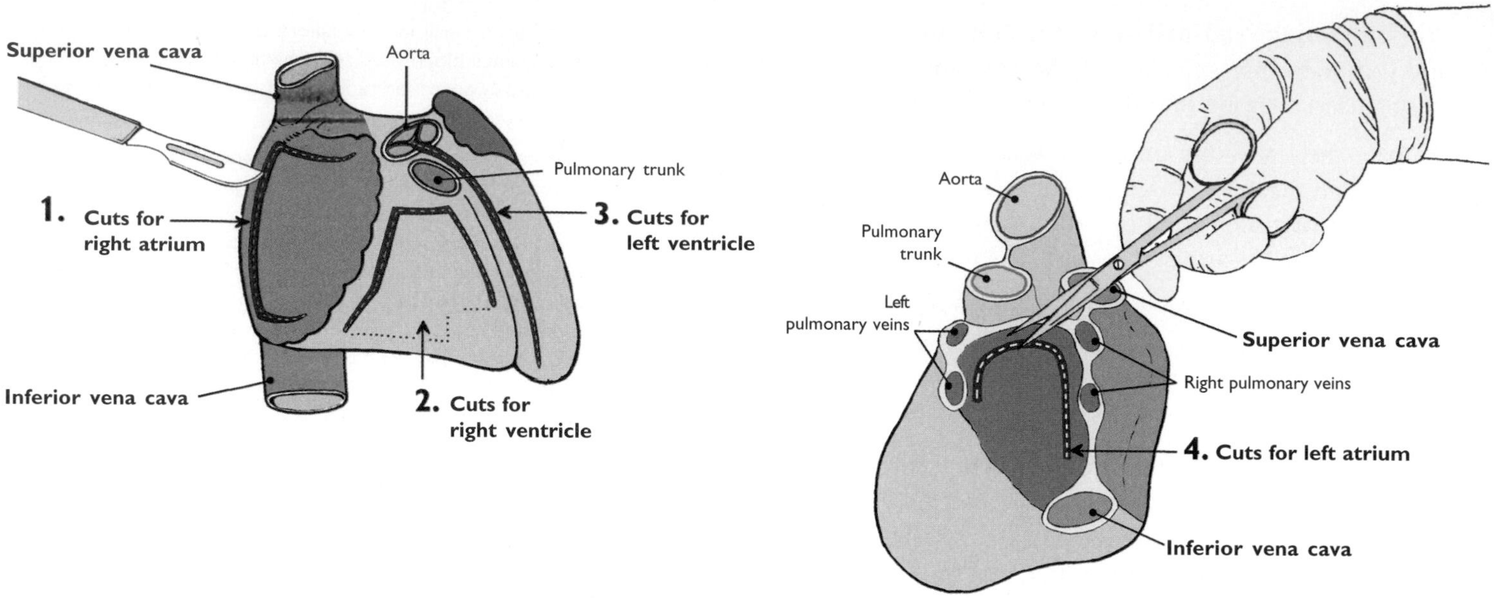

Figure 1.32. Incisions for opening the chambers of the heart.

Right Atrium. Open the right atrium in the following manner (Fig. 1.32):

- Make a short cut through the tip of the right auricle. Next, cut with scissors through the atrial wall from the initial incision toward the inferior vena cava.
- Then, cut horizontally superior to the inferior vena cava, almost to the coronary groove.
- Turn the flap of the atrial wall, and open the right atrium widely.
- Remove blood clots, and wash the area thoroughly with cold water.

Observe the following features (Fig. 1.33):

- A smooth posterior atrial wall (*Note:* "posterior" in reference to the anatomical position of the heart).
- A rough anterior atrial wall; it has comb-like parallel ridges, the **pectinate muscles**.
- The posterior and anterior walls are separated by a vertical ridge, the **crista terminalis.**
- The smooth posterior part receives the following veins: **superior vena cava, inferior vena cava, and coronary sinus.**
- **Valve of coronary sinus;** it guards the opening of the coronary sinus that empties into the right atrium between the opening of the inferior vena cava and the atrioventricular orifice.

Grant's 1.55
Rohen 240
A.D.A.M. 2.23
Netter 208
Clemente 207
A.V.A. 3: 1.13.23

Grant's 1.55B
Rohen 270
Netter 217
Clemente 221, 223

Grant's 1.60
Netter 213
Clemente 215-218

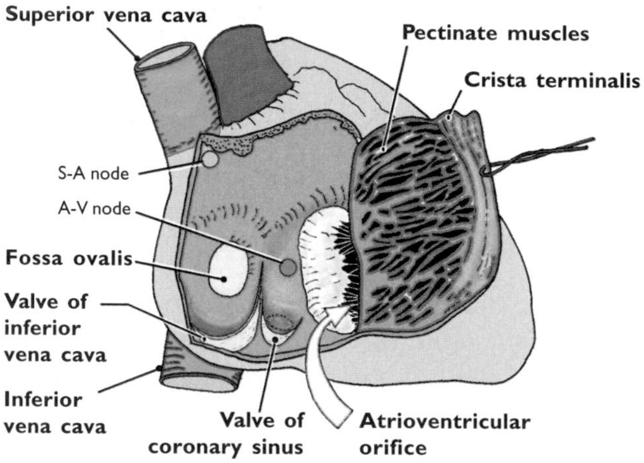

Figure 1.33. Interior of right atrium. The approximate locations of nodes of the conduction system are indicted by yellow and green dots.

- The large **atrioventricular or tricuspid orifice**, leading anteriorly to the right ventricle.
- **Fossa ovalis**, an oval depression of the interatrial wall.

Clinical Correlation: The **fossa ovalis** is the remnant of the fetal **foramen ovale.** In regard to the fetal circulation, it is significant that the blood flow from the inferior cava is directed toward the fossa ovalis, while blood from the superior part of the body via the superior vena cava is directed toward the tricuspid orifice.

Parts of the specialized **conduction (or conducting) system** of the heart are topographically related to the right atrium. These structures are too small to be visible in gross dissection. However, in view of their clinical importance, familiarize yourself with their approximate locations. Point a probe to the vicinity of two parts of the conduction system (Fig. 1.33).

1. **Sinuatrial node** (S-A node). It lies in the crista terminalis at the junction between right atrium and superior vena cava. It is supplied by the nodal artery.

2. **Atrioventricular node** (A-V node). It lies in the lower part of the interatrial septum, near the coronary sinus opening.

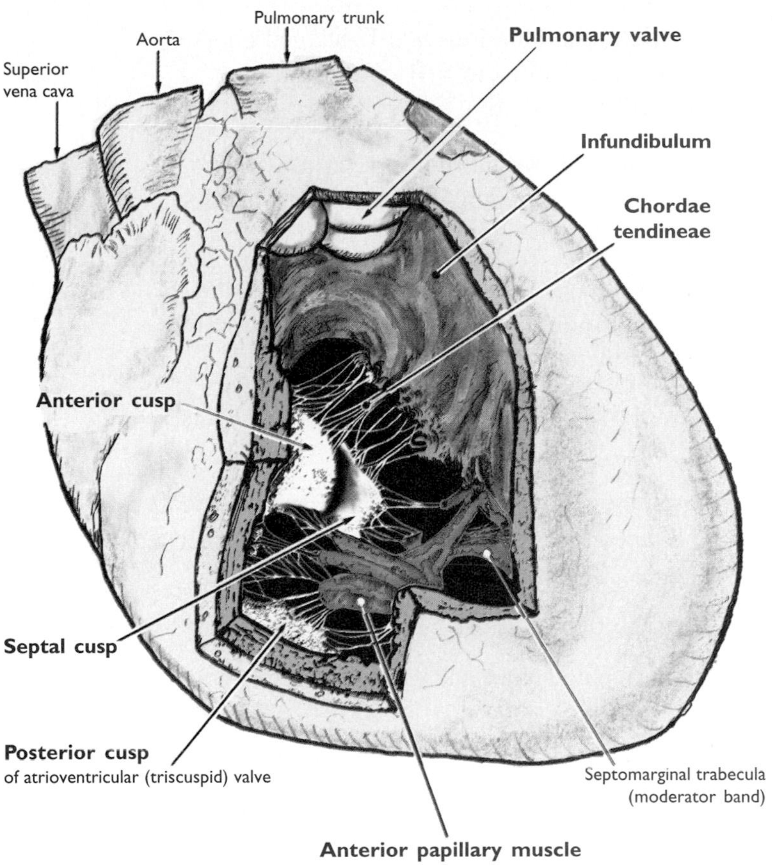

Figure 1.34. Interior of right ventricle.

Right Ventricle. Open the right ventricle in the following manner (Fig. 1.32):

- Pass a blunt instrument or your little finger into the pulmonary trunk (artery). Determine the level of the pulmonary valves.
- Make a short transverse incision into the right ventricular wall inferior to the level of the pulmonary valves.
- Insert your finger through the opening, and guide the scissors for the following cuts: 1 cm away from and parallel to the coronary groove toward the inferior border of the heart. Next, cautiously from the left end (anatomical position) of the initial transverse incision, about 2 cm from and parallel to the anterior interventricular groove, toward the inferior border of the heart.
- Turn the flap of right ventricular wall, and open the chamber widely.
- Remove blood clots. Use considerable care to avoid damage to the delicate chordae tendineae. Rinse the right ventricle thoroughly with cold water.
- Observe the following features (Fig. 1.34):
- The **right atrioventricular orifice**. It is situated dorsally, and it is large enough to admit the tips of three (average-sized) fingers.
- This orifice contains **three cusps**, hence the name **tricuspid valve**. The cusps are continuous with one another at their bases. Toward the edges, they are arranged as **anterior, septal**, and **posterior cusps.** Small secondary cusps may be present and may obscure the general arrangement.
- The **chordae tendineae**. Observe that these tendinous strands pass from the margins and ventricular surfaces of the cusps into the apices of papillary muscles (the strands are arranged like the cords of a parachute.)

⇦
GRANT'S 1.56
ROHEN 240, 243
A.D.A.M. 2.24
NETTER 208
CLEMENTE 207, 208

- **Papillary muscles**. The **anterior papillary muscle** is the largest and most prominent. Its chordae tendineae are attached to the anterior and posterior cusps. The other papillary muscles are much smaller and irregular in disposition. They are designated **posterior** and **septal.** The septal papillary muscles are very small and multiple. Each papillary muscle controls the adjacent sides of cusps.
- The interior wall of the right ventricle is roughened by muscular ridges and bridges. These are known as the **trabeculae carneae** (L. *trabs*, wooden beam; *carneus*, fleshy).
- Septomarginal trabecula (moderator band), stretching from the interventricular septum to the base of the anterior papillary muscle.

⇦
GRANT'S 1.56B
NETTER 211
CLEMENTE 213

- The **orifice of the pulmonary trunk** (pulmonary orifice). The cone-shaped portion of the chamber inferior to the orifice is the **conus arteriosus or infundibulum**. Within the right ventricle, the blood takes a U-shaped course in passing from the orifice of entrance to the orifice of exit.

- The **valve of the pulmonary trunk** (pulmonary valve) consists of three semilunar valvules of cusps: an *anterior*, a *right*, and a *left*.

Left Atrium. Observe the entrances of the **four pulmonary veins** into the right and left sides of the atrium. Proceed as follows:

- Leave the openings of the pulmonary veins intact.
- Open the left atrium by means of an inverted U-shaped incision through the posterior wall (Fig. 1.32).
- Turn the flap inferiorly.
- Remove blood clots, and wash thoroughly with cold water.

Observe the following features:

- The **left atrioventricular or mitral orifice** opening through the inferior half of the anterior wall into the left ventricle.
- The opening of the tubular left auricle.
- The site of closure of the **foramen ovale**, situated anteriorly and to the right (anatomical position of heart) and usually defined by a curved ridge.
- The atrial wall is smooth, except for small pectinate muscles in the left auricle.

Left Ventricle. Note that during the following procedure some blood vessels will be cut. Open the left ventricle in the following manner (Fig. 1.32):

- Make a cut 1 cm to the left (anatomical position) of and parallel to the anterior interventricular groove.
- Expect that the thickness of the wall is about 1 to 1.5 cm.
- Start the cut near the apex and extend it to the root of the aorta.
- Guide the cut with a finger passing from the left atrium through the left atrioventricular orifice into the left ventricle.

⇦ *Grant's 1.58* Rohen 241 A.D.A.M. 2.19 Netter 210 Clemente 196, 208

⇨ *Grant's 1.57* Rohen 240 A.D.A.M. 2.25 Netter 209 Clemente 209, 210

⇦ *Grant's 1.60* Rohen 240 A.D.A.M. 2.25 Netter 209 Clemente 209

- Extend the incision along the entire length of the ascending aorta. Try to avoid cutting the leaflets of the aortic valve.
- During the prescribed cut, the left coronary artery or its branches as well as the great cardiac vein must be severed.
- Open the left ventricle and the length of the ascending aorta widely.
- Remove blood clots. Use considerable care to avoid damage to the delicate chordae tendineae. Rinse the left ventricle thoroughly with cold water.

Observe the following features (Fig. 1.35):

- The left ventricular cavity is cone-shaped in outline and circular on cross section.
- Compare left and right ventricles and note that, by contrast, the right ventricle is crescent-shaped on transverse section (Fig. 1.36). The interventricular septum is convex toward the right chamber because the pressure is higher on the left arterial than on the right venous side.

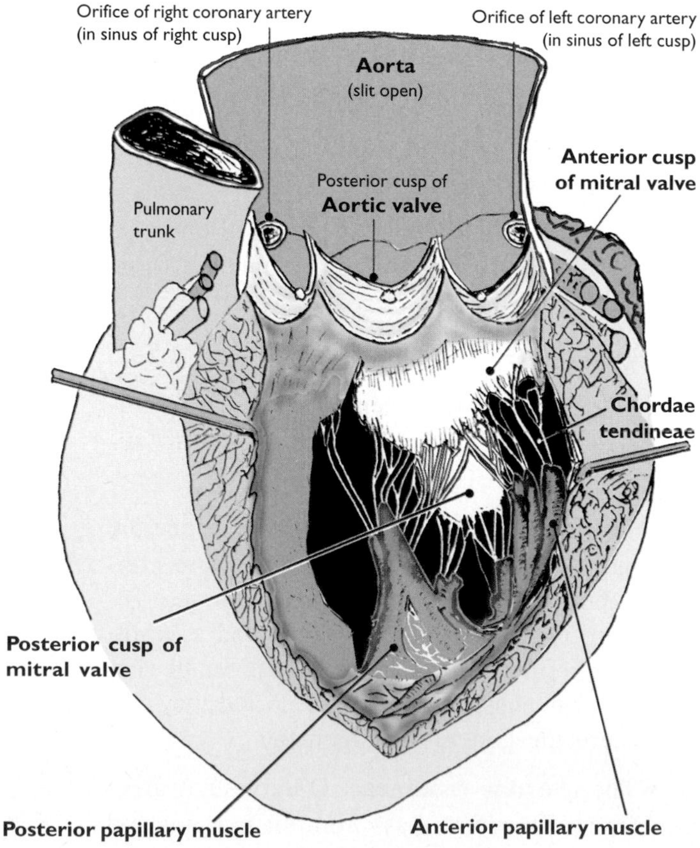

Figure 1.35. Interior of left ventricle.

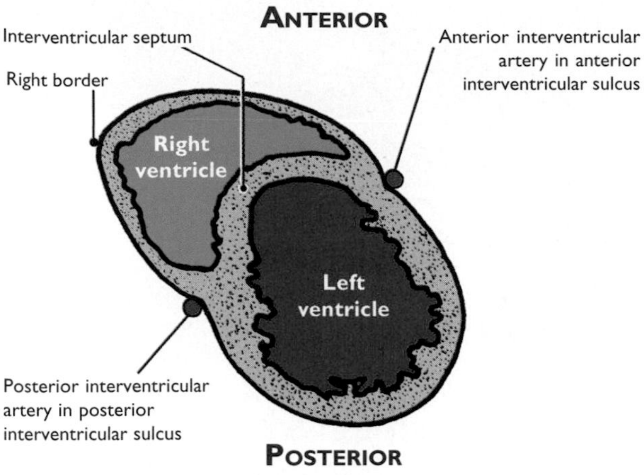

Figure 1.36. Horizontal section through right and left ventricles.

- The muscular wall is about 1 to 1.5 cm in thickness, but much thinner at the apex. In the normal (not necessarily in the diseased) heart, the left ventricular wall is about three times as thick as the right one.
- The **left atrioventricular or mitral orifice** (Fig. 1.35).
- The **left atrioventricular valve (bicuspid or mitral valve)**, consisting of an **anterior cusp** and a **posterior cusp**. The larger anterior cusp intervenes between the atrioventricular and aortic orifices.
- **Chordae tendineae**, attached to two papillary muscles, *anterior* and *posterior*.
- **Trabeculae carneae.**
- **Aortic valve**, composed of three semilunar cusps: **right cusp**, **left cusp**, and posterior or **noncoronary cusp**. Observe the **nodule**, a small fibrous thickening at the middle of the free margin of each cusp.
- Probe the orifices of the **two coronary arteries** and study their relation to the two coronary valvules.
- The thick and extensive **muscular part of the interventricular septum.**
- The **membranous part of the interventricular septum**, about the size of a fingernail. It is situated just inferior to the attached margins of the right coronary and noncoronary cusps of the aortic valve. Palpate this thin, smooth, and fibrous structure between your index fingers, one in each ventricle.

Clinical Correlation: The thin **membranous interventricular septum** adjoins the atrial septum. During development, the membranous interventricular septum closes last. It may be the site of a congenital defect, the membranous ventricular septal defect (VSD). This defect is often seen in combination with other cardiac anomalies.

GRANT'S 1.60
NETTER 213
CLEMENTE 215-218

Review the **conducting system** of the heart. The atrioventricular (AV) bundle passes from the AV node to the membranous part of the interventricular septum. Subsequently, it divides into **right and left bundle branches** on either side of the muscular part of the interventricular septum. The right bundle branch connects via the septomarginal trabecula to the anterior papillary muscle. Damage to the conducting system (e.g., bundle branch block) results in various forms of cardiac arrhythmias. The dissection of the conducting system is extremely difficult.

GRANT'S 1.53B
ROHEN 254
A.D.A.M. 2.27
NETTER 203
CLEMENTE 194

Review of Relations. Examine the posterior aspect of the pericardial sac and the openings of the eight major vessels. The field of dissection should compare with that of Figure 1.28 or a similar atlas illustration. Place the dissected heart back into the remaining portion of the pericardial sac. Make sure that it is properly placed in its anatomical position. Identify the major vessels in the heart, and observe their former connections to the cut vessels in the interior of the pericardial sac:

- Superior vena cava;
- Inferior vena cava;
- Two right and two left pulmonary veins;
- Ascending aorta;
- Pulmonary trunk.
- In addition, identify the ligamentum arteriosum. What happens if this structure fails to close postnatally?

GRANT'S 1.57
NETTER 211
CLEMENTE 210

Moisten the entire region well with preservative fluid and cover the properly prepared specimen.

***Clinical Observation,* Heart:** Did you notice any abnormal fluids (e.g., blood) in the pericardial sac? Assess the size of the heart. Is it abnormally enlarged? Compare its size to that of the fist of the corresponding cadaver. Measure the thickness of the myocardium of the right and left ventricles; is there a difference? Observe the distribution pattern of the coronary arteries. Are the coronary arteries anomalous? Examine the lumina of the coronary arteries, particularly near the origin from the ascending aorta. Is the lumen patent, or is there narrowing or even occlusion of the lumen? Is there evidence of coronary bypass surgery? If you find coronary pathology, look for evidence of myocardial infarction (MI). Relatively fresh and large infarcts may present as bluish discolorations, whereas an old and healed infarct may appear as whitish scar tissue. In severe cases, the entire thickness of the ventricular wall may be involved. Are the heart valves smooth or damaged? Are the papillary muscles and the attached chordae tendineae intact? Did you discover a pacemaker lead? If so, where was the intracardiac electrode tip located?

Posterior Mediastinum

Orientation

Review the boundaries of the **posterior mediastinum** (Fig. 1.24). It is that portion of the mediastinum anterior to the bodies of the inferior eight thoracic vertebrae (T5 through T12) and posterior to the pericardium. Thus, it is logical to approach the structures in the posterior mediastinum through the posterior wall of the pericardial sac. Review the interior of the **pericardial sac** (Fig. 1.28). Pay special attention to the posterior wall of the sac and the oblique pericardial sinus. The esophagus, the descending aorta, and the mediastinal portions of both lungs are closely related to the pericardial sac.

GRANT'S 1.54
ROHEN 255
A.D.A.M. 2.29-2.32
NETTER 218, 219
CLEMENTE 187, 189
A.V.A. 3: 1.08.56

Temporarily, place the heart back into the opened pericardial sac. Examine its topographic relations to the esophagus. Note that the esophagus lies immediately posterior to the left atrium and part of the left ventricle. Next, temporarily place both lungs back onto their respective pleural cavities. Verify that the mediastinal portions of both lungs lie posterior to the heart. Having observed these important anatomical relations, you may now remove the lungs and the heart.

Clinical Correlation: The topographic relations between heart and esophagus have clinical implications. The posterior aspect of the heart can be best evaluated radiographically when the esophagus is filled with radiopaque material.The esophagus lies immediately posterior to the left atrium and part of the left ventricle. An enlargement of these chambers will indent the barium-filled esophagus and displace it posteriorly.

Certain heart murmurs in the left atrial area (regurgitant murmurs in mitral valve insufficiency) can be recorded with the aid of a small microphone channeled into the esophagus posterior to the heart.

Posterior Mediastinal Structures

Remove the posterior wall of the pericardial sac in the area of the oblique sinus (Fig. 1.37). Now, examine the posterior

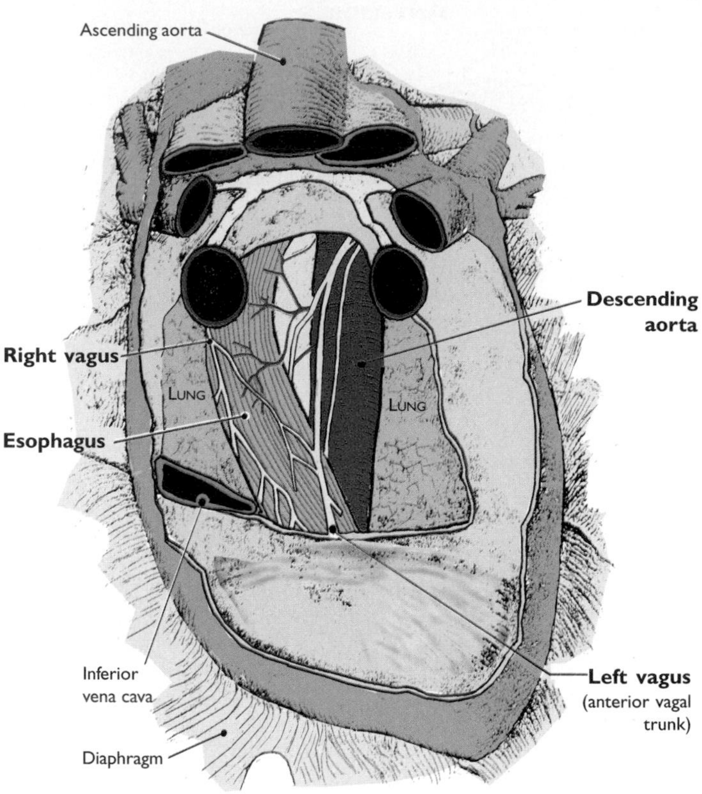

Figure 1.37. Window in the posterior wall of the pericardial sac allows access to the structures in the posterior mediastinum.

relations of the heart. Most anteriorly and slightly to the right is the **esophagus,** a collapsed muscular tube. To expose the structures in the posterior mediastinum, proceed as follows:

GRANT'S 1.37, 1.38
ROHEN 256
A.D.A.M. 2.29 - 2.32
NETTER 220
CLEMENTE 229, 237

- Remove the remainder of the pericardial sac, but leave intact the portion adhering to the diaphragm. Now you have wide access to the posterior mediastinum.
- Clean the **esophagus.** Pay special attention to the **two vagal nerves** and their relations to the esophagus.
- Identify and clean the **right vagus** posterior to the root of the right lung. Follow the nerve to the esophagus and verify that the vagal fibers separate and spread out on the esophagus as the **esophageal plexus** (Fig. 1.38).

GRANT'S 1.38
ROHEN 261
A.D.A.M. 2.29
NETTER 219
CLEMENTE 189
A.V.A. 3: 1.17.23

- Identify the **left vagus** as it crosses the left side of the aortic arch. Use a probe and bluntly dissect the nerve.
- Confirm that the concavity of the aortic arch is connected to the left pulmonary artery by a stout, obliquely set cord, the **ligamentum arteriosum.**

- Find and clean the **left recurrent laryngeal nerve**, a branch of the left vagus nerve, as it courses immediately posterior to the ligamentum arteriosum.

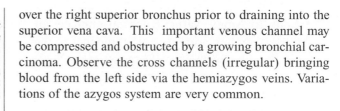

GRANT'S 1.37, 1.73, 1.74
ROHEN 261
A.D.A.M. 2.31
NETTER 218, 226
CLEMENTE 233-235
A.V.A. 3: 1.14.05

- Next, trace the left vagus posterior to the root of the left lung, and follow it to the esophagus.
- Verify the following (Fig. 1.38): Close to the diaphragm, the bundles of the esophageal plexus combine to form the two **vagal trunks**, an *anterior* and a *posterior* one. Due to the rotation of the gut during development, the bundles from the left vagus swing around to the anterior surface of the esophagus. The bundles from the right vagus come to lie dorsal to the esophagus. The vagal trunks pass through the diaphragm together with the esophagus to supply the stomach and other parts of the intestinal tract.

GRANT'S 1.70
ROHEN 261
A.D.A.M. 2.35
NETTER 220, 228, 229
CLEMENTE 236, 237
A.V.A. 3: 1.17.23

Before the next dissection step, study the **azygos system of veins**. Note that the intercostal veins on the right side are tributaries to the azygos vein (Fig. 1.38). Pay special attention to the fact that the azygos vein arches over the right superior bronchus prior to draining into the superior vena cava. This important venous channel may be compressed and obstructed by a growing bronchial carcinoma. Observe the cross channels (irregular) bringing blood from the left side via the hemiazygos veins. Variations of the azygos system are very common.

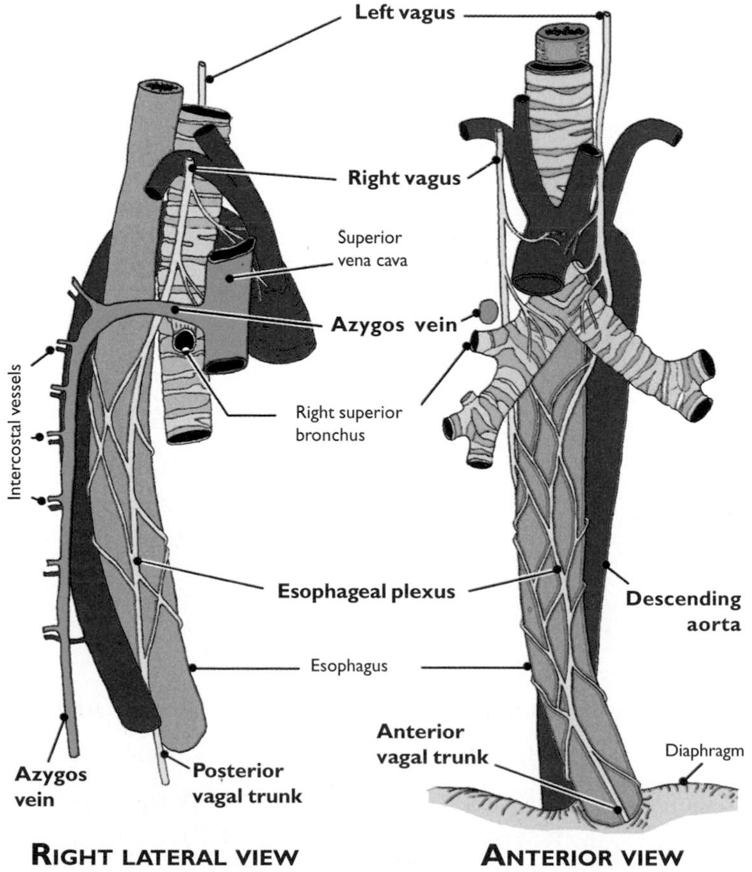

Figure 1.38. Right and left vagus nerve, esophageal nerve plexus, and vagal trunks. Azygos vein and related structures.

Turning back to the cadaver and to the posterior mediastinum, proceed as follows:

- Pull the esophagus to the left and expose the **azygos vein** on the right.
- Identify the vein as it arches superior to the root of the right lung.
- Follow the azygos vein caudally to the diaphragm. Note that the **intercostal veins** on the right side are tributaries to the azygos vein. Clean all vessels.

Another structure coursing in the posterior mediastinum is the **thoracic duct**.

GRANT'S 1.69, 1.71
ROHEN 261
A.D.A.M. 2.13
NETTER 226, 227
CLEMENTE 233, 234

To identify it, proceed as follows:

- Pull the esophagus to the left and explore the interval between the **azygos vein** and the **descending aorta**. In this interval, identify the **thoracic duct**. The duct is a thin-walled, pale, and easily torn structure.
- Carefully free the fragile thoracic duct from the surrounding fatty areolar tissue. Commonly, the duct may be plexiform in the posterior mediastinum; i.e., you may find a network of several small ducts instead of one large thoracic duct. The thoracic duct traverses the **diaphragm** together with the descending aorta.

Clinical Correlation: The delicate thoracic duct may be injured and torn as a complication of thoracic surgery, chest trauma, or tumor infiltration. As a result, chyle (fatty lymphatic fluid) accumulates in the posterior mediastinum, leading to a so-called "widening of the mediastinum" that can be visualized on chest radiographs. The milky chylous fluid may gradually leak from the mediastinum into the pleural cavities. There, by means of a pleural tap, it may be aspirated into a syringe. The amounts of extravasated chyle may be considerable.

Demonstrate the remaining structures in the **posterior mediastinum**. Proceed as follows:

- Identify the **descending aorta.** Clean it from the surrounding fatty areolar tissue.
- Demonstrate the **descending aorta** throughout its length.

Grant's 1.68
Netter 196
Clemente 231
A.V.A. 3: 1.09.07

- Look for small, variable arterial branches of the descending aorta. Identify branches to the esophagus and trachea. Demonstrate at least one pair of **posterior intercostal branches**. In addition, note at least one of the several **bronchial arteries** as they arise from the descending aorta.

Grant's 1.70, 1.71
Netter 198, 228
Clemente 233
A.V.A. 3: 1.19.26

- Next, using a probe, isolate the relatively thick **thoracic greater splanchnic nerve** on the right and on the left. Note that the nerve receives fibers from the 5th through the 10th thoracic sympathetic ganglia.
- Attempt to find the much smaller **thoracic lesser splanchnic nerve** just lateral to the greater thoracic splanchnic nerve. The lesser thoracic **splanchnic nerve** is formed by fibers from the 10th and 11th thoracic sympathetic ganglia.
- Follow the thoracic greater and lesser splanchnic nerves inferiorly. Note that they pierce the crus of the diaphragm. Their course in the abdomen will be explored later.

> ***Dissection Note:*** The **sympathetic trunks** lie posterior to each lung and *not* between the mediastinal pleurae. Therefore, the sympathetic trunks are *not* contained in any subdivision of the mediastinum. However, some of its branches, the splanchnic nerves, turn medially and anteriorly and thus become part of the posterior mediastinum.
>
> As a variation, the **thoracic splanchnic nerves** are sometimes fused. Be aware of the general plan of sympathetic nerve distribution to the viscera (Fig. 1.19).

Grant's 1.22C
Rohen 269
Netter 230
Clemente 169, 170

Review the classic anterior, middle, and posterior mediastinal subdivisions (Fig. 1.24). Study a transverse section through the heart and lungs, and identify the mediastinal subdivisions in this section.

Superior Mediastinum

Orientation

Review the boundaries of the **superior mediastinum** (Fig. 1.24). They are:

- Superiorly, superior aperture of thorax (i.e., superior entrance into thorax bounded by manubrium, 1st thoracic vertebra, and the two 1st ribs);
- Posteriorly, thoracic vertebrae 1 through 4;
- Anteriorly, manubrium of sternum;
- Laterally, mediastinal pleurae of the two lungs.
- Inferiorly, a plane from sternal angle to intervertebral disc T4-T5; this plane is just superior to the limit of the pericardium.

Superior Mediastinal Structures

Dissection of Superior Mediastinal Structures. Gain wider access to the area by removing (with pliers or a saw) the inferior portion of the manubrium. Leave the first sternocostal joints and the sternoclavicular joints intact.

> ***Dissection Note:*** Some instructors prefer to remove the sternum and the anterior portion of the first ribs to have unobstructed access to the superior mediastinum. Please check with your instructor.

Grant's 1.62
Rohen 248
Netter 200
Clemente 163

Thymus and Great Veins. Proceed with dissection as follows:

- Identify the **thymus**. In the adult cadaver, it is represented by a (functionally inactive) fatty mass that lies immediately posterior to the manubrium. Do not overlook the thymus just because it resembles fat. Note its venous drainage.
- Remove the thymus but do not damage the left brachiocephalic vein that lies posterior to it.

Clemente 281

> ***Clinical Correlation:*** In the newborn, the thymus is a broad, lobulated, active glandular structure that can be readily visualized on a routine chest radiograph. In the infant and child, the thymus is a prominent, active organ that reaches inferiorly into the anterior mediastinum. After puberty, the organ undergoes involution, and it may be scarcely recognizable in old age, having been replaced by fibrous tissue and fat.

Grant's 1.37, 1.74
Rohen 259, 261
A.D.A.M. 2.37
Netter 201, 226
Clemente 194, 234
A.V.A. 3: 1.11.55

Now, clean the **great veins**.

- At the right margin of the manubrium, the **two brachiocephalic veins** (innominate veins) meet to form the **superior vena cava.**
- Follow the superior vena cava inferiorly to the root of the right lung. Notice that the azygos vein drains into the superior vena cava.
- Cut the superior vena cava just superior to the entrance of the azygos vein.
- Reflect the great veins superiorly and expose the **arch of the aorta** (Fig. 1.39).

Arch of Aorta and Branches. The aortic arch, by definition, begins and ends at the

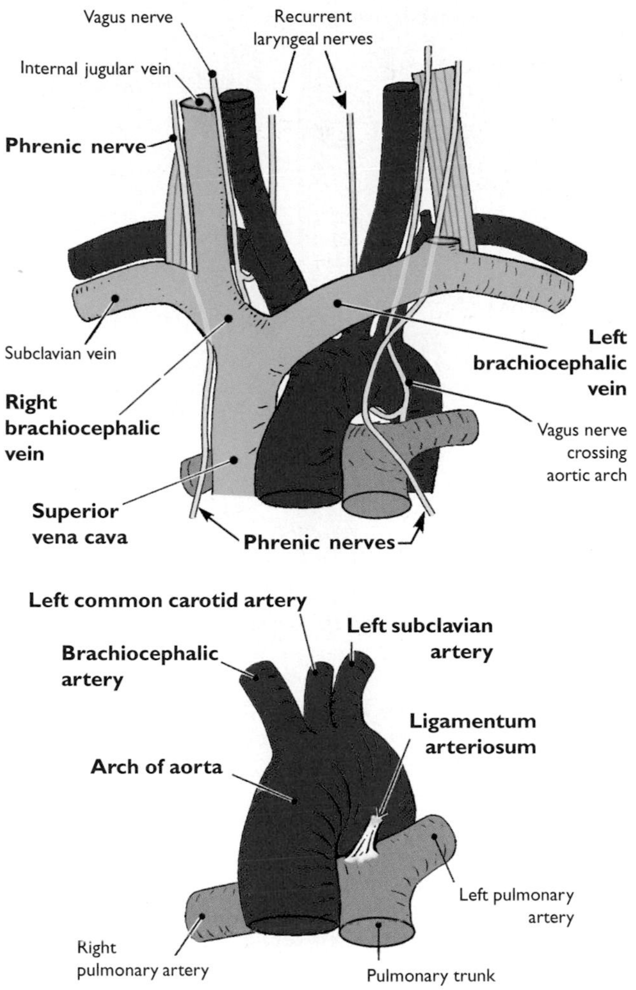

Figure 1.39. Arch of the aorta and related vessels and nerves.

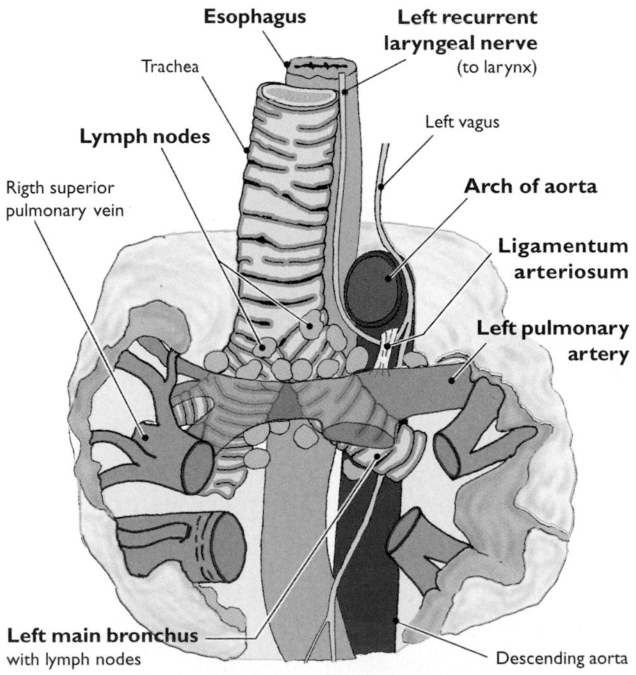

Figure 1.40. Principal structures that are closely related to the aortic arch (*normal anatomy*).

GRANT'S 1.63, 1.67
ROHEN 261
A.D.A.M. 2.13, 2.14
NETTER 225
CLEMENTE 194
A.V.A. 3: 1.06.07

same level: this is the sternal angle anteriorly, and the intervertebral disc T4-T5 posteriorly. Observe that the aorta arches over the left bronchus and then becomes the descending aorta. Demonstrate the aortic arch and the three great arteries arising from it. Identify:

- **Brachiocephalic trunk** (innominate artery), arising from the summit of the aortic arch.
- **Left common carotid artery.**
- **Left subclavian artery.** It lies immediately posterior to the left common carotid artery.
- Verify that the aortic arch passes from anterior to posterior.

GRANT'S 1.64
A.D.A.M. 2.17, 2.29
NETTER 201
CLEMENTE 194, 199
A.V.A. 3: 1.05.26

- Confirm that the concavity of the aortic arch is connected to the left pulmonary artery by a stout, obliquely set cord, the **ligamentum arteriosum**.
- Note that the aorta arches superior to (over) the left main bronchus and then becomes the descending aorta (Fig. 1.40).
- Verify that the following principal structures are closely related to the arch of the aorta (Fig. 1.40): **left pulmonary artery**, **ligamentum arteriosum**, **left recurrent laryngeal nerve**, and **left main bronchus** together with its related lymph nodes. The **esophagus** lies on the right side of the **aortic arch**.

Clinical Correlation: The area between the concavity of the aortic arch and the left pulmonary artery is of considerable clinical importance (Fig. 1.40). Bronchogenic carcinoma developing and malignantly growing in the area of the left main bronchus will invade the regional lymph nodes. The considerably enlarged lymph nodes, in turn, compress and impair the left recurrent laryngeal nerve, leading to paralysis of the left vocal cord in the larynx with associated persistent hoarseness. Conversely, an aneurysm (cirumscribed and pulsating dilation in advanced arterial disease) of the arch of the aorta may exert severe pressure on the left main bronchus, the esophagus, and the left recurrent laryngel nerve. This condition will most likely produce the "symptom complex" of breathing problems, difficulty in swallowing, and hoarseness.

GRANT'S 1.51, 1.52

There may be variations in the origins of arterial branches from the aortic arch. The vessels arising from the arch of the aorta can be demonstrated radiographically. Thus, abnormalities within these arteries as well as variations in the origins of the branches of the aortic arch can be detected. In addition, abnormalities of the aortic arch itself can be visualized radiographically. The aortic arch is also crossed by two slender **cardiac nerves** that are difficult to find. Often these nerves are mistaken for connective tissue. They arise in the neck from the sympathetic trunk and from the vagus and pass to the superficial cardiac plexus

GRANT'S 1.45, 1.64
NETTER 198
CLEMENTE 237

situated just to the right of the ligamentum arteriosum. These nerves also contain sensory fibers that carry the sensation of pain.

Left Phrenic Nerve and Left Vagus. The aortic arch is crossed by two nerves that descend vertically from the neck into the thorax: the **left phrenic nerve** and the **left vagus**. Identify and clean these structures (Figs. 1.38, 1.39):

GRANT'S 1.38, 1.63
ROHEN 253, 254
A.D.A.M. 2.35, 2.37
NETTER 200, 214
CLEMENTE 190, 192
A.V.A. 3: 1.17.09

- Locate the **left phrenic nerve** between the **subclavian artery** and **subclavian vein.**
- Demonstrate that it crosses the aortic arch.
- Clean the entire length of the nerve. Follow it anterior to the **root of the left lung.**
- Restore its approximate position on the left side of the (now removed) pericardial sac. Demonstrate its entry point into the **diaphragm.**
- Next, locate the **left vagus.** Find it in the angular interval between the **left common carotid** and **subclavian arteries.**

GRANT'S 1.64
NETTER 214
A.V.A. 3: 1.18.03

- Trace the left vagus across the left side of the aortic arch and clean it.
- Because it descends to the esophagus, it passes posterior to the root of the left lung, i.e., posterior to the left main bronchus (Fig. 1.41).
- Find and clean the **left recurrent laryngeal nerve.** Locate it immediately posterior to the ligamentum arteriosum. Follow it for a short distance superiorly. Later, the nerve will be followed to its termination in the larynx.

GRANT'S 1.70
NETTER 198, 214, 215, 228
CLEMENTE 237

Right Phrenic Nerve and Right Vagus (Figs. 1.38, 1.39). Proceed with dissection as follows:

GRANT'S 1.37, 1.63
ROHEN 253, 254
A.D.A.M. 2.35, 2.37
NETTER 200, 214
CLEMENTE 190, 237
A.V.A. 3: 1.16.35

- Identify and clean the **right phrenic nerve** as it descends lateral to the **superior vena cava**, anterior to the **root of the right lung**, lateral to the (now removed) pericardial sac, and lateral to the **inferior vena cava.**
- Note that the **right vagus** takes a course along the right side of the **trachea** and toward the posterior aspect of the root of the right lung (Fig. 1.41). Define small branches of the vagus that cross the trachea anteriorly; these are cardiac branches on their way to the deep cardiac plexus.

GRANT'S 1.64, 1.67
NETTER 197

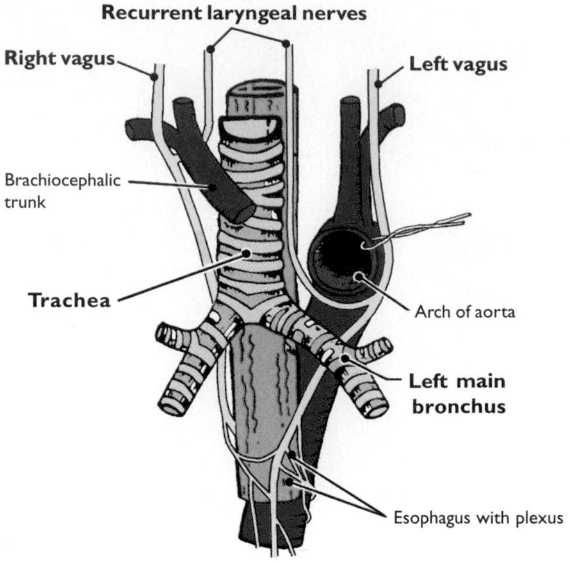

Figure 1.41. Right and left vagus, their recurrent laryngeal nerve branches, and their relations to trachea and esophagus.

Clinical Correlation: The right recurrent laryngeal nerve (a branch of the right vagus) cannot be demonstrated because it loops around the right subclavian artery that is beyond the boundaries of the superior mediastinum. In contrast, the left recurrent laryngeal nerve, with its close relation to the aortic arch, traverses the superior mediastinum. Thus, in cases of mediastinal tumors, the left recurrent laryngeal nerve is likely to be compromised, resulting in paralysis of the left vocal cord (with associated hoarseness).

Observe a number of fine branches from both vagi and sympathetic trunks as they course toward an area between the aortic arch and the bifurcation of the trachea. This is the site of the **deep cardiac plexus** that is much more extensive than the superficial cardiac plexus. Review the nerve supply of the thoracic contents.

Trachea and Related Structures. Pay special attention to the following clinically important structures:

- Demonstrate and clean the **tracheobronchial lymph nodes** on both sides of the trachea and in the vicinity of its bifurcation (Fig.1.40).
- This mass of pigmented nodes fills the angle within the fork of the trachea and intervenes between the right pulmonary artery and esophagus.
- Isolate the trachea in the superior mediastinum (Fig. 1.41). Be careful; do not damage nerve branches adhering to it.
- Identify the **bifurcation of the trachea.**

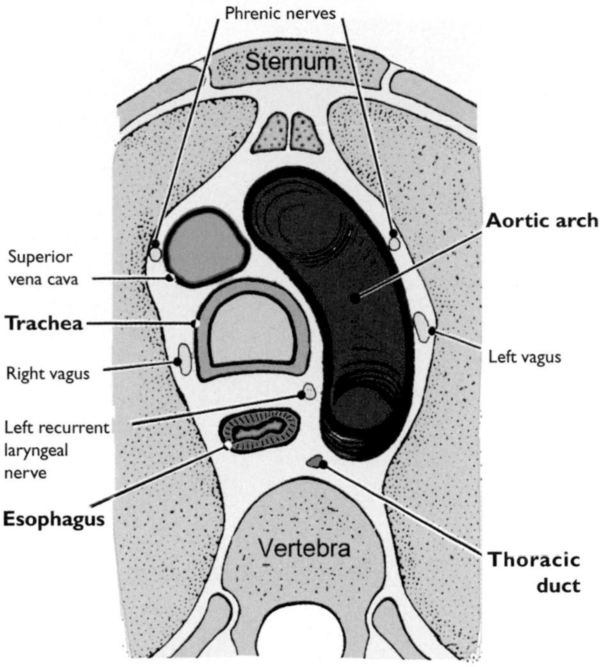

Figure 1.42. Transverse section through superior mediastinum at the level of the aortic arch.

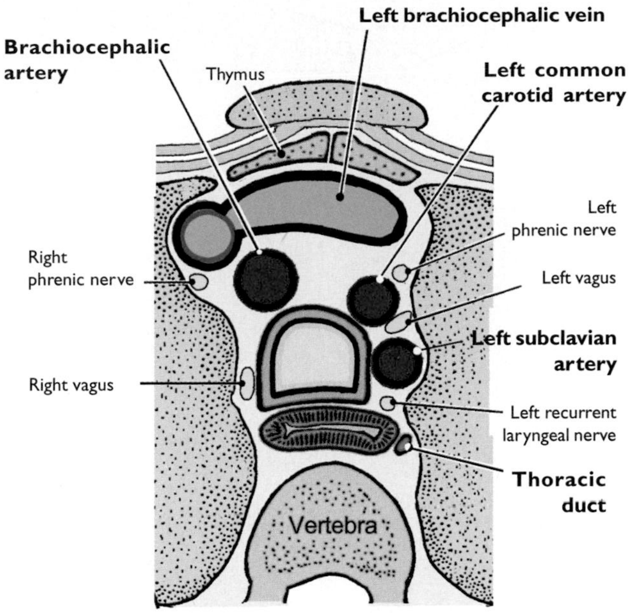

Figure 1.43. Transverse section through superior mediastinum superior to (above) the aortic arch.

- Study the strategic location of the **bifurcation of the trachea.** Review the four major structures topographically related to the bifurcation, sequentially from deep to superficial: lymph nodes at the tracheal bifurcation, pulmonary arteries, ascending aorta and arch of aorta, and brachiocephalic veins forming the superior vena cava.

GRANT'S 1.61, 1.65
ROHEN 256
A.D.A.M. 2.13
NETTER 194, 195, 198
CLEMENTE 233

- Palpate the anterior and posterior surface of the trachea near its bifurcation. Identify individual **tracheal rings.** Note that these "rings" are imperfect: only the anterior two-thirds of the circumference consists of cartilage. Posteriorly, the tracheal tube is completed by a musculofibrous membrane.

GRANT'S 1.65
A.D.A.M. 2.12
NETTER 190

- With scissors, incise the right main bronchus. Carry the incision to the tracheal bifurcation. Identify the **carina.** It is a ridge on the inside of the tracheal bifurcation.

Clinical Correlation: During bronchoscopy, the **carina** serves as an important landmark. It stands between the superior ends of the right and left main bronchi. Lymph nodes closely related to the tracheal bifurcation are often referred to as carinal nodes.

Foreign bodies (paper clips, small metal objects, etc.) are usually aspirated into the right main bronchus. Understand why:

(a) the right main bronchus is more vertical, shorter, and wider than the left one; (b) the carina is usually positioned slightly to the left of the median plane.

- Examine the right main bronchus. Compare its diameter and angle of descent with that of the left main bronchus. Note the rings of cartilage in the bronchial tree.

CLEMENTE 168

Correlation and Review. Correlate your gross anatomical observations in the superior mediastinum with suitable transverse sections:

- First, study a **transverse section at the level of the aortic arch** (Fig. 1.42). There are four parallel and vertically running structures: **esophagus, trachea, left recurrent laryngeal nerve,** and **thoracic duct.**
- Observe that the left recurrent laryngeal nerve lies in the interval between trachea and esophagus. The left vagus is related to the aortic arch, whereas the right vagus is applied to the lateral aspect of the trachea.
- Next, study a **transverse section superior to the level of the aortic arch** (Fig. 1.43). Note that the four parallel and vertically running structures are the same as in the more inferior transverse section.

GRANT'S 1.65
A.D.A.M. 2.11
NETTER 190
CLEMENTE 180

- Identify the three major arteries that arise from the aortic arch: **brachiocephalic, left common carotid,** and **left subclavian.**

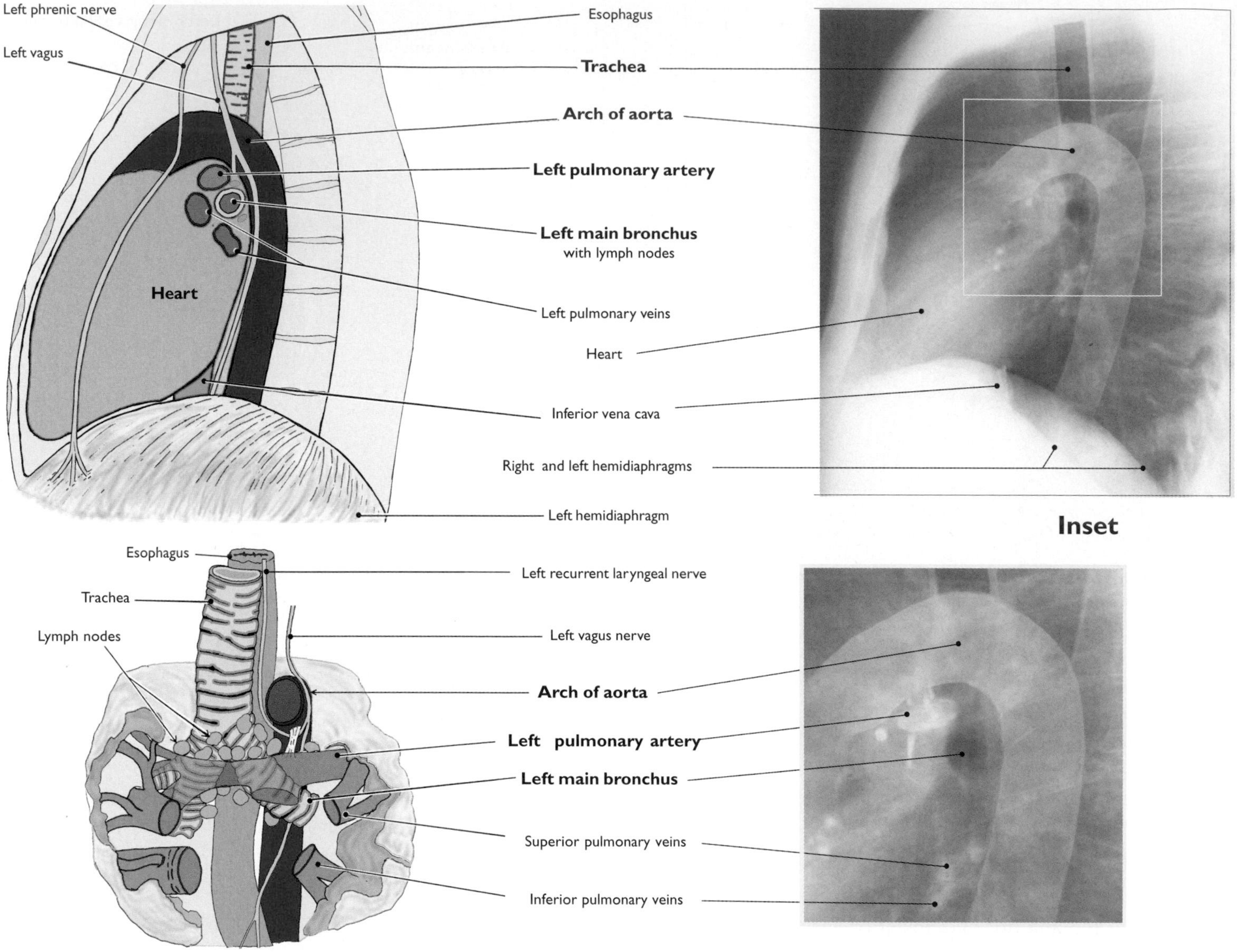

Figure 1.44. Radiograph of the left lateral chest (*digitally enhanced*) and related anatomical structures.

- Although you probably did not see the **thoracic duct** in the superior mediastinum, note its location just to the left and posterior to the esophagus. Note the thoracic duct on transverse section (Fig. 1.43).

> ***Clinical Correlation:*** Review the superior vena cava and its tributaries. Compression (obstruction) of this large vessel leads to a characteristic aggregate of signs and symptoms known as the **superior vena cava syndrome.** Obstruction of the superior vena cava most often is caused by malignant disease of the chest such as bronchogenic carcinoma. In most cases, tumors of the right lung are responsible for compression of this right-sided vessel. Blood from the upper limbs, head, and neck cannot freely drain to the heart; it must find its way to the heart via collateral venous drainage. As a result, the upper torso, head, and neck show evidence of increased blood volume such as grossly distended veins and capillary leakage.

⇦
GRANT'S 1.73, 1.74
NETTER 226
CLEMENTE 234
A.V.A. 3: 1.12.15

You have now finished the dissection of the main structures located in the posterior and superior mediastinum. Prepare the specimen for review:

- Keep all dissected structures moist with preservative fluid to avoid deterioration.
- Return the thoracic viscera (heart, lungs) into the chest cavity for reference.
- Ask your instructor if additional procedures should be followed.

The superior mediastinum is only an arbitrary subdivision. Many vital structures on their way to or from the neck pass through this space. Therefore, this region will be reviewed again during dissection of the neck.

Clinical Correlation: At this point, you should have a sound knowledge of the anatomy of the thorax. This understanding is absolutely essential when attempting to read routine chest films, a requirement for every physician.

Test your knowledge. First, refer to a **posterior-anterior (PA) radiograph** of the thorax. Identify bony structures such as the vertebral column (superimposed on the sternum), the clavicles, and the obliquely set ribs. Note that the right hemidiaphragm is positioned higher (due to the large liver) than the left one. Inferior to the left hemidiaphragm, air in the fundus of the stomach can be frequently seen. Note the well aerated (and therefore darker) lung fields with streaks of pulmonary vessels at each hilus. Define the outlines of the heart. Pay special attention to the position of the aortic arch.

⇦
GRANT'S 1.24
CLEMENTE 159

The **lateral view of a chest radiograph** is more challenging (Fig. 1.44). Identify the vertebral column, the ribs (right and left superimposed), and the sternum. Note the heart and the partially superimposed hemidiaphragms. Define the faint outlines of the ascending aorta, the aortic arch, and the descending aorta. Identify the area between the concavity of the aortic arch and the left pulmonary artery. This area is referred to clinically as the aortic-pulmonary (AP) window. Here, the left main bronchus can be seen. Usually, it is filled with air and, therefore, relatively dark on the negative chest film. In bronchiogenic carcinoma, infiltrated and enlarged cancerous lymph nodes may encroach on the space of the AP window and cause significant clinical symptoms (e.g., respiratory distress to due interference with the drainage of pulmonary blood vessels; cough due to irritation of the bronchial system; hoarseness due to compression of the left recurrent laryngeal nerve).

GAPP Tests. You are now encouraged to test your newly acquired knowledge of the anatomy of the thorax by taking GAPP Tests 1 through 4 on the following pages. For good reasons, the various structures are shown in black and shades of gray, just as they would present themselves radiographically on film or on a monitor screen. The use of color would give the answers away. However, you are encouraged to color the images yourself after you have positively identified the various structures. Correlate numbers with corresponding letters. The offered tests will increase your ability to assess the human anatomical substrate in its three-dimensional form. This skill will serve you well throughout your professional career.

TEST 1

GAPP

GROSS ANATOMY PRACTICAL PRIMER

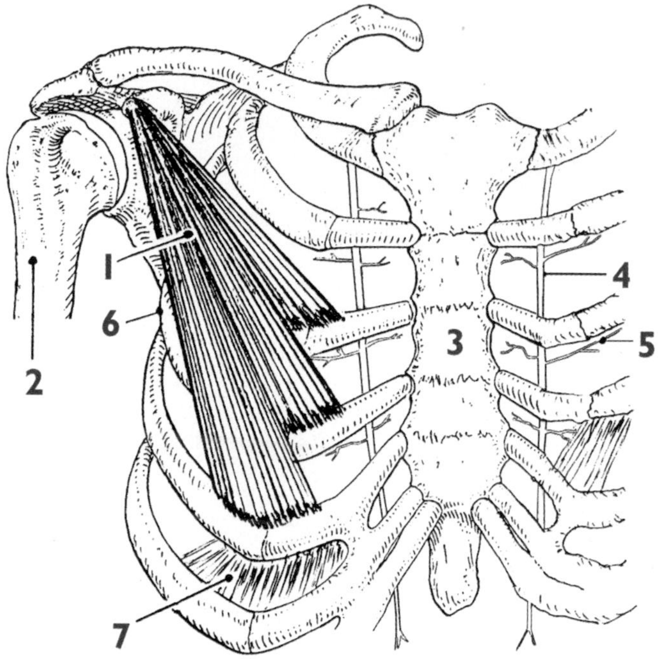

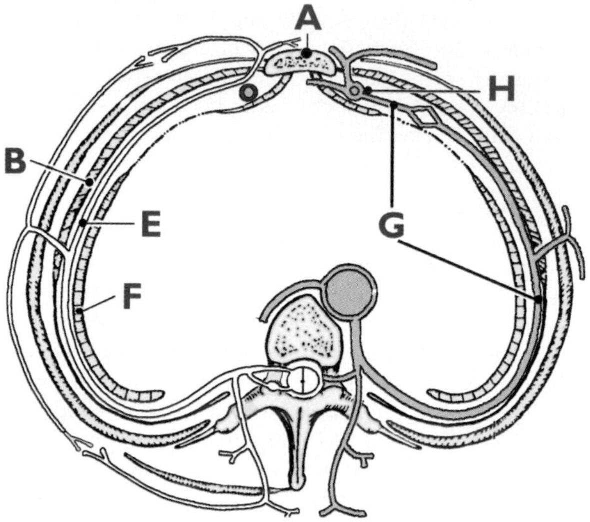

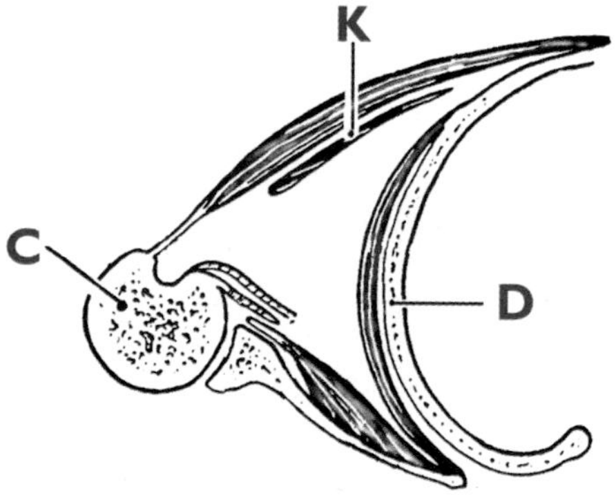

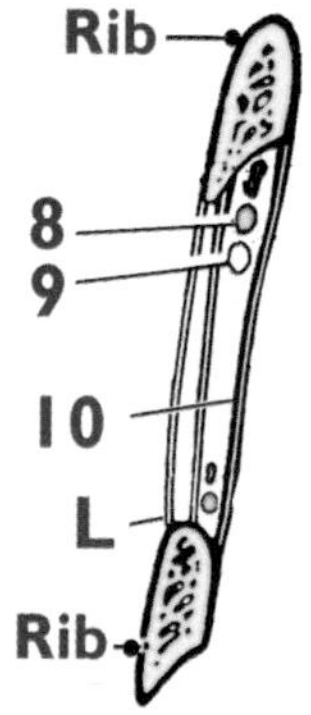

TEST YOUR 3-DIMENSIONAL CONCEPTUALIZATION.
MATCH THE NUMBERS WITH CORRESPONDING LETTERS:

1 ___	6 ___
2 ___	7 ___
3 ___	8 ___
4 ___	9 ___
5 ___	10 ___

GAPP TEST: IF YOU MADE AN ERROR, REVIEW AND GAIN A BETTER UNDERSTANDING OF THE CONCERNED 3-DIMENSIONAL ANATOMICAL CONCEPT. GAPP KEY: 1-K; 2-C; 3-A; 4-H; 5-G; 6-D; 7-B; 8-G; 9-E; 10-F.

TEST 2

GAPP
GROSS ANATOMY PRACTICAL PRIMER

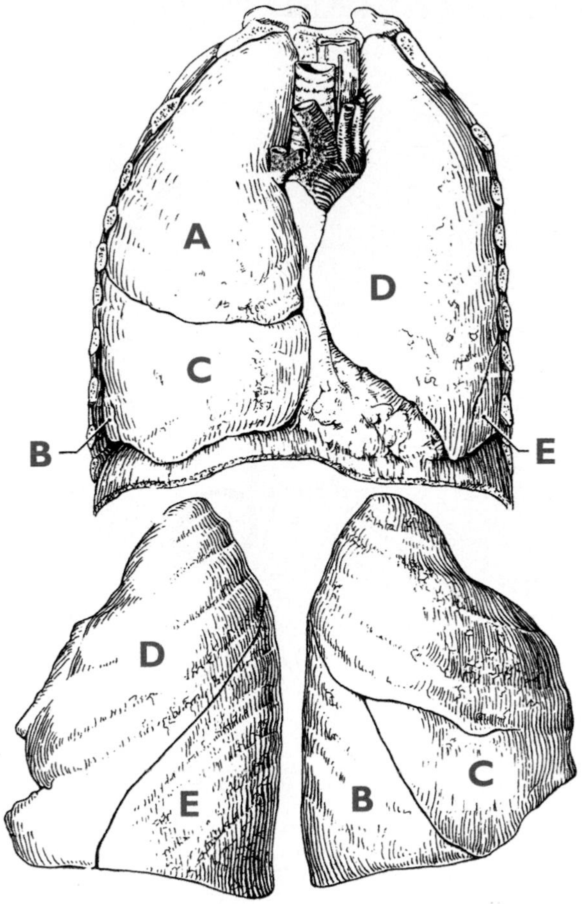

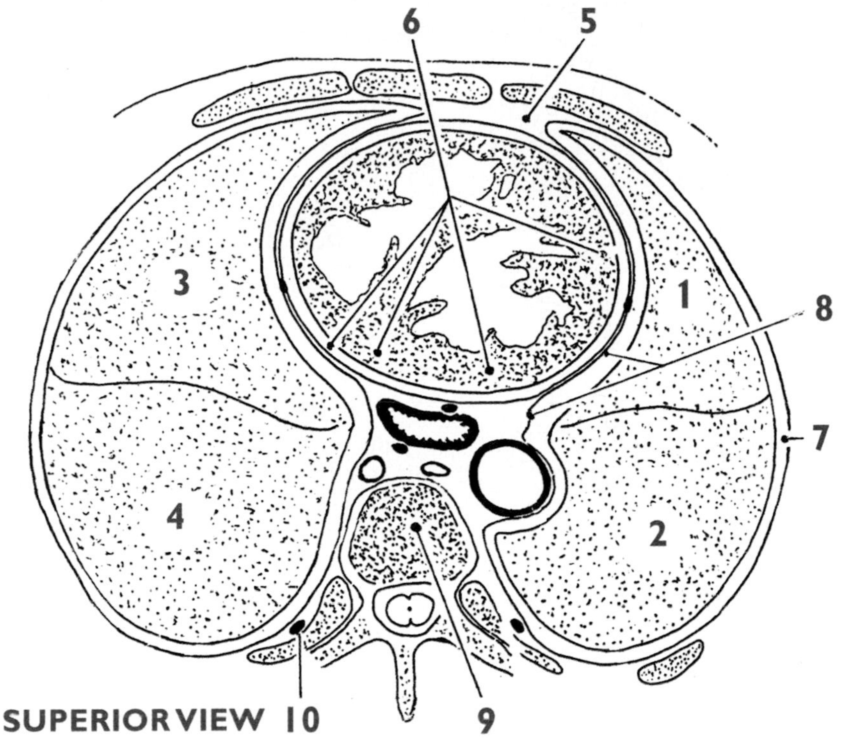

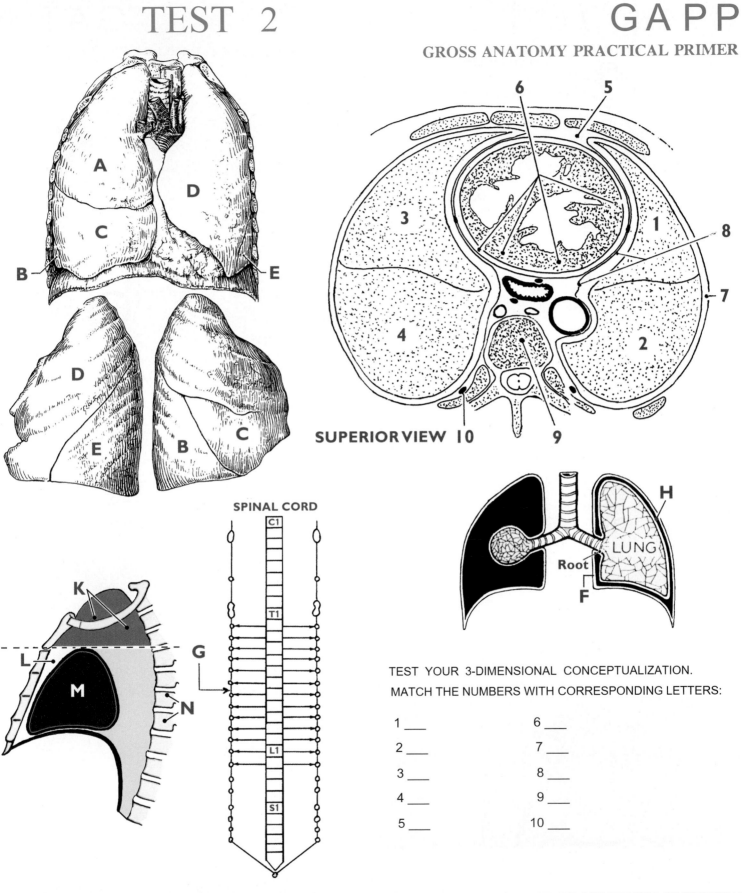

SUPERIOR VIEW

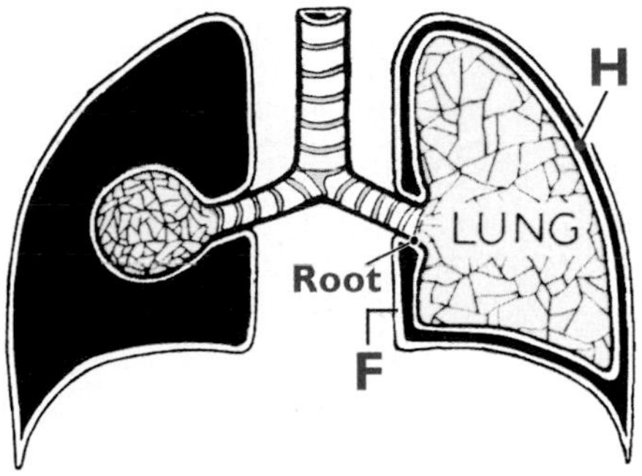

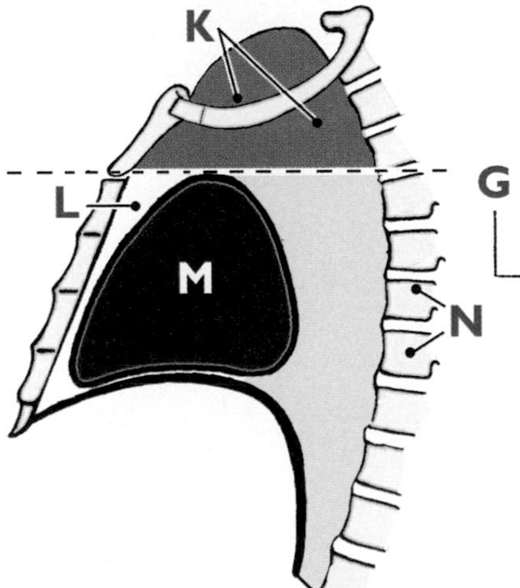

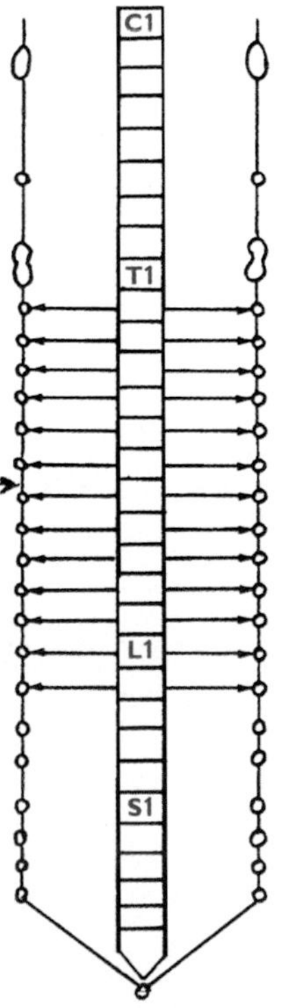

TEST YOUR 3-DIMENSIONAL CONCEPTUALIZATION.
MATCH THE NUMBERS WITH CORRESPONDING LETTERS:

1 ___	6 ___
2 ___	7 ___
3 ___	8 ___
4 ___	9 ___
5 ___	10 ___

GAPP TEST: IF YOU MADE AN ERROR, REVIEW AND GAIN A BETTER UNDERSTANDING OF THE CONCERNED 3-DIMENSIONAL ANATOMICAL CONCEPT. GAPP KEY: 1-D; 2-E; 3-C; 4-B; 5-L; 6-M; 7-H; 8-F; 9-N; 10-G.

TEST 3

GAPP

GROSS ANATOMY PRACTICAL PRIMER

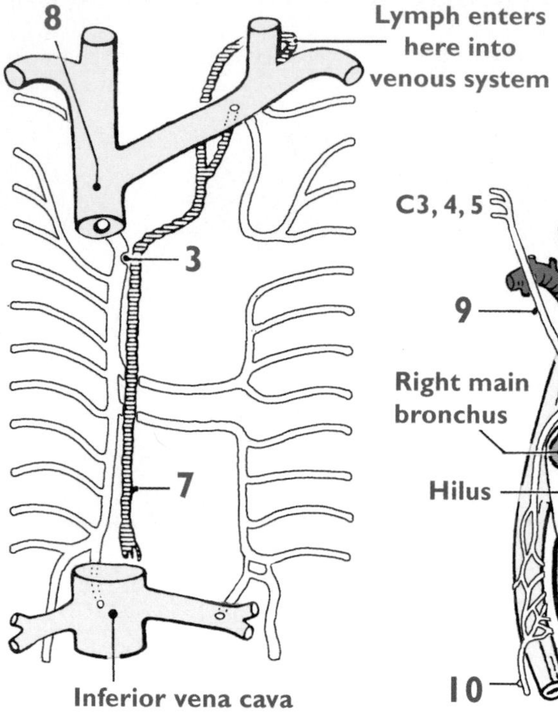

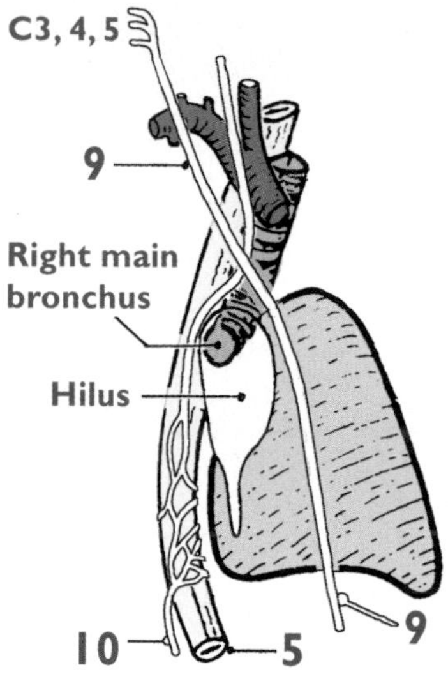

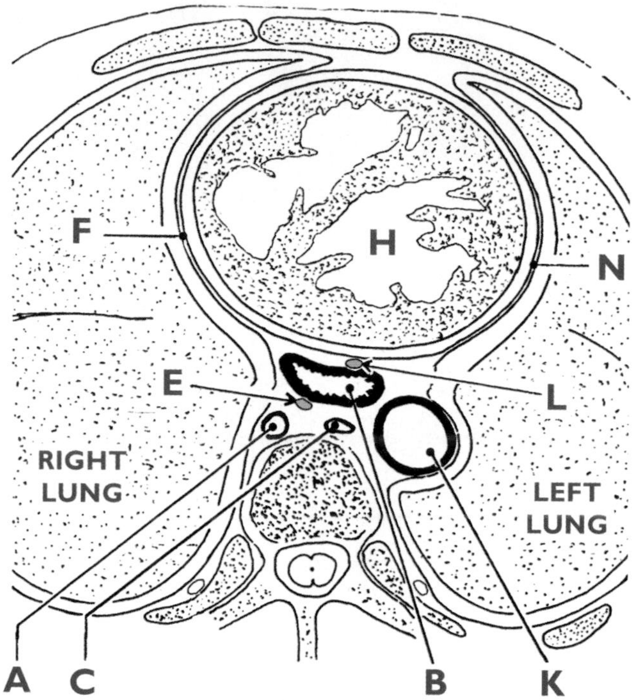

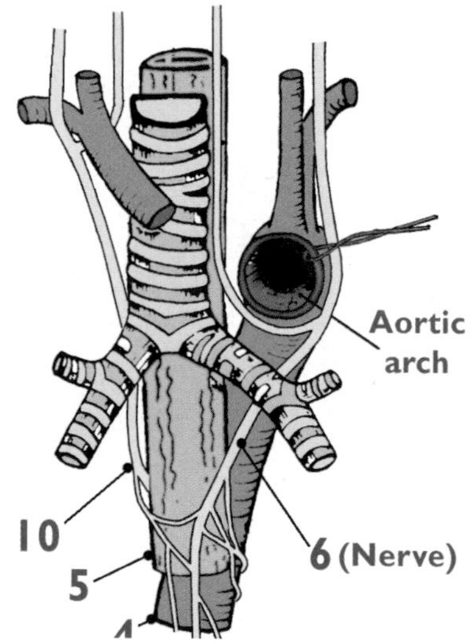

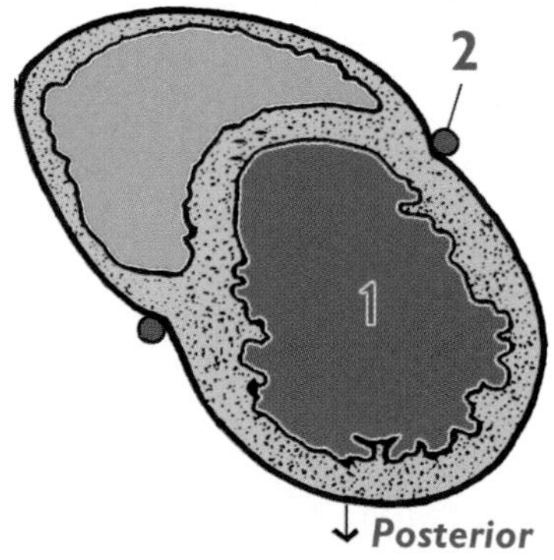

TEST YOUR 3-DIMENSIONAL CONCEPTUALIZATION.
MATCH THE NUMBERS WITH CORRESPONDING LETTERS:

1 ___	6 ___
2 ___	7 ___
3 ___	8 ___
4 ___	9 ___
5 ___	10 ___

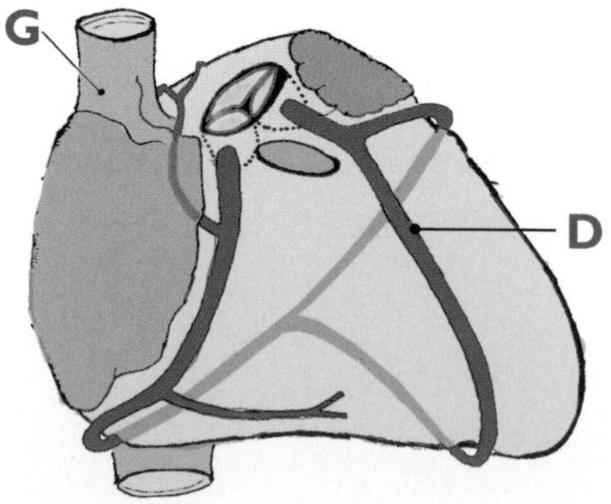

GAPP TEST: IF YOU MADE AN ERROR, REVIEW AND GAIN A BETTER UNDERSTANDING OF THE CONCERNED 3-DIMENSIONAL ANATOMICAL CONCEPT. GAPP KEY: 1-H, 2-D, 3-A, 4-K, 5-B, 6-L, 7-C, 8-G, 9-F, 10-E.

TEST 4

GAPP

GROSS ANATOMY PRACTICAL PRIMER

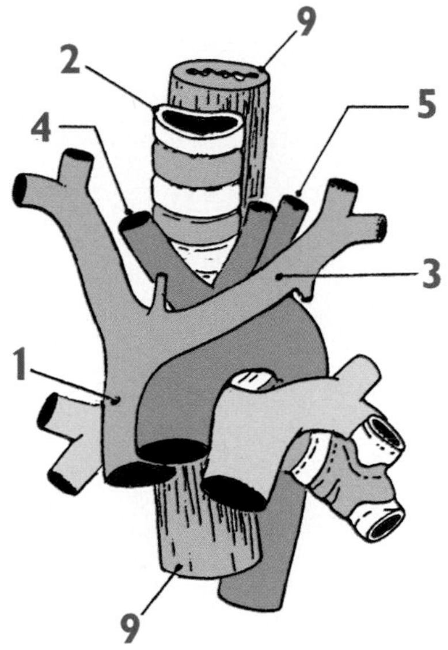

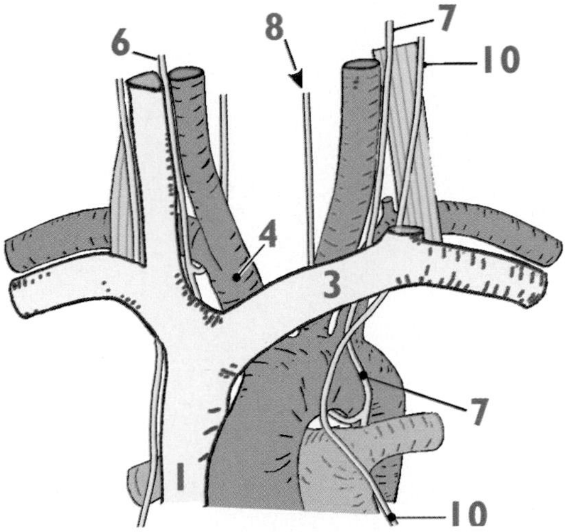

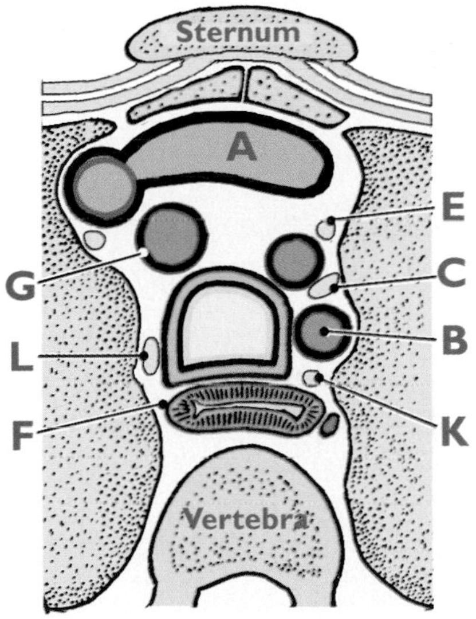

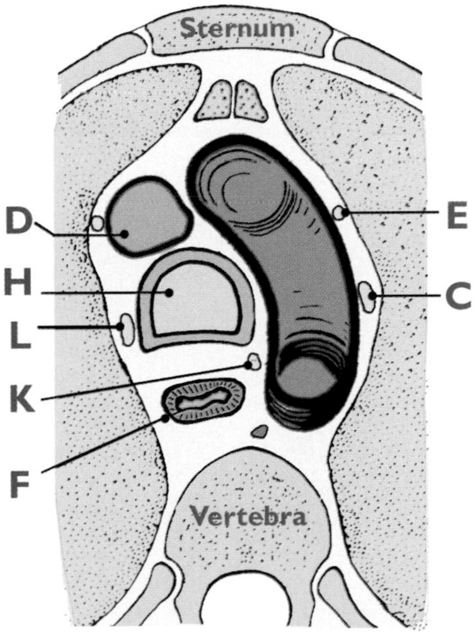

TEST YOUR 3-DIMENSIONAL CONCEPTUALIZATION.

MATCH THE NUMBERS WITH CORRESPONDING LETTERS:

1 ___	6 ___
2 ___	7 ___
3 ___	8 ___
4 ___	9 ___
5 ___	10 ___

GAPP TEST: IF YOU MADE AN ERROR, REVIEW AND GAIN A BETTER UNDERSTANDING OF THE CONCERNED 3-DIMENSIONAL ANATOMICAL CONCEPT. GAPP KEY: 1-D; 2-H; 3-A; 4-G; 5-B; 6-L; 7-C; 8-K; 9-F; 10-E.

Chapter 2
The Abdomen

Grant's Atlas of Anatomy, 10th Ed.:	*Grant's Fig. #*
Rohen, Color Atlas of Anatomy, 4th Ed.:	Rohen Page #
A.D.A.M. Student Atlas of Anatomy:	A.D.A.M. Plate #
Netter, Atlas of Human Anatomy, 2nd Ed.:	Netter Plate #
Clemente, Anatomy, 4th Ed.:	Clemente Fig. #
Acland's Video Atlas of Human Anatomy	A.V.A. Vol: hr.min.sec

Anterior Abdominal Wall

General Remarks

The contents of the abdominal cavity are protected anteriorly and laterally by the anterior abdominal wall. This wall consists of several layers. From superficial to deep, these layers are (Fig. 2.1):

Grant's 2.7
Rohen 198, 201
Netter 235
Clemente 256

1. Skin
2. Superficial fascia:
   a. fatty layer (of Camper)
   b. membranous layer (of Scarpa)
3. External oblique muscle
4. Internal oblique muscle
5. Transversus muscle
6. Transversalis fascia
7. Extraperitoneal fatty areolar tissue
8. Peritoneum

On each side of the midline, the three flat muscles (external oblique, internal oblique, and transversus) are reinforced by a longitudinal strap-like muscle, the rectus abdominis. This muscle is enclosed in a sheath produced by the aponeuroses of the three flat muscles.

Grant's 2.6A
Rohen 199
A.D.A.M. 1.38, 1.39
Netter 234, 235
Clemente 255
A.V.A. 3: 1.38.34

The ventral rami of the lower six thoracic nerves enter and supply the abdominal wall. Note that T10 supplies the skin around the umbilicus. Three nerves (T7, T8, T9) supply the region superior to the umbilicus; and three nerves (T11, T12, L1) supply the region inferior to the umbilicus.

Grant's 2.3A
Rohen 203
Netter 240
Clemente 246
A.V.A. 3: 2.02.40

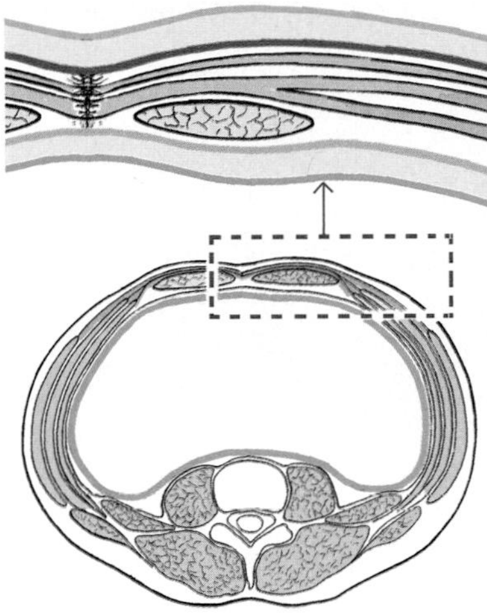

Figure 2.1. Layers of the lower anterior abdominal wall. The numbered layers correspond to the listing in the text.

In the male, the testes are housed in a special outpouching of the anterior abdominal wall, the scrotum. The scrotum consists of skin and superficial fascia that is void of fat. Each testis is connected to intrapelvic structures via the ductus deferens. The duct and its associated vessels and nerves constitute the major components of the spermatic cord. This cord traverses the abdominal wall through an obliquely set canal, the inguinal canal. The inguinal canal is of great clinical importance since loops of intestine may herniate through it. Therefore, this region of the anterior abdominal wall should be studied with particular attention.

In the female, the inguinal canal is relatively small. It contains the round ligament of the uterus, a tape-like structure corresponding in position to the spermatic cord of the male.

Landmarks and Surface Anatomy

Palpate the following (Fig. 2.2):

- **Xiphisternal junction,** at the inferior end of the body of the sternum;
- **Costal margin**, consisting of the upturned ends of cartilages 7 to 10;

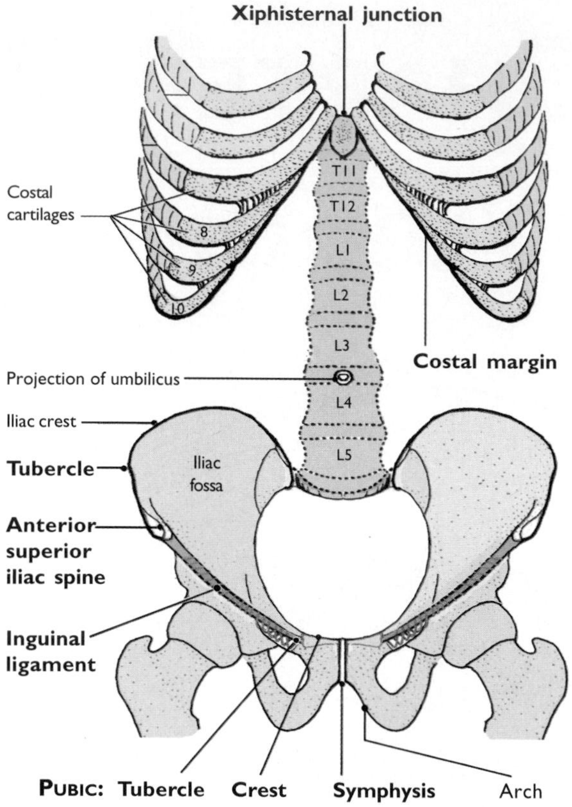

Figure 2.2. Landmarks and boundaries of the anterior abdominal wall.

- **Pubic symphysis**, marking the lowest limit of the anterior abdominal wall in the median plane;
- **Pubic crest**, extending laterally from the symphysis;
- **Pubic tubercle**, at the lateral end of the pubic crest;
- **Inguinal ligament**, stretching from the pubic tubercle to the anterior superior iliac spine;
- **Anterior superior iliac spine**, at the anterior end of the iliac crest;
- **Tubercle of the crest**, at the most lateral point of the crest.

◁
GRANT'S 2.2C
ROHEN 183
A.D.A.M. 1.3
NETTER 231
CLEMENTE 282, 284
A.V.A. 3: 1.37.42

Division of Abdominal Wall. Familiarize yourself with the commonly used divisions of the abdomen. For descriptive purposes, the abdominal wall is divided into quadrants or regions. Figure 2.3 shows the division of the abdomen into four quadrants by means of a horizontal plane passing through the umbilicus and a vertical median plane. This simple abdominal division is suitable for general localizations of abdominal problems. More specific localizations require the division of the abdomen into nine regions (Fig. 2.4). This clinical method of subdivision utilizes the two midclavicular planes and two horizontal planes (subcostal and transtubercular).

◁
A.D.A.M. 3.1, 3.2
NETTER 251

Demonstrate the nine abdominal regions on the cadaver abdomen. With a black grease pencil and on the abdominal wall only, indicate the two midclavicular lines (stretching

◁
A.D.A.M. 3.1
NETTER 251

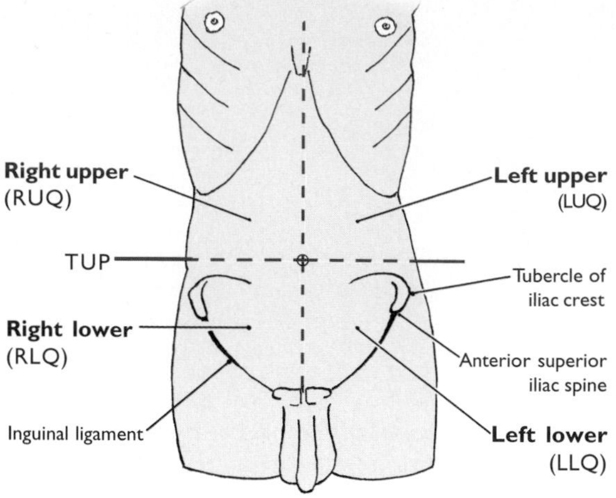

Figure 2.3. Division of the anterior abdominal wall into four quadrants. The division planes are the median plane and the transumbilical plane (TUP).

from midpoint of clavicle to midpoint of inguinal ligament). Next, mark the subcostal plane by joining the most inferior points of the costal margins. Denote the transtubercular line by joining the right and left tubercles of the iliac crests.

Clinical Observations and Correlation. Watch for evidence of trauma (gunshot wounds; stab wounds; collections of blood [hematomas]). Note old surgical scars and recent (unhealed) incisions, suture material or metal clips, if present.

Abdominal incisions are carefully made to access structures in the wall or within the abdominal cavity. With excellent anatomical knowledge, the surgeon tries to avoid permanent injuries to muscles and nerves. Commonly used abdominal incisions include: midline (median) incisions, traversing one or more of either the epigastric, umbilical, or hypogastric regions; paramedian incisions; obliquely set subcostal incisions; and suprapubic incisions in the hypogastric region. Are any of these incisions or scars present? If so, you may speculate what the surgeon might have done. A median incision through the linea alba avoids major blood vessels and nerves; it affords wide access to the abdominal cavity. A subcostal incision on the right is most often used for open gallbladder surgery (cholecystectomy), whereas barely visible round scars around the umbilicus may suggest closed or laparoscopic cholecystectomy. The spleen is often approached through a left subcostal incision. Suprapubic incisions afford access to pelvic organs such as the bladder or the uterus (C-section; hysterectomy). An oblique incision, approximately at the meeting point of umbilical region and right inguinal region, is frequently used for appendectomy. A scar in one or both inguinal regions may be indicative of previous hernia surgery. Are there any hernias? Look for them in the umbilical region and both inguinal regions. Lineae albicantes (white "stretch marks") are often found in obese people; or they may be an indication of previous pregnancies.

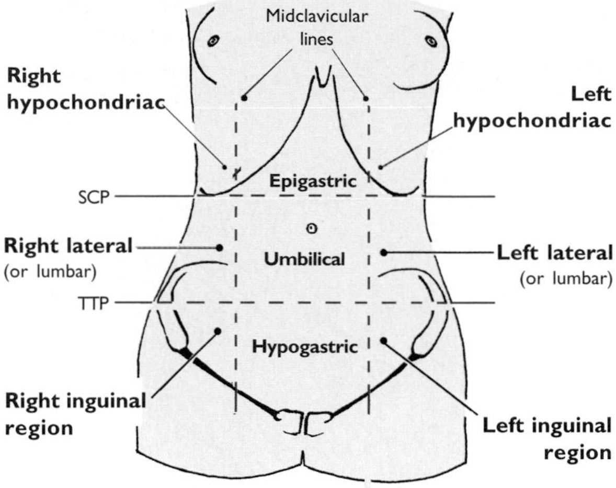

Figure 2.4. Subdivision of the anterior abdominal wall into nine regions by using the subcostal plane (SCP), the transtubercular plane (TTP), and the two midclavicular lines.

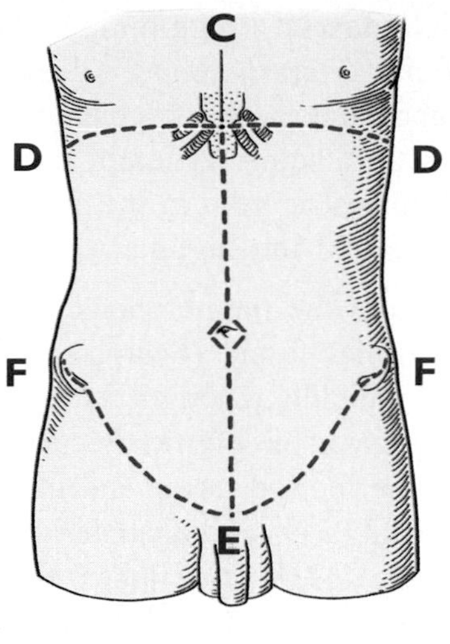

Figure 2.5. Skin incisions.

Before you begin ...

The three flat muscles (external oblique, internal oblique, transversus) will be studied, particularly in the important inguinal region. The composition and contents of the rectus sheath will be explored. Finally, the anterior abdominal wall will be reflected in such a manner that (a) full access to the contents of the abdominopelvic cavity is ensured; and (b) most components of the abdominal wall can be repositioned for future studies. These studies include a review of the inguinal canal and of the various layers of the abdominal wall.

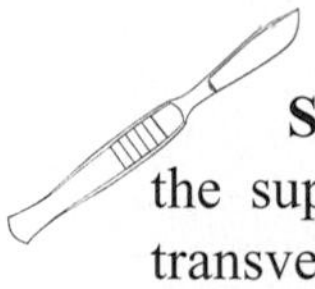

Skin Incisions. Place the cadaver into the supine position (face up). Put a block transversely beneath the lumbar region of the back. This procedure stretches the anterior abdominal wall. Make the following skin incisions according to Figure 2.5:

- Make a midline skin incision from the xiphisternal junction (C) to the symphysis pubis (E), encircling the umbilicus.
- If not already done during the dissection of the thorax, make a transverse incision from point (C) until stopped by the table (D).
- From point (E), cut along the pubic crest. Below the course of the inguinal ligament, extend the incision to the anterior superior iliac spine and along the iliac crest (E to F).
- Reflect the skin of the abdomen laterally.

Fascial Arrangements, Cutaneous Nerves

The **superficial layer of the superficial fascia (Camper's fascia)** may contain various amounts of fat. The **membranous, deep layer of the superficial fascia (Scarpa's fascia)** lies superficial to the aponeurosis of the external oblique (Fig. 2.6). It is mainly composed of fibrous tissue. It is unique in that it is continuous with the superficial perineal fascia (Colles' fascia) and dartos fascia which surrounds the shaft of the penis and the scrotal sac. In the lower abdominal wall, Scarpa's fascia is separated from the underlying aponeurosis of the external oblique only by the deep investing fascia of the external oblique (all muscles have an investing fascia). Sometimes it is difficult to separate the deep investing fascia of the external oblique from Scarpa's fascia. This fascial arrangement must be understood to appreciate certain clinical conditions in which Scarpa's fascia and the aponeurosis of the external oblique are forcefully separated and a potential space is created between the two; see Clinical Correlation (boxed material).

FASCIAL ARRANGEMENTS OF ANTERIOR ABDOMINAL WALL

NAME OF STRUCTURE:	ALSO KNOWN AS:	SPECIAL FEATURES:
Skin (cutis)	Epidermis + Dermis (corium)	Skin of scrotum is wrinkled because of underlying dartos musculature
Superficial layer of the superficial fascia (Subcutaneous tissue)	Camper's fascia	Contains small blood vessels and nerves; does not extend into scrotum or penis
Deep layer of superficial fascia	Scarpa's fascia	Continuous with dartos fascia of the penis and scrotum; continuous with the superficial perineal fascia (Colles' fascia)
Aponeurosis of the external oblique muscle	Obliquus abdominis externus	Potential space between aponeurosis of this muscle and Scarpa's fascia

Superficial fascia. Probe through the fat of the superficial fascia (Camper's fascia). This layer of subcutaneous tissue contains superficial nerves and veins. Attempt to find the superficial epigastric vein in the area between the umbilicus and the inguinal region.

⇦
Grant's *2.6A*
Rohen 198
A.D.A.M. 1.37
Netter 232
Clemente 247, 264

Next, explore the membranous, deep layer of the superficial fascia (Scarpa's fascia) by making an incision through the superficial fascia as indicated in Figure 2.6. Reflect the margins of the incised tissue and identify the fatty superficial fascia and its underlying membranous layer. Insert your index finger into the potential space between Scarpa's fascia and the aponeurosis of the external oblique (blue arrow #1 in Fig. 2.6).

With gentle, sweeping movements of the finger verify that the finger can be freely pushed into a number of directions: laterally, superiorly, and medially to some extent. Demonstrate that the finger can be pushed far inferiorly into the scrotal sac and toward the perineum (blue arrow #2 in Fig.2.6). In contrast, your finger cannot be pushed into the thigh (blue arrow #3 in Fig. 2.6). The reason for this important anatomical fact is that Scarpa's fascia ends inferiorly by being attached to the fascia lata (i.e., deep fascia of the thigh) along a line 2 cm below the inguinal ligament (dotted line in Fig. 2.6).

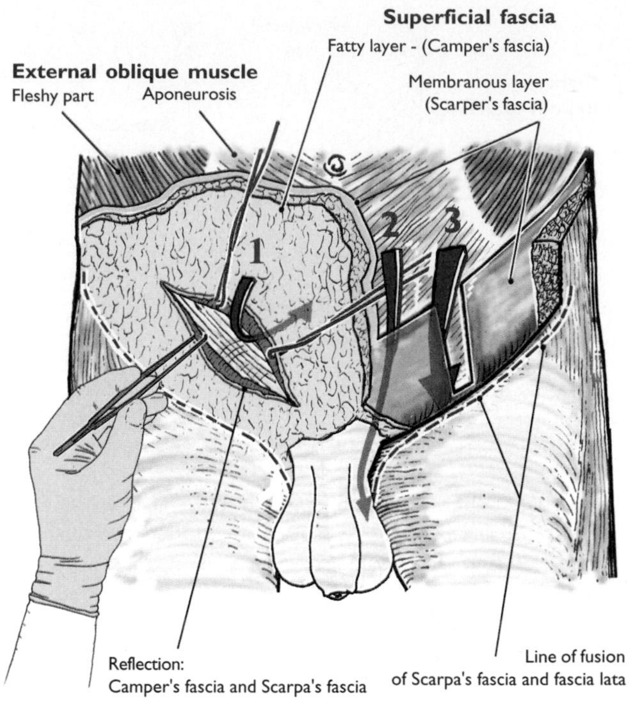

Figure 2.6. Incision of the superficial fascia to explore the potential space between the membranous layer (Scarpa's fascia) and the aponeurosis of the external oblique muscle.

The extent of the membranous, deep layer of the superficial fascia (Scarpa's fascia) is shown in Figure 2.7. Scarpa's fascia is unique in that it is continuous with the superficial perineal fascia (Colles' fascia) and dartos fascia which surrounds the shaft of the penis and the scrotal sac (Fig. 2.7A). In the lower abdominal wall, Scarpa's fascia can be easily separated from the underlying aponeurosis of the external oblique (red arrow in Fig. 2.7A), a fact that has important clinical implications.

⇦
A.D.A.M. 4.38
Netter 354

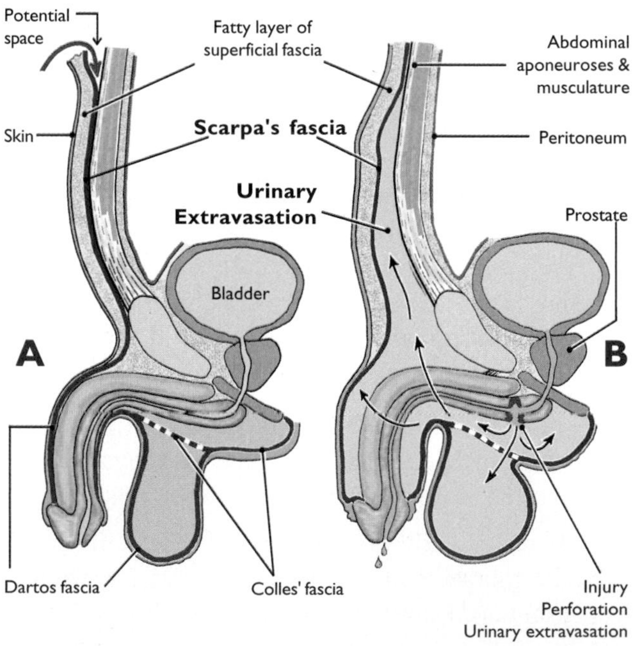

Figure 2.7. The membranous layer of the superficial fascia (Scarpa's fascia) and its continuation with the fasciae of the scrotum and perineum. *A*, normal fascial arrangements; the *red arrow* indicates the potential space between Scarpa's fascia and the aponeurosis of the external oblique. *B*, Extravasation of urine along fascial boundaries (following injury and perforation of the male urethra).

Clinical Correlation. The clinician must be aware of the fascial arrangements of the external genitalia and of the lower abdominal wall. If the penile urethra is injured (perineal injuries in car accidents; falling astride onto sharp objects such as fence poles, etc.), urine may escape from the urethra into the scrotum (Fig. 2.7B). From there, the extravasated urine may readily spread superiorly into the potential space of the lower abdominal wall between Scarpa's fascia and the aponeurosis of the external oblique. The clinical picture of this urinary extravasation may be dramatic with extensive, red edematous swelling of the scrotum, penis, and lower abdominal wall. Of course,

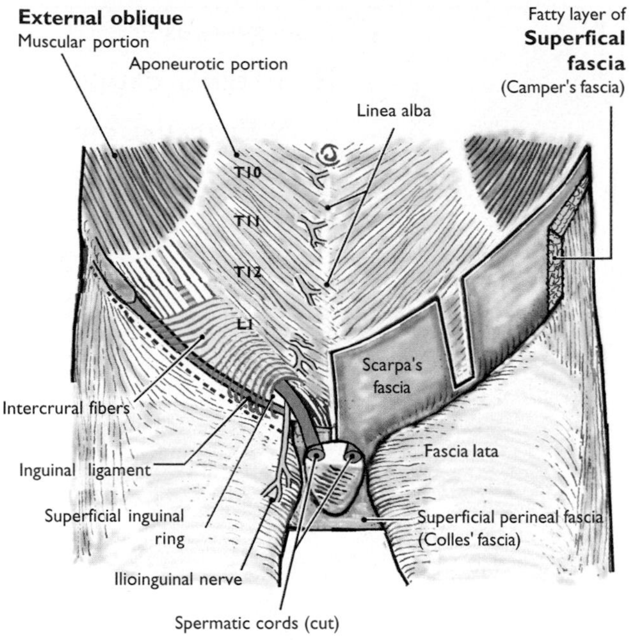

Figure 2.8. Scarpa's fascia and its continuation with Colles' fascia, external oblique, and superficial inguinal ring (penis and scrotum cut away).

> urinary extravasation into the thigh does not occur because of the inferior attachment of Scarpa's fascia to the fascia lata of the thigh.
>
> The right and left superficial epigastric veins are of potential clinical importance: The veins and their anastomoses with the lateral thoracic veins constitute important collateral venous channels to the upper part of the body. These collateral venous channels are utilized and engorged in patients whose venous blood cannot freely return to the heart (e.g., due to obstruction of the inferior vena cava or of the portal vein). Under these pathologic conditions, the superficial veins in the abdominal wall, especially around the umbilicus, become greatly dilated and tortuous. This phenomenon, known as caput medusae, is of important diagnostic value.

Cutaneous Nerves. Do not injure the underlying aponeurosis of the external oblique. Incise the superficial fascia 5 cm from the midline. Make this incision from the xiphoid process to the symphysis pubis. With the finger or the handle of a scalpel, detach the fascia medially for about 2.5 cm. Now, palpate the anterior cutaneous nerves. These nerves are in series with those in the thoracic region. The anterior cutaneous nerves of the abdomen are terminal twigs of the ventral rami T7 to L1. About 4 cm superior to the pubic crest, look for the anterior cutaneous branch of the iliohypogastric nerve (L1) (Fig. 2.8). Review the distribution of a spinal nerve.

⇦
GRANT'S 2.3A, 2.6A
ROHEN 204
A.D.A.M. 1.31
NETTER 240
CLEMENTE 248

⇦
GRANT'S 1.20
ROHEN 202, 204
A.D.A.M. 1.35
NETTER 241
CLEMENTE 13

⇨
GRANT'S 2.3
ROHEN 193
A.D.A.M. 1.37
NETTER 232, 237, 240
CLEMENTE 249
A.V.A. 3: 1.44.32

The fleshy fibers of the external oblique originate superior to the costal margin. Observe the fleshy digitations of the external oblique from each of the lower eight ribs (the upper four interdigitate with serratus anterior, the lower four with the latissimus dorsi). Between the digitations, observe the lateral cutaneous nerves (T7 to T12). Each nerve divides into a small posterior branch and a large anterior branch. The posterior branches turn posteriorly over the latissimus dorsi. The anterior branches descend, in the superficial fascia, in line with the fibers of the external oblique. Trace at least one anterior branch anteriorly to the abdominal wall.

⇨
GRANT'S 2.3A, 2.6A
ROHEN 195
NETTER 232
CLEMENTE 249
A.V.A. 3: 1.45.35

⇨
GRANT'S 2.7A
ROHEN 195
A.D.A.M. 1.39
NETTER 232, 237
CLEMENTE 249-252
A.V.A. 3: 1.41.05

Remove all remains of the superficial fascia. Clean the surface of the external oblique (Fig. 2.8). Clearly distinguish between the muscular and aponeurotic portion. Observe the curved line of union between these two portions. Notice the linea alba. It is a whitish groove in the midline of the abdominal wall, formed by interlacing fibers from the right and left sides. About halfway between the xiphoid process and the pubic symphysis, the linea alba is interrupted by the umbilicus.

Muscles of Anterior Abdominal Wall and Inguinal Region

The three paired, flat muscles of the anterior abdominal wall contribute to the formation of the inguinal canal. The inguinal region is of considerable clinical importance because inguinal hernias may occur here, particularly in males. Dissection of the inguinal region and its canal is difficult and often frustrating. Understand that the inguinal canal is an obliquely set tunnel that traverses the anterior abdominal wall. This tunnel runs parallel to and just superior to the medial half of the inguinal ligament. It is 3 to 5 cm in length. It extends between the superficial inguinal ring (an opening in the aponeurosis of the external oblique) and the deep (internal) inguinal ring (an opening in the transversalis fascia). During its course between these openings, the inguinal canal passes through the arched aponeurotic and muscular layers of the anterior abdominal wall formed by the three flat muscles (Fig. 2.9): external oblique (aponeurotic), internal oblique, and transversus abdominis (muscular). Thus, the inguinal canal can be likened to an arcade of three arches formed by the three flat abdominal muscles. The arches formed by the internal oblique and transversus abdominis are often fused and cannot be completely separated. In the male, the inguinal canal is traversed by the spermatic cord. The various abdominal layers make contributions to the spermatic cord as so-called "coverings" (for example, the external oblique contributes to the external spermatic fascia; the internal oblique contributes to the cremaster muscle).

In the female, the inguinal canal is less well defined; it contains the round ligament of the uterus. If you dissect a female cadaver, substitute in the text "round ligament" for "spermatic cord."

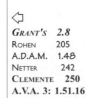

Dissecting instructions are provided for male cadavers. Dissection will proceed from superficial to deep. Each section of the canal (superficial inguinal ring and aponeurosis of external oblique; internal oblique; transversus abdominis; deep inguinal ring and transversalis fascia) will be clearly identified. If possible, review suitable prosections or museum specimens before beginning with your dissection.

External Oblique and its Contribution to the Inguinal Canal. The aponeurosis of the external oblique forms the first and most superficial arch (Arch A in Fig. 2.9) which is traversed by the spermatic cord. Carefully clean the aponeurosis of the external oblique in the inguinal region. Identify the following structures:

⇦
Grant's 2.8
Rohen 205
A.D.A.M. 1.37, 1.48
Netter 232, 240
Clemente 250, 251
A.V.A. 3: 1.51.00

- **Superficial inguinal ring.** It is, of course, subcutaneous. Delineate the arch-like, triangular aperture in the aponeurosis for the passage of the spermatic cord in the male (or for the passage of the round ligament in the female). The base of this triangular aperture is formed by the pubic crest; its sides are the medial and lateral crura.

- **Lateral (inferior) crus.** It is formed by the portion of the aponeurosis attaching to the pubic tubercle via the inguinal ligament. The spermatic cord rests on the inferior part of the lateral crus.

⇦
Grant's 2.8
Rohen 205
A.D.A.M. 1.48
Netter 242
Clemente 250
A.V.A. 3: 1.51.16

- **Medial (superior) crus.** It is that portion of the aponeurosis that diverges to attach to the pubic bone and crest medial to the pubic tubercle.

- **Intercrural fibers.** Lateral to the apex of the triangular gap. They prevent the crura from spreading apart.

- **Inguinal ligament** or Poupart's ligament. It forms the free inferior border of the aponeurosis of the external oblique. Notice and palpate its attachment to the anterior superior iliac spine and to the pubic tubercle.

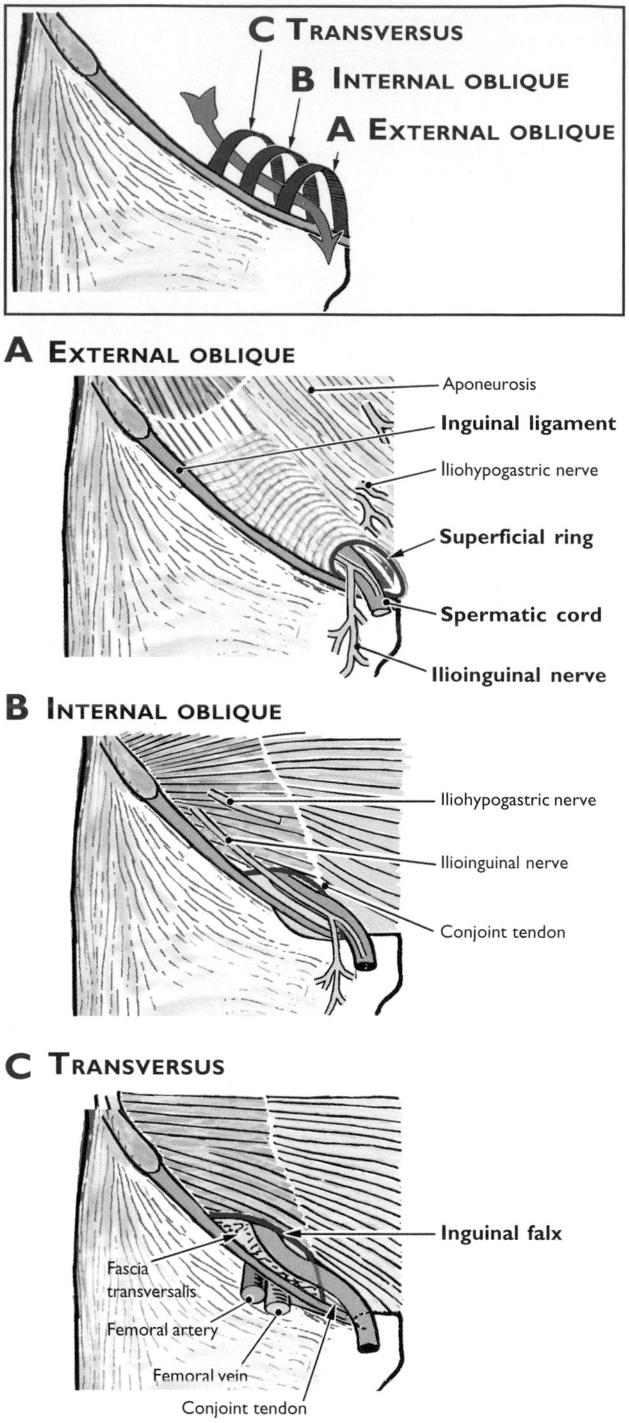

Figure 2.9. Contributions of the three flat abdominal muscles to the inguinal canal.

⇨
Grant's 2.6A
Rohen 205
Netter 240
Clemente 269
A.V.A. 3: 1.53.56

- Identify but do not disturb the **spermatic cord** (round ligament in the female) as it traverses the superficial inguinal ring (Fig. 2.9). Note the **ilioinguinal nerve** that emerges from the ring lateral to the spermatic cord. This nerve sends sensory twigs to the external genitalia and the medial aspect of the thigh. Do not destroy the proximal portion of the nerve (it will be used as a guiding structure for finding the plane between the internal oblique and the transversus abdominis).

Internal Oblique and its Contribution to the Inguinal Canal. To expose the next deeper muscle, the internal oblique, the aponeurosis of the external oblique muscle must be reflected. Proceed as follows:

- Split the fleshy fibers of the external oblique, starting the incision about 5 cm superior to the iliac crest and proceeding medially in the direction of the muscle fibers for approximately 10 cm.
- Insert two fingers into the incision, and separate the fibers of the external oblique from the fascia of the underlying internal oblique. Notice that the fibers of the internal oblique take a different direction.

⇦ *GRANT'S* 2.7A
ROHEN 205
A.D.A.M. 1.38
NETTER 242
CLEMENTE 254
A.V.A. 3: 1.50.55

- Enlarge the incision. Free the posterior (deep) surface of the external oblique as far as possible with your hand. Medially, the fingers cannot proceed beyond the rectus sheath, which is partially formed by the aponeurosis of the external oblique. Extend the incision inferomedially in the direction of the aponeurotic fibers of the external oblique. Cut as far as 2.5 cm superior to the superficial inguinal ring.
- Keep one hand as a guide in the plane between the two oblique muscles.
- Cut the external oblique: From the iliac crest superiorly, curving medially about 5 cm in front of the digitations of the serratus anterior, to a point corresponding approximately to the 5th costal cartilage.
- Reflect the inferior part of the divided external oblique inferiorly.
- Reflect the larger superior part of the muscle medially until stopped by the rectus sheath. Now, the anterior surface of the internal oblique is exposed.

⇦ *GRANT'S* 2.7A
ROHEN 205
NETTER 242
CLEMENTE 254
A.V.A. 3: 1.50.55

Examine the inferior portion of the internal oblique as it forms the **second arch of the arcade** (Arch B in Fig. 2.9). Use a probe and create a small gap between this arch and the traversing spermatic cord. Lateral to the spermatic cord, notice small muscle slips connecting the internal oblique with the spermatic cord. This is the muscular contribution of the internal oblique to the **cremaster muscle**.

⇨ *GRANT'S* 2.11, 2.12
ROHEN 206
A.D.A.M. 1.49, 1.50
NETTER 242, 243
CLEMENTE 253, 270
A.V.A. 3: 1.50.33

Verify that the fibers of the internal oblique become aponeurotic as they approach their insertion into the pubic crest and the pecten pubis just medial to the inguinal canal. At that point, the tendinous fibers of the internal oblique join the tendinous fibers of the transversus abdominis; this joint tendon is appropriately known as the **conjoint tendon**. Identify it.

⇨ *GRANT'S* 2.11
ROHEN 204, 206
NETTER 243
CLEMENTE 255
A.V.A. 3: 1.50.09

Transversus Abdominis and its Contribution to the Inguinal Canal. This muscle contributes to the **third and deepest arch of the arcade** (Arch C in Fig. 2.9). As pointed out earlier, the musculotendinous arches formed by the internal oblique and transversus abdominis are often fused and cannot be completely separated.

⇨ *GRANT'S* 2.6A
ROHEN 204
A.D.A.M. 1.38, 1.39
NETTER 240, 245

Additional Dissection Note: Check with your instructor to determine if you should attempt to separate the muscle fibers of the internal oblique from transversus abdominis. If you should, proceed as follows: Clean the anterior surface of the internal oblique and demonstrate the course of its muscle fibers. Do not injure the **ilioinguinal nerve**. Clean this nerve and follow it proximally to the point where it traverses the internal oblique. Now, use the nerve as a guiding structure to determine the plane between the internal oblique and the underlying transversus abdominis. The ilioinguinal nerve, a branch of L1, runs in the space between the two innermost muscles (Fig. 2.10). With a pair of scissors, split the internal oblique along its fiber course where it is traversed by the ilioinguinal nerve (about 2 to 3 cm above the inferior border of the muscle). Insert your finger into the plane between the internal oblique and the transversus abdominis. Push the finger inferiorly and separate the inferior borders of the two muscles. The inferior free edge of the transverse abdominis forms the inguinal falx, below which the abdominal wall is unsupported by muscle. Difficulties will be encountered if the two muscles are fused inferolaterally.

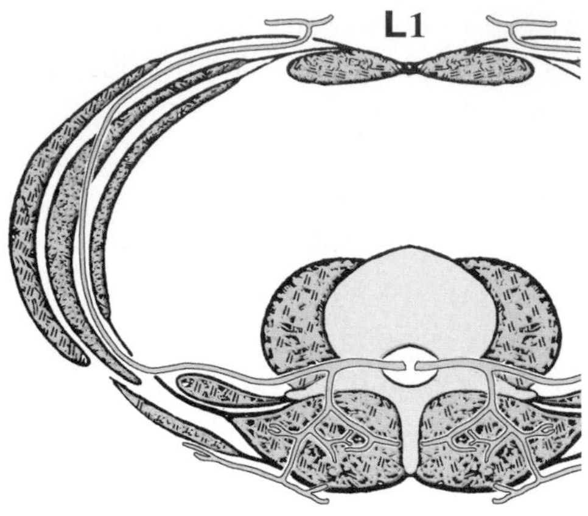

Figure 2.10. Course of ventral nerve ramus L1 in abdominal wall.

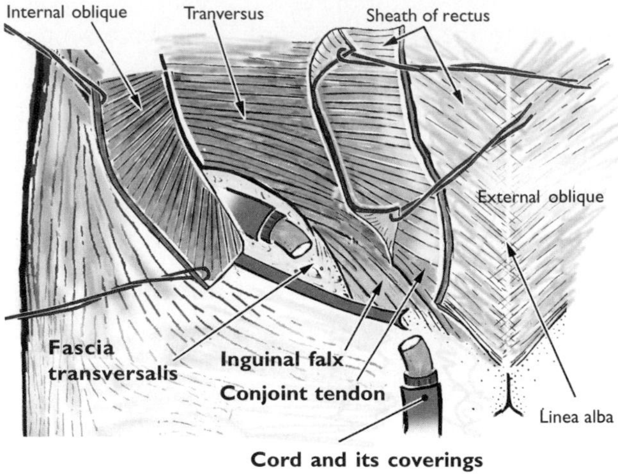

Figure 2.11. Inguinal falx and fascia transversalis.

At any rate, the tendinous portions of the internal oblique and the transversus abdominis are always fused medial to inguinal canal where they insert, as the **conjoint tendon**, into the pubic crest and pecten pubis (Fig. 2.11). Verify this fact in the cadaver.

Grant's *2.11, 2.12*
Rohen 206
A.D.A.M. 1.49, 1.50
Netter 242, 243
Clemente 253, 270
A.V.A. 3: 1.50.33

Deep Inguinal Ring and Transversalis Fascia. Pull the free inferior margin of the transversus abdominis (or the margin of the fused internal oblique and the transversus) anteriorly and superiorly. Sweep the handle of the scalpel or a probe between it and the underlying **fascia transversalis** (Fig. 2.11). This fascia is the internal investing layer which lines the entire abdominal wall. It is somewhat transparent. Through it, you can see some yellowish extraperitoneal fat and areolar tissue. The next deeper layer is the peritoneum, which cannot be seen at this time. Roll the spermatic cord laterally and observe the **inferior epigastric vessels** shining through the fascia transversalis. Just lateral to these inferior epigastric vessels is the **internal opening of the inguinal canal, the deep inguinal ring**. Push a probe medially along the spermatic cord toward the deep inguinal ring. This orifice will be examined again later from its inner aspect during dissection of pelvic structures.

Grant's *2.14A, 2.15*
Rohen 206, 208
Netter 243, 245
Clemente 266, 270
A.V.A. 3: 1.47.50

Grant's *2.15B*
Rohen 207
Clemente 279

Grant's *2.12*
Rohen 206
Netter 243, 245
Clemente 266, 270
A.V.A. 3: 2.01.52

Grant's *2.15C*
Rohen 207

Review the walls of the inguinal canal (Fig. 2.9):

- *Anterior:* Mainly the aponeurosis of the external oblique;
- *Inferior* (floor): Inguinal ligament and lacunar ligament, i.e., fibers of the medial end of the inguinal ligament that are rolled under the spermatic cord and attach to the pubic pecten;
- *Superior* (roof): Arches of the internal oblique and the transversus abdominis;
- *Posterior:* Fascia transversalis, reinforced medially by the conjoint tendon.

Grant's *2.12*
Rohen 206
A.D.A.M. 1.51, 152
Netter 243, 245
Clemente 266, 270
A.V.A. 3: 1.51.28

Clinical Correlation. The inguinal canal is like an arcade of three arches traversed by the spermatic cord (Fig. 2.12). During standing, coughing, or vigorous straining, the abdominal muscles contract. The arched fleshy fibers of the internal oblique and transversus cause the roof of the canal to become lower and taut. The action is essentially that of a half-sphincter.

An enlarged or congenitally patent inguinal canal is a potential channel through which abdominal viscera may protrude. The protruding viscera are contained in a hernial sac, which is an outpouching of the peritoneal membrane. Hernias through the inguinal canal are called **indirect hernias**. Indirect inguinal hernias are located lateral to the inferior epigastric vessels.

Great and prolonged increase in intra-abdominal pressure may eventually produce an outward bulging of a sac whose walls are composed of peritoneum, extraperitoneal fat, and fascia transversalis. If this sac (hernial sac) protrudes medial to the inferior epigastric vessels, the condition of a **direct inguinal hernia exists**.

The elicitation of the **cremasteric reflex** is part of every routine physical examination in the male patient. When the skin on the inner side of the thigh is scratched, the testicle on the same side is drawn upward. The afferent fibers of this reflex are carried in the ilioinguinal and genitofemoral nerves. Sensory (afferent) fibers of these nerves supply the skin of the scrotum and the adjacent inner side of the thigh. Motor fibers of the genital branch of the genitofemoral nerve supply the cremaster muscle (efferent reflex arc). Centrally in the spinal cord, the reflex involves segments L1 and L2.

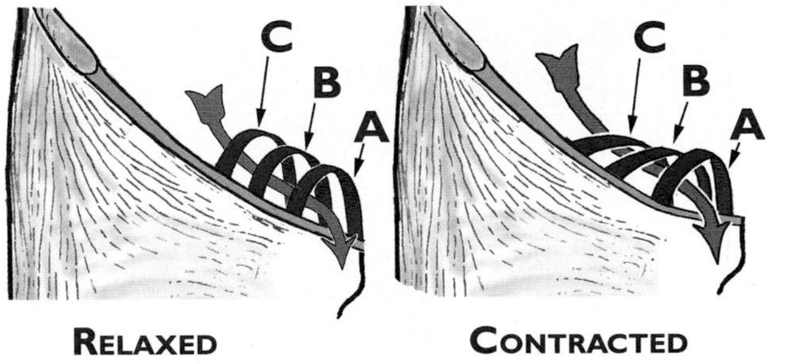

Figure 2.12. The inguinal canal resembles an arcade of three arches (*A, B, C*) traversed by the spermatic cord (*red arrow*). The muscular arches (*B, C*) can contract and narrow the canal whereas the aponeurotic arch (*A*) remains open.

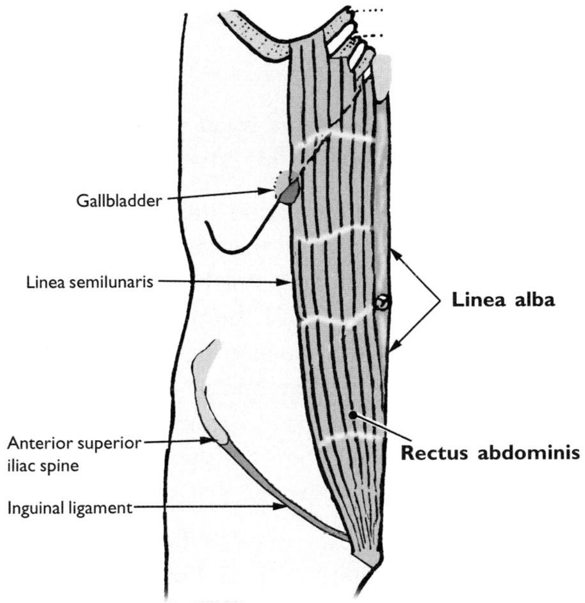

Figure 2.13. Rectus abdominis.

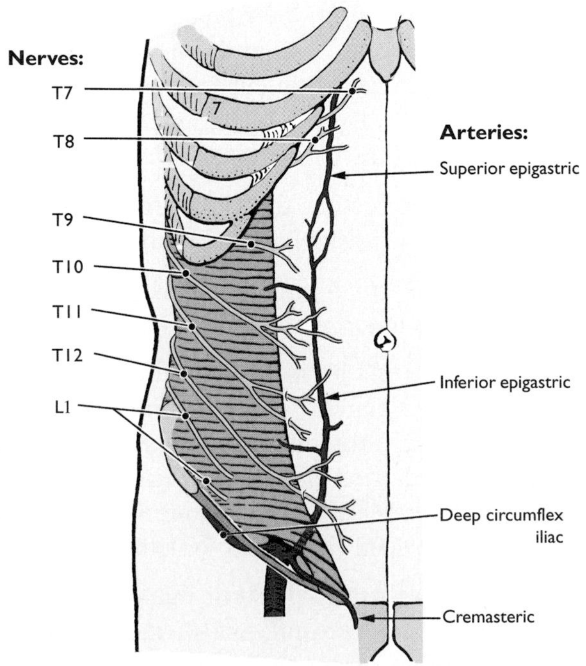

Figure 2.14. Nerves and arteries within the rectus sheath.

GRANT'S 2.6A
ROHEN 202, 203
A.D.A.M. 1.39
NETTER 233
CLEMENTE 253
A.V.A. 3: 1.38.33

Rectus Abdominis (Fig. 2.13). Reposition the cut halves of the external oblique. Outline the approximate location of the **rectus abdominis**. Note that the muscle is three times as wide superiorly as it is inferiorly. The fleshy fibers of the rectus are inserted into the cartilages of ribs 5 to 7. Inferiorly, the muscle arises from the symphysis and body of the pubis. On the anterior surface of the inferior part of the rectus abdominis you may find a small triangular muscle, the pyramidalis. It is functionally unimportant. Now, open the **rectus sheath** vertically to display its contents:

- Inferior to the umbilicus, keep the vertical incision about 12 mm from the midline.
- Superior to the umbilicus, make the vertical incision about 25 mm from the midline.
- Observe that the rectus sheath is firmly attached to the rectus muscle at the three **tendinous insertions**. Sever these connections with a scalpel.
- Carefully mobilize the rectus muscle with your hands, but do not remove it. Note that the anterior branches of six spinal nerves (T7 to T12) pierce the rectus sheath laterally. These nerves enter and supply the muscle (Fig. 2.14).

GRANT'S 2.7A
ROHEN 202 - 204
A.D.A.M. 1.39
NETTER 240
CLEMENTE 258
A.V.A. 3: 2.02.40

- In its middle, divide the rectus muscle transversely. Carefully reflect the two halves superiorly and inferiorly, respectively.
- On the posterior (deep) surface of the inferior half, observe the large **inferior epigastric vessels**.
- On the posterior (deep) surface of the superior half, note the smaller **superior epigastric vessels**.

GRANT'S 2.7A
ROHEN 202 - 204
A.D.A.M. 1.39
NETTER 234, 236, 238, 239
CLEMENTE 260

Clinical Correlation: The superior and inferior epigastric arteries and veins anastomose (Fig. 2.14). If the venous blood from the inferior part of the body cannot return freely to the heart (obstruction of inferior vena cava), the anastomosing inferior and superior epigastric veins provide an important collateral venous channel to the superior part of the body. Conversely, collateral arterial circulation via the superior and inferior epigastric arteries provides channels for arterial blood flow to the lower part of the body if the aorta is occluded (e.g., in coarctation of aorta).

Study the rectus sheath (Fig. 2.15). Examine the posterior layer or wall of the sheath. Identify the **arcuate line**, midway between the symphysis pubis and the umbilicus. At the level of the arcuate line, the inferior epigastric vessels enter the rectus sheath. Verify this.

Grant's 2.7
Rohen 204
A.D.A.M. 1.39
Netter 236, 238, 239
Clemente 255
A.V.A. 3: 1.40.22

The aponeuroses of the three flat abdominal muscles contribute to the formation of the rectus sheath. Inferior to the arcuate line, all aponeurotic layers pass ventral to the rectus (Fig. 2.15A); only the transversalis fascia remains dorsal to the muscle. Superior to the level of the arcuate line, the aponeurosis of the internal oblique splits: Together with the aponeurosis of the transversus it forms the posterior layer; together with the aponeurosis of the external oblique, it forms the anterior layer of the rectus sheath (Fig. 2.15B).

The **linea alba** is formed by decussating fibers of the aponeuroses of the right and left flat abdominal muscles (external oblique; internal oblique; transversus). Superior to the umbilicus, the linea alba is a band, about 2 cm wide (Fig. 2.13). Inferior to the umbilicus (Fig. 2.11), it is a thin line since the two recti muscles come into contact with each other. The linea alba is a raphe or decussation, and therefore it is extensile.

Grant's 2.10A
Rohen 195
A.D.A.M. 1.39
Netter 233-235, 241
Clemente 249-252
A.V.A. 3: 1.41.06

Inferior to the arcuate line, remove the transversalis fascia. Remove the extraperitoneal fat and areolar tissue, and thus expose and identify the peritoneum. Do not incise this gray membrane.

Reflection of the abdominal wall. The objective is to reflect the anterior abdominal wall in such a way that (a) full access to the contents of the abdominopelvic cavity is ensured; and (b) most components of the abdominal wall can be repositioned for future studies. Proceed in the following manner:

- Detach the fleshy fibers of the rectus from ribs 5 to 7, severing the superior epigastric vessels in the process.
- At the level of the xiphoid process and just left to it, make a vertical incision (about 3 cm long) through the linea alba, keeping on the left side about 1 cm from the midline (to preserve the obliterated umbilical vein). Be careful not to injure the contents of the abdominal cavity.
- Place the index finger of one hand through the incision into the abdominal cavity. With your finger, pull the anterior abdominal wall anteriorly, thereby creating a gap between abdominal wall and abdominal contents.

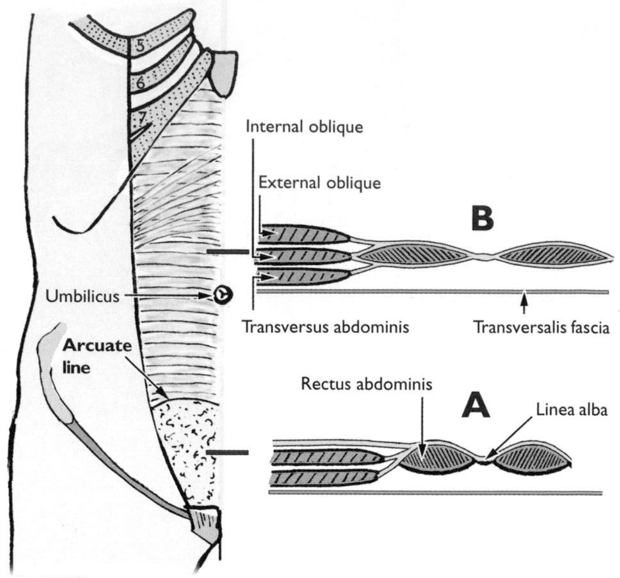

Figure 2.15. Posterior wall of rectus sheath (*left*), and transverse sections of rectus sheath at two different levels (*A* and *B*).

- Now, it is safe to extend the vertical incision inferiorly. Cut around the umbilicus on the left side so that it remains attached to the right side of the abdominal wall. Inferior to the umbilicus, continue the incision on the left, about 5 mm from the midline and as close as possible to the left rectus sheath (to preserve the obliterated urachus). Continue the vertical incision to the symphysis pubis.
- Subsequently, place one hand into the left side of the abdominal cavity to separate abdominal wall from abdominal contents. With the scalpel in the other hand, detach the left abdominal wall from the rib cage. Starting at the xiphoid process, follow the inferior border of rib 10; then carry the cut to the left iliac crest. Reflect the left side of the anterior abdominal wall inferiorly.

Before reflecting the right side of the abdominal wall, establish the following facts:

Grant's 2.18
Rohen 280
A.D.A.M. 3.5
Netter 252, 270
Clemente 286

- The **falciform ligament** spans the space between the anterior abdominal wall and liver.
- Contained in the inferior free margin of the falciform ligament is the **ligamentum teres**. This is the obliterated umbilical vein that, in the fetus, carries blood from the umbilical cord to the liver. Make sure that your dissecting partners have seen these two structures.
- Now, detach the falciform ligament from the anterior abdominal wall and sever the ligamentum teres.

- Subsequently, reflect the right side of the anterior abdominal wall in the same manner as the left side.

Review the various layers of the **abdominal wall**. At the rib cage, observe the attachments of the three severed, flat abdominal muscles:

- The origin of the **external oblique** from the external surface of the lower ribs;
- The insertion of the **internal oblique** into the inferior surface of the lower ribs;
- The origin of the **transversus abdominis** from the inner surfaces of the lower ribs.

GRANT'S 2.6, 2.7
ROHEN 198 - 204
A.D.A.M. 1.37 - 1.39
NETTER 232 - 235
CLEMENTE 247-257
A.V.A. 3: 1.41.41

Examine the peritoneal aspect of the umbilical region. The obliterated remains of fetal structures radiate from the umbilical region. They are:

- The obliterated umbilical vein or **ligamentum teres** of the liver;
- The obliterated allantoic duct (urachus) or **median umbilical ligament**, in the midline ascending from the apex of the bladder;
- The obliterated umbilical artery or **medial umbilical ligament**, one on each side.

GRANT'S 2.18B
NETTER 236
CLEMENTE 261, 262

Scrotum, Spermatic Cord, and Testis

The scrotum, spermatic cord, and testis are closely related to the inguinal canal. Their dissection is appropriate at this time. The scrotum is essentially a cutaneous outpouching of the anterior abdominal wall with all its layers (Fig. 2.16). Therefore, a finger can be pushed from the subcutaneous tissue of the anterior abdominal wall into the scrotal sac (in the female, into the labia majus). Realize that the scrotum is divided into right and left halves. During development, the two testes (testicles) descend into their respective scrotal halves and are anchored to it inferiorly by a fibrous band, the gubernaculum testis. The superficial fascia of the scrotum is void of fat. It contains a layer of involuntary (smooth) muscle fibers, the dartos. When contracting under the influence of cold temperature, this muscle significantly decreases the surface area of the scrotum, thus maintaining the best temperature for the testes. In contrast, the dartos relaxes at higher temperatures, renders the scrotal skin thin with an increased surface area, and thus regulates the optimal temperature for testicular function.

GRANT'S 2.14A, 2.15A
ROHEN 206
A.D.A.M. 1.49 - 152
NETTER 361
CLEMENTE 273

LAYERS OF THE ABDOMINAL WALL	CORRESPONDING LAYERS IN SCROTUM
1. Skin	1. Skin
2. Superficial fascia a) fatty (Camper) b) membranous (Scarpa)	2. Dartos muscle and fascia
3. External oblique	3. External spermatic fascia
4. Internal oblique	4. Cremaster muscle
5. Transversus	
6. Fascia transversalis	6. Internal spermatic fascia
7. Extraperitoneal fatty tissue	7. Areolar tissue with localized collections of fat
8. Peritoneum	8. Tunica vaginalis

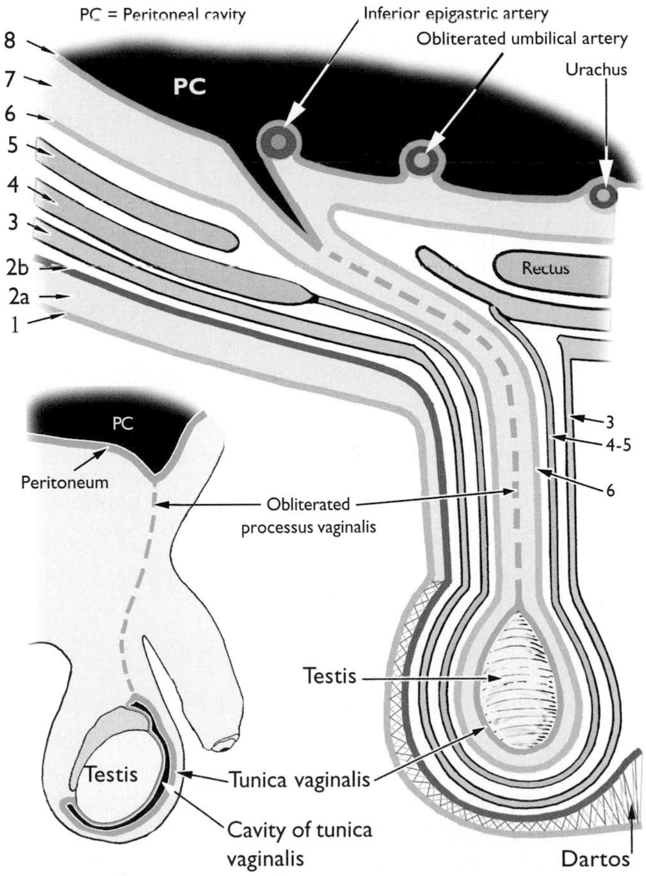

Figure 2.16. Layers of the anterior abdominal wall prolonged into the scrotum. In this section, the scrotum has been raised to the horizontal position. The numbered layers correspond to the table above.

Exposure of Spermatic Cord and Testis

Free the cord from the surrounding fat. Push your index finger into the scrotal sac so that the finger intervenes between testis medially and scrotal wall laterally.

- With the finger in this position, make an incision halfway down the scrotum, through the skin, dartos, and superficial fascia.
- Free the testis and cord from the surrounding areolar tissue.
- In the superior part of the scrotum and within the cord, palpate a firm tubular structure. This is the ductus deferens, which can be easily exposed here during the surgical procedure of vasectomy (see Clinical Correlation below).
- Snip the band of tissue that anchors the inferior pole of the testis to the scrotum. This is the gubernaculum testis.
- Shell the spermatic cord with the attached testis out of the scrotum.
- Observe that the scrotal sac is divided into two pouches by a median septum.
- Verify that the superficial fascia of the scrotum is void of fat.

Spermatic Cord. The main purpose of the spermatic cord is to provide a conduit to and from the testis. Thus, in its center, the spermatic cord contains the following constituents or components (Fig. 2.17):

- The ductus (vas) deferens, a thick-walled muscular tube that transports sperm;
- The testicular artery supplying the testis with blood;
- Numerous testicular veins forming the pampiniform venous plexus;
- Autonomic nerve fibers, including pain fibers, running with the blood vessels;
- Lymph vessels.

Coverings of the Cord. The constituents of the cord are surrounded by three fascial layers, the coverings, that have been derived from the anterior abdominal wall (Fig. 2.16). Understand that the investing fascia of the external oblique aponeurosis contributes to external spermatic fascia; the internal oblique muscle contributes to the musculature of the cremasteric fascia; the internal spermatic fascia is derived from the fascia transversalis. Study and understand a transverse section through the spermatic cord (Fig. 2.17).

Grant's 2.17
Rohen 206, 321
A.D.A.M. 149 - 152
Netter 361
Clemente 271-274
A.V.A. 3: 1.52.26

Spermatic Cord. Carefully incise the tubular coverings of the cord longitudinally. Identify and demonstrate:

- **External spermatic fascia**, the thin outermost covering;
- **Cremasteric fascia**, the middle covering; it is areolar and contains loops of cremaster muscle;
- **Internal spermatic fascia**, the filmy innermost covering of the spermatic cord.
- In the center of the spermatic cord, explore the constituents of the cord.

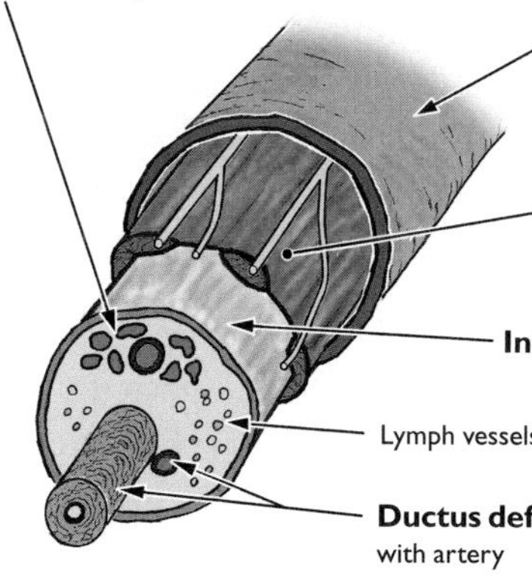

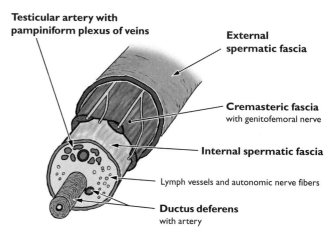

Figure 2.17. Schematic transverse section through the spermatic cord and its components.

- Initially, identify the **ductus (vas) deferens** by palpation; it is hard and cord-like in consistency. Using a probe and forceps, free a portion of the duct. Look for the small deferent artery that clings to it.
- Free a larger artery, the **testicular artery**, which runs with the **pampiniform plexus** of veins.
- Trace the ductus deferens superiorly into the inguinal canal and toward the deep inguinal ring. Note that it hooks around the lateral side of the inferior epigastric vessels (Fig. 2.18). Note the long course (about 45 cm) of the ductus deferens from the testicle to the prostate.

Grant's 2.11
Rohen 206, 208
A.D.A.M. 152
Netter 243 - 245
Clemente 270, 273
A.V.A. 3: 1.52.54

Grant's 2.14A, 2.15A
Rohen 206
A.D.A.M. 1.49 - 1.52
Netter 245
Clemente 271
A.V.A. 3: 1.53.13

Clinical Correlation. The ductus deferens can be easily palpated and surgically exposed in the superior part of the scrotum (Fig. 2.19). During the relatively simple surgical sterilization procedure of **vasectomy**, the right and left deferent ducts are located here, exposed, and severed. As a precaution (to prevent reconnection), a small segment of each duct is excised. Sperm production in the testes continues; however, the sperms cannot reach the prostate and urethra. Therefore, the ejaculate no longer contains sperms.

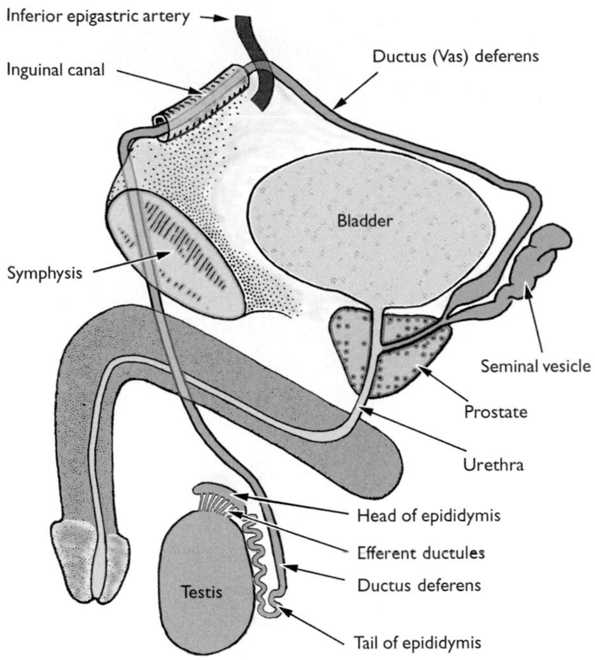

Figure 2.18. Male urogenital system: testis, ductus deferens, prostate, and urethra.

GRANT'S 2.17
ROHEN 321
A.D.A.M. 4.13, 4.15
NETTER 362
CLEMENTE 275

Testis (Fig. 2.20). A major portion of each testis is surrounded by the **tunica vaginalis testis**. The tunica vaginalis is a closed serous sac (potential space) of peritoneal origin. During development, the descending testis and epididymis invaginate into the posterior wall of this sac. Deep to the tunica vaginalis is the **tunica albuginea**, the dense, white connective tissue capsule of the testis. The sperms are generated in the **seminiferous tubules**. They pass through a network of canals, the **rete testis**, and through **efferent ductules** to the head of the epididymis (Figs. 2.18, 2.20). The **epididymis** is attached to the superior and posterolateral surface of the testis. It contains the highly convoluted **duct of the epididymis**, which is continuous with the **ductus (vas) deferens**.

GRANT'S 2.17E
NETTER 362
CLEMENTE 276, 278

Dissect the testis in the following manner:

- Carefully remove any superficial areolar tissue that may adhere to the **tunica vaginalis testis**.
- Demonstrate the extent of the sac by injecting air or water into it (using syringe and fine needle). Observe that the (artificially distended)

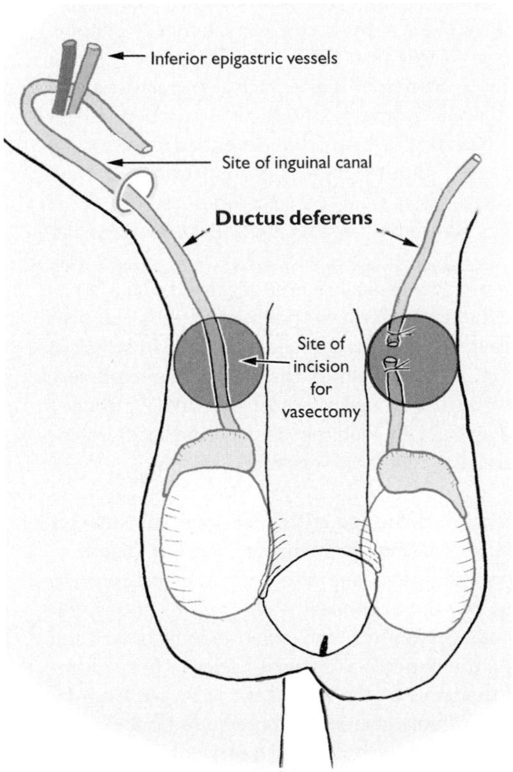

Figure 2.19. Superficial location of the ductus (vas) deferens in the superior part of the scrotum. Sites of incisions for bilateral vasectomy.

Dissection Note: Feel free to practice the vasectomy procedure on one side of the cadaver (Fig. 2.19). Leave the ductus deferens of the other side intact. Divide the ductus deferens, inspect its lumen, and appreciate the thickness of its muscular wall.

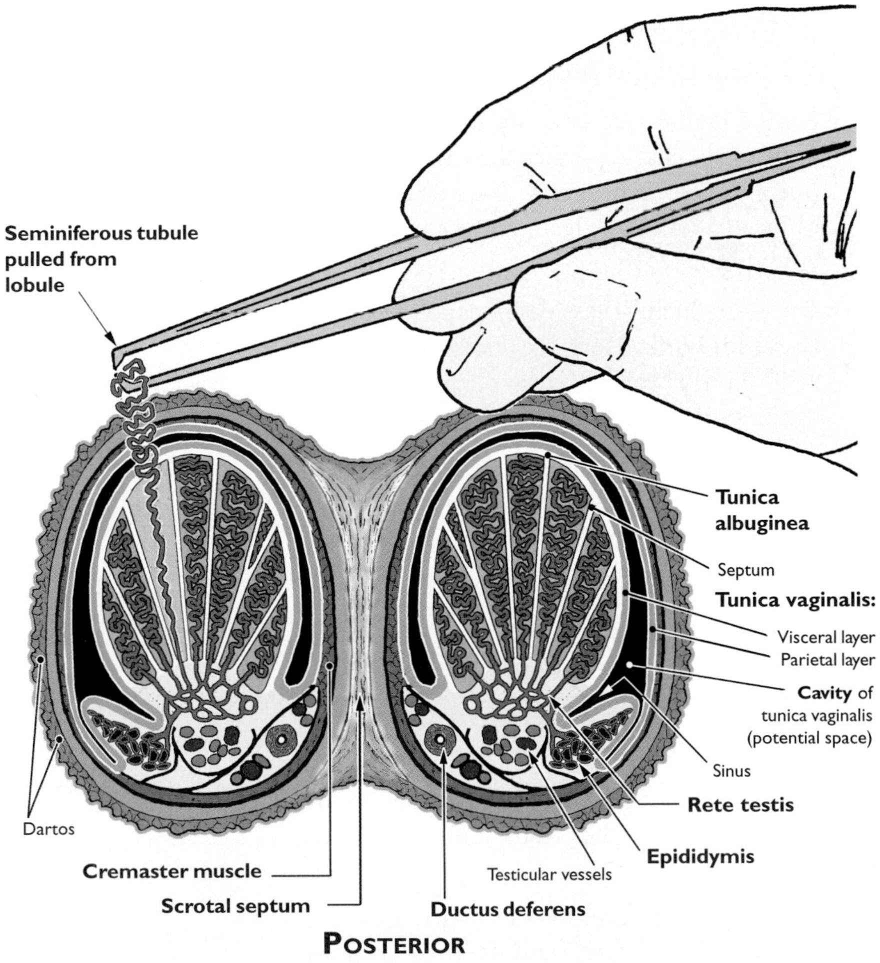

Figure 2.20. Horizontal section through right and left halves of scrotum. Seminiferous tubule being pulled from lobule of testis (schematic; enlarged).

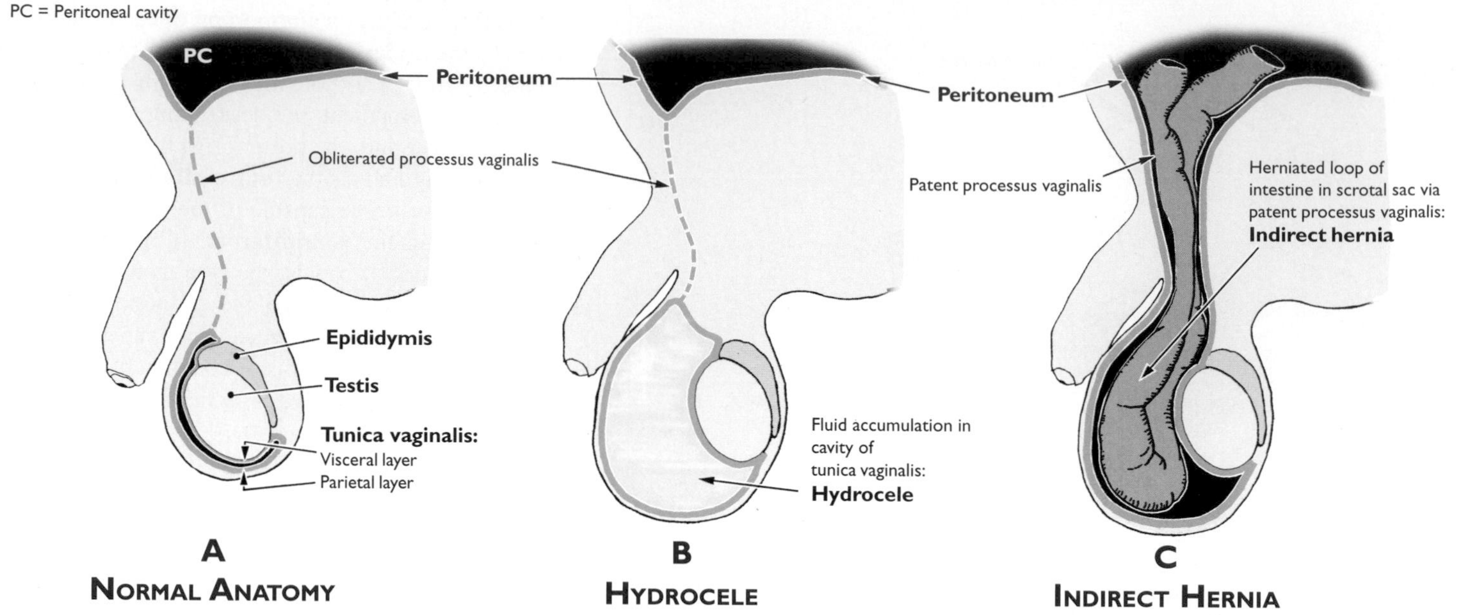

Figure 2.21. Processus vaginalis and tunica vaginalis. Normal anatomy and pathologic conditions.

cavity covers the anterior, medial, and lateral surfaces of the testis (but not its posterior surface).

- Incise the tunica vaginalis testis and inspect the interior of the serous sac.
- On the lateral side, identify the sinus of the epididymis that separates the testis from the **body of the epididymis**. The visceral layer of the sac covers the testis and the head of the epididymis.
- Trace the ductus (vas) deferens to the **tail of the epididymis**. Here, the duct is thin-walled and easily torn. Unravel part of the epididymis.
- With a probe, free some of the 15 to 20 fine **efferent ductules** between the superior pole of the testis and the **head of the epididymis**.
- Trace blood vessels to and from the testis.
- Incise the anterior aspect of the testis longitudinally from its superior to its inferior pole.
- Note the thickness of its fibrous capsule, the **tunica albuginea**.
- Look for fibrous strands or septa that divide the interior of the testis into numerous lobules.
- Tease some of these lobules apart, and note the fine thread-like **seminiferous tubules** (Fig. 2.20).

⇦
GRANT'S 2.17B
NETTER 361
CLEMENTE 274

⇦
GRANT'S 2.17D
NETTER 362
CLEMENTE 275

⇨
GRANT'S 2.15B
NETTER 379

⇦
GRANT'S 2.17A,C
NETTER 361, 362, 372
CLEMENTE 275, 277

⇨
GRANT'S 2.16
A.D.A.M. 4.21, 4.22
NETTER 379
CLEMENTE 243, 490

Clinical Correlation. Under pathologic conditions, the potential space of tunica vaginalis testis may be enlarged and distended by blood (hematocele) or serous fluid (hydrocele; Fig. 2.21B). A hydrocele can eventually become as large as or larger than a fist. Taking into account the topographic relations of tunica vaginalis and testis, understand that, in hydrocele, the testis is surrounded anteriorly and on both sides by the distended cavity of the tunica vaginalis. During physical examination of the hydrocele, the testis can only be palpated posterior to the swelling; i.e., where it is *not* covered with tunica vaginalis.

An enlarged or congenitally patent inguinal canal is a potential channel through which abdominal viscera may protrude. The protruding viscera are contained in a hernial sac, which is an outpouching of the peritoneal membrane. Hernias through the inguinal canal are called **indirect hernias** (Fig. 2.21C). Indirect inguinal hernias are located lateral to the inferior epigastric vessels.

The **lymphatic drainage of the scrotal sac and its contents** is of clinical importance. Realize that lymphatics from the penis and also from the scrotum (an outpouching of the abdominal wall) drain to nodes that receive lymph vessels from the lower abdominal wall and lower limb: the superficial inguinal nodes. Thus, inflammation of the penis or the scrotal sac will most likely be associated with enlargement of these superficial inguinal nodes. In contrast, **lymphatics from the right and left testes** drain into deeply positioned right and left lateral nodes, respectively. Subsequently, these lateral nodes empty into the preaortic lymph nodes. Testicular tumors, spreading along lymph vessels, will involve lateral and preaortic nodes. These latter nodes cannot be palpated on physical examination. However, they can be evaluated with CT or MRI scans; pathologically enlarged lymph nodes can be demonstrated in this manner.

Peritoneum and Peritoneal Cavity

Orientation

The **peritoneum** is a thin, translucent, serous membrane. To understand its complexities, certain fundamental facts must be appreciated (Fig. 2.22):

- The peritoneum lines the **walls** of the abdominal cavity; there, it is known as **parietal peritoneum.**
- It forms a completely closed sac or cavity, the **peritoneal cavity** (in the female, the uterine tubes open into the peritoneal cavity and create two small communications with the outside).

⇦
GRANT'S 2.20
ROHEN 274
A.D.A.M. 3.3
CLEMENTE 291
A.V.A. 3: 1.47.37

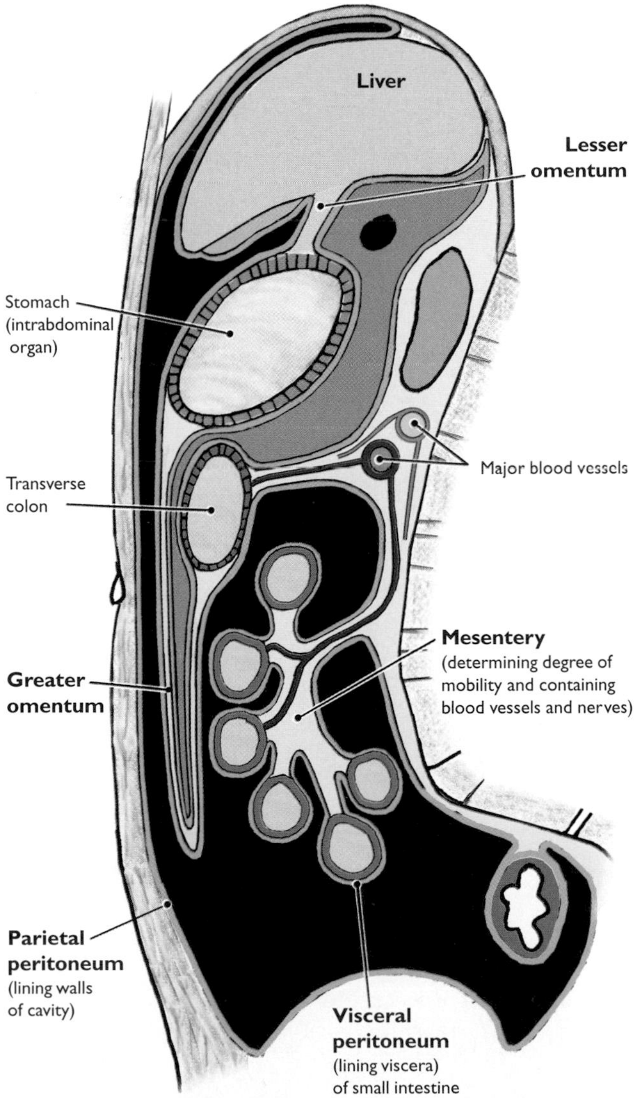

Figure 2.22. Peritoneum (green), peritoneal cavity **(black)**, and omental bursa (gray).

- An organ that invaginates the peritoneal sac is invested in peritoneum. The outer investment of the organ is the serous coat or **visceral peritoneum** of the organ. In general, this applies to the gastrointestinal system.
- **Retroperitoneal organs** remain behind (retro) the sac and are merely covered in front with peritoneum. In general, this applies to the urinary system.
- Two layers of peritoneum are attached to each of the two curvatures of the stomach. The **lesser omentum** is attached to the *lesser* curvature of the stomach, and the **greater omentum** is attached to the *greater* curvature.
- The mobility of an abdominal organ depends to a great extent on its peritoneal covering.
- **Mesenteries** are two layers of peritoneum that "sling" the intestine from the posterior abdominal wall. Vessels and nerves travel to and from the intestine between the two layers.
- All other double layers and folds of peritoneum are called **peritoneal ligaments.**
- **Folds or plicae** may be produced by blood vessels and ducts lifting the peritoneum off the body wall.
- Everywhere within the peritoneal cavity, peritoneum is in contact with peritoneum. The cavity is merely a potential space containing a small amount of lubricating serous fluid. Thus, intraabdominal organs can move upon each other without significant friction.

Clinical Correlation: Under certain pathologic conditions, the potential space of the peritoneal cavity may be distended into an actual space containing up to several liters of fluid. This accumulation of serous fluid in the peritoneal cavity is known as ascites. Also, other substances (e.g., blood from a ruptured spleen, bile from a ruptured bile duct, pus from a burst abscess, or fecal matter from ruptured intestine) may accumulate in the abdominal cavity and cause very serious conditions.

Inspection of Abdominal Cavity and Viscera

Dissection Note: Work will be more pleasant and efficient if you clean the entire surface of the peritoneal cavity with a damp sponge. Always keep the cavity and its contents moist with mold-deterrent preservative fluid.

Inspect the abdominal cavity. Do not dissect at this time. Study the dispositions of various organs and of the peritoneum. You may encounter pathologic conditions (e.g., cancer; enlarged liver or spleen; etc.). As a result of old inflammatory processes, *adhesions* (strands of fibrous tissue) may exist between the opposing surfaces of peritoneal membranes. These adhesions must be broken down with your gloved fingers.

Identify the following structures (Fig. 2.23):

Grant's 2.18A
A.D.A.M. 3.5, .3.6
Netter 252
Clemente 286

- **Greater omentum**. It is attached to the caudal border of the greater curvature of the stomach. Spread out this apronlike structure to appreciate its size and extent. It covers anteriorly the transverse colon and extends inferiorly to cover portions of the small intestine. Expect to find considerable variations in size and thickness. In emaciated cadavers, it may be very thin. In obese cadavers, the greater omentum contains a considerable amount of fat and, therefore, it may be of remarkable thickness and weight. Observe these variations in different cadavers. Be aware that the greater omentum has mobility and can wrap itself around inflamed areas to wall them off and prevent spread of infection. In that way, adhesions are created. These must be broken down, using your fingers or blunt dissection.
- **Diaphragm,** forming the roof of the abdomen.
- **Liver,** divided into a **right** and a **left lobe** by the **falciform ligament.** This ligament connects the liver to the diaphragm and to the anterior abdominal wall in the median plane. Place your opened hand into the potential space between diaphragm and right lobe of liver.
- **Gallbladder**. It is attached to the visceral (inferior) surface of liver. It reaches beyond the sharp inferior border of the liver.

Grant's 2.2A, 2.19A
Rohen 273
A.D.A.M. 3.5
Netter 258
Clemente 292

- **Stomach or gaster.** It may be dilated and conspicuous or contracted and less evident. Identify the long and convex **greater curvature**. Verify that the greater omentum is attached to it. Observe the right concave border of the stomach. This is the **lesser curvature.** It is connected to the liver by the lesser omentum. Verify this by gently lifting up the liver.

Grant 2.2A, 2.19A
A.D.A.M. 3.5
Netter 258
Clemente 292

- **Spleen or lien.** It lies posterior to the stomach in contact with the diaphragm. It is connected to the left part of the greater curvature of the stomach by two layers of peritoneum.
- Reflect the greater omentum cranially over the costal margin and thereby uncover the following structures (Fig. 2.24):

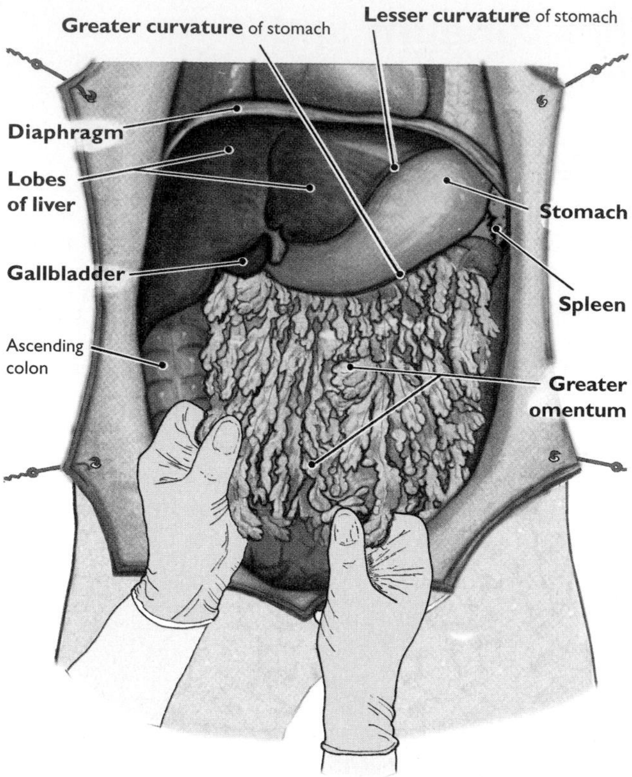

Figure 2.23. Spread out the greater omentum to appreciate its size and its relations to abdominal organs.

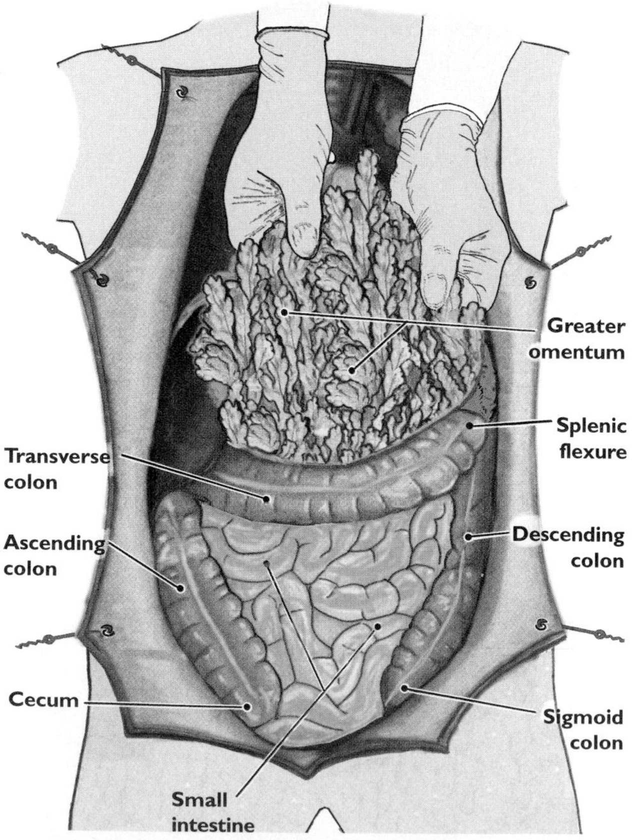

Figure 2.24. Reflect the greater omentum superiorly to expose the small and large intestine.

- **Small intestine.** The mobile coils of the jejunum and ileum are visible (combined length approximately 6 meters or nearly 20 feet). The small intestine terminates by emptying into the cecum, a large blind pouch of the large intestine (Fig. 2.25A).
- **Large intestine**. It frames the small intestine on three sides:

GRANT'S 2.1A, 2.2A
ROHEN 273
A.D.A.M. 3.5
NETTER 252, 253
CLEMENTE **287**

GRANT'S 2.2A, 2.62A
ROHEN 273
A.D.A.M. 3.5
NETTER 252, 253
CLEMENTE **287**

GRANT'S 2.2
ROHEN 272

GRANT'S 2.19A
A.D.A.M. 3.9, 3.10
NETTER 258
CLEMENTE **299**

1. On the right side, the **cecum** and the **ascending colon.**
2. Superiorly, the **transverse colon.**
3. On the left side, the **descending colon** and the **sigmoid colon.**

In the abdomen, follow the **alimentary canal (GI tract)** from its beginning to its end (Fig. 2.25). Certain parts of the GI tract are not immediately accessible (e.g., duodenum, pancreas) and, therefore, cannot be demonstrated at this time. Study the names and general dispositions of the parts of the GI tract from proximal to distal ends.

Detailed inspection of the small intestine. There are three parts: **duodenum, jejunum,** and **ileum.**

Duodenum. The exit from the stomach is the **pylorus.** The pyloric portion of the stomach is immediately succeeded by the **duodenum**, which has four parts (Figs. 2.25B, 2.26). The first portion of the duodenum is mobile. The hepatoduodenal ligament attaches to it. Verify this by gently lifting up the liver. Ascertain that the lesser curvature of the stomach and the first 3 cm of the duodenum are the attachment sites for the **lesser omentum**, which continues to the liver. Demonstrate the two parts of the lesser omentum (Fig. 2.26): the **hepatogastric ligament** (from liver to stomach) and the **hepatoduodenal ligament** (from liver to duodenum).

The remainder of the duodenum is inaccessible at the present time. The duodenum is C-shaped and molded around the head of the pancreas (Fig. 2.25B). Because of its

A

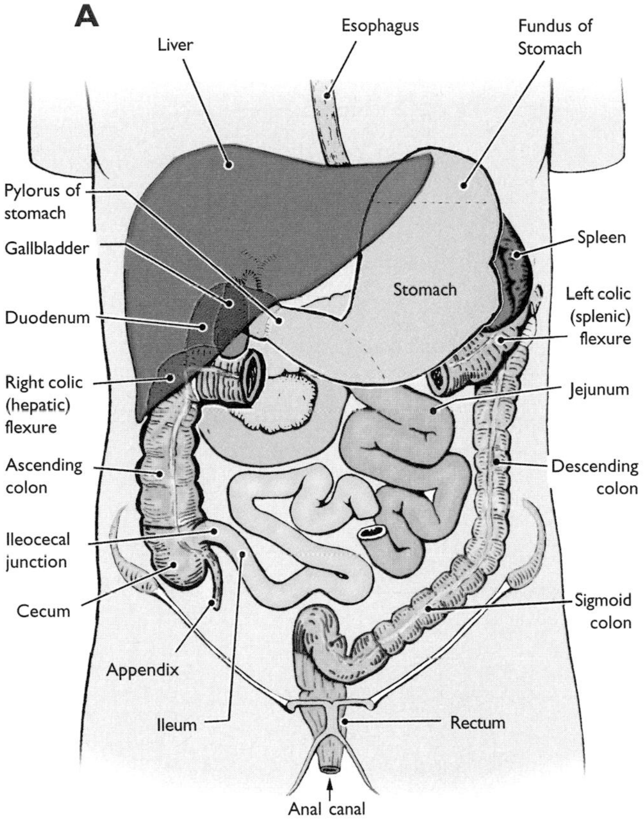

B

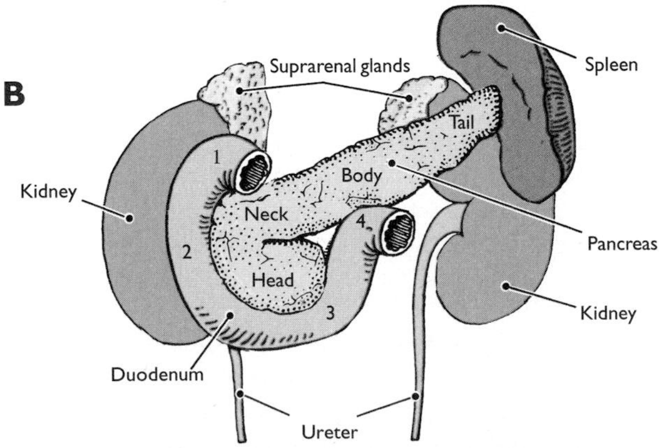

Figure 2.25. ***A***, Diagram of digestive system and disposition of abdominal organs (transverse colon removed). ***B***, Spleen, pancreas, and duodenum are uncovered by removal of the stomach. The four parts of both duodenum and pancreas are indicated.

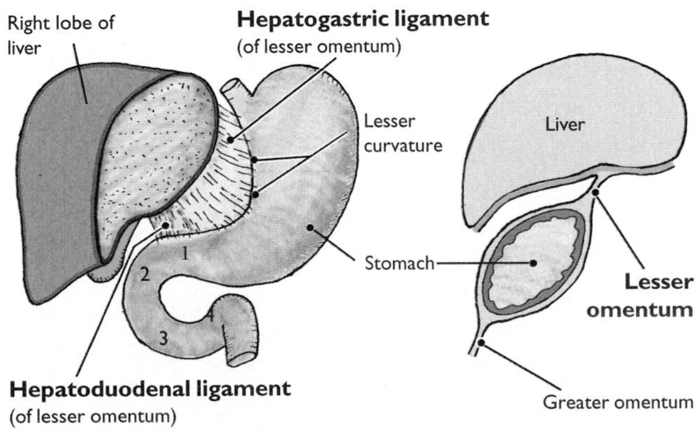

Figure 2.26. Diagram of lesser omentum and its attachments. Left lobe of liver removed.

shape, the superior (1st) part and the ascending (4th)part are only about 5 cm apart. Find the termination of the duodenum at the **duodenojejunal junction,** in the following manner (Fig. 2.27): Pull the mobile small intestine to the right side, then follow the jejunum proximally as far as possible. Find the point where the immobile duodenum ends and the mobile jejunum begins. This is the duodenojejunal junction. Push your finger to the left of the junction and explore the duodenal fossae (*blue arrows* in Fig. 2.27). If these fossae are enlarged or anatomically altered, loops of intestine can herniate into it. Just to the left of your exploring finger runs the inferior mesenteric vein.

⇦
GRANT'S 2.62B
ROHEN 284
A.D.A.M. 3.20
NETTER 253
CLEMENTE 327

⇦
A.D.A.M. 3.15
NETTER 253
CLEMENTE 328

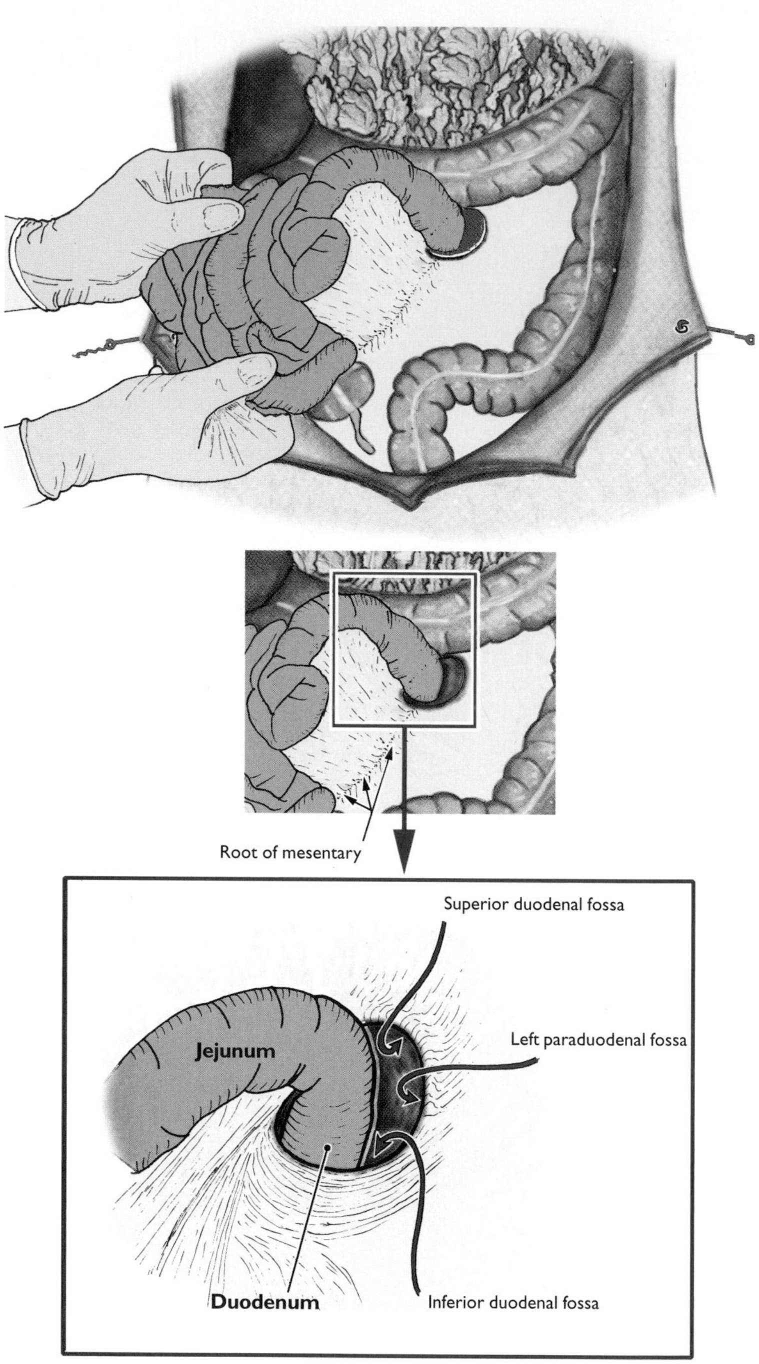

Figure 2.27. To find the duodenojejunal junction, pull the mobile small intestine to the right side. The *INSET* shows the duodenal fossae to the left of the junction.

Immediately succeeding the duodenum is the mobile part of the small intestine. Pull the small intestine to the left side (Fig. 2.28). Follow the jejunum proximally as far as possible and once more identify the duodenojejunal junction. What holds this junction in place and prevents it from sagging? Refer to the insert of Figure 2.28 and note that the ascending (4th) part of the duodenum is suspended by the **suspensory ligament of the duodenum** (ligament of Treitz). This is a fibromuscular ligament that arises from the right crus of the diaphragm, descends and crosses to the opposite side, and anchors the intestine at the duodenojejunal junction. This structure will be reviewed again during the dissection of the diaphragm at the end of this chapter. Palpate (but do not dissect) the duodenum through the parietal peritoneum.

Jejunum and Ileum. Turn again to the mobile part of the small intestine. It consists of **jejunum** (proximal 2/5) and **ileum** (distal 3/5). The ileum empties into the **cecum** at the **ileocecal orifice** or **junction** (Fig. 2.25). The distance between the duodenojejunal junction and ileocecal junction is about 15 to 20 cm in the adult. Yet, the total length of small intestine accommodated between these two points is about 20 ft (or 6 m). Find out how this is possible. Verify that the **root of the mesentery** of the mobile part of the small intestine stretches diagonally across the posterior wall from the duodenojejunal to the ileocecal junction (Fig. 2.27). This root is only 15 to 20 cm long. However, the **intestinal border of the mesen-**

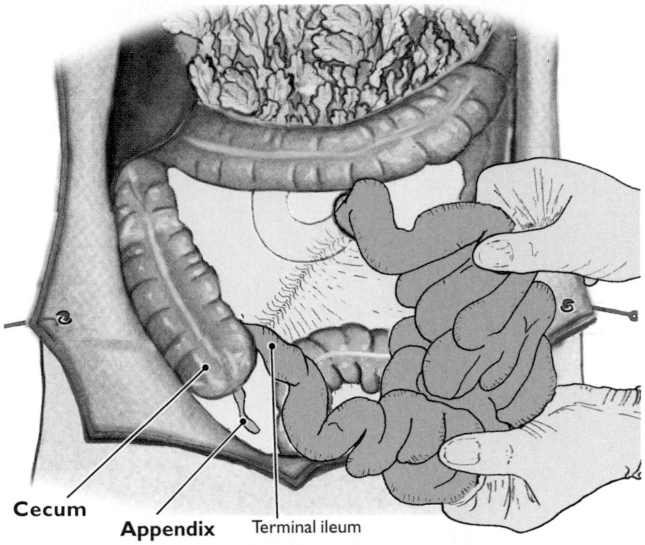

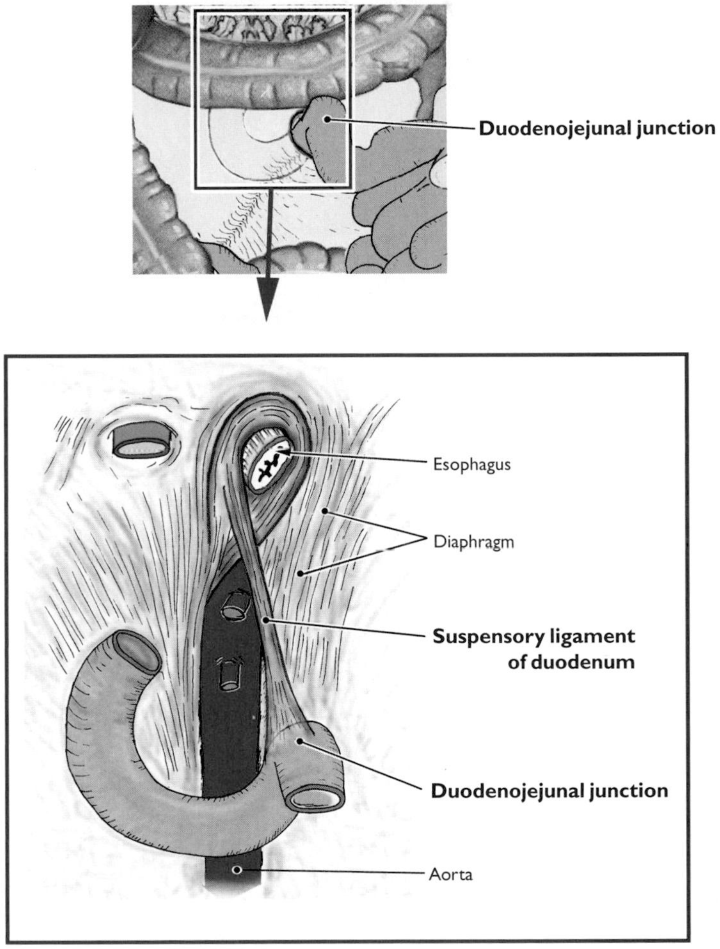

Figure 2.28. The duodenojejunal junction is suspended by the suspensory ligament of the duodenum (ligament of Treitz).

tery is elaborately ruffled to accommodate the substantial length of jejunum and ileum. The small intestine is so convoluted and mobile that you can pass many feet of it through your hands without knowing whether you are proceeding to its duodenal end or its cecal end. However, by placing a hand on each side of the mesentery and drawing the fingers anteriorly from root to intestinal border, the convolutions are locally untwisted and the direction of the gut becomes obvious.

⇦
GRANT'S 2.62B
ROHEN 284, 298
A.D.A.M. 3.7
NETTER 254, 334, 340
CLEMENTE 327

Detailed inspection of the large intestine (Figs. 2.25, 2.28). It consists of **cecum** with attached **appendix, colon** (ascending; transverse, descending; sigmoid), **rectum,** and **anal canal.** Observe the following features:

- **Cecum** (L. *caecus*, blind); extends inferiorly beyond the ileocecal junction into the right iliac fossa. The length of its mesentery, i.e., the degree of its mobility, varies considerably.

⇨
GRANT'S 2.65 - 2.67
ROHEN 287
A.D.A.M. 3.25
NETTER 264 - 266
CLEMENTE 335, 339

- **Vermiform appendix** (L. *vermis*, worm; *forma*, shape; *appendere*, to hang on); opens into the cecum inferior to the ileocecal orifice; may occupy any position consistent with its length; most commonly found retrocecal, i.e., posterior to the cecum (Fig. 2.29); its mesentery is a triangular fold of peritoneum, the mesoappendix.

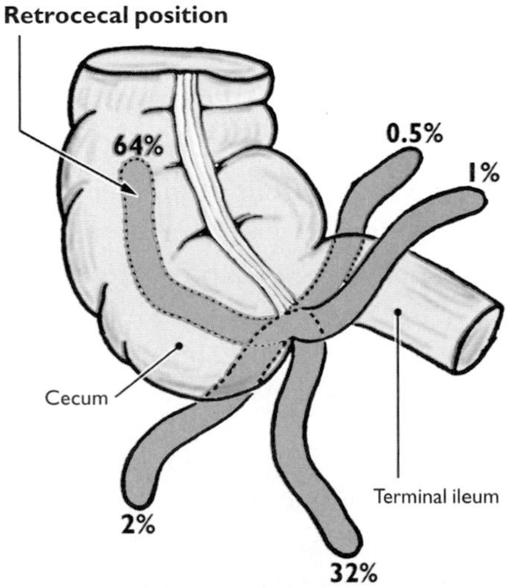

Figure 2.29. Various positions of vermiform appendix (most commonly retrocecal).

- **Ascending colon** (Gr. *kolon*, large intestine; hollow); has no mesentery; therefore, it is attached to the posterior abdominal wall; ascends to the liver where it makes a right-angle bend. This is the **right colic flexure or hepatic flexure** (Fig. 2.25).

- **Transverse colon;** extends transversely from **right colic flexure** to **left colic flexure or splenic flexure.** The left colic flexure is attached to the diaphragm by the **phrenicocolic ligament,** which also forms a shelf to support the spleen. The left colic flexure is at a more superior level and a more posterior plane than the right colic flexure. Between the two flexures, the transverse colon is freely movable. Its mesentery, the **transverse mesocolon,** is connected to the inferior border of the pancreas (Fig. 2.30). Also adherent to the transverse colon is the apronlike **greater omentum**.

- **Descending colon;** descends from the sharply curved left colic flexure to the pelvic brim. It is of smaller caliber than the ascending colon. Its posterior surface is attached to the posterior abdominal wall (Fig. 2.25).

- **Sigmoid colon** (resembling the Greek letter *sigma*); it has a long mesentery and, therefore, considerable freedom of movement. Identify the point where the mesentery, the **sigmoid mesocolon,** ends. Here, the sigmoid colon is continuous with the rectum.

- **Rectum** (L. *rectus*, straight). The rectum is only partially covered with peritoneum. Its relation to other pelvic structures will be studied later.

- The outer longitudinal muscular coat of the large intestine is concentrated into three narrow bands, the **teniae coli.** The three teniae begin at the appendix. The free tenia of the descending colon is easily visible (Fig. 2.31).

- Because the teniae are shorter than the other layers of the colon, they cause the formation of characteristic sacculations called **haustra** (plural: *haustra*; singular: *haustrum* (Fig. 2.31). Appreciate a view of the haustra in a double-contrast radiograph of the large intestine.

- **Appendices epiploicae** (omental tags) are small bags of fat that hang from the colon throughout its length (Fig. 2.31).

⇦
GRANT'S 2.52
A.D.A.M. 3.20
NETTER 255, 257
CLEMENTE 333, 334

⇦
GRANT'S 2.2, 2.62A
ROHEN 286 - 290
A.D.A.M. 3.5 - 3.7
NETTER 254
CLEMENTE 327, 331

⇦
GRANT'S 2.64
A.D.A.M. 3.28
CLEMENTE 342

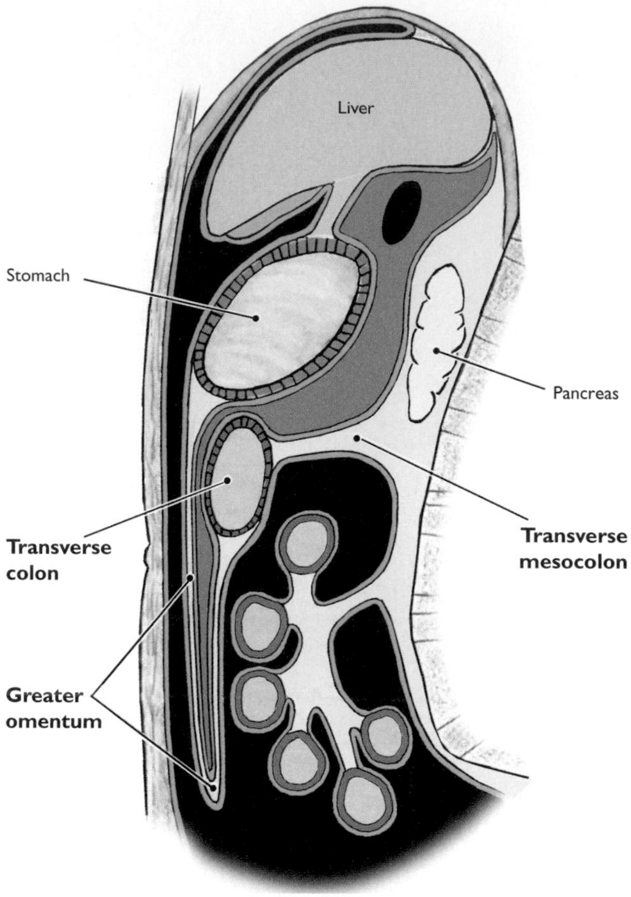

Figure 2.30. Transverse colon and its mesentery.

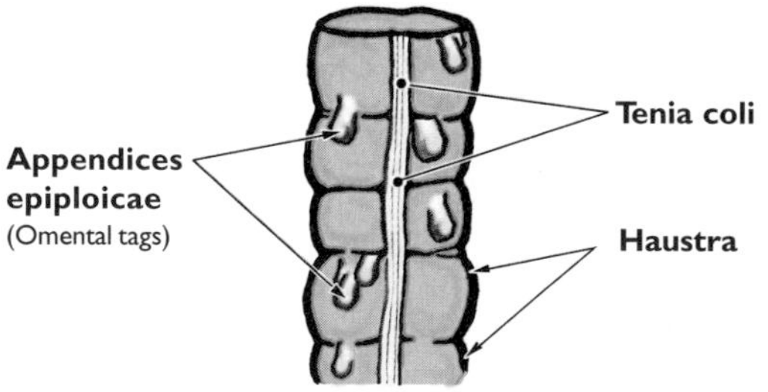

Figure 2.31. Segment of colon showing appendices epiploicae (omental tags), haustra, and one of the three teniae.

Clinical Correlation: Correlate your gross anatomical observations with a suitable magnetic resonance image. Study radiographs of the large intestine. Identify the rectum and the various portions of the colon. Realize that the contrast material (barium) is infused into the large intestine via the rectum (barium enema). Note that the contrast material usually does not enter the small intestine. This fact is due to a normally competent ileocecal valve.

⇦ *GRANT'S 2.64* A.D.A.M. 3.28 CLEMENTE 342

Liver and related structures. Return the greater omentum to its original position (Fig. 2.23). Inspect and study the upper abdominal viscera and their disposition in the abdominal cavity.

Liver or Hepar (Gr. *hepar*, liver). It is the largest organ in the male and non-pregnant female, weighing 1.2 to 1.6 kg. Note that its **right lobe** appears six times as large as the **left.** Observe the two surfaces of the liver, the diaphragmatic surface and the visceral surface.

⇦ *GRANT'S 2.18* ROHEN 287 A.D.A.M. 3.5 NETTER 252 CLEMENTE 310

- The **diaphragmatic surface** is in contact with the diaphragm. It is very extensive, convex, and smooth.
- The **visceral surface** is in contact with viscera (stomach, duodenum, colon, right kidney). It is concave and irregular, facing inferiorly, to the left, and posteriorly.

⇦ *GRANT'S 2.32* ROHEN 292 A.D.A.M. 3.15 NETTER 258 CLEMENTE 308

Pull the sharp inferior margin of the liver anteriorly, expose the visceral surface (Fig. 2.32), and observe two important structures:

- The **porta hepatis**; it is the "doorway" to the liver. Identify it by looking for a 5 cm transverse fissure through which vessels, ducts, and nerves enter and exit (Fig. 2.34).
- The **gallbladder**; study its four contact relations: liver, duodenum, colon, and anterior abdominal wall (Figs. 2.33, 2.34). If the gallbladder is absent (cholecystectomy), take note of it; look for postsurgical adhesions around the gallbladder bed.

⇦ *GRANT'S 2.36B* NETTER 276

Clinical Correlation. The four contact relations of the gallbladder are of clinical importance. An inflamed gallbladder can become adherent to and fuse with topographically related structures, notably the colon and/or the duodenum with which the gallbladder is in close contact (Figs. 2.33, 2.34). The *INSET* of Figure 2.34 shows how the

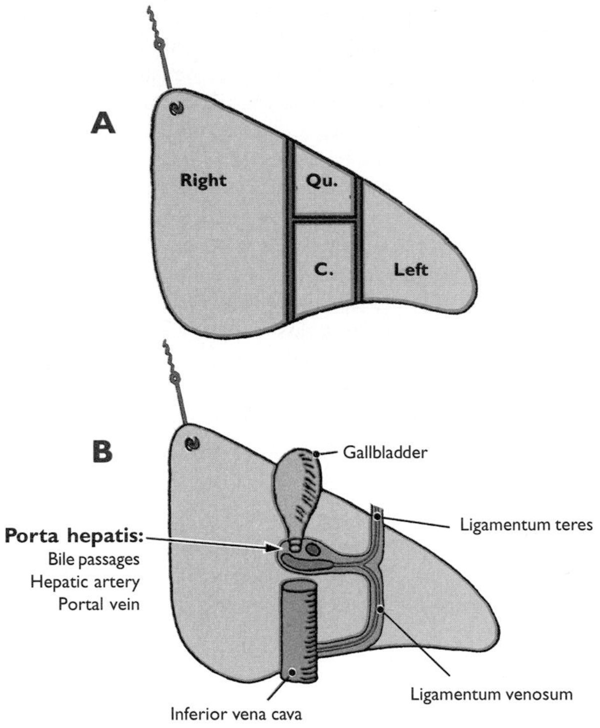

Figure 2.32. Elevated and exposed visceral surface of the liver. ***A***, H-shaped fissures and sulci defining the four lobes. ***B***, Porta hepatis with bile passages and blood vessels at the transverse fissure.

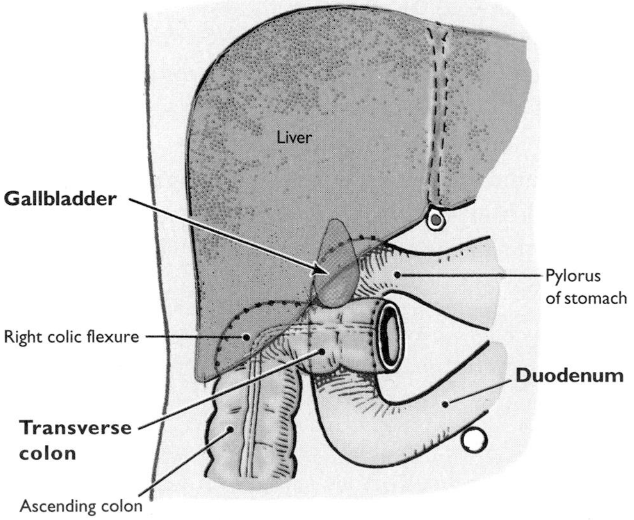

Figure 2.33. Interrelations of gallbladder, duodenum, and transverse colon (anterior view).

normal anatomy can be distorted by disease processes. An impacted gallstone may obstruct the normal drainage of bile from the gallbladder. Over time, the gallbladder may become dilated and inflamed. Chronic inflammation may lead to tissue fusion at the contact points (abdominal wall, colon, duodenum). The tissue boundaries between the diseased gallbladder and the GI tract may break down producing a fistula (cholecystoenteric fistula) through which bile or gallstones can enter the GI tract. For example, a large single gallstone could perforate into the duodenum and pass through the jejunum and ileum all the way to the ileocecal valve. If it cannot pass through this narrow valve, bowel obstruction (gallstone ileus) will result, with disastrous consequences. Conversely, air or gas from the GI tract can enter the gallbladder through a cholecystoenteric fistula. This air can be visualized radiographically; it is an important diagnostic sign.

Realize that the size of the gallbladder varies from patient to patient (subject to subject). Gallbladders can be very small or very large. This is a variation of normal. Study radiographs of the biliary passages and the gallbladder.

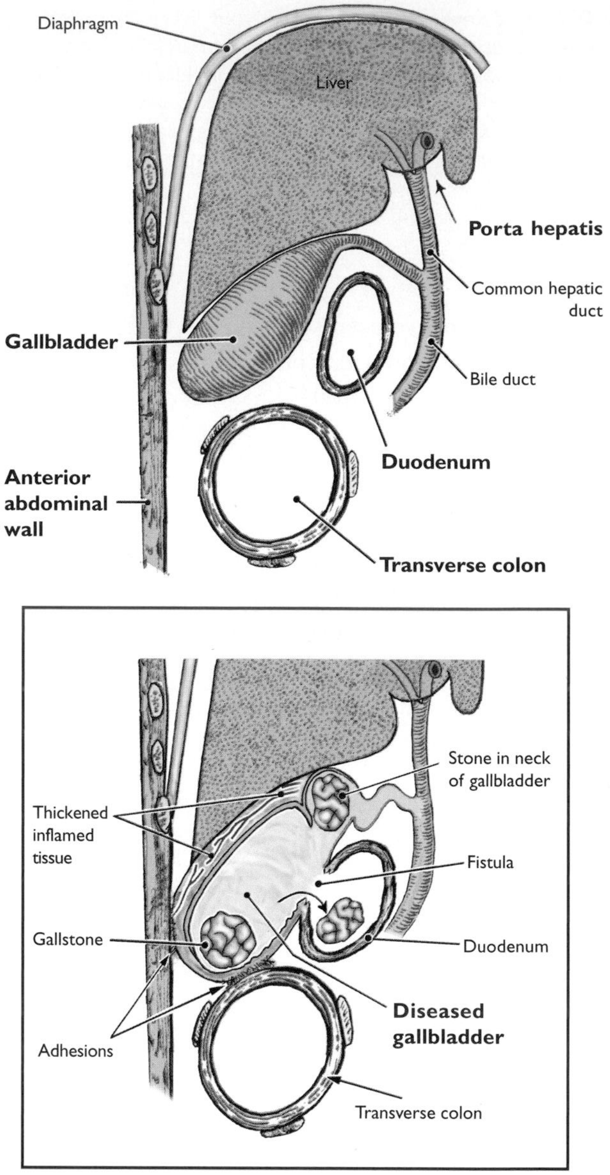

Figure 2.34. Interrelations of gallbladder, duodenum, and transverse colon (sagittal view). Inset depicts several pathological sequelae of chronic gallbladder disease.

GRANT'S 2.26, 2.38
ROHEN 279
CLEMENTE 314, 315

Hepatoduodenal Ligament (Figs. 2.26, 2.35A). Once again, identify the **lesser omentum** as it stretches from the lesser curvature of the stomach and from the initial portion of the duodenum to the visceral surface of the liver. Focus your attention on the right free margin of the lesser omentum, the **hepatoduodenal ligament.** Between the two peritoneal layers of this ligament are the structures that pass to the porta hepatis: **hepatic artery, portal vein, bile passages,** autonomic nerves, and lymphatics. Stand on the right side of the cadaver. With the hand palm up, place your index finger behind (dorsal to) the hepatoduodenal ligament in the direction of the *arrow* shown in Figure 2.35A. Your finger will pass through the **omental foramen** (epiploic foramen; foramen of Winslow) into the **omental bursa or lesser sac**. Anterior to your finger is the hepatoduodenal ligament with its important contents.

GRANT'S 2.19
ROHEN 292
A.D.A.M. 3.9 - 3.11
NETTER 258, 271
CLEMENTE 299

Omental Bursa and Peritoneal Reflections

GRANT'S 2.19 - 2.21
ROHEN 291 - 293
A.D.A.M. 3.3, 3.21, 3.32
NETTER 255, 256
CLEMENTE 291, 303

Omental Bursa. The exploration of the **omental bursa** (lesser sac) will be easier if **its anterior wall, the lesser omentum,** is partially removed: Break through the filmy membrane that stretches between the lesser curvature of the stomach and liver. Leave the hepatoduodenal ligament and its contents undisturbed. Place your hand into the widely opened lesser sac and study its extent.

- Direct your fingers inferiorly (*blue arrow* in Fig. 2.35B) They will pass posterior to the stomach and, at the same time, anterior to the pancreas and transverse mesocolon. Then, the fingers will pass toward the **inferior recess** that lies between the two double layers of the gastrocolic ligament, the apronlike part of the greater omentum.

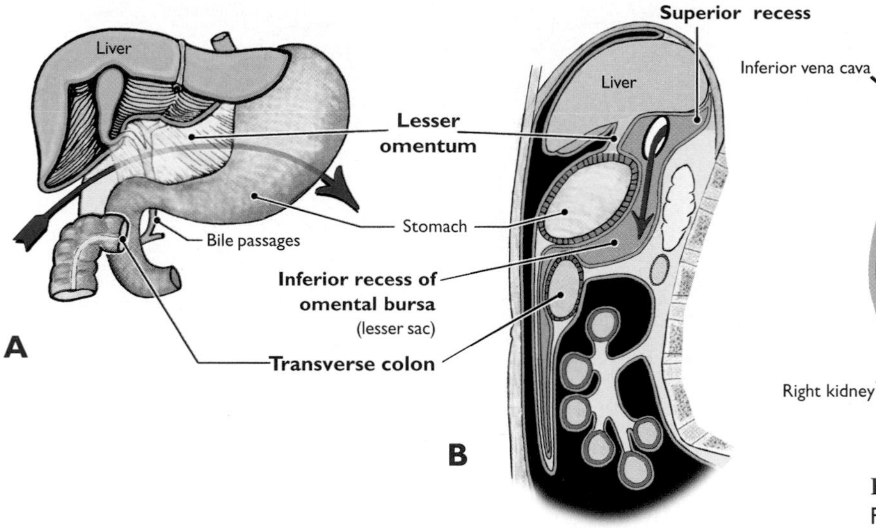

Figure 2.35. Entrance into omental bursa (lesser sac) through omental (epiploic) foramen. *A,* The blue line of the arrow passes through the omental bursa and posterior to the stomach. *B,* Walls of the omental bursa in sagittal section.

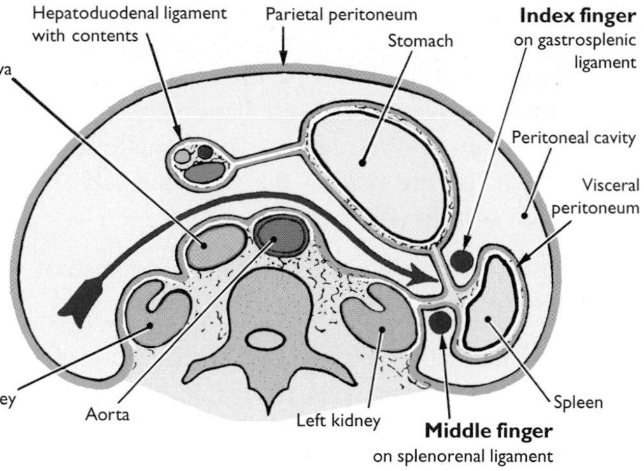

Figure 2.36. Horizontal extent of omental bursa (lesser sac). Fingers are positioned to palpate the "pedicle" of the spleen.

> ***Clinical Correlation:*** Normally, these two double layers fuse during fetal development; as a result, the inferior recess is obliterated (Fig. 2.35B). Understand that the greater omentum is composed of four layers of peritoneum.
>
> If the greater omentum is incised between the transverse colon and the stomach, surgical access can be gained to the omental bursa (lesser sac). This procedure is employed in surgical approaches to the pancreas.

- Pass your middle finger superiorly in the median plane between the liver and the posterior aspect of diaphragm (Fig. 2.35B). Your finger is now in the **superior recess** of the omental bursa. Palpate the structures bordering this superior recess: Posterior to your finger is the diaphragm; anteriorly, the caudate lobe of the liver; to the left, the abdominal portion of the esophagus; to the right, the large inferior vena cava.
- Push your finger to the far left and examine the horizontal extent of the omental burse (Fig. 2.36). Here, the peritoneal attachments of the spleen are the boundaries of the lesser sac.

Attachments of the Spleen. Examine the peritoneal attachments of the spleen (Fig. 2.36):

⇦
GRANT'S 2.21
NETTER 256
CLEMENTE 303

- Stand on the right side of the cadaver and push your right hand between diaphragm and spleen until the spleen lies scooped in the palm.
- Pass your *right middle finger* dorsal to the spleen until stopped by the **splenorenal ligament,** that stretches from the spleen to the left kidney.

⇨
GRANT'S 2.18
ROHEN 280
A.D.A.M. 3.5
NETTER 252
CLEMENTE 301

- Now, place your left fingers into the far left portion of the lesser sac and palpate the intervening splenorenal ligament.
- Next, leave your left hand in the omental bursa, place the *right index finger* between greater curvature of stomach and spleen, and palpate the intervening **gastrosplenic ligament**. Understand that these two ligaments, splenorenal and gastrosplenic, suspend the spleen between the kidney and the stomach. They form a pedicle (stalk) that transmits blood vessels to and from the hilus of the spleen.

From your observations and from the diagram in Figure 2.36 it should be obvious that:

- The splenorenal and gastrosplenic ligaments are double layers of peritoneum;
- Their inner layers are continuations of the peritoneum of the omental bursa (lesser sac);
- Their outer layers are continuations of the peritoneum of the peritoneal cavity (greater sac);
- Both ligaments form the left boundary of the omental bursa;
- The spleen itself is covered with peritoneum of the greater sac.

Attachments of the Liver. Provide better access to the hepatic region by cutting the right costal cartilages 6 and 7 near the xiphisternal junction and by partially incising the diaphragm. Now, examine the **peritoneal attachments of the liver** (Fig. 2.37):

- Identify the **falciform ligament of the liver**.

- Place your right hand between the diaphragm and the left lobe of the liver; simultaneously, place your left hand between the diaphragm and the larger right hepatic lobe. Your hands are now in the right and left anterior **subphrenic recesses.**
- Verify that the hands cannot meet because of the intervening falciform ligament.
- The hands can be pushed dorsally for a considerable distance between the diaphragm and the diaphragmatic surface of the liver until stopped by the reflections of the peritoneum from the liver onto the diaphragm (Fig. 2.37).

These peritoneal reflections from liver onto diaphragm leave an irregular triangular area of the liver *without* peritoneal covering. Therefore, this uncovered area is called the **bare area** of the liver (Fig. 2.37). The peritoneal reflections around the bare area are called the **coronary ligament**. The peritoneal fold attaching the left tip of the left hepatic lobe to the diaphragm is the **left triangular ligament.** Palpate it. The superior reflection of the coronary ligament is continuous with the falciform ligament. The inferior part of the coronary ligament is reflected onto the diaphragm and the right kidney; therefore, it is alternatively called the **hepatorenal ligament** (Fig. 2.37).

⇦
GRANT 'S 2.31
ROHEN 281
A.D.A.M. 3.17
NETTER 270
CLEMENTE 309 - 311

Inferior to the hepatorenal ligament is a potential peritoneal space, the **hepatorenal recess** (pouch of Morrison). This recess is bounded by the liver, the right kidney, the colon, and the duodenum.

> ***Clinical Correlation:*** The hepatorenal recess (of Morrison) is of surgical importance. It lies at the lowest point of the peritoneal cavity when the subject is recumbent (Fig. 2.38). Thus, pathological fluids may accumulate there. In the recubent position, another low point in peritoneal cavity is the rectovesical recess in the male or the rectouterine recess in the female. Pathological material can be transported from one recess to another, depending on the position of the patient.
>
> The subphrenic recesses, particularly the right recess, are a common site for abscess formation (accumulation of pus). A subphrenic abscess may penetrate the diaphragm and enter the pleural cavity; this is a grave complication.

Peritoneal Gutters (Fig. 2.39). The mesentery of the mobile small intestine, the ascending colon, and the descending colon are attached to the posterior abdominal wall in a characteristic fashion. As a result, **four gutters** exist that can conveniently conduct materials (ascites, inflammatory material, blood, bile, etc.) from one point of the peritoneal cavity to another (see also Fig. 2.57).

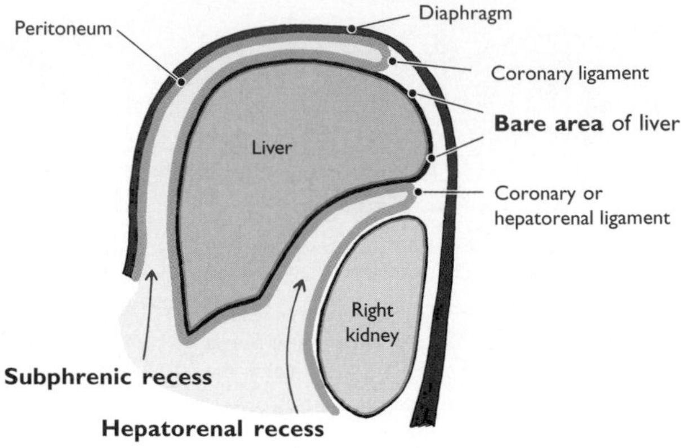

Figure 2.37. Paramedian section through diaphragm, liver, and right kidney. Subphrenic recess and hepatorenal recess or pouch (of Morrison).

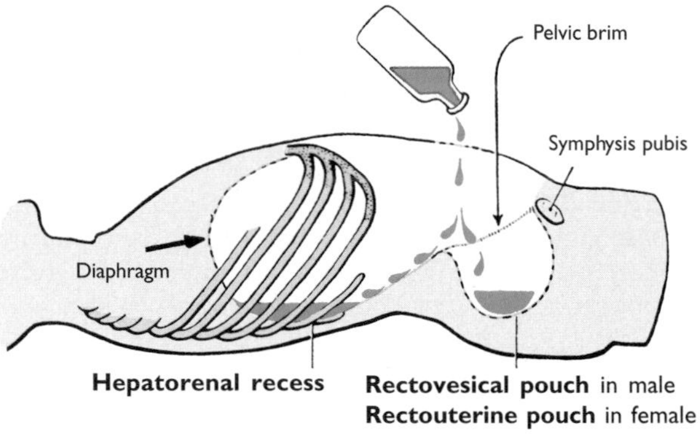

Figure 2.38. The most dorsal (posterior) parts of the peritoneal cavity. Fluids may collect in the recesses (pouches) when the subject lies recumbent.

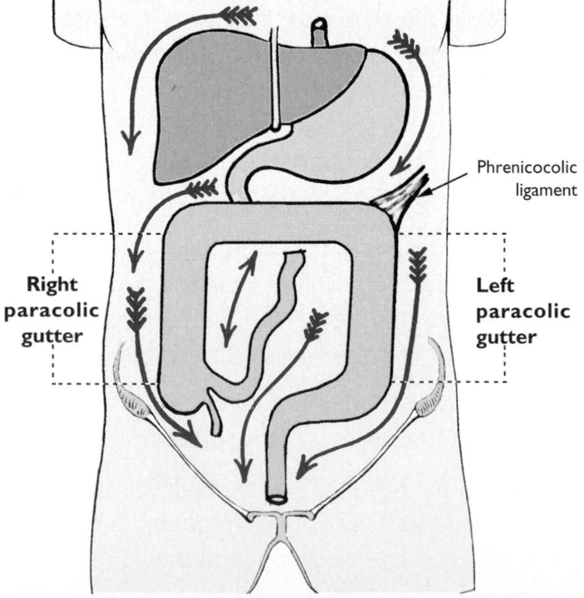

Figure 2.39. The four gutters in the peritoneal cavity. The *blue arrows* indicate the channels along which pathologic materials can be transported into the pelvic portion of the abdominopelvic cavity.

Identify in the cadaver:

- The **right lateral (paracolic) gutter,** to the right of the ascending colon; it may conduct fluid from the omental bursa via the hepatorenal pouch into the pelvis.
- The **left lateral (paracolic) gutter** to the left of the descending colon; it is closed cranially by the phrenicocolic ligament.
- The **gutter to the right of the mesentery;** it is closed cranially and caudally.
- The **gutter to the left of the mesentery;** it opens widely into the pelvis.

GRANT'S 2.52
A.D.A.M. 3.20
NETTER 255, 257
CLEMENTE 333, 334

Clinical Correlation. The **paracolic gutters** are of considerable clinical importance. They provide the pathways for flow of ascites and for the spread of intraperitoneal infections. Infectious material in the abdomen can be transported along these gutters into the pelvis; conversely, infections arising in the pelvis may extend superiorly. In a similar manner, the paracolic gutters can provide pathways for the spread of tumor deposits (seeded metastases).

Before you begin ...

Do *not* dissect at this time. Just understand that the following steps and procedures are planned: The vessels and ducts connecting the porta hepatis with other abdominal structures will be demonstrated. Next, the branches of the three unpaired abdominal arteries (celiac; superior mesenteric; inferior mesenteric) will be followed to their fields of supply. Similarly, the venous drainage of the GI tract into the portal venous system will be studied. Subsequently, the entire GI tract will be removed as a unit together with its three unpaired organs (liver; pancreas; spleen).

Bile Passages, Celiac Trunk, and Portal Vein

The following dissection requires time, patience, and adequate preparation on your part. Insert your finger into the omental (epiploic) foramen. Anterior to your finger lies the remaining free edge of the lesser omentum, the **hepatoduodenal ligament**, with its **contents: bile passages, hepatic artery, portal vein, autonomic nerves,** and **lymphatics.**

To aid dissection and to provide a clearer field, replace the finger with white paper or other bright material (Fig. 2.40). Remove the

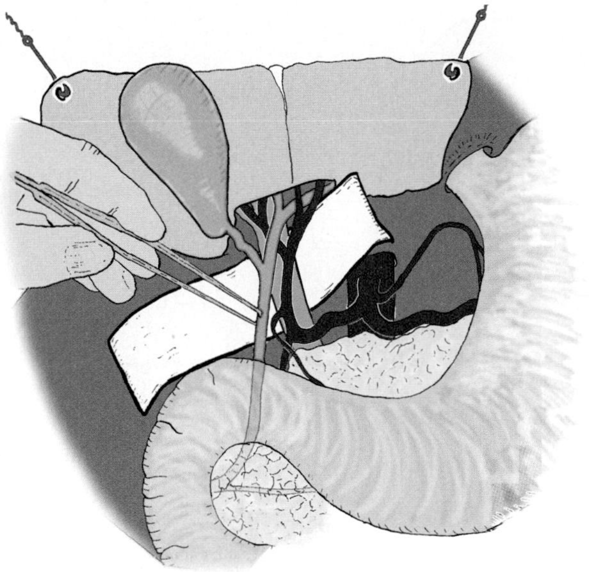

Figure 2.40. The main structures contained in the hepatoduodenal ligament: bile passages, hepatic artery, and portal vein. The forceps are pulling on the bile duct. The paper strip passes through the omental foramen.

GRANT'S 2.36
ROHEN 294, 295
A.D.A.M. 3.11, 3.14
NETTER 271, 276, 282
CLEMENTE 292

peritoneum from the hepatoduodenal ligament until the **bile duct** is exposed. The bile duct has the caliber of a pencil. It is thin-walled and usually empty and collapsed. By careful dissection, establish that the bile duct is connected to the gallbladder via the **cystic duct**. Follow the bile passages toward the liver and identify the **common hepatic duct,** and the rather short **right and left hepatic ducts** (Fig. 2.41). Be mindful of the possible variations of the cystic and hepatic ducts. Study radiographs of the biliary passages.

GRANT'S 2.39, 2.41
NETTER 277

Note that the structures in the hepatoduodenal ligament are surrounded and accompanied by a substantial network of **autonomic nerve fibers** that originate from the celiac ganglia (at the root of the celiac artery). To simplify the field of dissection, you may discard these nerves. Look for at least one of several **hepatic lymph nodes** located around the bile duct and the portal vein. Focus your attention on blood vessels. Carefully free the **hepatic artery proper,** which lies on the left side of the bile duct (Fig. 2.41) Follow the common hepatic artery to the celiac trunk, a very short unpaired vessel which originates directly from the abdominal aorta immediately inferior to the diaphragm (Fig. 2.42A) At the superior border of the first portion of the duodenum, the **common hepatic artery** divides into the **gastroduodenal artery** and the

GRANT'S 2.98D
NETTER 295

GRANT'S 2.28, 2.29, 2.34
ROHEN 294, 295
A.D.A.M. 3.12, 314
NETTER 282, 283
CLEMENTE 292
A.V.A. 3: 1.56.54

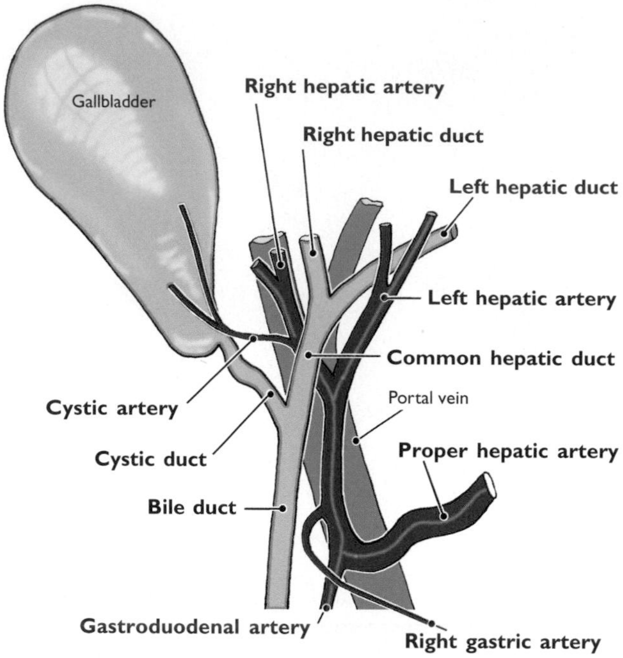

Figure 2.41. Close-up of structures contained in the hepatoduodenal ligament. Tributaries of bile duct and branches of common hepatic artery.

hepatic artery proper. Clean the hepatic artery and its branches (Fig. 2.41):

- **Right gastric artery,** to the lesser curvature of the stomach;
- **Left hepatic artery,** to the left lobe of the liver;
- **Right hepatic artery,** to the right lobe of the liver;
- **Cystic artery** (Fig. 2.43), a slender branch, usually arising from the right hepatic artery.

GRANT'S 2.43, 2.44
NETTER 288

Clinical Correlation: Surgeons must be aware of common variations in the **hepatic and cystic arterial supply**. If the arterial distribution in the cadaver does not conform with the usual pattern (Figs. 2.41, 2.42) consider alternate possibilities. Variations in the origin and course of the hepatic artery are common (40%). In about 12% of the cases, the right hepatic artery is aberrant or "replaced" and arises as a separate vessel from the superior mesenteric artery. The left hepatic artery may be "replaced," i.e., it may take origin from the left gastric artery. The right and left hepatic arteries may also originate separately from the celiac trunk.

There may be *accessory* right or left hepatic arteries; these are vessels that are additional to those arteries originating according to the usual standard pattern. Surgeons must be aware of these variations. The blood supply of the liver may be seriously disturbed (liver necrosis) following unintended ligation of arteries solely supplying certain parts of the liver. For example, during gastrectomy (surgical removal of the stomach) a "replaced" left hepatic artery (originating from the left gastric artery) could be unintentionally ligated, thus endangering the entire blood supply to the left lobe of the liver.

GRANT'S 2.35
NETTER 288

Cystic artery. Because of the enormous surgical importance of the gallbladder, its blood supply must be well understood by surgeons. Usually, the cystic artery arises from the right hepatic artery (Fig. 2.43). It may run anterior (75%) or posterior (13%) to the common hepatic duct. Less frequent variations (about 12%) include the origin of the cystic artery from the left hepatic artery, the hepatic artery proper, the gastroduodenal artery, the celiac trunk, and even directly from the aorta. Blood supply of the gallbladder from two different cystic arteries (double cystic artery) is possible. Generally, the cystic artery is related to the **cystic triangle**, which is defined by the cystic duct, the hepatic duct, and by the liver.

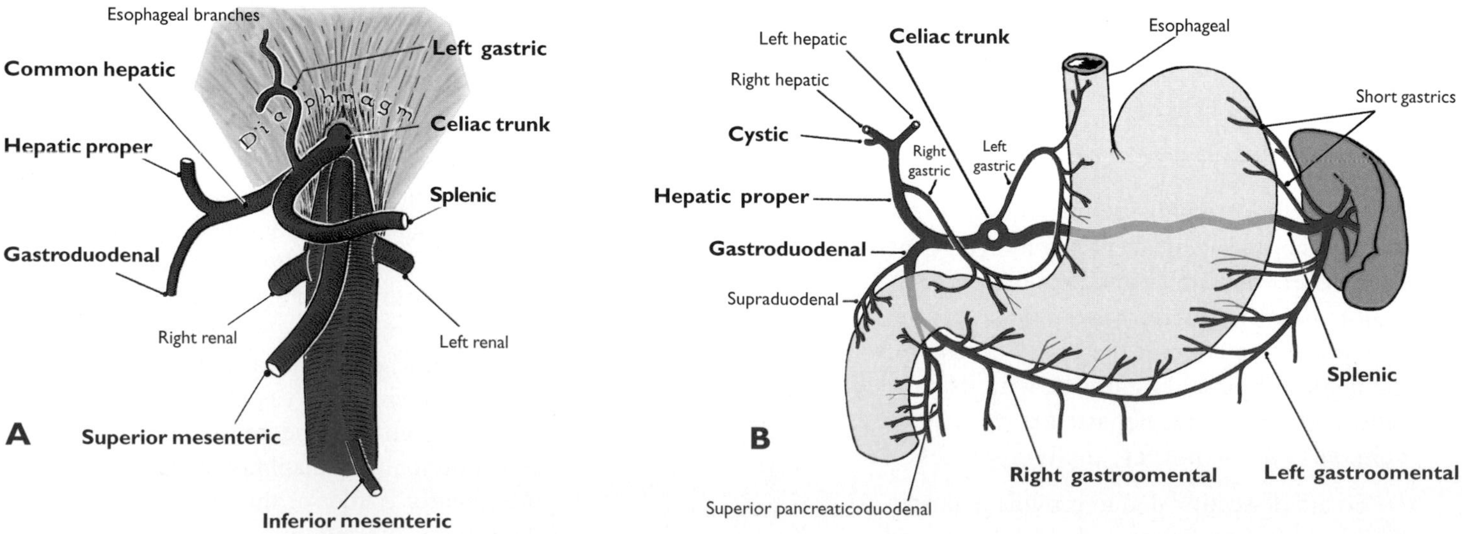

Figure 2.42. ***A***, Branches of the abdominal aorta. ***B***, Celiac trunk and its branches.

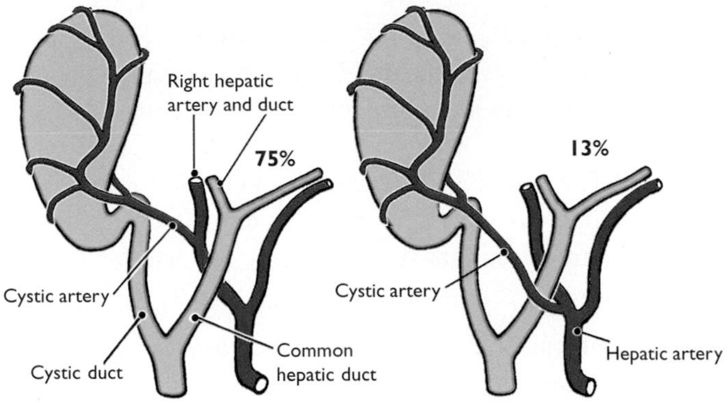

Figure 2.43. The cystic artery arises from the right hepatic artery. It may run posterior (75%) or anterior (13%) to the common hepatic duct.

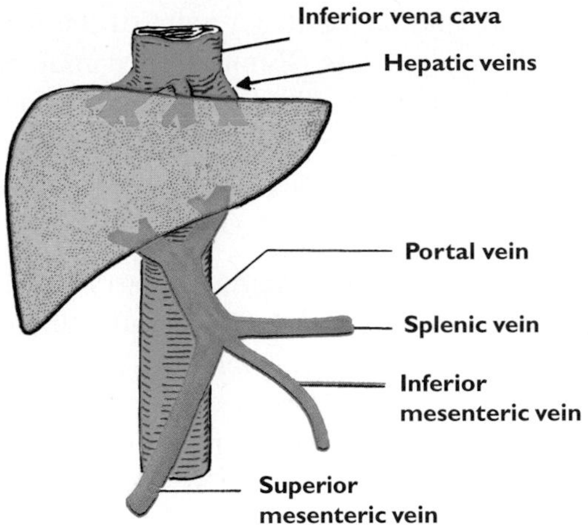

Figure 2.44. Portal vein and its tributaries.

> Study a celiac arteriogram, and compare it with a diagram of branches of the celiac trunk. Note that the contrast material has reached the liver via the hepatic arteries. The splenic artery is characteristically tortuous.

GRANT'S 2.28
A.D.A.M. 3.12
CLEMENTE 297

Dissect the two other branches of the celiac trunk (Fig. 2.42):

- The large **splenic artery**. Follow it only for 2 to 3 cm along the superior border of the pancreas. Do not dissect it further at this time.
- The **left gastric artery**. Follow it to the lesser curvature of the stomach. Observe that it anastomoses with the **right gastric artery** to form an arterial arch along the lesser curvature.

GRANT'S 2.29
ROHEN 295
A.D.A.M. 3.12
NETTER 283
CLEMENTE 293

Along the greater curvature of the stomach, examine the right and left gastroepiploic arteries that often form an arterial arch (Fig. 2.42):

GRANT'S 2.29
ROHEN 294
A.D.A.M. 3.11
NETTER 282
CLEMENTE 292

- Clean the **right gastroomental artery.** Follow it posterior to the first part of the duodenum where it arises from the gastroduodenal artery.
- Next, carefully clean the **left gastroomental artery.** Follow it through the fatty greater omentum toward the spleen.
- Leave the gastroomental arteries attached to the greater curvature of the stomach, but sever the greater omentum (gastrocolic ligament) just inferior to these arteries. The greater omentum remains attached to the transverse colon.
- Pull the stomach superiorly. Understand why the detachment of the greater omentum from the stomach provides wide access to the omental bursa (Fig. 2.35).

GRANT'S 2.49, 2.50
ROHEN 282, 283
A.D.A.M. 3.15
NETTER 293, 294
CLEMENTE 298

- Observe that the pancreas is readily accessible. Palpate it.
- Let your partner pull the spleen anteriorly while you are tracing the left gastroomental artery to the hilus of the spleen and to the splenic artery (Fig. 2.42B).
- Next, complete the dissection of the **splenic artery.** Observe that it contributes branches to the body and tail of the pancreas.
- Look for short gastric branches from the splenic artery to the fundus of the stomach.

Portal Vein and Its Tributaries. Review the portal venous system (Fig. 2.44). The portal vein carries venous blood from the abdominal portion of the GI tract, the spleen, and the pancreas to the liver for metabolic processing. By definition, the portal vein begins at the junction of the splenic vein and the superior mesenteric vein. The drainage point of the inferior mesenteric vein varies. Most often, the inferior mesenteric vein joins the splenic vein; however, it may also drain directly into the portal vein or into the superior mesenteric vein.

GRANT'S 2.52, 2.55
ROHEN 283
A.D.A.M. 3.15
NETTER 292
CLEMENTE 293

Dissect and examine the tributaries to the portal venous system.

- Using your fingers, carefully mobilize the tail and then the body of the pancreas.
- Note that the **splenic vein** lies inferior to the splenic artery.
- Follow the splenic vein to the **portal vein**.

GRANT'S 2.51
A.D.A.M. 3.12
NETTER 283
CLEMENTE 293

- At this location, identify the **superior mesenteric vein.** Note that it is the largest tributary of the portal vein.

- Now, find the drainage point of the **inferior mesenteric vein**. Remember, it may empty into either the splenic vein or the superior mesenteric vein, or it may join the portal vein at the junction of the splenic and superior mesenteric veins (Fig. 2.44).

- Look for the **gastric veins** that carry blood from the esophagus and the lesser curvature of the stomach to the portal vein.

◁
GRANT'S 2.49, 2.50
ROHEN 282
A.D.A.M. 3.15, 3.16
NETTER 293, 294
CLEMENTE 295

> ***Clinical Correlation:*** Portal hypertension (i.e., portal venous pressure above 20 cm H_2O) may result from suprahepatic causes (e.g., heart failure), intrahepatic causes (e.g., cirrhosis), or infrahepatic causes (e.g., portal vein thrombosis; tumor compression of portal vein). As a consequence of portal venous hypertension, the portal venous blood cannot freely drain, the esophageal and gastric veins become engorged, dilated, and eventually varicose. Rupture and extensive bleeding from these **esophageogastric varices** is an alarming and serious complication of portal venous hypertension. An understanding of the anatomy of the portal venous system is a prerequisite for intelligent diagnosis and treatment. Esophageal varices can be demonstrated radiographically.

◁
GRANT'S 2.50B

Superior and Inferior Mesenteric Vessels

Superior mesenteric artery (SMA). This artery is an unpaired vessel that arises from the abdominal aorta about 1 cm caudal to the celiac trunk (Fig. 2.42A). It has about the same diameter as the celiac trunk. The objective is to demonstrate the extensive field supply of the superior mesenteric artery: Duodenum (except its superior portion); jejunum; ileum; cecum with appendix; ascending colon; and approximately one-half of the transverse colon.

◁
GRANT'S 2.68
ROHEN 284, 285
A.D.A.M. 3.23 - 3.25
NETTER 286, 287
CLEMENTE 329

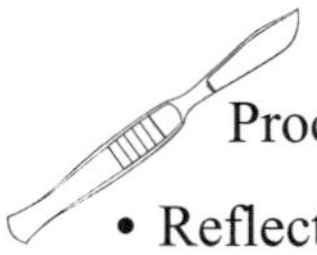

Proceed in the following manner:

- Reflect tail and body of the pancreas to the right.

▷
GRANT'S 2.69, 2.71
A.D.A.M. 3.26
CLEMENTE 330

- Carefully free the origin and initial portion of the **superior mesenteric artery.**

- Note the dense nervous network surrounding the vessel. This is the **superior mesenteric plexus of nerves.** Remove it to the extent necessary.

▷
GRANT'S 2.68
ROHEN 284, 285
A.D.A.M. 3.23, 3.25
NETTER 286, 287
CLEMENTE 329

- Follow the superior mesenteric artery to the point where it crosses anterior to the inferior (3rd) part of the duodenum. Realize that this vascular arrangement can potentially compress the third part of the duodenum between superior mesenteric vessels and the dorsally positioned abdominal aorta.

◁
GRANT'S 2.55A
A.D.A.M. 3.25
NETTER 284
CLEMENTE 316

- The **superior mesenteric vein** lies immediately to the right of the artery. It drains the same area that is supplied by the artery.

Next, follow the superior mesenteric vessels (arteries and veins) to the various parts of the small and large intestine. Use the following approach:

- Lift the transverse colon, with the attached greater omentum, superiorly over the chest margin and retain it there.

- Draw the small intestine to the left, and have your partner stretch the mesentery taut.

- Palpate the superior mesenteric vessels just to the right of the duodenojejunal junction.

- Then, using scissors or two pairs of blunt forceps, expose and clean the vessels between the two layers of the mesentery (Fig. 2.45). Now, identify and follow the branches of the superior mesenteric artery.

The branches of the superior mesenteric artery are named according to the structures that they supply:

- **Intestinal arteries,** 15 to 18 arteries to jejunum and ileum; arteries unite to form loops or arches from which straight terminal branches arise. These are the **vasa recta** that pass alternately to opposite sides of the jejunum and ileum (Figs. 2.45, 2.46, 2.47). The vasa recta do not anastomose within the mesentery; thus, "windows" appear between the vessels (Fig. 2.46). In the ileum, the arterial loops and arches become more complex, and the vasa recta become progressively shorter (Fig. 2.47). Demonstrate a few arterial arches and vasa recta in the jejunum and ileum. Study a superior mesenteric arteriogram.

- **Ileocolic artery** (Fig. 2.48); passes to the right iliac fossa; supplies cecum and appendix (appendicular artery); anastomoses with ileal branches and with the right colic artery.

- **Right colic artery**, arises from either the superior mesenteric or the ileocolic artery; supplies ascending colon; anastomoses with neighboring arteries.

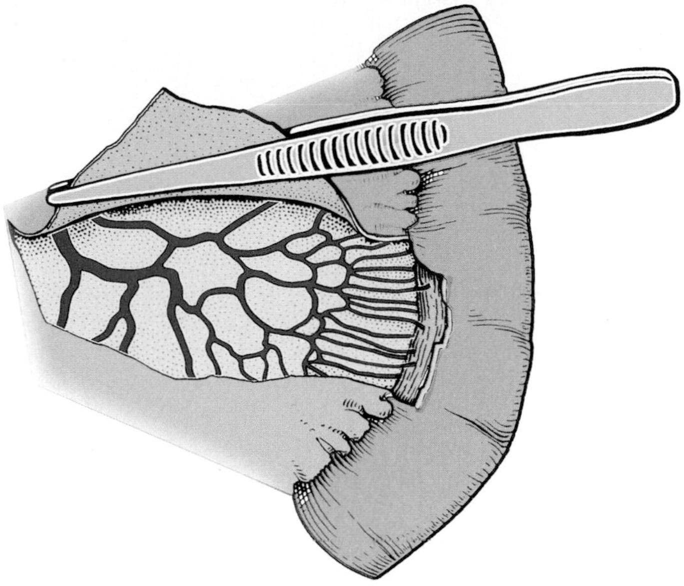

Figure 2.45. Exposure of blood vessels contained in the mesentary.

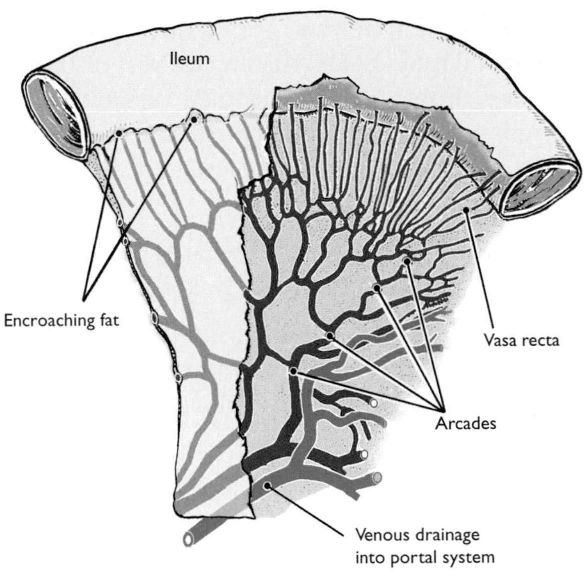

Figure 2.47. Vessels of the ileum.

• **Middle colic artery**; supplies the right half of the transverse colon; anastomoses with neighboring arteries.

GRANT'S 2.98A, C
NETTER 296, 297

The tributaries of the **superior mesenteric vein** correspond to the branches of the superior mesenteric artery. Identify the superior mesenteric vein and trace it to the **portal vein**.

GRANT'S 2.49
ROHEN 285
A.D.A.M. 3.29
NETTER 2.91, 292
CLEMENTE 329, 331

The mesentery contains a large aggregate of **lymph nodes** (numbering between 100 and 200). In most cases, these nodes are small. However, if there had been prior inflammatory or malignant bowel disease, some of the nodes can be of substantial size. Make an attempt to identify these clinically important nodes along the branches (tributaries) of the superior mesenteric vessels. Eventually, larger lymphatic vessels lead into the **superior mesenteric nodes** that are located near the point of origin of the superior mesenteric artery from the abdominal aorta.

GRANT'S 2.72
ROHEN 284, 285
A.D.A.M. 3.25
NETTER 287
CLEMENTE 331

Inferior mesenteric artery (IMA). This artery is an unpaired vessel that arises from the abdominal aorta, about 3 cm superior to the aortic bifurcation (Fig. 2.42A). The inferior mesenteric artery is much smaller than the superior mesenteric artery. The objective is to demonstrate the field of supply of this artery:

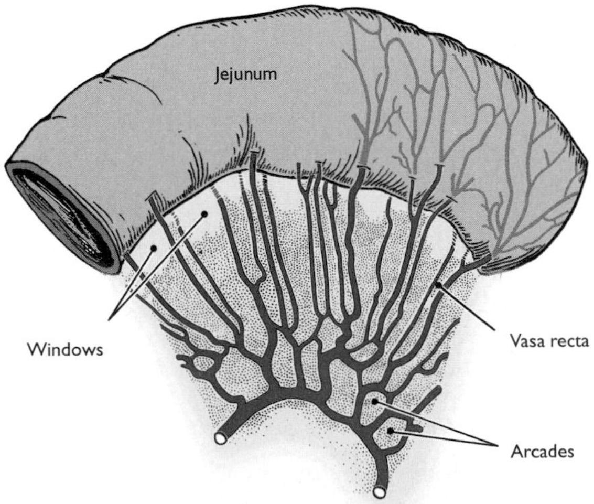

Figure 2.46. Arteries of the jejunum.

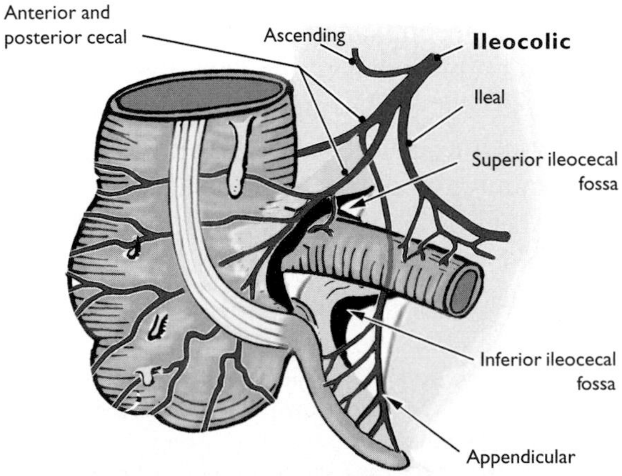

Figure 2.48. Branches of the ileocolic artery.

left half of transverse colon; descending colon; sigmoid colon; the greater part of the rectum. First, palpate and then dissect the origin of the inferior mesenteric artery. It is surrounded by the inferior mesenteric plexus of nerves.

Trace the artery toward the large intestine, and identify its branches (Fig. 2.49):

- **Left colic artery**; runs toward the left colic flexure; supplies the descending colon and the left half of the transverse colon; anastomoses with the middle colic artery.
- **Sigmoid arteries**; usually four branches that form arches.
- **Superior rectal artery**; supplies the proximal part of the rectum; divides into a right and a left branch that descend on either side of the rectum.
- Finally, study an inferior mesenteric arteriogram.

GRANT'S 3.12A
A.D.A.M. 4.53
NETTER 369
CLEMENTE 453

GRANT'S 2.73
CLEMENTE 332

Clinical Correlation: The branches of the superior and inferior mesenteric arteries form a series of anastomosing loops along the colon. The result is a continuous **marginal artery** (of Drummond) situated along the wall of the large gut (Fig. 2.50). There are areas where the anastomoses are insufficiently developed, and hence there is less effective collateral circulation (*asterisk* * in Fig. 2.50). This fact is of clinical importance in cases of mesenteric artery occlusion (thrombosis; embolism).

The tributaries of the **inferior mesenteric vein** correspond to the branches of the inferior mesenteric artery. Identify the inferior mesenteric vein and trace it to the **portal vein**. The inferior mesenteric vessels are accompanied by lymph vessels and **lymph nodes** that drain into the **inferior mesenteric nodes** around the root of the inferior mesenteric artery. Identify one representative node in the mesentery. If there had been prior cancer of the rectum or the sigmoid colon, the inferior mesenteric nodes are probably pathologically enlarged.

GRANT'S 2.53
ROHEN 282, 283
A.D.A.M. 3.29
NETTER 292
CLEMENTE 331

GRANT'S 2.98C
NETTER 297

Clinical Correlation: The **superior rectal vein** originates from the rectal venous plexus. The rectal venous plexus is also drained by the middle and inferior rectal veins that, in turn, empty into the caval system of veins. In portal venous hypertension, blood flow in the superior rectal vein may be reversed. Portal blood may be carried to the rectal plexus and, from there, shunted into the caval system. The resulting increased blood flow and pressure in the rectal venous plexus leads to the development of hemorrhoids. Thus, in case of hemorrhoids, the physician must always evaluate the condition of the portal venous system.

The portal venous system has no valves. This fact explains why the blood flow in the portal system can be easily reversed.

GRANT'S 2.53
A.D.A.M. 4.54
NETTER 370
CLEMENTE 455

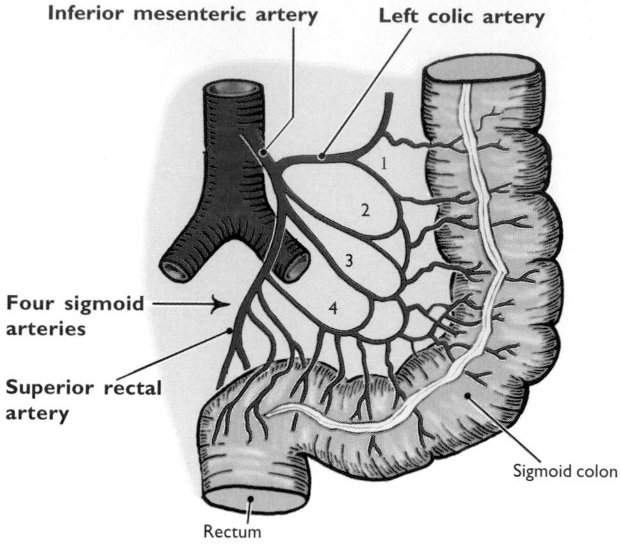

Figure 2.49. Branches of the inferior mesenteric artery.

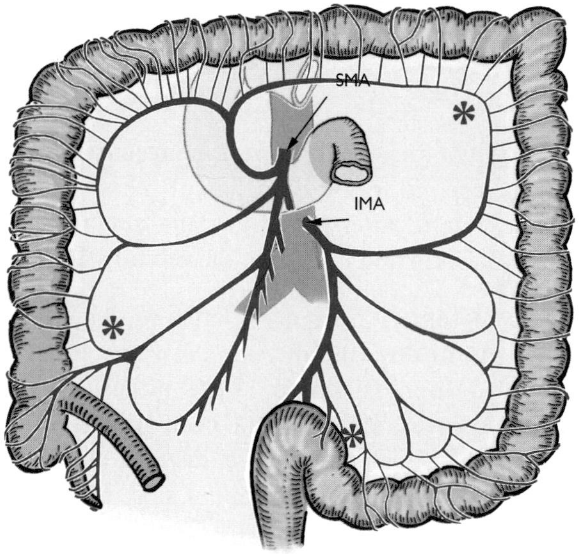

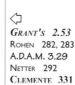

Figure 2.50. Arterial supply of the colon by the superior mesenteric artery (SMA) and the inferior mesenteric artery (IMA). The asterisks **(*)** denote three weak areas in the marginal anastomoses.

Removal of the GI Tract

> ***Dissection Note:*** The removal of the GI tract requires skill and a good understanding of the involved anatomical structures. Some instructors favor only partial removal of organs. In many cases, only every other cadaver is eviscerated while other specimens remain intact for review purposes. Please, check with your instructors.

Unless otherwise specified, prepare for removal of the entire GI tract together with its three unpaired organs (liver; pancreas; spleen). This ***en bloc extirpation*** offers several advantages:

- No essential structures will be destroyed. The unity of the GI tract remains intact.
- The removed GI tract can be placed on a separate table or tray for convenient and more accessible examination. The student will be able to study the GI tract repeatedly and in detail, even while fellow students are engaged in the dissection of other areas.
- Once placed on a table or tray, the student will have the challenging task to lay out the viscera in their *characteristic anatomical configuration*. This exercise alone is a valuable and impressive learning experience.
- The knowledge gained from this *en bloc* extirpation and examination will prepare the student well for subsequent pathology and autopsy exposure. Pathologists routinely remove organ systems *en bloc*. Often, the viscera of the neck and thorax are removed as a block together with the upper part of the GI system (stomach, duodenum, liver, pancreas, and spleen) while the bulk of the small and large gut is separated at the duodenojejunal junction (at the suspensory muscle of the duodenum, also known as the ligament of Treitz) and remains in the abdomen for practical reasons. However, complete *en bloc* extirpations are also employed in pathology. We have opted for complete removal of the GI tract to maintain continuity of the GI tract and to expose the posterior abdominal wall and to facilitate access into the pelvis.
- If so desired, the entire GI tract can be placed back into the abdominal cavity, and topographic relations with other structures can be reestablished.

En bloc **Removal of GI Tract.** Proceed with the en bloc extirpation in the following manner:

- Tie two strings about 2.5 cm apart tightly around the **rectum.** Cut the rectum between the two strings to prevent escape of its contents.
- Cut the **inferior mesenteric artery** close to the abdominal aorta. Leave a short stump attached to the aorta for future reference of this vessel. At the same time, you will also cut through autonomic nerve fibers originating in the inferior celiac ganglion.

GRANT'S 2.76
A.D.A.M. 3.32
NETTER 254, 257
CLEMENTE 333, 334

- Cut through the V-shaped **mesentery of the sigmoid colon**. Keep to its lateral side in order *not* to damage the inferior mesenteric vessels or the left ureter.

GRANT'S 2.52
A.D.A.M. 3.20
NETTER 255, 257
CLEMENTE 333, 334

- With your fingers, detach the **descending colon** from the posterior abdominal wall. At the left colic flexure, cut through the **phrenicocolic ligament**. The phrenicocolic ligament provides a shelf for the spleen. Thus, after sectioning the ligament, the **spleen** is sufficiently mobilized.
- Detach the **ascending colon** from the posterior abdominal wall. Keep to its lateral side to protect the vessels supplying the colon.
- Pull the transverse colon with the attached greater omentum caudally, and expose the **origin of the superior mesenteric artery.** Sever this vessel close to the abdominal aorta. In doing so, you will also cut through autonomic nerve fibers arising from the superior mesenteric ganglion. If the right hepatic artery arises from the superior mesenteric artery (12%), be sure to include it in this section.
- Sever the **celiac trunk** at its origin from the aorta. Make sure to include all its branches. By necessity, you will also cut through autonomic nerve fibers originating from the celiac ganglia.

GRANT'S 2.92, 2.93
A.D.A.M. 2.41
NETTER 181
CLEMENTE 363

- Tie a string around the **esophagus** close to the diaphragm. If the thorax has already been dissected, tie the string around the esophagus within the thorax just superior to the diaphragm. Cut the esophagus and the vagal nerves superior to the string (to avoid escape of gastric contents). Using blunt dissection, free the distal portion of the esophagus from the esophageal hiatus of the diaphragm and pull it into the abdominal cavity. (If the thorax has not been dissected as yet, cut the tied esophagus just inferior to the diaphragm). Free the **stomach** completely so that it is only attached to the duodenum and blood vessels. Cut vagal branches to the celiac plexus of nerves.
- The **duodenojejunal junction or flexure** is held in place by a fibromuscular band, the **suspensory muscle of the duodenum** (ligament of Treitz). This structure (Fig. 2.51) passes from

the posterior aspect of the ascending part of the duodenum and the duodenojejunal flexure to the right crus of the diaphragm. Palpate this supporting structure and sever it close to the duodenojejunal junction. With your fingers, detach the **duodenum** and **pancreas** from the posterior abdominal wall. Do *not* damage the bile passages or vessels of the pancreaticoduodenal region.

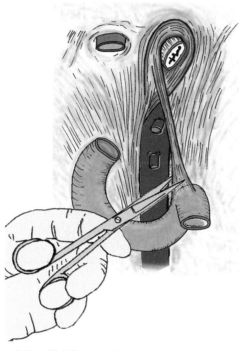

Figure 2.51. Mobilize the duodenojenjunal junction by cutting through the suspensory ligament of the duodenum.

NETTER 253
CLEMENTE 210, 211

GRANT'S 2.2
ROHEN 272
A.D.A.M. 3.5
NETTER 252
CLEMENTE 282

GRANT'S 2.49, 2.50A
ROHEN 282, 283
A.D.A.M. 3.15
NETTER 293, 294
CLEMENTE 298

- Identify the **inferior vena cava** as it approaches the dorsal surface of the liver. Lift the liver anteriorly and superiorly, and follow the inferior cava to the point where it is attached to the dorsal surface of the liver. At this level, cut through this large vessel as close to the liver as possible.

- The last organ to be mobilized is the **liver:** incise the **falciform ligament** between the diaphragm and the diaphragmatic surface of the liver. Cut the **left triangular ligament** and then the anterior portion of the **coronary ligament**. Forcibly, pull the liver inferiorly with one hand and **cut the inferior vena cava** at the point where it pierces the diaphragm. Cut along the remaining portion of the coronary ligament. Observe the hepatorenal ligament as you cut through it.

- Finally, **remove the detached GI tract together with the liver, the pancreas, and the spleen.** Carefully lift the organs out of the abdominal cavity. Avoid tearing the fragile inferior mesenteric vein; thus, support the weight of the sigmoid colon and the descending colon with one hand. Place the organs on a tray or table, and arrange them in their *characteristic anatomical configuration*. This is an instructive exercise that will contribute greatly to your understanding of the disposition of the GI tract and its three unpaired organs (liver; pancreas; spleen). Now, the various organs, their interconnections, and their blood vessels can be conveniently examined in greater detail.

Detailed Examination of GI Tract and Its Unpaired Organs

Place the removed GI tract on a tray or table, and arrange them in their *characteristic anatomical configuration*. Now, trace the **main tributaries to the portal vein**:

- Splenic vein;
- Superior mesenteric vein;
- Inferior mesenteric vein.
- Clean these vessels and the portal vein. Make a special effort to trace **esophageal and gastric veins** to the portal vein. Does your cadaver specimen have esophageogastric varices?

GRANT'S 2.31A
NETTER 270
CLEMENTE 309, 311
A.V.A. 3: 2.00.15

Clean the **celiac trunk.** Observe strands of **autonomic nerve fibers** accompanying the celiac trunk and its branches. These fibers are derived from the celiac plexus of nerves. Review and then clean all **branches of the celiac trunk** (Fig. 2.42B):

GRANT'S 2.29
ROHEN 284, 285
A.D.A.M. 3.12
NETTER 284
CLEMENTE 292

- **Splenic artery.** Verify that it sends branches to the body and to the tail of the pancreas (Fig. 2.52B).

GRANT'S 2.92, 2.93
A.D.A.M. 1.41
NETTER 181
CLEMENTE 363

GRANT'S 2.98B
NETTER 299
CLEMENTE 308

- Look for **lymph nodes** along the course of the splenic artery. These nodes receive lymphatic drainage from the tail of the pancreas and from the spleen, hence the term **pancreaticosplenic nodes**.

- **Left gastric artery.**
- **Common hepatic artery.** Identify the division of this artery into the **hepatic artery proper** and the **gastroduodenal artery**.
- Now, follow the **gastroduodenal artery** to the duodenum and pancreas. Note that it contributes to anterior and posterior **pancreaticoduodenal arches** (arcades), which lie in the angle between the duodenum and pancreas (Fig. 2.52A). These are the anterior and posterior **superior pancreatoduodenal arteries** that supply the proximal part of the duodenum and pancreas with blood from the celiac trunk.
- Similarly, the distal half of the duodenum is supplied with blood from the **superior mesenteric artery** (Fig. 2.52).

⇦
GRANT'S 2.29
ROHEN 284, 285
A.D.A.M. 3.12
NETTER 284, 285
CLEMENTE 293, 316

Pick up the severed end of the **superior mesenteric artery**.

- Verify that this sizeable artery crosses the duodenum ventrally near the junction of the third and fourth portions of the duodenum (Fig. 2.53).
- Clean and follow the branches of the superior mesenteric artery to the head of the pancreas and the three distal portions of the duodenum that are molded around the head of the pancreas.
- Identify the anterior and posterior **inferior pancreatoduodenal arteries** that form part of the two pancreaticoduodenal arches (Fig. 2.52A).
- Review the rich and complex dual blood supply of the duodenum and pancreas by branches of both the celiac trunk and the superior mesenteric artery.

Review the **bile passages** (Fig. 2.54). Turn the duodenum and pancreas slightly as to make their posterior surfaces accessible.

⇦
GRANT 2.55, 2.57
ROHEN 278, 279
A.D.A.M. 3.14, 3.15
NETTER 276, 284, 285
CLEMENTE 312 - 317

- Follow the **bile duct** (common bile duct) to a groove on the posterior surface of the head of the pancreas.
- With probe and scissors, carefully free the duct from surrounding pancreatic tissue. Follow it to the point where it passes obliquely through the wall of the descending (sec-

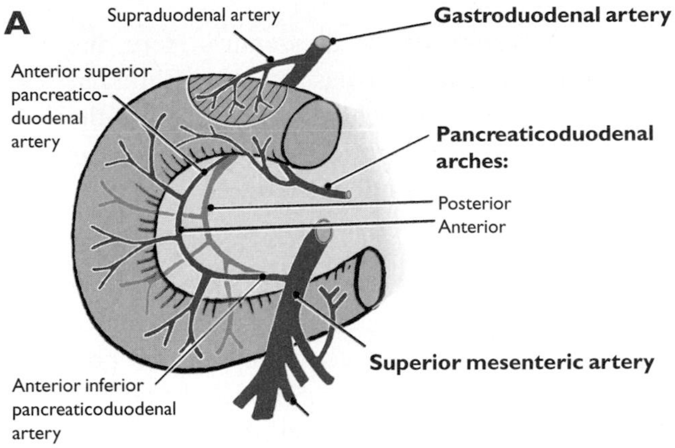

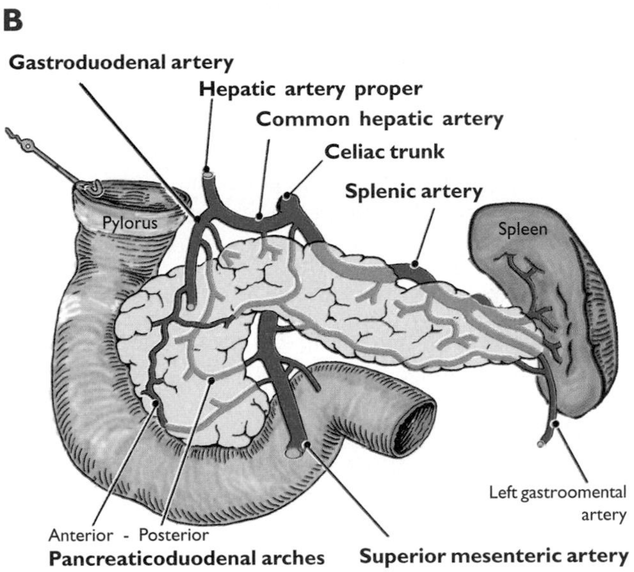

Figure 2.52. Dual blood supply of the duodenum and pancreas from the celiac trunk and the superior mesenteric artery.

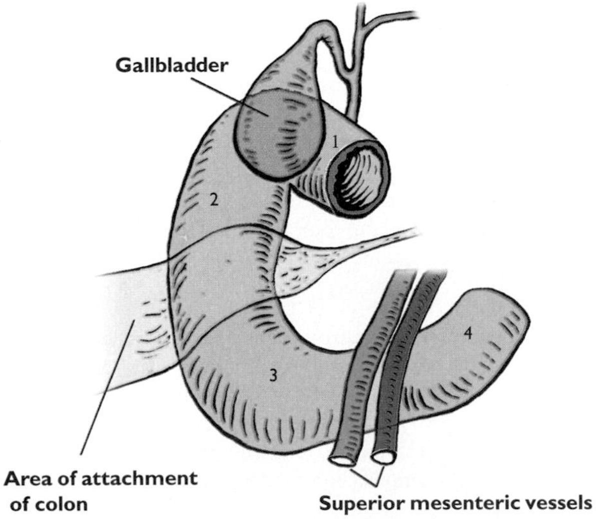

Figure 2.53. Three structures are related to the duodenum: gallbladder, colon, and superior mesenteric vessels.

ond) portion of the duodenum. Here, the common bile duct has its own sphincter, known as choledochus. The opening of the common bile duct into the duodenum is at the **major duodenal papilla**.

- Take great care to preserve the **main pancreatic duct** that usually joins the terminal portion of the bile duct (Fig. 2.54). Notice that the wall of the common terminal portion (or common channel) of both the bile duct and the pancreatic duct is thickened. This is due to a smooth sphincter muscle, the **sphincter of the hepatopancreatic ampulla** (Spincter Oddi).

- Follow the main pancreatic duct for 5 cm into the substance of the pancreas. Note numerous small ducts that drain into the main duct. In addition, an accessory duct may open separately into the duodenum.

- Open the duodenum by a 5 cm incision just opposite the entrance of the bile duct.

- Observe the **major duodenal papilla** and the hood-like **plica** that covers it. If an accessory pancreatic duct is present, there may be a minor duodenal papilla about 2 cm superior to the major papilla. Be aware of the variability of pancreatic ducts.

> ***Clinical Correlation:*** The bile passages and the pancreatic ducts can be demonstrated radiographically. This can be accomplished by *endoscopic retrograde cholangiography* and *pancreatography (ERCP)*. A fiberoptic endoscope is passed through the patient's mouth, esophagus, and stomach into the second portion of the duodenum. Under visual control, the major duodenal papilla is cannulated, and a radiopaque dye is injected in a retrograde manner (i.e., in the opposite direction of the usual flow of fluids). In this manner, the pancreatic and biliary systems can be evaluated radiographically. Correlate your gross anatomical knowledge of these systems with a suitable image obtained with ERCP.
>
> Gallstones may pass through the common bile duct and get impacted at the major duodenal papilla. On occasion, the sphincter of the hepatopancreatic ampulla (Sphincter Oddi) needs to be incised to relieve an obstruction at the papilla. Subsequent reconstructive surgery of the ampulla and papilla may be necessary.
>
> The variability of the pancreatic ducts is clinically important. To understand it fully, study a diagram of the development of the pancreatic ducts.

◁ *GRANT'S 2.55, 2.57*
ROHEN 278, 279
A.D.A.M. 3.14, 3.15
NETTER 276, 284, 285
CLEMENTE 312 - 317

◁ *GRANT'S 2.58*
ROHEN 279
A.D.A.M. 3.14
NETTER 276 - 279
CLEMENTE 318

◁ *GRANT'S 260*
NETTER 280
CLEMENTE 318 - 324

◁ *GRANT'S 2.40*

◁ NETTER 278

◁ *GRANT 'S 2.60*
NETTER 280
CLEMENTE 318 - 324

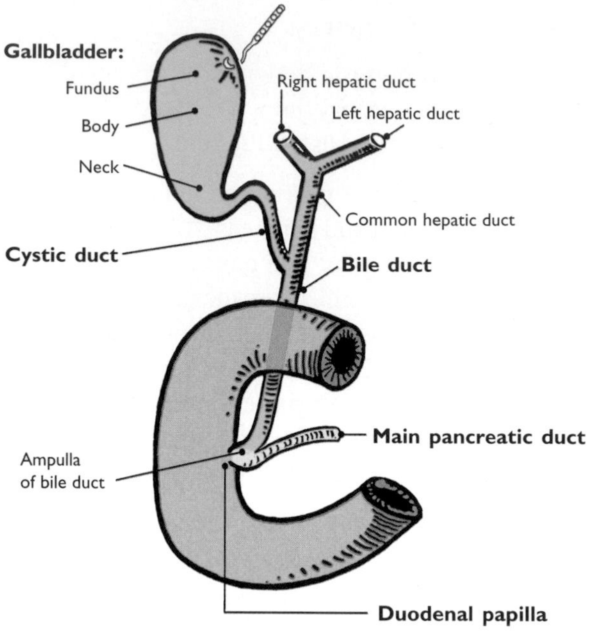

Figure 2.54. Extrahepatic bile passages.

Examine the **bile duct** throughout its entire length (Fig. 2.54). Does your cadaver specimen have a gallbladder? Is there evidence that a cholecystectomy had been performed prior to death?

- If the gallbladder is present, take note of its size and shape.

- Follow the **cystic duct** to the **gallbladder.**

- In addition to the previously identified cystic artery (Fig. 2.43), notice fine blood vessels around the cystic duct and other parts of the bile passages (Fig. 2.55). These are the tiny veins that drain the gallbladder and the extrahepatic bile passage.

- With probe and forceps, carefully remove part of the fundus of the gallbladder from its bed. Notice numerous small veins that plunge directly from the gallbladder into the liver (Fig. 2.55). A magnifying glass is helpful in a more detailed examination of these tiny vessels.

> ***Clinical Correlation:*** The small veins of the gallbladder and extrahepatic bile passages are of surgical importance. Immediately after cholecystectomy (removal of the gallbladder), the surgeon must overcome the problem of blood oozing from the gallbladder bed. In addition, oozing of blood from the network of small veins associated with the bile passages must be controlled. Study Figure 2.55 and realize that the venous blood from the gallbladder and the bile passages reaches either the portal vein or is directly drained into the liver.

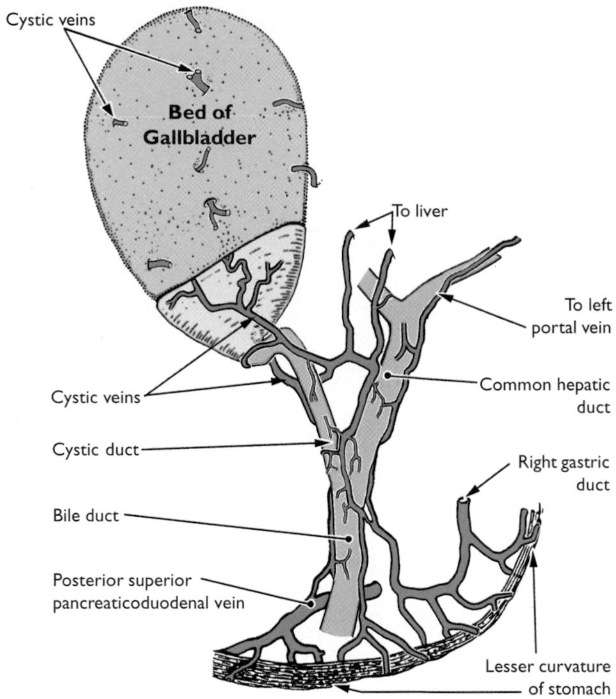

Figure 2.55. Veins of the gallbladder and extrahepatic bile passages.

Incise the gallbladder and examine its contents. Is bile present? How much? Are there gallstones? Observe the characteristic honeycombed mucosa of the gallbladder. Be aware of variations.

GRANT'S 2.41, 2.57
ROHEN 279
NETTER 276, 277
CLEMENTE 312, 313

Next, examine the **liver.** Note that its sharp inferior border separates the visceral from the diaphragmatic surface. On the posterior aspect, observe the triangular, granulated **bare area.** Here, the liver was attached to the diaphragm. Around the bare area, note the peritoneal reflections of the **coronary ligament.**

GRANT'S 2.31
ROHEN 281
A.D.A.M. 3.19
NETTER 270
CLEMENTE 309 - 311

Examine the **visceral surface** of the liver. H-shaped fissures and sulci define four lobes (Fig. 2.56). The transverse fissure is the site of the porta hepatis.

- Observe the **four lobes of the liver**: right, left, quadrate, and caudate. Note the H-shaped deep fissures and wide sulci:
- **Right sagittal fossa**, posteriorly forming a groove for the inferior vena cava (IVC), and inferiorly forming the shallow bed for the gallbladder.
- **Left sagittal fissure**, accommodating the ligamentum venosum posteriorly, and the round ligament (ligamentum teres) inferiorly.
- **Transverse fissure**, the **porta hepatis**.

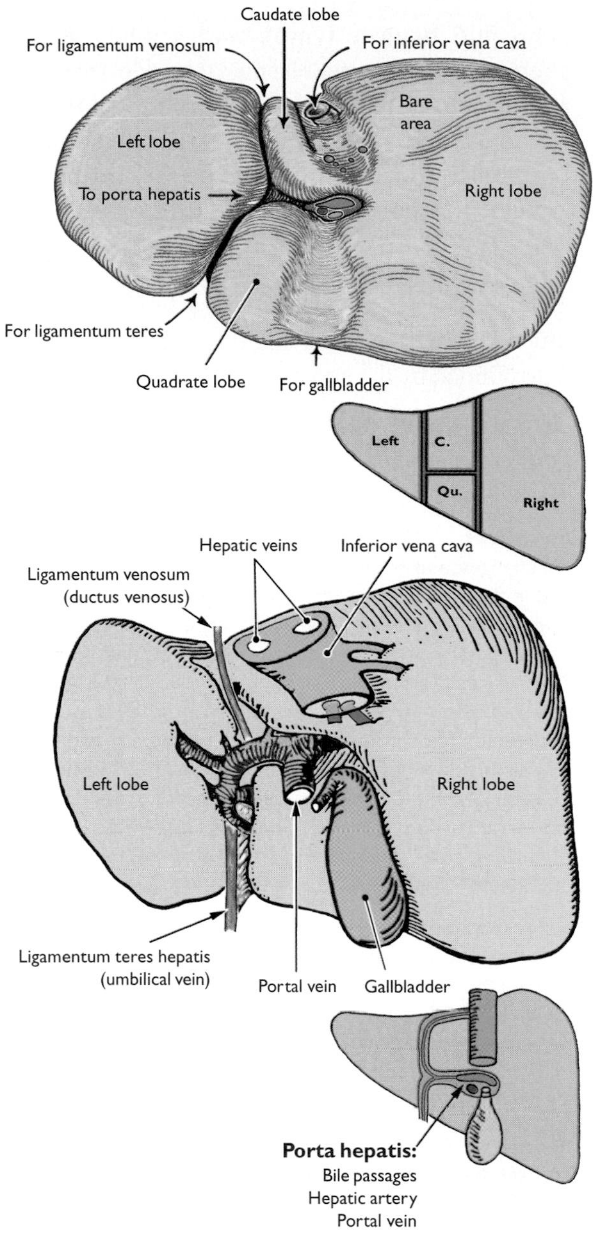

Figure 2.56. Posteroinferior view of liver. The H-shaped fissures and sulci define the four lobes of the liver (right, left, quadrate, and caudate). The fissures and sulci contain certain structures: inferior vena cava, gallbladder, ligamentum venosum, and ligamentum teres. The horizontal fissure is the site of the porta hepatis.

GRANT'S 2.42
ROHEN 281
NETTER 273
A.V.A. 3: 2.01.01

Review all structures passing through the porta hepatis (bile passages; hepatic artery; portal vein). Examine the small segment of **inferior vena cava** that is attached to its groove. Note that the two or three large **hepatic veins** drain directly into it (Fig. 2.56). Be fully aware of the difference between portal vein and hepatic veins.

The liver has a substantial lymphatic drainage. At the porta hepatis, several lymph vessels drain into **hepatic lymph nodes**. Make an attempt to find a representative node (usually not larger than a small bean) around the bile duct and portal vein. From there, the lymphatics drain into the **celiac nodes** around the root of the celiac artery.

Grant's 2.98D
Netter 298

Section part of the liver and observe:

- Branches of portal vein, hepatic artery, and bile ducts (stained green) lying together and being surrounded by the perivascular fibrous capsule.
- Hepatic veins, unaccompanied (lying alone) and having no capsule.

Grant's 2.50
Rohen 281
Netter 273

Clinical Correlation: The liver is subject to many pathologic changes, and some of these are likely to be encountered in the gross anatomical laboratory. The liver may be smooth and considerably enlarged. This happens most often in passive liver congestion due to cardiac insufficiency (cardiac liver). In contrast, the liver may appear small and show a regular formation of small nodules throughout. Such a finding is most likely a case of liver cirrhosis (frequently the result of alcoholism). Metastatic (secondary) tumors are often encountered. These vary in appearance. You may find numerous small white nodules bulging over the surface, or you may find an occasional single large node.

The liver can be subdivided into segments, similar to those in the lung. Each segment contains its own branch of the hepatic artery, bile duct, and portal vein. This segmentation is of surgical relevance since parts of a diseased liver can be removed segmentally without indiscriminately interrupting the functionally important triad of hepatic artery, bile duct, and portal vein.

The patency of portal triads and particularly of hepatic veins can be readily assessed with an ultrasound scan.

Grant's 2.45, 2.46
Rohen 281
A.D.A.M. 3.17, 3.18
Netter 272

Spleen. Sizes and weights vary considerably. Observe:

Grant's 2.54
Netter 281

- **Hilus;** for entrance and exit of splenic vessels;
- **Borders;** anterior and superior borders are sharp and often notched; posterior and inferior borders are rounded;
- **Visceral surface;** divided according to contact areas with other viscera: gastric, renal, pancreatic, and colic;
- **Diaphragmatic surface;** convex and smooth.

Place your hand into the (now empty) left hypochondriac region, where the spleen was located. Study the topographic relationship of spleen to ribs 9, 10, and 11 (Fig. 2.57). Push a probe horizontally through the 9th intercostal space, about 2 to 3 cm posterior to the midaxillary line. The instrument passes through the pleural cavity and through the diaphragm into the abdominal cavity and then into the spleen (Fig. 2.57).

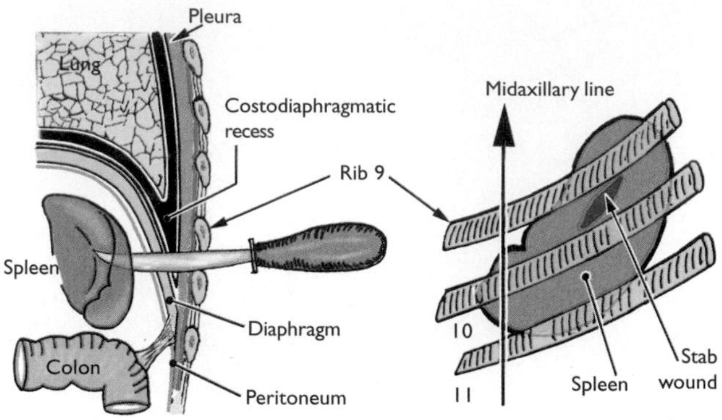

Figure 2.57. Topographic relations of the spleen. A knife pushed through the 9th intercostal space, just posterior to the midaxillary line, will penetrate the pleural cavity, diaphragm, peritoneal cavity, and spleen.

Clinical Correlation: The above mentioned topographic relations are of great importance in evaluating stab wounds and injuries associated with displaced rib fractures. Because of the profuse bleeding from an injured (ruptured) spleen into the abdominal cavity, an emergency splenectomy may have to be performed.

An abnormal enlargement of the spleen (splenomegaly) is often encountered during a routine physical examination. Reasons for splenomegaly include passive congestion in hepatic and heart disease, blood disorders of various types, and infestation with parasites.

The anterior notched border of the spleen can often be visualized on plain radiographic films. Verify the close relationship between spleen and colon. The anterior notched border of the spleen can occasionally produce a characteristic scalloping of the colonic surface near the left (splenic) flexure. A pathologically enlarged spleen may indent the fundus or the greater curvature of the stomach. This fact is useful in diagnostic radiology.

In about 10 to 20% of cases, one or more small "accessory spleens" may exist. They are usually located in the splenic hilus or along the splenic vessels. Does the cadaver you are working on have an accessory spleen?

Interior Organ Inspection. The interior of representative portions of the GI tract should be inspected. Study prosected specimens and specially prepared museum specimens. If these are not available, use the removed GI tract of the cadaver and observe the following:

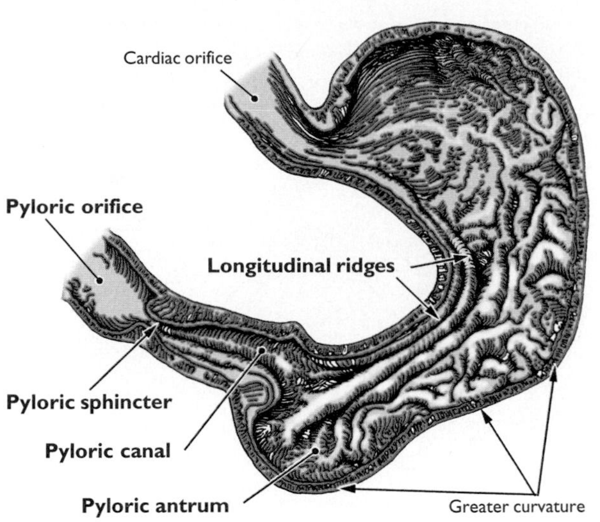

Figure 2.58. Interior of the stomach.

Stomach. (Fig. 2.58) Starting at the abdominal portion of the esophagus, open the stomach along its greater curvature. Extend the cut into the first portion of thc duodenum. Wash the mucosa clean. Proceed as follows:

- Observe **longitudinal ridges** along the lesser curvature;
- Note the **pyloric antrum** and **canal**;
- Pay special attention to the **pyloric sphincter**;
- Assess the diameter of the **pyloric orifice**.

GRANT'S 2.65
CLEMENTE 338

Duodenum. If not already done, open the duodenum by a 5 cm incision just opposite the entrance of the bile duct.

- Observe the **major duodenal papilla** and the hood-like **plica** that covers it.
- If an accessory pancreatic duct is present, there may be a minor duodenal papilla about 2 cm superior to the major papilla.
- Identify the pronounced folds of mucosa, the **plicae circulares**.

GRANT'S 2.26
A.D.A.M. 3.22
CLEMENTE 304

GRANT'S 2.65, 2.67
ROHEN 287
NETTER 264, 265
CLEMENTE 335

Jejunum. Open and clean a small portion of the jejunum. Look for tall, closely packed plicae circulares.

GRANT'S 2.63
NETTER 267
CLEMENTE 341

Ileum. Make two openings in the ileum, one in its proximal portion, and one about 30 cm from the terminal ileum. Observe:

- There are relatively few plicae circulares in the upper part;
- In its lower part, the plicae are virtually absent.

GRANT'S 2.64
A.D.A.M. 3.28
CLEMENTE 342

- Look for a Meckel's diverticulum. In 2% of cases, a diverticulum of various length (remnant of yolk stalk) can be found within 100 to 160 cm (about 3 to 5 feet) of the ileocecal valve.
- Study radiographs of the upper gastrointestinal (GI) system and the small intestine.

GRANT'S 2.24
ROHEN 276
A.D.A.M. 3.21
NETTER 259
CLEMENTE 296

Ileocecal region. Open the cecum. Clean the region with a sponge and water. Study the ileocecal orifice, the ileocecal valve, and the orifice of the vermiform appendix. Section the appendix and examine its interior surface. Be aware of the varied locations of the vermiform appendix.

GRANT'S 2.58
ROHEN 279
A.D.A.M. 3.14
NETTER 262
CLEMENTE 296

Colon. Open a representative portion of the transverse colon, preferably one with prominent **haustra** (sacculations). Clean the mucosa. Between the haustra and on the inner aspect, note the crescentic mucosal folds, the **plicae semilunares**. Correlate your gross anatomical observations with a suitable radiograph.

Store the detached GI tract with its three unpaired organs in a plastic bag for future reference. Make sure the specimen is well moistened with preservative fluid.

Posterior Abdominal Structures

Orientation, Inspection, and Palpation

GRANT'S 2.63
NETTER 263

The posterior abdominal viscera are situated in the **retroperitoneal space**; i.e., in the space between parietal peritoneum and the muscles and bones of the posterior abdominal wall (Fig. 2.59). In this retroperitoneal space lie the paired kidneys with their excretory ducts (ureters), the paired suprarenal glands, the aorta, the inferior vena cava, and the abdominal portion of the bilateral sympathetic trunks. All these structures are contained in the loose areolar connective tissue of the retroperitoneal space.

Clinical Correlation: The retroperitoneal space is not at all rigidly confined but is capable of accommodating considerable volume changes. This may acutely occur when an artery ruptures. The amount of blood loss into the retroperitoneal space can be substantial and life threatening.

The connective tissue of the retroperitoneal space may proliferate, a condition known as retroperitoneal fibrosis. Its mass may become so bulky that it compresses the blood vessels, nerves, and ureters that course within the retroperitoneal space, thus causing considerably symptoms, including pain and interference with the urinary system.

Dissection Note: A practical point: It is impossible to dissect nerves and vessels in a pool of liquefied fat. Work will be more efficient and pleasant if you sponge clean the colic gutters, the pouches, and the posterior abdominal region. Always keep the specimen moist with mold-deterrent preservative fluid.

Palpate the kidneys and the suprarenal (adrenal) glands. They lie lateral to the vertebral column at the levels of vertebrae T12 to L3. Palpate and identify the abdominal aorta and its bifurcation. To the right of the aorta observe the inferior vena cava (IVC). Before beginning with the dissection, review the posterior abdominal viscera and their clinically important ventral relations.

- Point your finger to the inferior part of the **right kidney.** Here, it was in contact with the right colic flexure.
- About three-fourths of the ventral surface is still covered with parietal peritoneum. Here, the right kidney was in contact with the visceral surface of the liver.
- Place your finger on the medial border of the right kidney. Here, it was in contact with the descending portion of the duodenum.
- Examine the **left kidney** and its relations. At about the middle of its ventral surface, it was in contact with the tail of the pancreas.
- Inferior to this pancreatic area is a region that was in contact with the left colic flexure.

Before you begin ...

The following approach to the region will be taken: The parietal peritoneal covering of the posterior abdominal wall will be removed. This procedure will completely expose the abdominal aorta and its branches, and the inferior vena cava and its tributaries. The kidneys will be shelled out of their fatty capsules. Next, their vessels and excretory ducts (ureters) will be studied. After ventral reflection of the kidneys and removal of the fatty renal capsule, the posterior abdominal wall will be accessible. Its muscles will be studied. Then, the lumbar plexus of nerves will be examined. Finally, the roof of the abdominal cavity, the diaphragm, will be studied.

Grant's 2.76
Rohen 298
A.D.A.M. 3.32
Netter 311
Clemente 343, 346

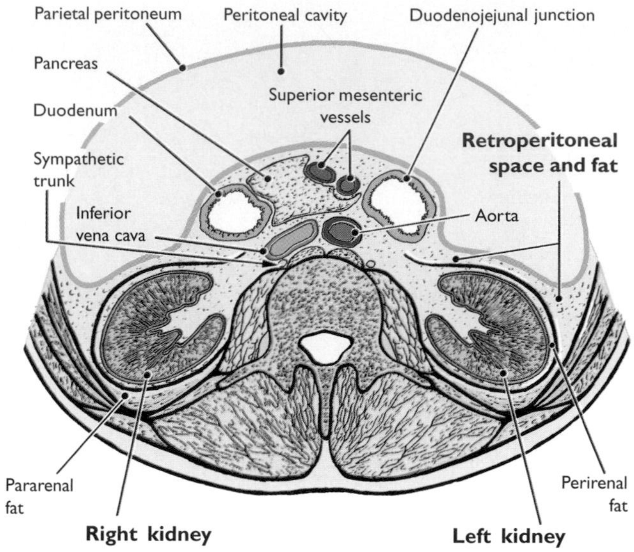

Figure 2.59. Transverse section of abdomen at the level of the kidneys. Retroperitoneal structures include the kidneys, aorta, inferior vena cava, and sympathetic trunks.

Vessels. The testicular (male) and ovarian (female) vessels are small and easily damaged or lost; the corresponding veins are usually much larger. Observe these vessels shining through the parietal peritoneal covering. Remove all remnants of parietal peritoneum. Gently pull on the membrane and separate it from the underlying connective tissue. Vessels and ducts can now be identified and cleaned.

Grant's 2.77A
A.D.A.M. 3.32
Netter 311
Clemente 345

In the **male cadaver,** note that the testicular vessels cross the ureter. The ureter must *not* be damaged during dissection. Pick up the testicular vessels at the deep inguinal ring. Free them and follow them superiorly. Observe:

Grant's 2.77A
Rohen 310, 311
A.D.A.M. 3.31
Netter 311, 372
Clemente 345

- The **left testicular vein** drains into the **left renal vein.**
- The **right testicular vein** drains directly into the **inferior vena cava (IVC).**
- The **right** and **left testicular arteries** originate directly from the aorta, inferior to the origin of the renal arteries.

In the **female cadaver,** dissect the corresponding **ovarian vessels**. They cross the external iliac vessels very close to the ureter.

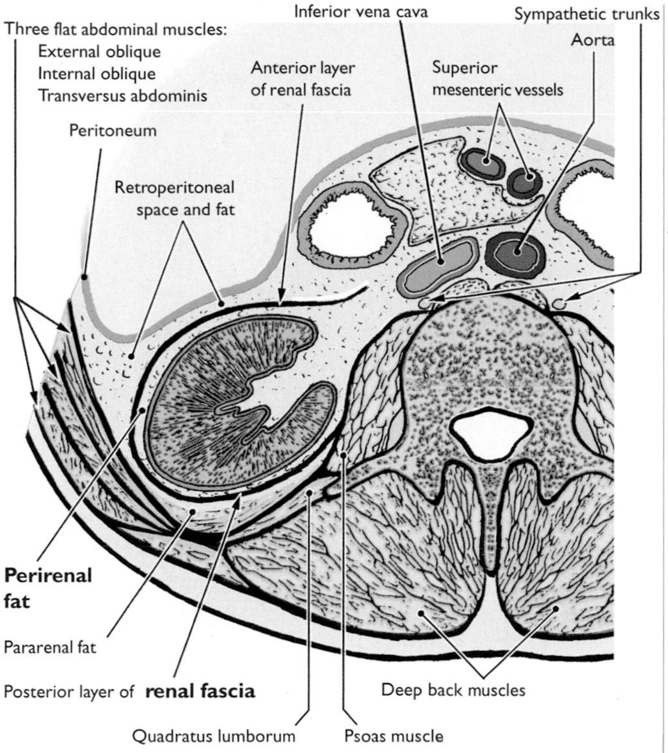

Figure 2.60. Transverse section at the hilus of the right kidney.

Kidneys and Suprarenal Glands

GRANT'S 2.77A
ROHEN 307
A.D.A.M. 3.31, 3.33
NETTER 314
CLEMENTE 345

Kidneys (L. *renes*, kidneys). The relation of the kidney to adjacent structures can be best appreciated on transverse section (Fig. 2.60). Each kidney is embedded in a substantial mass of fat, the **perirenal fat or adipose (fatty) capsule.** Most of the fat lies lateral and posterior to the organ. The **renal fascia** encloses both the kidney and its fatty capsule. The anterior layer of the renal fascia runs with the renal vessels and becomes very thin as it approaches the aorta and inferior vena cava. The posterior layer of the renal fascia blends with the fasciae of two muscles of the posterior abdominal wall, the quadratus lumborum and the psoas. The kidneys are not rigidly fixed to the posterior abdominal wall. In fact, in the living subject, they move slightly up and down during respiration.

With your fingers, shell out the kidneys from the renal fascia and fatty capsule. The superior pole is separated from the suprarenal gland by a thin layer of fat. Carefully pass your fingers between kidney and suprarenal gland and separate the two organs. Leave all blood vessels intact.

Note the characteristic bean shape of the kidney. The approximate measurements of an adult kidney are: length, 11 to 12 cm; breadth, 5 to 8 cm; thickness, 3 to 4 cm. The weight of each kidney varies from 120 to 170 g. In one of 400 cases, you may find a "horseshoe" kidney. This is an anomaly.

Left kidney. Proceed as follows:

- Dissect the **left renal vein** from the IVC to the hilus of the left kidney.
- Observe and clean venous tributaries: **left testicular vein** in the male or the **ovarian vein** in the female, and **venous channels from the left suprarenal gland.**
- To have full access to the renal artery, cut the left renal vein close to the IVC and reflect it toward the left.
- Now, find the **left renal artery.** Follow this large vessel to the renal hilus. Usually, the artery divides into two branches before it enters the kidney. Accessory renal arteries are common.
- Observe fine branches to the ureter and to the suprarenal gland. The renal arteries are accompanied by autonomic nerve fibers. Identify strands of autonomic nerves surrounding the left renal artery.

GRANT'S 2.95
A.D.A.M. 3.37
NETTER 314, 322
CLEMENTE 344

Left Renal Pelvis and Ureter. Reflect the left kidney anteriorly and toward the right. At the most posterior part of the hilus, identify the **renal pelvis** and its inferior continuation, the **ureter.** Follow and dissect the ureter. Observe:

GRANT'S 2.90
A.D.A.M. 3.33
NETTER 324
CLEMENTE 344, 345

GRANT'S 2.77A
ROHEN 311
A.D.A.M. 3.31
NETTER 311
CLEMENTE 345

- **Abdominal part of ureter**; crosses the psoas major muscle; runs obliquely posterior to the testicular (ovarian) vessels. Verify that the superior portion of the right ureter runs lateral to the IVC.
- **Pelvic part of ureter;** dissect it for a short distance along the wall of the pelvic cavity. Its junction with the urinary bladder will be seen later.

Right Kidney. Proceed as follows:

GRANT'S 2.77A
ROHEN 307
A.D.A.M. 3.31, 3.33
NETTER 314
CLEMENTE 345

- Dissect the relatively short right renal vein from IVC to the hilus of the right kidney.
- Since the left renal vein was severed earlier, the IVC can easily be reflected inferiorly and slightly to the right. This procedure will expose the **right renal artery** (or arteries).
- Identify the **renal pelvis,** and follow the **ureter** inferiorly.
- Observe the relations between right ureter, right testicular (ovarian) vessels, and psoas muscle.

> ***Clinical Correlation:*** If the right ureter passes posterior to the IVC, it is called "retrocaval ureter." This condition may interfere with proper drainage of urine from the right kidney.

GRANT'S 2.86C

Muscles. Next, reflect the kidneys and remove the substantial fatty renal capsule and the renal fascia by forcibly pulling it off the posterior abdominal wall. Clean the posterior abdominal wall, and sponge the entire area clean. Identify the following muscles of the posterior abdominal wall (Fig. 2.61)

GRANT'S 2.77A, 2.91
ROHEN 311, 312
A.D.A.M. 3.33, 5.25
NETTER 311, 462
CLEMENTE 345, 360
A.V.A. 3: 1.33.40

- **Transversus abdominis**
- **Quadratus lumborum**
- **Psoas major**
- Identify the **diaphragm** and the floating **12th rib**.

Now, study the topographic relations between kidneys and the posterior abdominal wall. Verify that the dorsal surface of each kidney is in contact with the diaphragm, psoas major, quadratus lumborum, and the posterior tendinous portion of the transversus abdominis. The superior pole of the right kidney lies at the level of the 12th rib. The left kidney is positioned somewhat higher; its superior pole lies at the level of the 11th rib (Fig. 2.61). The liver is responsible for "pushing" the right kidney down (and the right lung up).

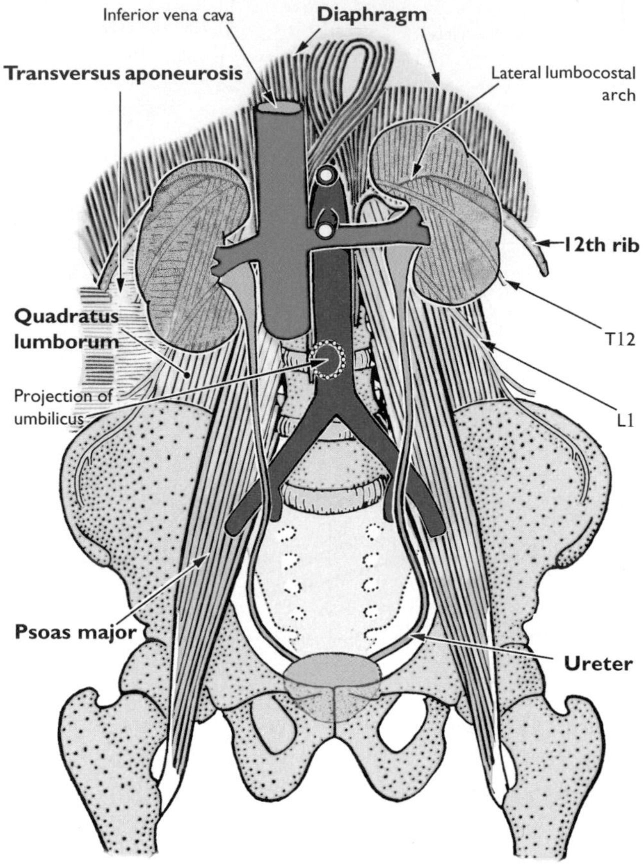

Figure 2.61. Posterior relations of the kidneys.

> ***Clinical Correlation:*** The traditional surgical approach to the kidney is the lumbar renal or retroperitoneal approach. Lumbar nephrectomy (extirpation of kidney via the retroperitoneal lumbar route) is indicated when contamination of the peritoneal cavity is likely (inflammatory renal disease, calculi). The lumbar approach to the kidney is an optional exercise described in Appendix I. The transabdominal approach to the kidney is mainly employed for surgery of the renal vessels and kidney transplants.
>
> In renal transplantation, the donor kidney is transplanted into the lower abdomen. The donor renal vessels are connected to the recipient's external iliac vessels. The ureter of the donor kidney is sutured into the urinary bladder.
>
> The arterial distribution in the kidney is of surgical importance. Usually, the renal artery divides into an anterior and posterior branch. These branches supply the anterior and posterior halves of the kidney, respectively. There are no anastomoses. Thus, there are no large vessels in the longitudinal plane of the kidney. Surgical procedures along this plane (nephrotomy) offer the advantage of minimal hemorrhage. Study a corrosion cast of a segmental artery. Correlate the renal arterial distribution with a renal arteriogram.

GRANT'S 2.80
A.D.A.M. 3.35
NETTER 313, 315
CLEMENTE 355, 356

Kidney on Section (Fig. 2.62). Do *not* sever the kidneys from their vessels or ureters. Divide the left kidney into anterior and posterior halves by splitting it longitudinally along its convex, lateral border. Identify and observe:

GRANT'S 2.87 - 2.89
NETTER 312

- **Fibrous capsule,** which can be easily stripped off;
- **Renal cortex;** the outer one-third;
- **Renal medulla,** consisting of **renal pyramids** and **renal columns**;

GRANT'S 2.81, 2.82
NETTER 315

- **Renal papillae;** in groups of two or three, projecting into small cups, the calyces minores;
- **Calyces minores,** uniting to form two or three **calyces majores;**

GRANT'S 2.84A
CLEMENTE 350

GRANT'S 2.84B
CLEMENTE 351

- The major calyces unite to form the **renal pelvis,** which leads to the **ureter.**

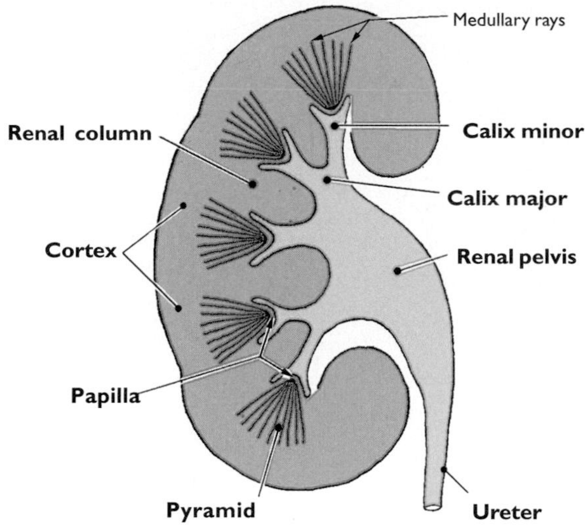

Figure 2.62. Schema of macroscopic structure of kidney on longitudinal section.

> ***Clinical Correlation:*** Study the renal collecting structures in a pyelogram. Normally, the renal pelvis is found at the level of the spinous process L1. Be aware of variations.
>
> Kidney stones (renal calculi) are formed in the kidney and renal pelvis. Small stones may spontaneously pass through the ureter into the bladder. This process is usually associated with considerable pain (ureteric colic). Larger stones may have to be removed surgically or they may be subjected to crushing (lithotripsy).

GRANT'S 2.77A, 2.95
ROHEN 311, 312
A.D.A.M. 3.31
NETTER 314
CLEMENTE 345, 348, 349

Suprarenal (Adrenal) Glands (Fig. 2.63). The suprarenal glands are friable and very easily torn. They are closely related to the superior poles of the kidneys. Only a film of fatty tissue intervenes between kidney and suprarenal gland. These glands deteriorate rapidly after death. Depending on the quality of body embalmment, they may or may not be well preserved. The right and left adrenal glands differ in gross morphology and their topographic relationships.

Verify that the **right adrenal gland** is roughly triangular in shape, has only a loose attachment to the superior pole of the right kidney, and lies just posterior to the inferior vena cava. Observe that the **left adrenal gland** is semilunar in shape and is closely adjacent to the superior and medial border of the left kidney (occasionally extending to the level of the renal hilus). Numerous arteries supply the suprarenal glands (Fig. 2.63). Fine superior suprarenal branches are derived from the **inferior phrenic arteries**. Branches to the middle portion of the glands usually arise directly from the **aorta** just superior to the celiac trunk.

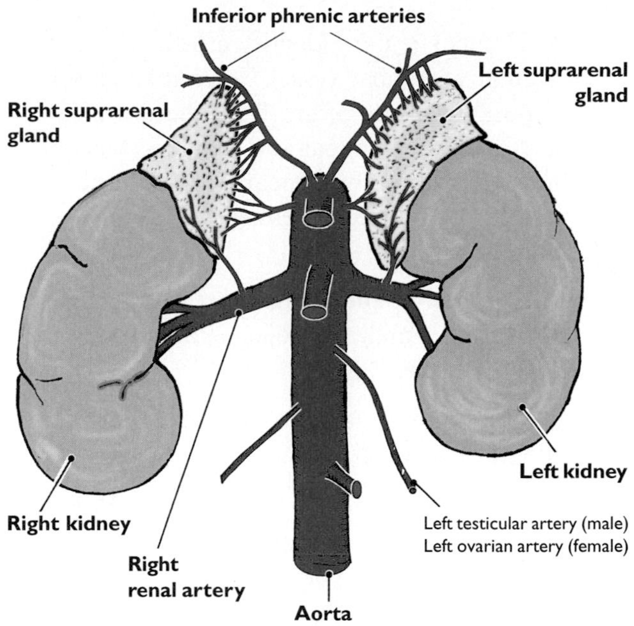

Figure 2.63. Multiple arterial blood supply of the suprarenal glands.

GRANT'S 2.86
ROHEN 3.36
NETTER 316
CLEMENTE 354, 358, 359

Inferior suprarenal branches originate from the respective **renal arteries**. The venous blood from the left and right adrenal glands empties, respectively, into the left renal vein and into the inferior vena cava. The suprarenal glands receive numerous sympathetic nerve fibers. Section one gland, and distinguish between cortex and medulla.

> ***Clinical Correlation:*** The kidneys and adrenal glands have a separate embryonic origin. Therefore, the development and position of the adrenal glands is usually unaffected by renal abnormalities or anomalous renal positions. The adrenal glands develop in their normal position just lateral to the celiac trunk.
>
> The adrenal glands can usually be well demonstrated and morphologically evaluated by computed tomography (CT).

GRANT'S 2.100B
ROHEN 309
A.D.A.M. 1.23, 1.24
NETTER 311, 320
CLEMENTE 364
A.V.A. 3: 1.55.43

Review the abdominal aorta and its branches. Identify (Fig 2.63):

- **Branches to the GI tract and its three unpaired organs** (celiac; superior mesenteric; inferior mesenteric);
- **Branches to the three paired organs** (suprarenal; renal; testicular or ovarian);
- **Branches to the walls** of the abdominal cavity (phrenic; lumbar). Realize that there are four paired **lumbar arteries** that are responsible for the segmental blood supply of

the lumbar region. Identify at least one representative lumbar vessel. Trace it as closely as possible to its origin from the dorsal aspect of the abdominal aorta. Notice that the lumbar arteries disappear in the depth of muscles positioned on either side of the vertebral column.

- **Bifurcation of abdominal aorta,** at the level of L4. The umbilicus projects just superior to the bifurcation (Fig. 2.61).
- **Common iliac arteries,** which divide into internal and external iliac arteries.

Review the **inferior vena cava (IVC)** and its tributaries .Recapitulate the **porto-caval system**.

Grant's 2.100B
Rohen 309
A.D.A.M. 1.23, 1.24
Netter 311, 320
Clemente 364
A.V.A. 3: 1.58.01

Posterior Abdominal Wall

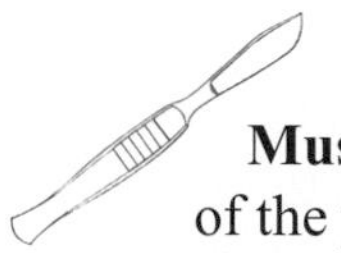

Muscles. Once again, identify the muscles of the posterior abdominal wall (Fig. 2.64). Clean the muscles and study their extent:

- **Psoas major;** arises from lumbar vertebrae (sides; intervertebral discs; transverse processes); ventral to the psoas major, observe the long flat tendon of the psoas minor and the geni-tofemoral nerve.
- **Iliacus;** is fan-shaped; occupies the extensive iliac fossa; iliacus and psoas form a functional unit; thus, they are referred to as **iliopsoas.** The iliopsoas is the most powerful flexor of the thigh. It is inserted into the lessser trochanter of the femur.
- **Quadratus lumborum;** thick, rhomboidal muscular sheet, running from iliac crest to lumbar transverse processes and rib 12; flexes vertebral column.
- **Transversus abdominis**; running horizontally posterior to the oblique borders of the quadratus lumborum.

Grant's 2.50A, 2.101
Rohen 282
A.D.A.M. 1.25, 1.26, 3.15
Netter 293
Clemente 298
A.V.A. 3: 2.00.13

Nerves of the Posterior Abdominal Wall (Fig. 2.65). These are ventral rami of T12 to L5 that are derived from the **lumbar nerve plexus**. Carefully remove the fascia from the posterior abdominal muscles to expose the nerves. Expect to find variations. The usual pattern is as follows:

Grant's 2.91
Rohen 429, 447
A.D.A.M. 5.22, 5.25
Netter 462, 463
Clemente 364, 365
A.V.A. 3: 2.03.32

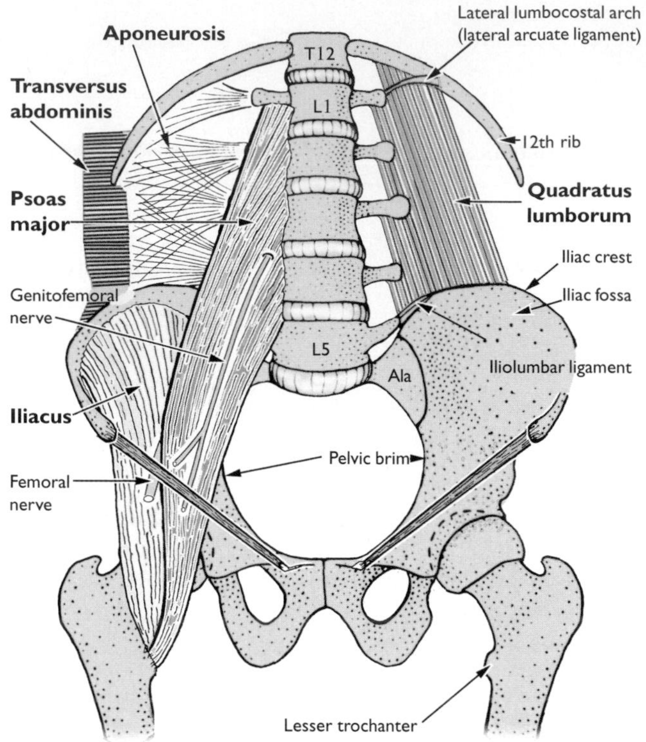

Figure 2.64. Muscles of the posterior abdominal wall.

- **Subcostal nerve** (T12); about 1 cm caudal to rib 12.
- **Iliohypogastric** and **ilioinguinal nerves** (L1); descending steeply in front of the quadratus lumborum. Frequently, the two nerves arise from a common trunk and do not separate until they reach the transversus abdominis muscle. Positively identify the ilioinguinal nerve. Locate it again at the anterior abdominal wall.Trace it back from the superficial inguinal ring to the plane between internal oblique and transversus abdominis. Establish its continuity at the posterior abdominal wall. *Note:* Variations of these two nerves are common. Occasionally, the ilioinguinal nerve is absent.
- **Genitofemoral nerve**; piercing the anterior surface of the psoas. It supplies a small portion of skin inferior and medial to the inguinal ligament as well as the cremaster muscle.
- **Lateral cutaneous nerve of thigh**; it passes deep to the inguinal ligament near the anterior superior iliac spine. This nerve supplies the lateral aspect of the thigh with sensory fibers.

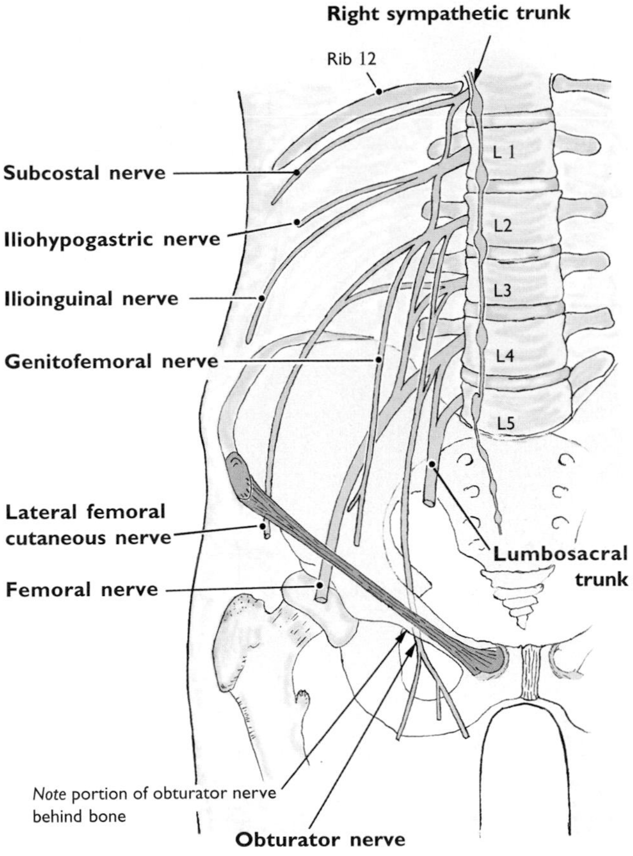

Figure 2.65. Lumbar plexus of nerves.

- **Femoral nerve** (L2, L3, L4); large nerve lying in the angle between psoas and iliacus, and then deep to the inguinal ligament; provides motor and sensory contributions to the anterior and medial thigh.

- **Obturator nerve** (L2, L3, L4); at the medial border of the psoas. Find the nerve in the following manner: For necessary orientation, identify the obturator foramen in the skeleton. Palpate the obturator groove from inside the pelvis. Now, palpate the obturator groove from inside the pelvis in the cadaver. This is precisely the point where the obturator nerve passes from the pelvis into the thigh. Within the pelvis, free the nerve with a probe and follow it superiorly to the medial border of the psoas.

- **Lumbosacral trunk**. This large trunk consists of ventral rami of part of L4 and all of L5. The trunk runs caudally to the sacral plexus. The large and flat lumbosacral trunk is tightly applied to the ala of the sacrum. It is difficult to see with the psoas muscle in place.

GRANT'S 2.95
A.D.A.M. 3.31, 8.19
NETTER 300 -311, 322
CLEMENTE 365
A.V.A. 3: 2.05.01

- **Sympathetic trunk**. Trace the continuity of the sympathetic trunk from the thoracic cavity to the abdominal cavity. Study the location of the sympathetic trunks on transverse section (Fig. 2.60). Look for rami communicantes passing from ganglia to lumbar nerves. **Review the autonomic nerve supply of the abdomen**.

Dissection Note: The origin of the nerves of the posterior abdominal wall from the lumbar plexus can only be studied after careful removal of the psoas major muscle. Since the nerves traverse the muscle at different depths, it is necessary to remove the psoas in a piecemeal manner. Ask you instructor if the psoas muscle should be removed on both sides.

Usually it is sufficient to demonstrate the lumbar plexus on one side only. Using fingers and forceps, peel away the psoas muscle and remove it gradually bit by bit. Study the **lumbar plexus** (Fig. 2.65). Identify the **lumbosacral trunk**.

Thoracic Diaphragm

GRANT'S 2.92
ROHEN 265
A.D.A.M. 2.41
NETTER 181
CLEMENTE 362, 363
A.V.A. 3: 0.52.20

Diaphragm (Figure 2.66) The diaphragm forms the roof of the abdominal cavity and the floor of the thoracic cavity. It is a dome-shaped structure and the principal muscle of respiration. Its right and left halves (the hemidiaphragms) are supplied by the respective right and left phrenic nerves that arise from spinal cord segments C3, C4, and C5.

GRANT'S 2.91
ROHEN 429, 447
A.D.A.M. 5.22, 5.25
NETTER 462, 463
CLEMENTE 364, 365
A.V.A. 3: 2.04.14

Clinical Correlation: The nerve supply of the diaphragm from cervical spinal cord segments explains why diaphragmatic respiration is paralyzed in cases of cervical cord injuries. A paralyzed hemidiaphragm cannot contract (descend); i.e., it remains high in the thorax, a fact that can be readily recognized on a radiographic chest film.

The central part of the diaphragm is tendinous (central tendon). The pericardial sac is attached to it. By necessity, there must be openings in the diaphragm to allow passage of structures between abdomen and thorax. Thus, there are openings for the inferior vena cava, the aorta, and the esophagus.

Dissect the abdominal aspect of the diaphragm (Fig. 2.66). Strip the parietal peritoneum and areolar tissue off its fleshy fibers. Identify:

- **Sternal part;**

- **Costal part;** from the inferior six ribs; interdigitating with transversus abdominis;
- **Lumbar part,** consisting of a **right crus** and a **left crus.**
- Identify the **right crus**. Just lateral to the esophageal hiatus, look for a muscle slip running in an inferomedial direction. This is the remaining portion of the suspensory muscle of the duodenum (Ligament of Treitz) that supports the duodenojejunal flexure (Fig. 2.51).
- Identify the **Left crus** (Fig. 2.66).
- Fleshy fibers from the **arcuate ligaments** (lumbocostal arches);
- **Medial arcuate ligament;** a tendinous arch providing a gap for the psoas muscle;
- **Lateral arcuate ligament;** across the superior portion of the quadratus lumborum;
- **Central tendon.**

Study the three large openings in the diaphragm (Figs. 2.66, 2.67). Readily identify the two openings from which the traversing structures have been removed: **vena caval foramen** and **esophageal hiatus.** The aorta (still in place) traverses the **aortic hiatus.** Identify the thoracic vertebral levels at which the openings in the diaphragm occur (Fig. 2.67). *Observe:* The higher the vertebral level, the more ventral is the hiatus (opening) in the diaphragm.

Study the nerve supply to the diaphragm (Fig. 2.68). In the thorax, follow the **right** and **left phrenic nerves** into the substance of the diaphragm. The phrenic nerves provide the entire motor supply to the diaphragm. In addition, the phrenic nerves are also responsible for most of the sensory (pain) fibers to both the abdominal and thoracic aspects of the diaphragm. The peripheral parts of the diaphragm receive sensory fibers from several intercostal nerves.

The **greater splanchnic nerves** traverse the crura of the diaphragm. To find them, proceed in the following manner:

- In the thorax, identify the greater splanchnic nerve on one side. Follow it to the diaphragm.

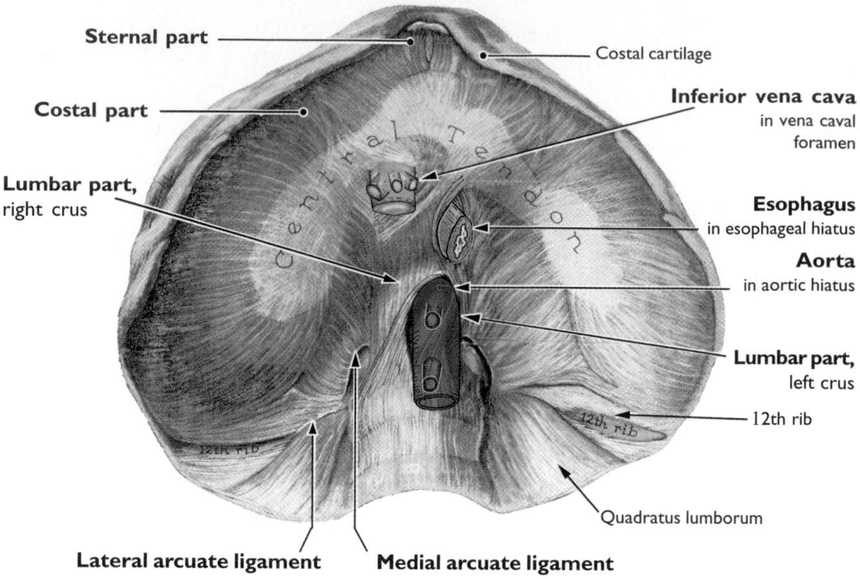

Figure 2.66. Diaphragm.

GRANT'S 2.92
ROHEN 265
A.D.A.M. 2.41
NETTER 181
CLEMENTE 362, 363
A.V.A. 3: 0.53.46

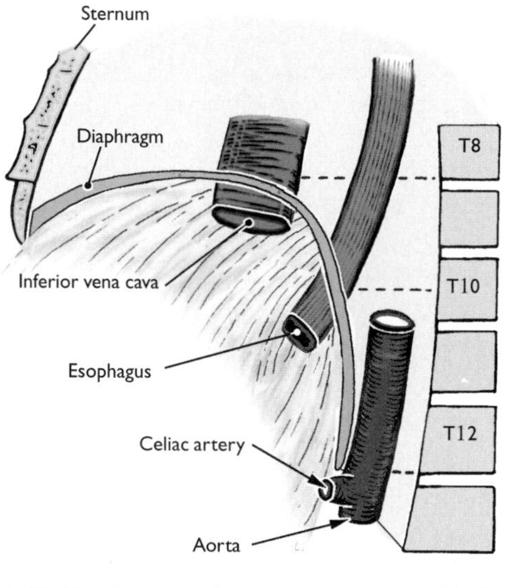

Figure 2.67. Diaphragm at levels of T8 through T12. The more superior the vertebral level, the more anterior is the opening in the diaphragm.

- Parallel to the nerve, push a probe through the diaphragm. Pick up the probe and splanchnic nerve at the abdominal aspect of the crura.
- Note that the main portion of the splanchnic nerve runs toward the celiac ganglion.
- Review the autonomic nerve supply of the abdomen.

A.D.A.M. 2.41
NETTER 181, 182

GRANT'S 1.82
NETTER 181
CLEMENTE 364
A.V.A. 3: 1.19.26

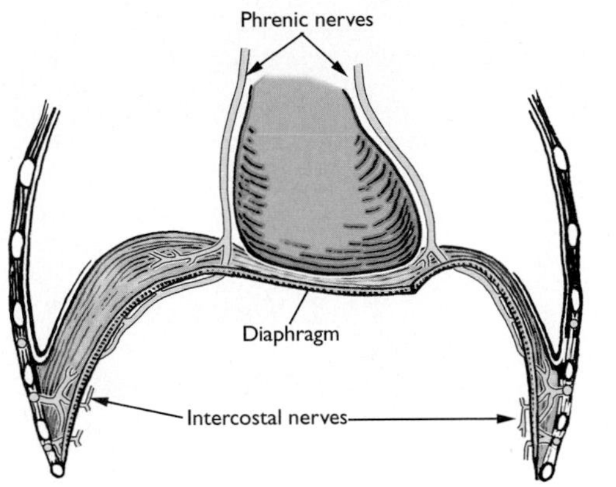

Figure 2.68. Nerve supply of the diaphragm.

Clinical Correlation: **Transverse sections through abdomen.** Integrate gross anatomical studies of the abdomen with transverse sectional anatomy. Use actual transverse sectional slices or plastic-embedded sliced specimens if available. Knowledge of transverse sectional anatomy is of considerable importance in view of the wide clinical use of computerized tomography (CT) and/or magnetic resonance images (MRI) for diagnostic purposes. Study abdominal transverse sections at three important levels: at the level of the liver and spleen, at the level of the renal vessels, and at the level of the inferior poles of the kidneys. Study the corresponding magnetic resonance images and appreciate the fact that significant structural information can be obtained in the living person with this technology. The physician must be able to analyze these transverse sectional images and to distinguish normal from abnormal. Remember that it is clinical convention to view transverse CT and MRI sections from inferior; thus, right-sided structures (e.g., liver) appear on the left side of the printed image.

⇦
GRANT'S 2.103
ROHEN 273, 300, 301
A.D.A.M. 3.4
NETTER 519 - 521
CLEMENTE 371 - 374

Other sections through abdomen. Using the technique of ultrasound, one can obtain various sections through parts of the abdomen, particularly through soft tissues and blood vessels. Although these images appear somewhat distorted in comparison with the actual anatomical field, they nevertheless can provide most valuable diagnostic information. Appreciate examples of abdominal ultrasound images.

TEST 5

GAPP
GROSS ANATOMY PRACTICAL PRIMER

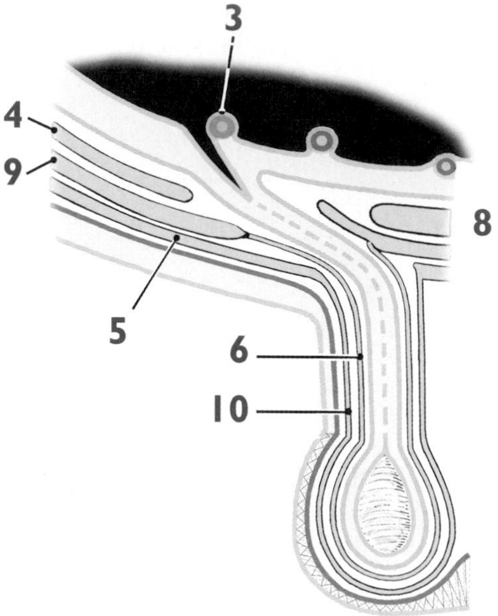

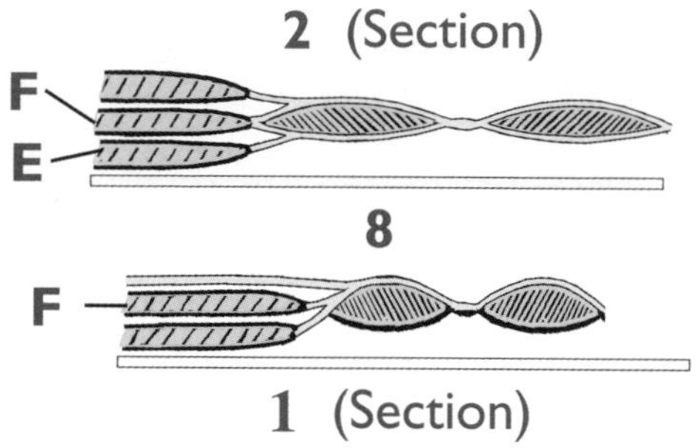

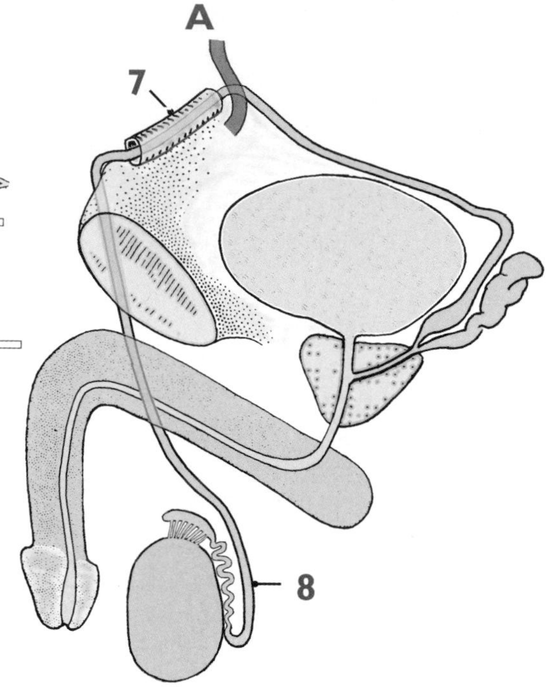

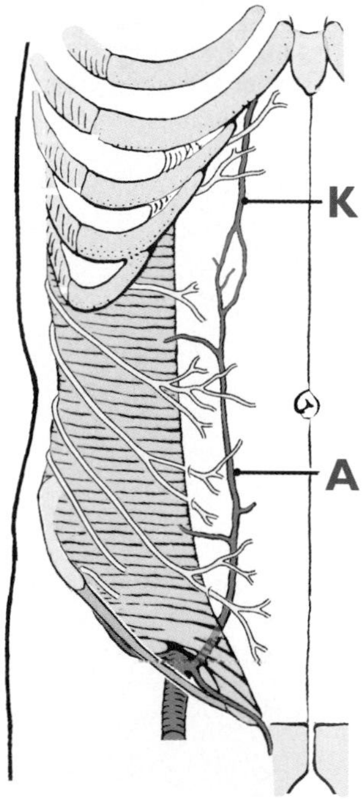

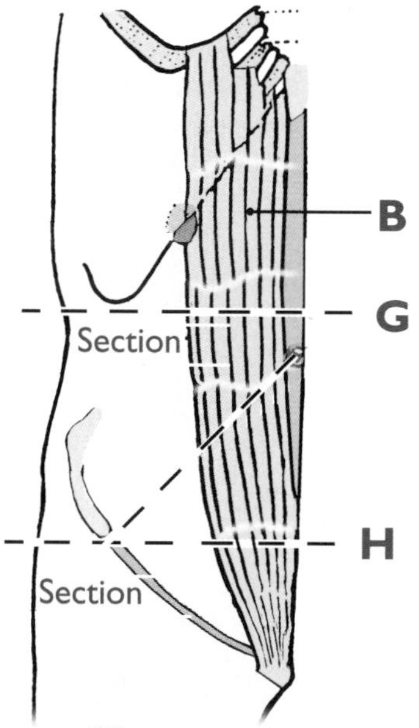

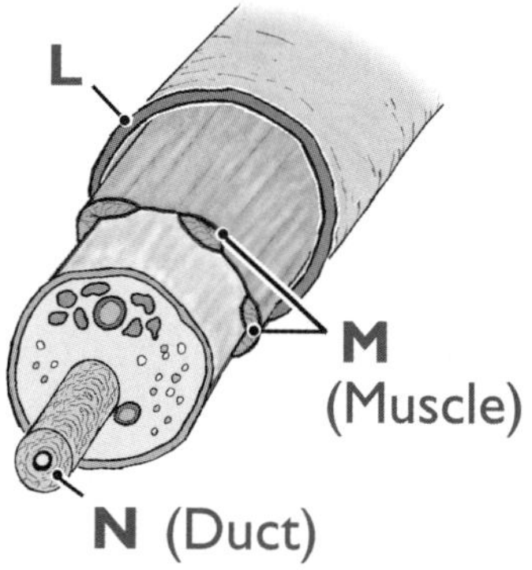

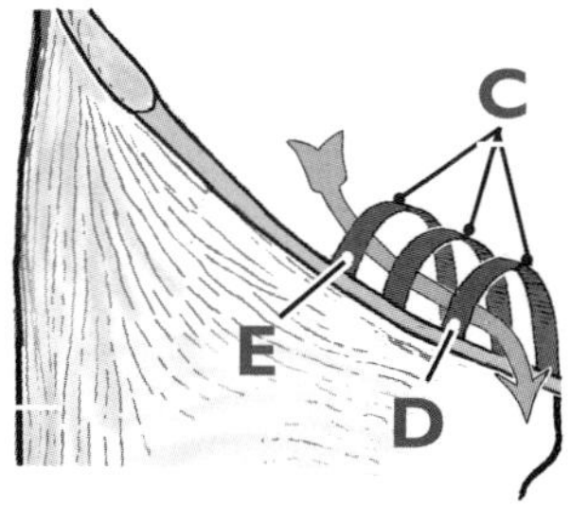

TEST YOUR 3-DIMENSIONAL CONCEPTUALIZATION.
MATCH THE NUMBERS WITH CORRESPONDING LETTERS:

1 ___	6 ___
2 ___	7 ___
3 ___	8 ___
4 ___	9 ___
5 ___	10 ___

GAPP TEST: IF YOU MADE AN ERROR, REVIEW AND GAIN A BETTER UNDERSTANDING OF THE CONCERNED 3-DIMENSIONAL ANATOMICAL CONCEPT. GAPP KEY: 1-H, 2-G, 3-A, 4-E, 5-D, 6-M, 7-C, 8-N, 9-F, 10-L.

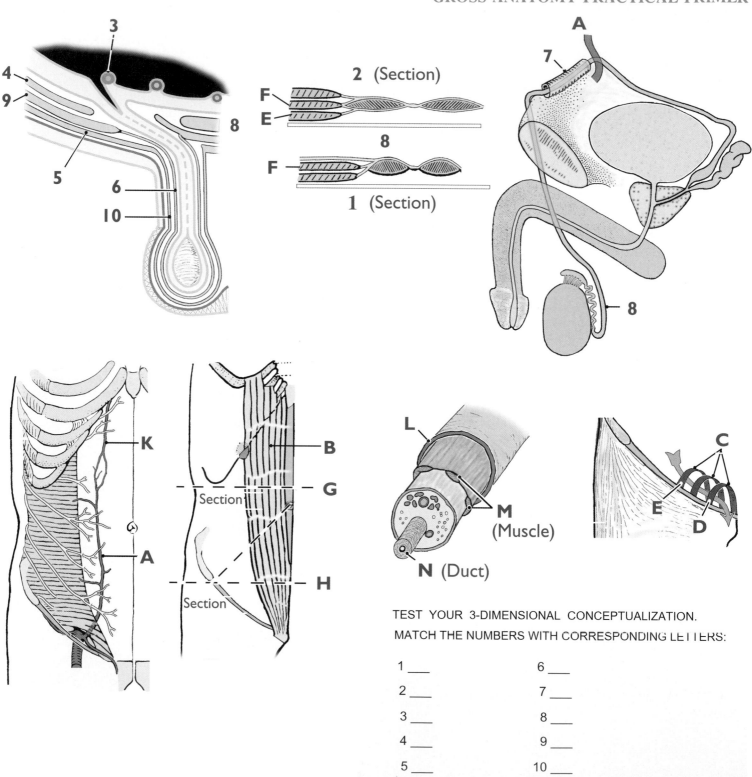

TEST 6

GAPP

GROSS ANATOMY PRACTICAL PRIMER

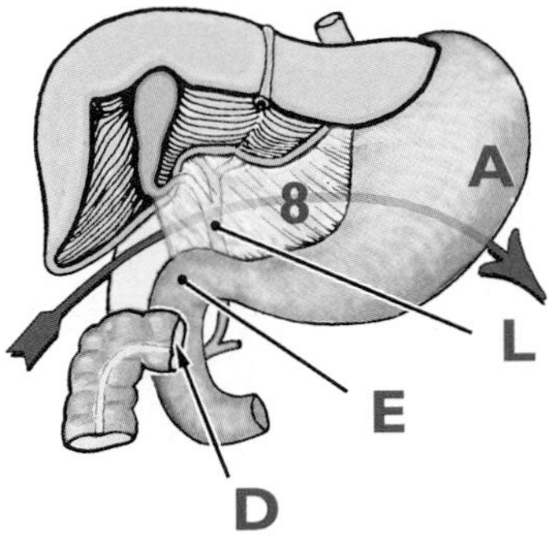

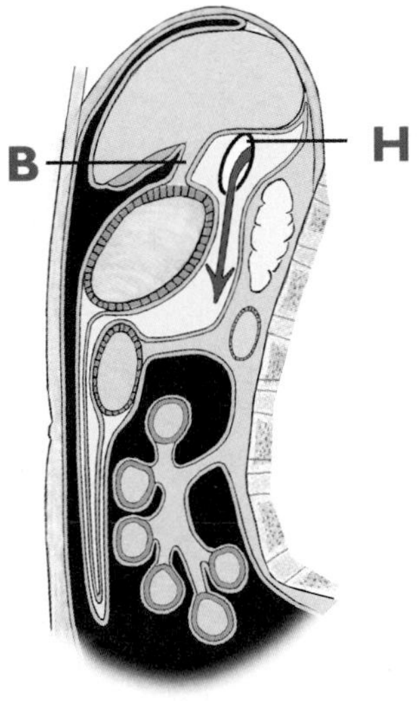

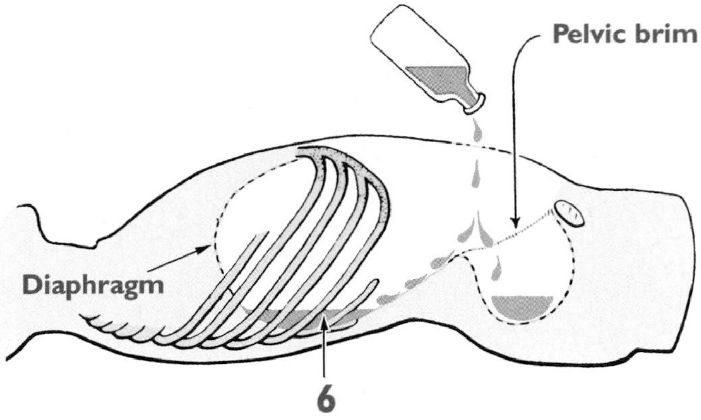

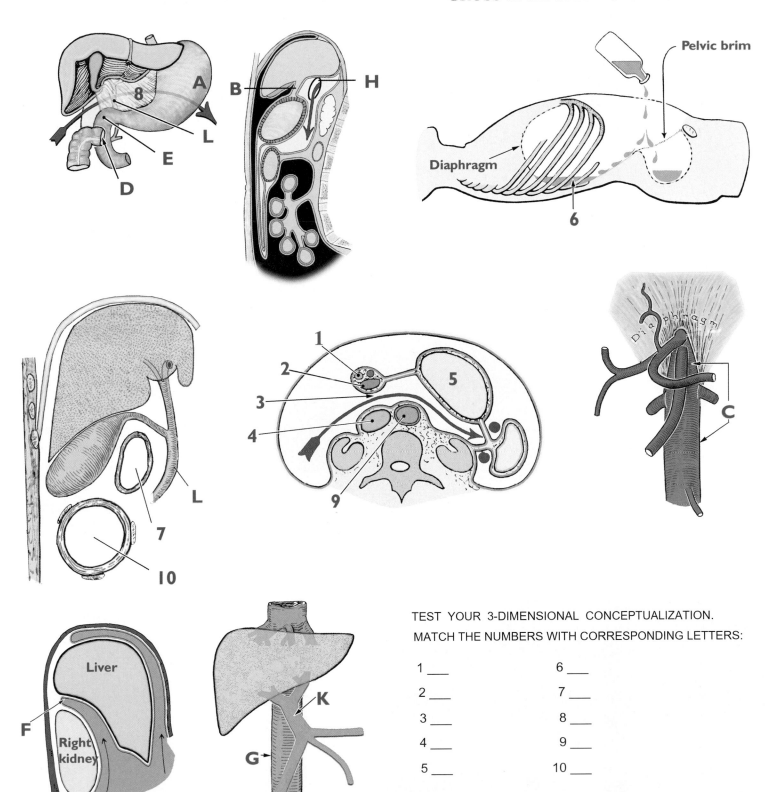

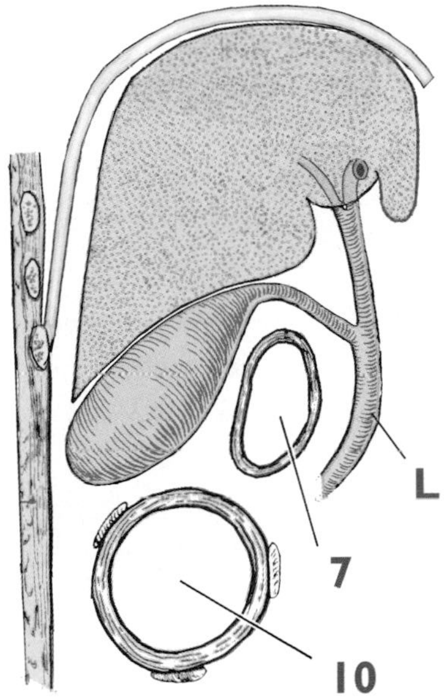

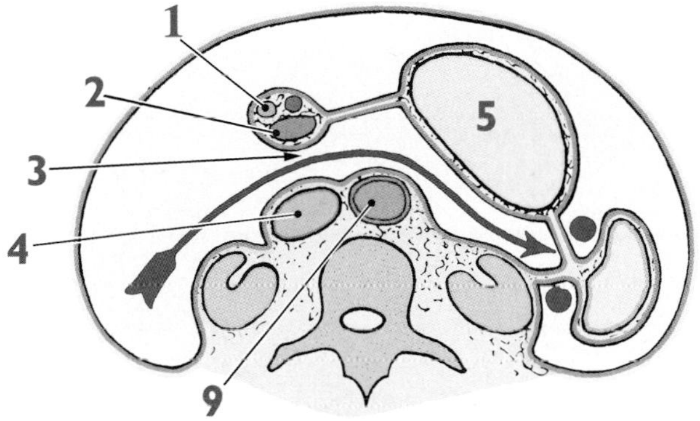

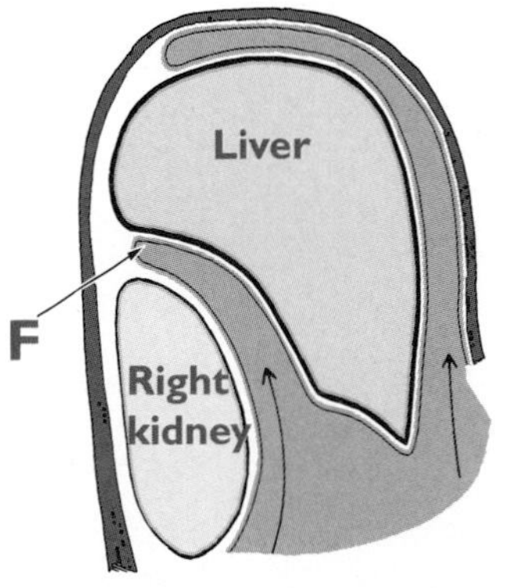

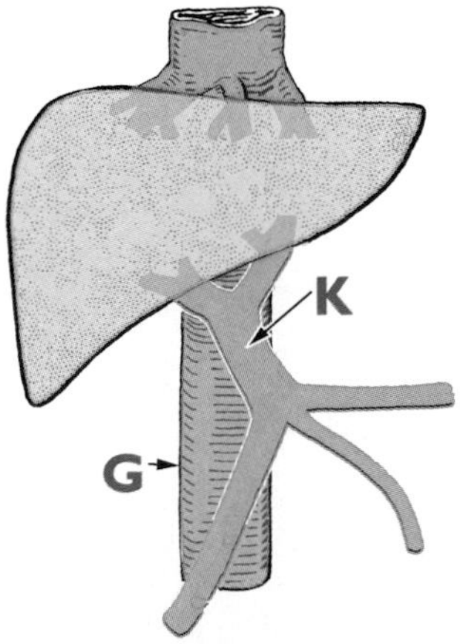

TEST YOUR 3-DIMENSIONAL CONCEPTUALIZATION.

MATCH THE NUMBERS WITH CORRESPONDING LETTERS:

1 ___ 6 ___

2 ___ 7 ___

3 ___ 8 ___

4 ___ 9 ___

5 ___ 10 ___

GAPP TEST: IF YOU MADE AN ERROR, REVIEW AND GAIN A BETTER UNDERSTANDING OF THE CONCERNED 3-DIMENSIONAL ANATOMICAL CONCEPT. GAPP KEY: 1-L, 2-K, 3-H, 4-G, 5-A, 6-F, 7-E, 8-B, 9-C, 10-D.

TEST 7

GAPP
GROSS ANATOMY PRACTICAL PRIMER

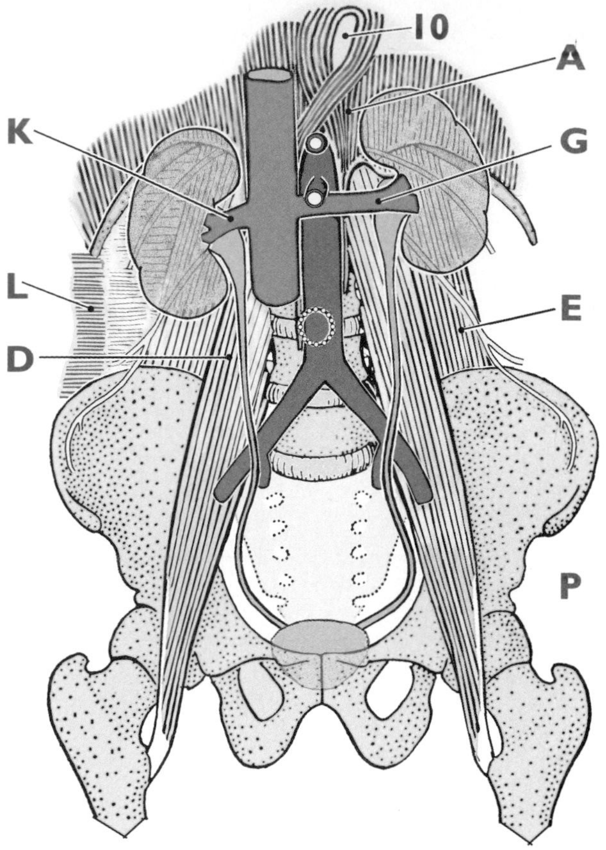

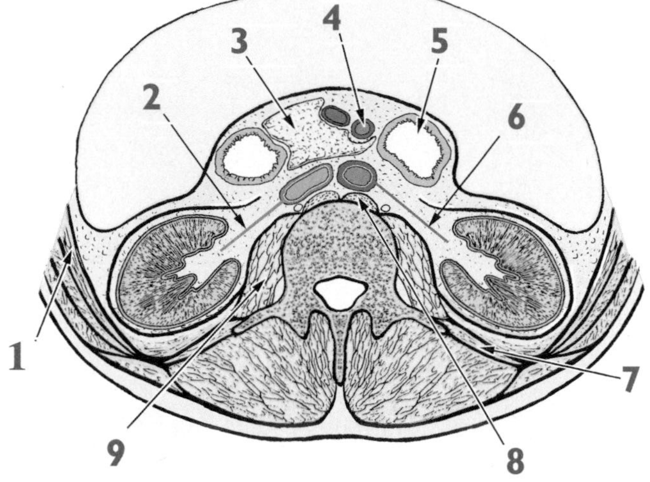

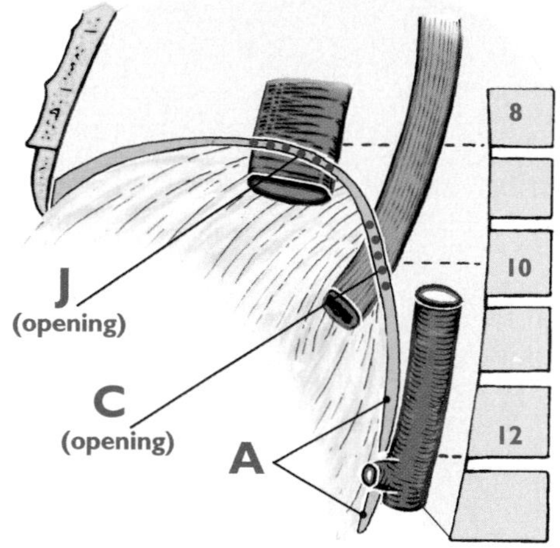

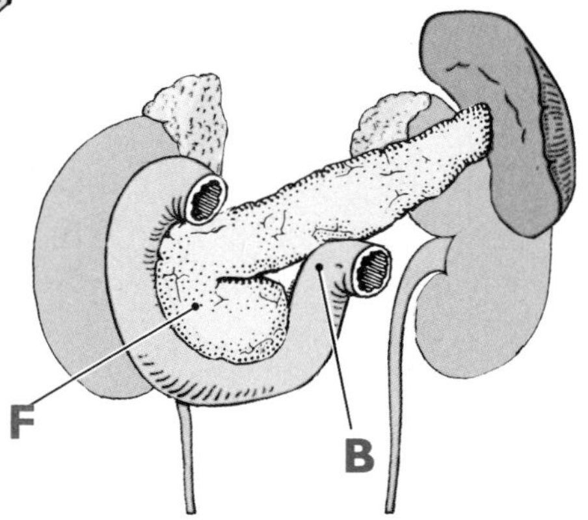

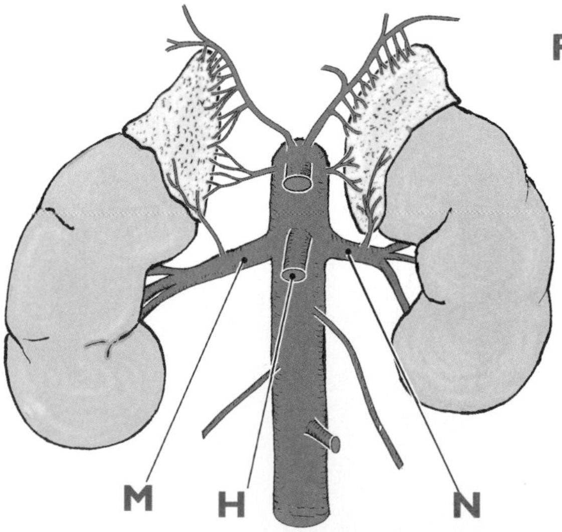

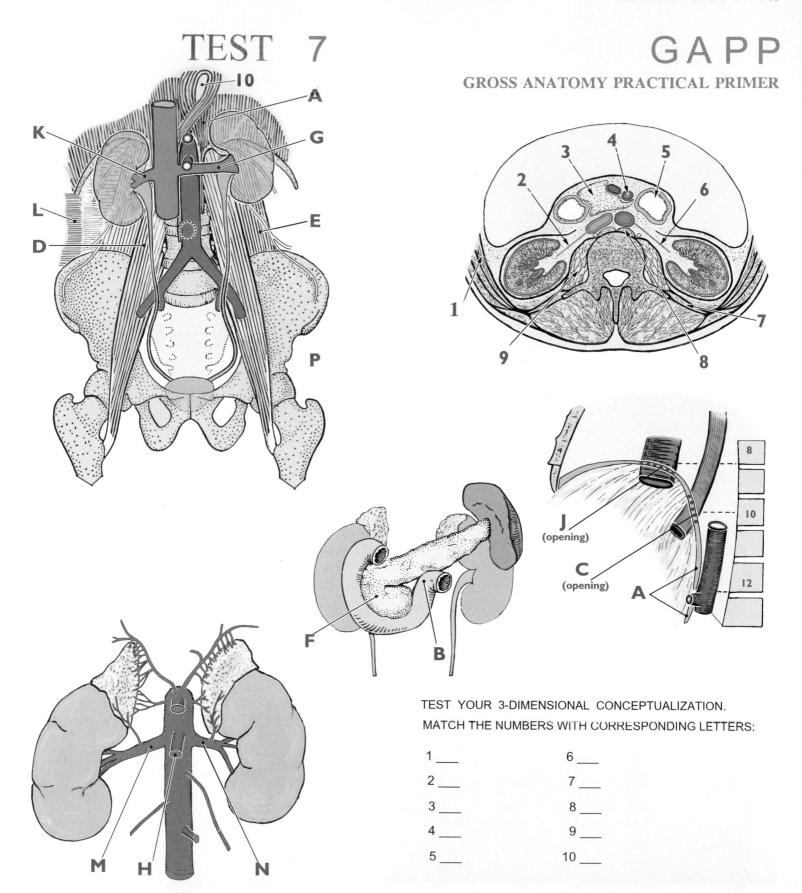

TEST YOUR 3-DIMENSIONAL CONCEPTUALIZATION.

MATCH THE NUMBERS WITH CORRESPONDING LETTERS:

1 ___	6 ___
2 ___	7 ___
3 ___	8 ___
4 ___	9 ___
5 ___	10 ___

GAPP TEST: IF YOU MADE AN ERROR, REVIEW AND GAIN A BETTER UNDERSTANDING OF THE CONCERNED 3-DIMENSIONAL ANATOMICAL CONCEPT. GAPP KEY: 1-L, 2-K, 3-F, 4-H, 5-B, 6-N, 7-E, 8-A, 9-D, 10-C.

Chapter 3

The Pelvis and Perineum

Grant's Atlas of Anatomy, 10th Ed.:	*Grant's* *Fig.* #
Rohen, Color Atlas of Anatomy, 4th Ed.:	Rohen Page #
A.D.A.M. Student Atlas of Anatomy:	A.D.A.M. Plate #
Netter, Atlas of Human Anatomy, 2nd Ed.:	Netter Plate #
Clemente, Anatomy, 4th Ed.:	Clemente Fig. #
Acland's Video Atlas of Human Anatomy	A.V.A. Vol: hr.min.sec

Orientation

Laboratory Approach

The dissection of the pelvis and perineum requires time, skill, and patience. Dissection is difficult because (1) only one or two students can work simultaneously on the spatially limited dissection field, (2) the topography of various anatomical structures is complex, and (3) there are considerable anatomical differences between male and female specimens.

The requirements for this anatomical region vary greatly from school to school. No singular dissection approach to the limited space of the pelvis and perineum will suffice to demonstrate all the complexities of this anatomical region. Therefore, during the initial dissection, the student can only obtain an overview of the pelvic and perineal structures. In the usual setting of an anatomical laboratory, specially prepared specimens of both male and female pelvic and perineal structures are available to complement the standard dissection and to augment the student's perception of this very complex region. It is possible that your teaching faculty may want to make changes in the dissection sequence or approach. Please check with your instructors.

The method presented in this chapter has been chosen because it has been used successfully in a number of schools. *Definitions, important landmarks* and the *anal region* are covered initially. Subsequently, the chapter is divided into two separate sections: (1) male pelvis and perineum and (2) female pelvis and perineum, taken into account with the differences between male and female specimens. Students are urged to exchange information in the dissection of specimens from the opposite sex. Obviously, students will be expected to demonstrate knowledge of both male and female anatomy in the pelvic and perineal regions.

The laboratory approach includes hemisection of the pelvis into a right and a left half. This procedure allows adequate access to various pelvic structures. One hemisected pelvis can be used to demonstrate the sacral nerves and the muscles of the true pelvis. The other hemisected pelvis should be used to dissect the viscera and the vasculature of the entire pelvis.

Grant's 3.1
Rohen 411
A.D.A.M. 4.5, 4.6
Netter 332
A.V.A. 3: 2.08.32

General Remarks and Definitions

The **pelvis** (L. *pelvis*, basin) is divided into the greater pelvis and lesser pelvis. By definition, the **pelvic brim** is the circumference of a plane dividing the pelvis into two portions (Fig. 3.1). The **greater pelvis** (pelvis major; false pelvis) is situated superior to the pelvic brim and is bounded on either side by the ilium. The **lesser pelvis** (pelvis minor; true pelvis) is situated inferior to the pelvic brim. The inlet to the pelvis minor is called the **superior pelvic aperture**. The **peritoneal cavity** extends into the lesser pelvis (hence the term "abdominopelvic cavity").

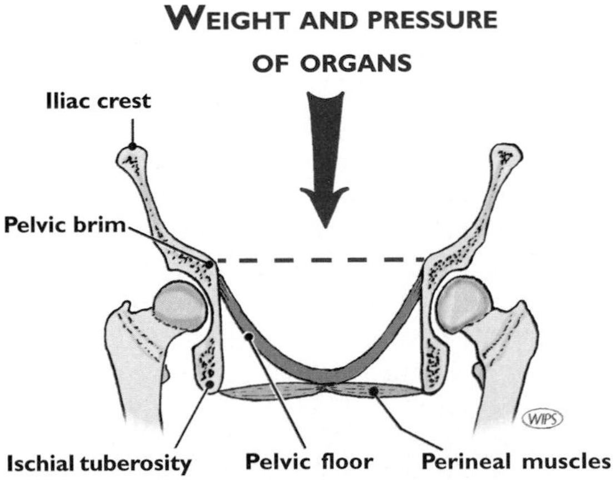

Figure 3.1. The pelvic floor on coronal section.

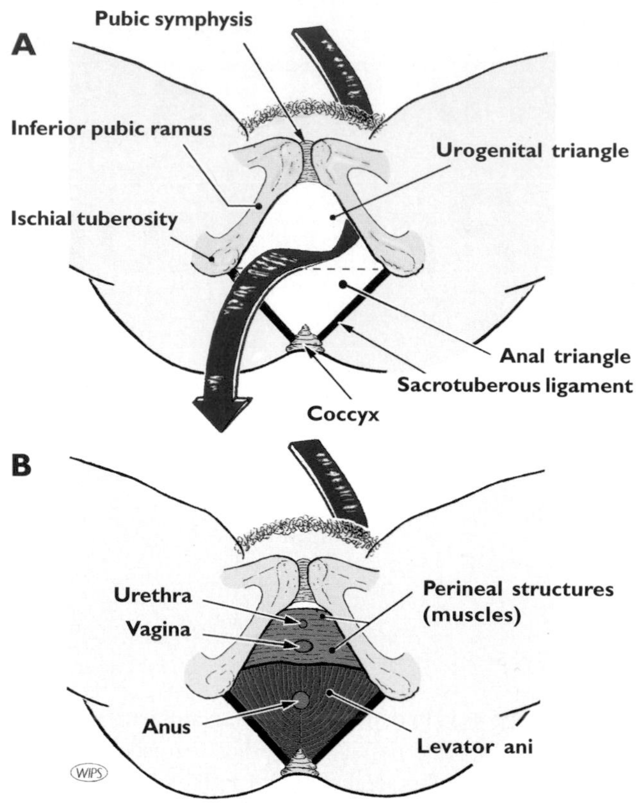

Figure 3.2. The inferior pelvic aperture and its floor. ***A***, In the articulated bony pelvis, the blue arrow passes freely from the abdominopelvic cavity through the open, diamond-shaped pelvic outlet. This aperture is divided into the urogenital and the anal triangles. ***B***, The inferior aperture is effectively closed by the pelvic floor (levator ani muscles) and overlying perineal structures. Note the openings for the urinary, genital, and GI systems.

The diamond-shaped **inferior pelvic aperture** or pelvic outlet is defined anteriorly by the **pubic symphysis**, laterally by the **ischial tuberosities**, and posteriorly by the **sacrum** and **coccyx** (Fig. 3.2). The pelvic outlet has a sturdy floor that prevents the abdominopelvic organs from falling through the opening (see *blue arrow* in Fig. 3.2A).

The **floor of the pelvis** is formed by muscles (Figs. 3.1, 3.2B). The principal organs contained in the pelvic cavity have their outlet in the median plane. They pass through the pelvic floor and are anchored to it. The GI tract (rectum / anus) lies posteriorly and passes through the **anal region** or **anal triangle**. The urinary system (urethra) lies anteriorly. The genital system (vagina in the female) takes an intermediate position. Both systems (urinary and genital) pass through the **urogenital region** or **urogenital triangle** of the pelvic floor. Together, the **anal triangle** and the **urogenital triangle** form the diamond-shaped **perineum** or perineal region that covers the pelvic outlet inferiorly (Fig. 3.2).

The walls of the pelvic cavity are in part lined with muscles (Fig. 3.3). No muscle crosses the pelvic brim. (If muscles crossed the pelvic brim, they would interfere with childbirth by partially obstructing the pelvic inlet.)

⇨
A.D.A.M. 4.37, 4.38
NETTER 341
A.V.A. 3: 2.27.43

⇨
GRANT'S 3.1, 3.3
ROHEN 409-414
A.D.A.M. 4.5, 4.6
NETTER 332
CLEMENTE 386-389
A.V.A. 3: 2.09.10

⇦
A.D.A.M. 4.6
NETTER 332
CLEMENTE 390
A.V.A. 3: 2.14.03

⇦
GRANT'S TABLE 3.2
A.D.A.M. 4.9
NETTER 334, 336
CLEMENTE 428
A.V.A. 3: 2.20.35

⇦
ROHEN 328, 342
A.D.A.M. 4.1, 4.2
NETTER 354
A.V.A. 3: 2.24.50

Pelvic Fascia (Fig. 3.3). The pelvic fascia consists of **two parts:** (1) **parietal pelvic fascia** and (2) **visceral pelvic fascia.** The intrapelvic surfaces of the muscles lining the walls of the pelvic cavity are covered with the **parietal pelvic fascia.** This fascia is firmly attached to the **pelvic brim** (which runs anteriorly toward the pubic symphysis). The parietal pelvic fascia is also continuous with the fascia lining both the superior and inferior surfaces of the muscles of the pelvic floor. The **visceral pelvic fascia** provides a fascial covering for the pelvic viscera (e.g., for the bladder). The space between parietal pelvic fascia and bladder, particularly posterior to the pubic region but also extending laterally, is called the **retropubic space.** This space contains extraperitoneal fat and areolar tissue, blood vessels, and nerves.

Important Landmarks

Refer to an articulated bony pelvis, preferably one with intact ligaments. Feel free to orientate the pelvis in such a manner that its position compares with that of the cadaver under dissection.

The **bony pelvis** (Fig. 3.4A) is formed by the:

- **Right hip bone** (os coxae) anteriorly and laterally on the right;
- **Left hip bone** (os coxae) anteriorly and laterally on the left;
- **Sacrum and coccyx,** parts of the vertebral column, interposed dorsally between the two hip bones.

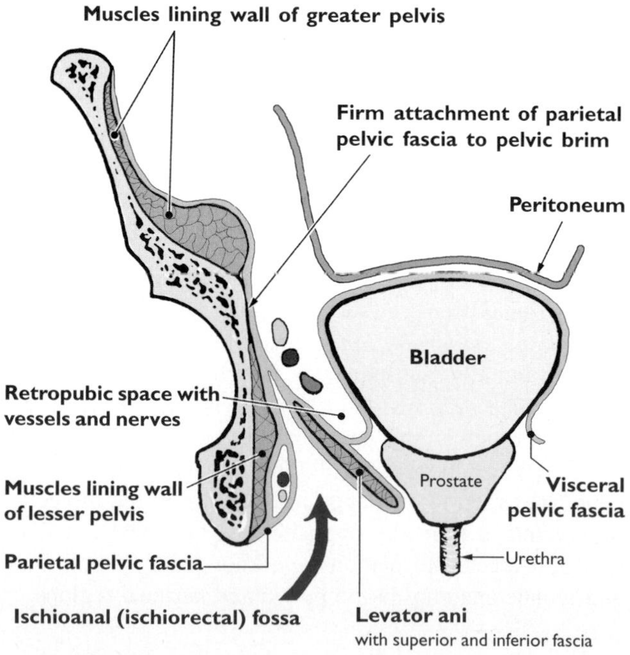

Figure 3.3. Diagram of pelvic fascia (male pelvis, coronal section).

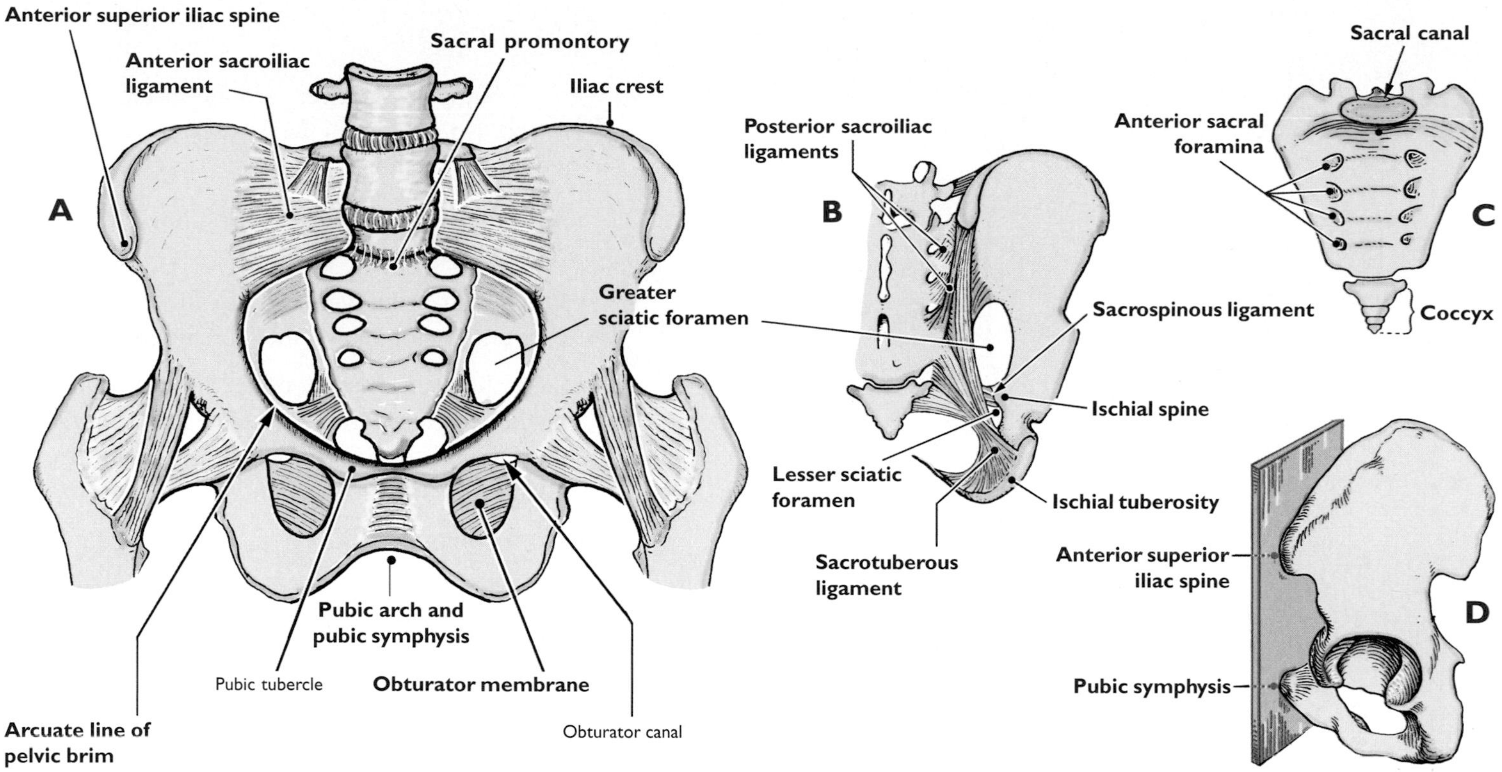

Figure 3.4. Bony landmarks and ligaments of the pelvis. ***A,*** Superior aperture and ligaments of female pelvis; ***B,*** Dorsal view of pelvis; ***C,*** Anterior surface of sacrum and coccyx; ***D,*** Pelvic orientation in standing position.

The **pelvic brim** surrounds the **pelvic inlet or superior aperture** of the pelvis. It extends from the **promontory** of the sacrum dorsally to the **symphysis pubis** ventrally. Distinguish the three parts of the pelvic brim: sacral part, iliac part, and pubic part.

The **obturator foramen** is closed by the **obturator membrane**. Superiorly, the obturator canal (for obturator nerve and vessels) traverses the membrane. Identify the **pubic arch**. Compare male and female pelvis. In the female, the pubic arch is much wider.

The **hip bone** (os coxae) consists of three parts: ilium, ischium, and pubis. These three elements meet at the acetabulum, the cup-shaped cavity for the head of the femur. On the hip bone identify the **ischial tuberosity** and the **ischial spine**. In the articulated pelvis, observe the **sacrospinous and sacrotuberous ligaments** (Fig. 3.4B). The sacrospinous ligament stretches from coccyx to ischial spine. The sacrotuberous ligament stretches from sacrum to ischial tuberosity. The sacrospinous and sacrotuberous ligaments form the partial boundaries for two foramina: the **lesser sciatic foramen** and the **greater sciatic foramen**.

On the **sacrum** (L. *sacer*, sacred), identify the ventral or pelvic surface (Fig. 3.4C), the **anterior sacral foramina** for the passage of ventral nerve rami S1 to S4, and the **promontory.** Superiorly, note the **sacral canal** which transmits spinal nerves S1 to S5 on their way to the sacral foramina. The **coccyx** (Gr. *kokkyx*, cuckoo; resembling a cuckoo's bill) consists of three to five rudimentary vertebrae. The **sacroiliac articulation** is a joint (synovial type) between the auricular surfaces of sacrum and ilium, held together by anterior sacroiliac ligaments (Fig. 3.4A) and posterior sacroiliac ligaments.

In the **erect posture** (anatomical position), the anterior superior iliac spines and the upper end of the symphysis pubis occupy the same vertical plane (Fig. 3.4D). In this position, the plane of the superior aperture (pelvic inlet) forms an angle of 50° to 60° with the horizontal plane. Verify this.

⇨
GRANT'S 3.1
ROHEN 409. 410
A.D.A.M. 4.5, 4.6
NETTER 331, 332
CLEMENTE 393
A.V.A. 3: 0.11.50

⇦
GRANT'S 3.1A, 3.1C
A.D.A.M. 4.4
NETTER 330
CLEMENTE 386, 388
A.V.A. 3: 2.11.00

⇦
GRANT'S 3.3A, 3.3C
NETTER 330, 331
CLEMENTE 391, 392
A.V.A. 3: 2.10.20

⇨
ROHEN 414
NETTER 332
CLEMENTE 383
A.V.A. 3: 2.09.34

Clinical Correlation: Familiarize yourself with some measurements of the female pelvis. These measurements are of obstetrical importance. Obtain an articulated female pelvis and observe the following:

- A line connecting the superior end of the symphysis pubis with the coccyx lies in the horizontal plane (in the anatomical position).
- At the **superior pelvic aperture or pelvic inlet**, identify the midsagittal line connecting the superior end of the symphysis pubis with the promontory of the

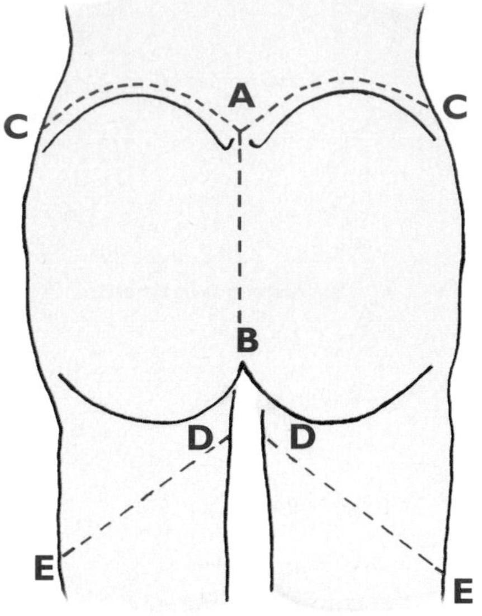

Figure 3.5. Skins incisions.

sacrum.This line indicates the plane of the pelvic inlet or brim.The plane of the pelvic inlet forms an angle of about 60° with the horizontal plane.

- **Transverse diameter** (~ 13.5 cm); it is measured across the greatest width of the superior aperture.
- A line connecting the lower end of the symphysis pubis with the tip of the coccyx is the **anteroposterior** or **conjugate diameter** (~ 10.5 to 11 cm). It indicates the **pelvic outlet** or the **inferior pelvic aperture.** The plane of the pelvic outlet forms an angle of about 15° with the horizontal plane.
- The transverse diameter (~ 11 cm) of the pelvic outlet is measured between the two ischial tuberosities.
- The pubic arch in the female is wide. The subpubic angle measures about 90°. In the male, the subpubic angle measures only about 60°.
- In addition to the pelvic parameters, study a radiograph of the pelvis.

Anal Region (Triangle)

Before you begin ...

Do not dissect at this time. Understand that the next objective is the study of the **anal region (triangle)** and its nerve and blood supply. By reflecting the gluteus maximus and partially exposing the gluteal region, it will be easier to trace nerves and blood vessels to the perineal region.

ROHEN 414
NETTER 332
CLEMENTE 383
A.V.A. 3: 2.08.38

GRANT'S 5.24B
ROHEN 454
A.D.A.M. 5.33
NETTER 461
CLEMENTE 504, 505
A.V.A. 3: 2.26.11

GRANT'S 5.28
ROHEN 455
A.D.A.M. 5.33
NETTER 461, 469
CLEMENTE 506
A.V.A. 3: 2.13.02

Skin Incisions

Turn the cadaver into the prone position (*face down*). Make skin incisions according to those shown in Figure 3.5:

- A median vertical cut from the lower lumbar region to the coccyx (*A* to *B*);
- From point *A* lateralward just above the iliac crest, until stopped by the table (*A* to *C*);
- From the medial aspect of the thigh (about 2.5 cm below the gluteal fold) to the lateral part of the thigh about 15 cm below the greater trochanter (*D* to *E*);
- From points *B* to *D*.

To save time, remove skin and subcutaneous fat in one piece (from skin down to deep fascia enveloping both the gluteus maximus and the thigh). This approach will destroy some of the cutaneous nerves of the gluteal region. Do not cut too deeply across the posterior aspect of the thigh (*D* to *E*); otherwise the posterior cutaneous nerve of the thigh will be injured.

Remove skin and subcutaneous tissue. Expose the **gluteus maximus** (Fig.3.6). Define the superior and inferior borders of this vast rhomboidal muscle. If the lower limb has already been dissected earlier, simply reflect the gluteus maximus laterally and proceed with the exploration of the anal region. Otherwise, reflect the gluteus maximus in the following manner:

- Detach its superior portion close to the ilium (see *dotted blue line* in Fig. 3.6).
- With a scalpel, cut through its fibers very close to their origin from the posterior surface of the sacrum and coccyx.
- Place your fingers under the inferior portion of the muscle. Note that it is attached to the **sacrotuberous ligament**. Using a pair of scissors, carefully detach the gluteus maximus from the sacrotuberous ligament. Do *not* cut the ligament.
- It is not necessary to reflect the muscle completely. Reflect the muscle laterally to the point where the inferior gluteal nerve and vessels enter it (i.e., near its "center").

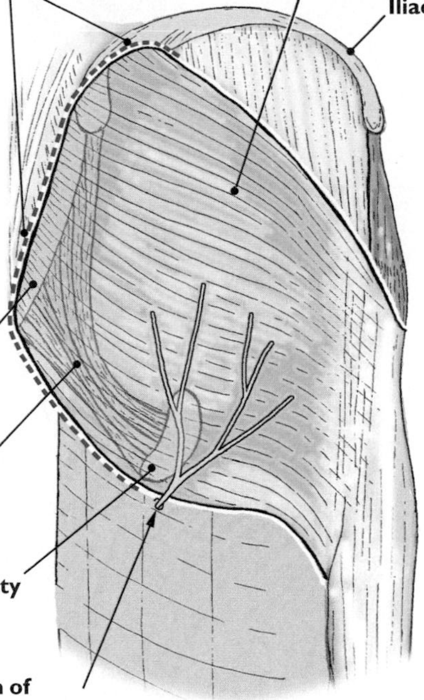

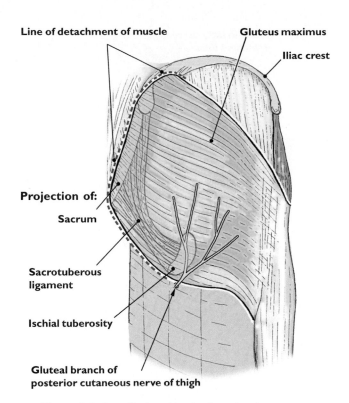

Figure 3.6. Partially detach and reflect the gluteus maximus muscle to expose the nerve and the vessels to the ischioanal fossa.

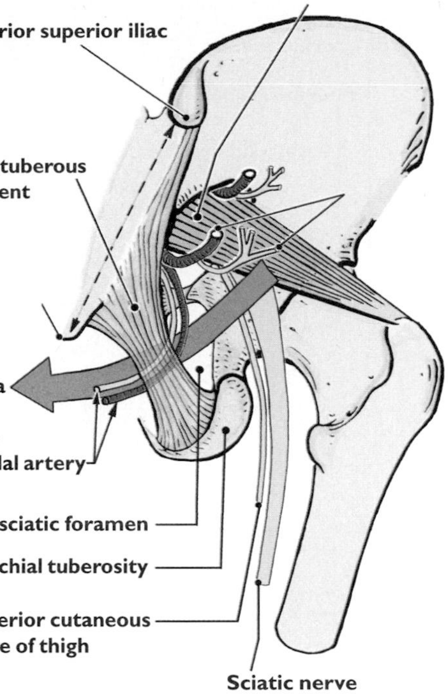

Figure 3.7. The *green arrow*, together with the pudendal nerve and internal pudendal artery, passes through the lesser sciatic foramen into the ischioanal fossa.

Refer to an articulated bony pelvis, preferably one with its ligaments intact.

- Hold this orientation specimen in such a manner that its position corresponds to the region under dissection.
- Identify the **greater and lesser sciatic foramina.**
- Palpate the **ischial spine** and **ischial tuberosity.** Now, approaching from the gluteal region, palpate the same structures in the cadaver.
- Force your finger through the greater sciatic foramen. Observe that your finger passes along with the piriformis muscle and the sciatic nerve.

Next, push your finger through the lesser sciatic foramen into the ischioanal (ischiorectal) fossa of the anal triangle. The finger runs in the same direction as the pudendal nerve and the internal pudendal vessels (see *green arrow* in Fig. 3.7). These vessels and nerve fibers supply the perineal structures.

⇦
GRANT'S 5.30
ROHEN 421
NETTER 331
CLEMENTE 391, 392
A.V.A. 3: 2.13.44

⇨
GRANT'S 3.39
ROHEN 328
A.D.A.M. 4.39
NETTER 364
CLEMENTE 457
A.V.A. 3: 2.19.41

Dissection Note: Before proceeding with the dissection of the ischioanal (ischiorectal) fossa and its contents, the anal canal should be distended and stabilized. This is best done by inserting a super-size tampon, along with its plastic insertion tube, into the anal canal. This procedure adds rigidity and stability to the anus and makes dissection of the anal triangle considerably easier.

Ischioanal (Ischiorectal) Fossa (Fig. 3.8)

The ischioanal fossa is a large, wedge-shaped space on either side of the anus. Its surfaces are formed by the fasciae of the obturator internus and levator ani. Its base is the skin of the perineum (skin of anal triangle). The ischioanal fossa is filled with soft fat. This tissue accommodates the distended rectum.

Clinical Correlation: Infections of the ischioanal (ischiorectal) fossa may result in the formation of an abscess. The abscess may spontaneously open into the rectum or through the skin into the perineal region. Surgeons must be aware of the fact that the right and left ischioanal fossae communicate via the deep postanal space (which lies posterior to the anus between superficial and deep external sphincter). As a result, an infection in one ischioanal fossa may eventually involve a semicircular area around the posterior aspect of the anus.

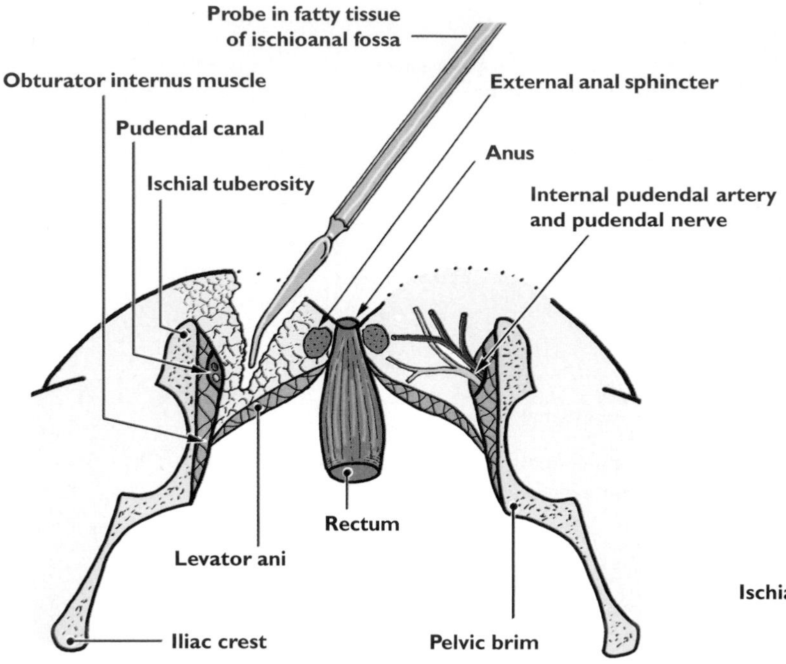

Figure 3.8. Ischioanal fossa and anus on coronal section (specimen in prone position).

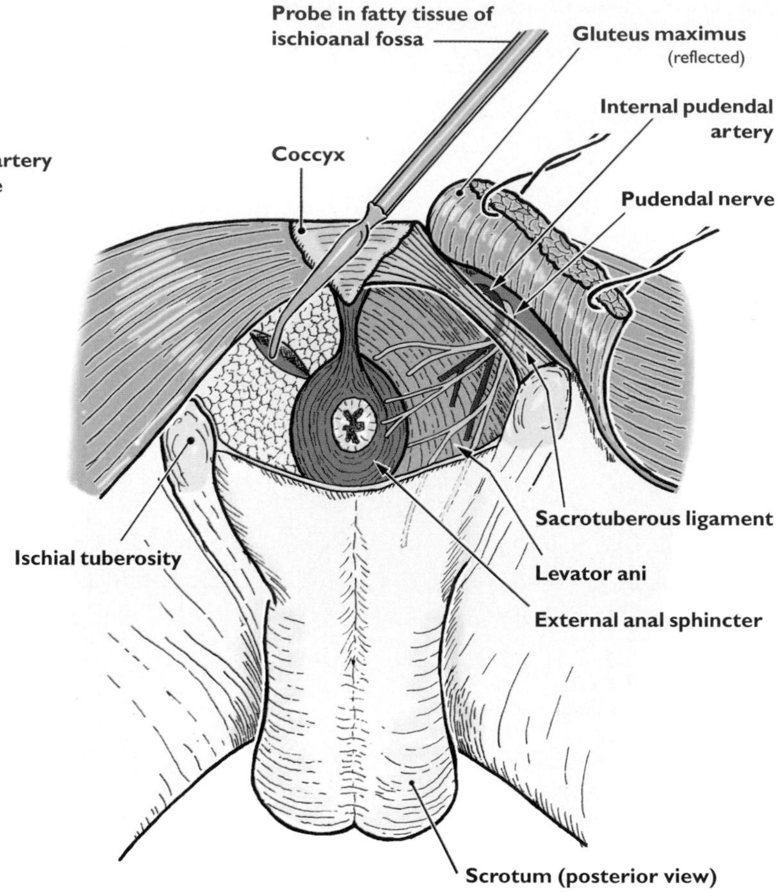

Figure 3.9. Ischioanal fossa and related structures (male cadaver in prone position).

Proceed in the following manner (Fig. 3.9):

- Incise the fat of the ischioanal (ischiorectal) fossa.
- With the blade directed toward the anus, start the incision roughly midway between ischial tuberosity and coccyx. Insert the blade approximately 4 cm deep. As the anus is approached, gradually withdraw the scalpel.
- Insert your finger or a probe into the incision (Fig. 3.9). Palpate the distinct strands of the **inferior rectal (hemorrhoidal) nerve** and **vessels.**
- Enlarge the opening with your finger. In a piecemeal fashion, remove the fat with a forceps.

Dry the area with paper towels.

- Observe vessels and nerves traversing the fossa from the lateral wall toward the anus (Fig. 3.9).

Clean the **sphincter ani externus** (external anal sphincter). It consists of three parts:

- The delicate subcutaneous part, encircling the anal orifice;
- The superficial part, anchoring the anus to the perineal body ventrally and to the coccyx posteriorly;

⇦
Grant's 3.39
Rohen 329
A.D.A.M. 4.41-4.44
Netter 3.82, 384
Clemente 427, 465

⇦
Grant's 3.39, 3.40A
Rohen 328
Netter 364-367
Clemente 426, 464
A.V.A. 3: 2.23.41

⇨
Grant's 3.39
Rohen 330
Netter 382, 384
Clemente 427, 465
A.V.A. 3: 2.29.23

- The deep part, forming a wide encircling band; it is fused with the levator ani (puborectal sling). During defecation, the puborectal sling and all parts of the sphincter ani externus relax.

Temporarily remove the stabilizing tampon from the anal canal. With a gloved hand, insert your middle finger into the rectum. At the same time, place the fingers of your other hand on the sphincter ani externus within the ischioanal fossa. Appreciate the thickness of this muscle. Subsequently, insert the tampon again into the anal canal (or use a new tampon).

Laterally and within the ischioanal fossa, clean the **fascia of the obturator internus**. The inferior portion of the obturator fascia is thickened. It splits to form a fibrous canal, the **pudendal canal** (Fig. 3.8). The canal contains the **pudendal nerve** and the **internal pudendal vessels**. These structures run along the ischiopubic ramus toward the urogenital triangle. Carefully incise the obturator fascia along the ischiopubic ramus and just ventral to the sacrotuberous ligament. With a probe, pick up the contents of the pudendal canal. Carefully push the probe into the canal. Then push forward along the ischiopubic ramus toward the inferior portion of the symphysis pubis. This is the course of the pudendal nerve and the internal pudendal vessels to the urogenital triangle and the dorsum of the penis (clitoris in the female). A detailed dissection of these structures will be performed later.

⇦
GRANT'S 3.39
ROHEN 330
A.D.A.M. 4.45
NETTER 384
CLEMENTE 427, 465
A.V.A. 3: 2.32.31

Male Pelvis and Perineum

General Arrangement

Study the general arrangement of the *soft parts* of the male pelvis (Fig. 3.10):

- The **perineum** is the area between the thighs.
- The perineal region is diamond-shaped and divided into two triangular areas, the **anal region** (or triangle) and the **urogenital region** (or triangle).
- The **anal canal** is located in the anal triangle. It pierces the levator ani muscle.
- The **urinary bladder** and **prostate** are supported by the muscular pelvic floor.
- The **male urethra** is long. It traverses the prostate gland, pierces the anterior portion of the urogenital triangle, and then traverses the penis.
- Parts of the penis and its erectile tissue are located in the urogenital triangle.

⇦
GRANT'S 3.37F
ROHEN 328
A.D.A.M. 4.1
NETTER 354
CLEMENTE 445
A.V.A. 3: 2.24.38

⇦
GRANT'S 3.6B
ROHEN 316
A.D.A.M. 4.35
NETTER 338
CLEMENTE 445

The anal region has already been studied (see earlier part of this chapter). Now the urogenital region (triangle) must be dissected.

Male Urogenital Region (Triangle)

The dissection of the male urogenital region will be done by using the so-called "traditional approach," which is preferred by many anatomists: The cadaver is in the supine position (face up). The thighs are widely stretched apart. The dissector sits or stands in front of the exposed perineal region (just as a urologist would). Usually, only one student can work on the region at a given time. The lighting must be excellent.

Place the cadaver in the supine position (face up). Stretch the thighs widely apart. This can be accomplished by using either wooden boards placed between the feet or by abducting the lower limbs with the aid of ropes.

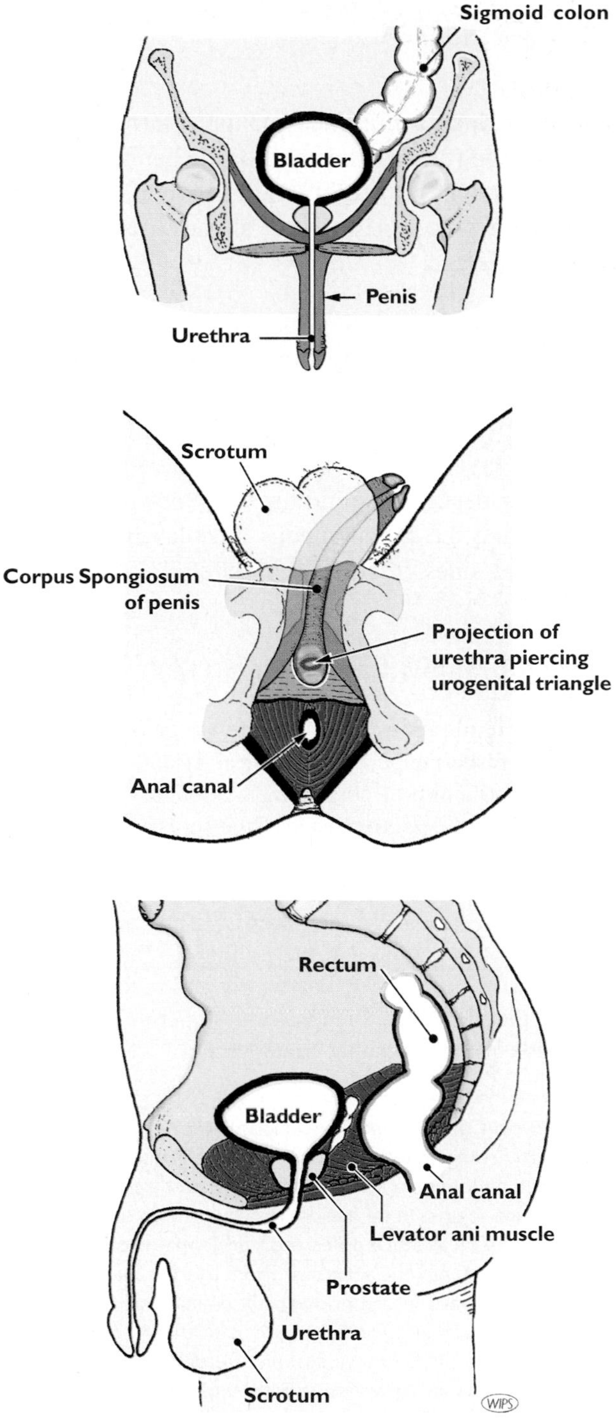

Figure 3. 10. General arrangement of male pelvic organs, pelvic floor, and perineum.

> ***Dissection Note:*** The scrotum has been dissected earlier together with the structures of the anterior abdominal wall, the spermatic cord, and the testes (see Chapter 2). Review this material.

Skin Incisions

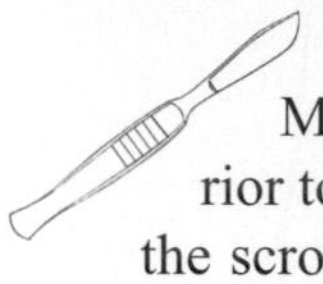

Make a midline incision. Start posterior to (below) the shaft of the penis. Split the scrotum into right and left halves. Carry the cut posteriorly to the already dissected anal triangle.

Reflect the skin flaps of the urogenital region. Note that the **superficial fascia** consists of two layers, a superficial fatty layer and a deeper membranous layer. Observe that the **fatty layer** is continuous with the subcutaneous tissue surrounding the anus posteriorly and the subcutaneous fatty layer of the medial sides of the thighs laterally.

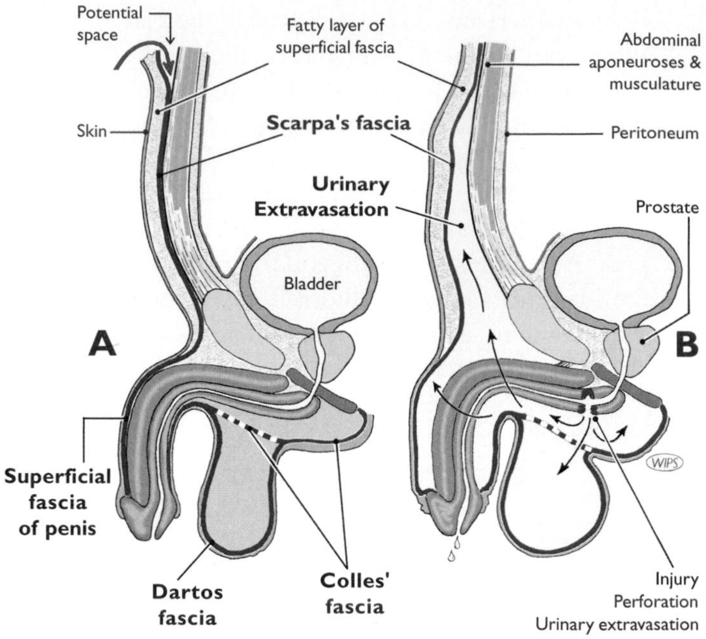

Figure 3.11. The superficial perineal fascia (Colles' fascia) is continuous with the superficial fascia of the scrotum (dartos fascia) and of the penis, and Scarpa's fascia of the lower abdominal wall. ***A,*** Normal fascial arrangements. ***B,*** Extravasation of urine along fascial boundaries following injury and perforation of the urethra.

Membranous Layer (Fig. 3.11A)

Grant's 3.39
A.D.A.M. 4.40
Netter 354
Clemente 469

The membranous layer of the superficial fascia (**Colles' fascia**; superficial perineal fascia) is an aponeurotic structure of considerable strength. It is continuous with the **dartos fascia** of the penis and scrotum, and the membranous layer of the superficial fascia (**Scarpa's fascia**) of the lower anterior abdominal wall. Note that the membranous layer is firmly attached to the rami of the pubic and the ischium as far posterior as the ischial tuberosity. Posteriorly and in the median plane, the membrane blends with the perineal body at the base of the urogenital triangle.

> ***Clinical Correlation:*** The clinician must be aware of the fascial arrangements of the external genitalia and of the lower abdominal wall. If the penile urethra is injured (perineal injuries in car accidents; falling astride onto sharp objects such as fence poles, etc.), urine may escape from the urethra into the scrotum. From there it may readily spread upward into the lower abdominal wall between Scarpa's fascia and the aponeurosis of the external oblique (Fig. 3.11B). The clinical picture of this urinary extravasation may be dramatic with extensive, red edematous swelling of the scrotum, penis, and lower abdominal wall. Urinary extravasation into the thigh does *not* occur because Scarpa's fascia ends by firm attachment to the fascia lata (i.e., the deep fascia of the thigh). This clinical picture can only be understood properly if one is mindful of the above-mentioned fascial arrangements.

Superficial Perineal Space

Incise the **membranous layer** of the superficial fascia (Colles' fascia) about 2 to 3 cm from the median plane.

Grant's 3.39
Rohen 329
A.D.A.M. 4.42
Netter 376, 382
Clemente 469

- With a probe, pick up the **posterior scrotal nerves** and vessels. Insert your fingertip deep to the fascia. Your finger is now in the **superficial perineal space** or **pouch.**
- Confirm the posterior extent of the space by placing a finger of the other hand into the ischioanal fossa. Observe that the posterior portion of the membranous layer is between both fingertips. The **contents of the superficial perineal pouch** include three paired muscles and portions of the penile erectile tissue: the crura and the bulb of the penis.

Grant's 3.39
Rohen 328, 329
A.D.A.M. 4.42
Netter 355
Clemente 469

Identify and clean the **three paired muscles** within the superficial perineal pouch (Fig. 3.12):

- **Superficial transverse perineal muscle** (transversus perinei superficialis), a slender muscle passing from ischial tuberosity to the perineal body or central tendon. This structure is a fibromuscular node in the median plane. At this node, several perineal muscles converge and interlace. Note branches of the pudendal nerve and the internal pudendal artery as they course from the pudendal canal into the urogenital triangle and on toward the pubic symphysis (Fig. 3.12).

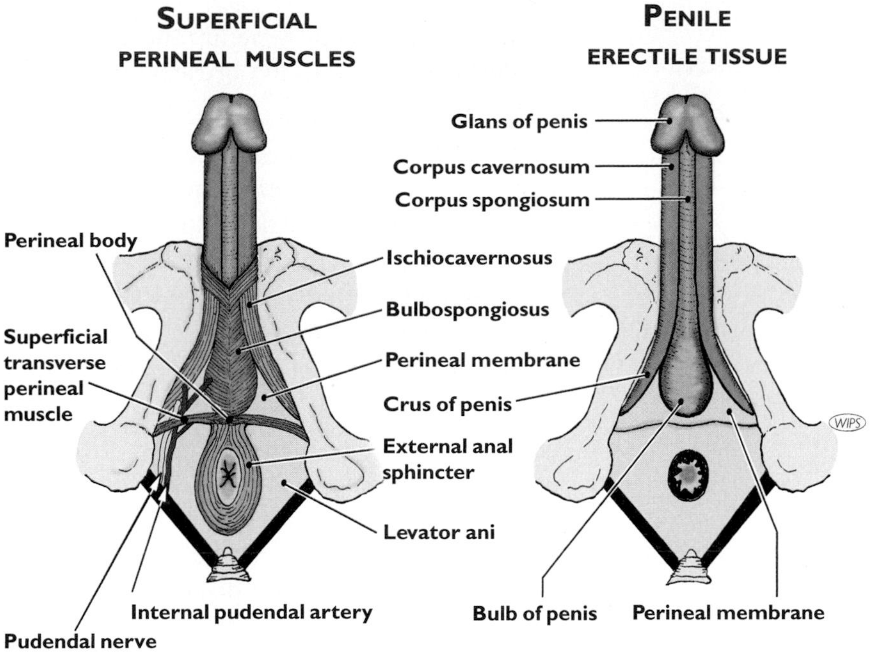

Figure 3.12. Contents of the superficial perineal space: superficial perineal muscles and part of the penile erectile tissue.

- **Ischiocavernosus**, arising from the ischial tuberosity and covering the crus of the corpus cavernosum on the same side. *Function:* it alters erection, once achieved, by forcing blood from the cavernous tissue of the crus of the penis into the distal part of the corpus cavernosum penis.

GRANT'S 3.43A
ROHEN 326
A.D.A.M. 4.21, 4.44
NETTER 354-356
CLEMENTE 469, 478

- **Bulbospongiosus**; The right and left muscles together are shaped like a feather. It arises from a median raphe and from the perineal body, and it encircles the bulb and the adjacent part of the corpus spongiosum penis. Raise the thin anterior, free border of the muscle. *Function:* the paired bulbospongiosi form a sphincter that empties part of the spongy urethra. Also, the bulbospongiosus alters erection, once achieved, by forcing blood from the spongy portion of the bulb into the distal part of the corpus spongiosum penis.

GRANT'S 3.37E, 3.39
ROHEN 329
A.D.A.M. 4.44
NETTER 355
CLEMENTE 469

Separate the three superficial perineal muscles from each other until a small triangular area comes into view. This is part of the **perineal membrane**. Next, remove the **three superficial perineal muscles**. Use the **perineal body** (or central tendon) as a reference point (Fig. 3.12).

GRANT'S 3.39
A.D.A.M. 4.44
NETTER 355, 356

- First, remove the slender **superficial transverse perineal muscle**, thereby fully exposing the posterior extent of the **superficial perineal space or pouch.**

GRANT'S 3.41, 3.42
ROHEN 326
NETTER 380
CLEMENTE 441, 467

- Next, split the **bulbospongiosus muscle** at its raphe and remove it, thereby exposing the **bulb of the penis** (bulb of corpus spongiosum; Fig. 3.12). Subsequently, clear away the **ischiocavernosus muscle** on both sides, thereby exposing the right and left **crura of the penis.**

- Study the components of the erectile tissues of the penis. The **glans penis** is the distal expansion of the corpus spongiosum. The glans (L., *glans*, acorn) is pierced by the spongy urethra.

Penis, Fascia, Vessels, and Nerves

Remove the skin of the penis (L. *penis*, tail) leaving the glans intact. The **superficial fascia** is devoid of fat. It contains superficial veins that drain to the inguinal region. Deep to the loose superficial fascia is the tight tubular investing sheath, the **deep fascia of the penis** (Buck's fascia) that holds the erectile tissue components together. Incise this deep fascia between the glans and the symphysis pubis. On the dorsum of the shaft of the penis identify the following (Fig. 3.13):

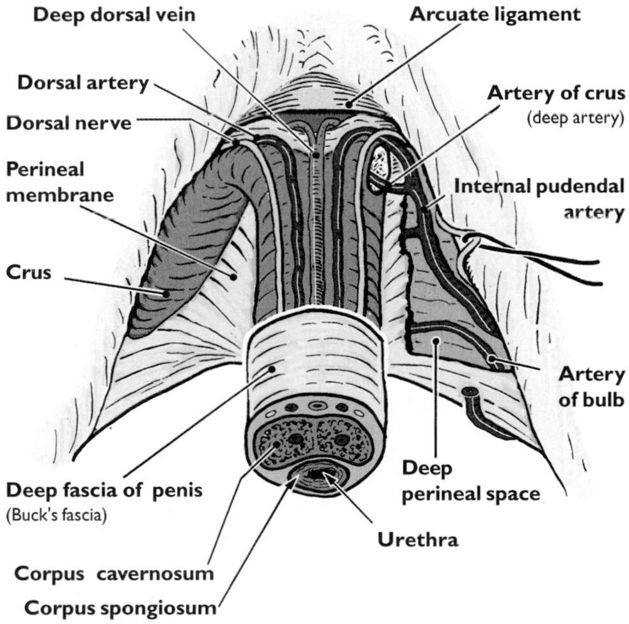

Figure 3.13. Portions of penis and related structures in the urogenital triangle.

- The unpaired **deep dorsal vein** of the **penis**. Follow it to where it passes just inferior to the symphysis pubis. Most of the blood from the penis drains through this vein into the prostatic venous plexus.

- The paired **dorsal arteries of the penis,** branches of the internal pudendal arteries.
- The paired **dorsal nerves of the penis,** branches of the pudendal nerves.

Spongy Urethra or Penile Urethra

The *entire* male urethra consists of three portions: prostatic, membranous, and spongy (see Fig. 3.14). At this point, only the **spongy (penile) portion** of the urethra will be examined. As the name implies, the spongy urethra runs within the corpus spongiosum penis. Examine the **external urethral orifice** near the tip of the glans penis. Push a probe into it. The next objective is to open the penile urethra in a longitudinal direction (Fig. 3.14):

- Push the probe deeper (more proximal) into the spongy urethra. Continue to split it until reaching the bulb of the corpus spongiosum. Here the urethra bends at almost a right angle and passes through the deep perineal space.

GRANT'S 3.41-3.43
ROHEN 327
CLEMENTE 467

GRANT'S 3.41
A.D.A.M. 4.35
NETTER 338
CLEMENTE 445

GRANT'S 3.43, 3.44
ROHEN 316
A.D.A.M. 4.35
NETTER 338
CLEMENTE 445

GRANT'S 3.37B
ROHEN 331
A.D.A.M. 4.48
NETTER 357
CLEMENTE 462

- Examine the mucous membrane of the spongy urethra. Note the orifices of tiny mucous glands.

Next, mobilize the penis by cutting the **suspensory ligament of the penis**, a triangular band attached anteriorly to the symphysis pubis (Fig. 3.15). Observe the **deep dorsal vein of the penis** passing inferior to the pubic arch into the pelvis.

- Cut the vein. Free the crura. Next, pull gently on the bulb and, using a sharp blade, detach it from the inferior surface of the urogenital diaphragm. In doing so, you are cutting through blood vessels to the penis and through the **urethra** at the junction of the spongy portion and the distal portion of the membranous urethra.
- Note that the short **membranous urethra** lies within the deep perineal space. It will be examined later.

Detach the **penis** entirely by cutting through the right and left dorsal nerves and dorsal arteries of the penis near the symphysis pubis.

Make two **transverse sections** through the glans penis:

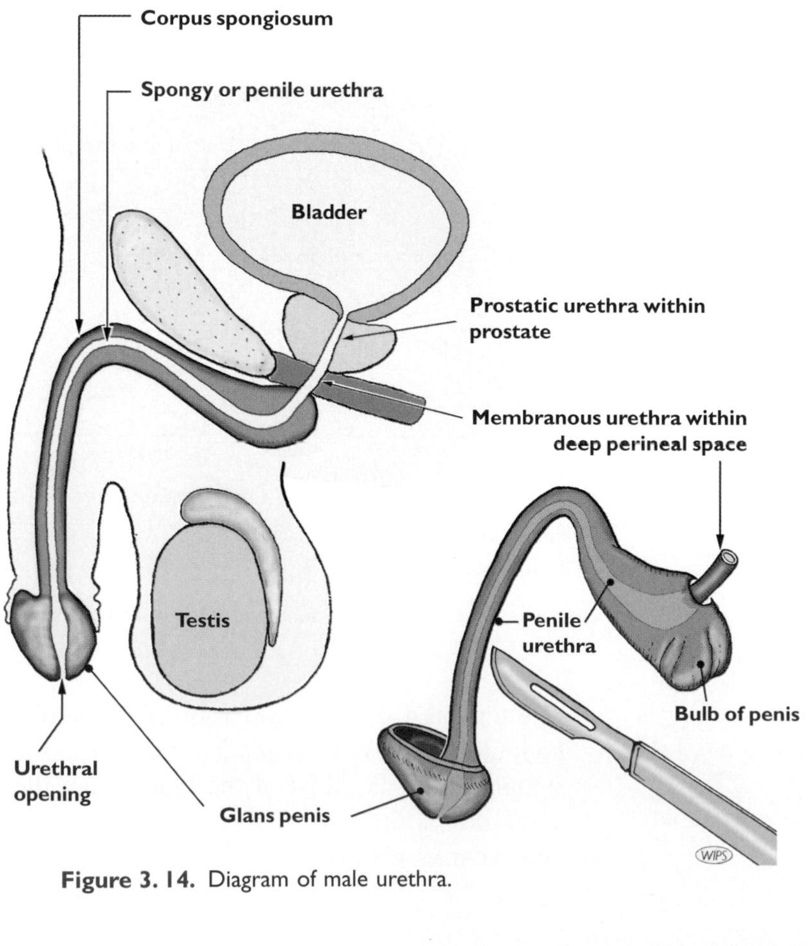

Figure 3.14. Diagram of male urethra.

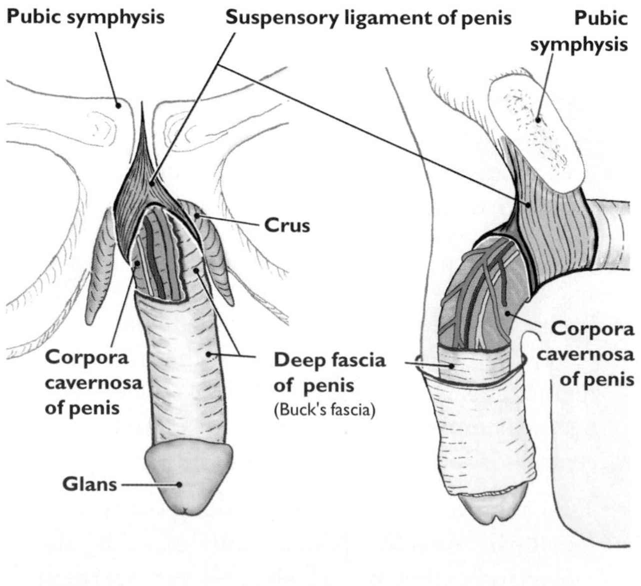

Figure 3.15. Suspensory ligament of penis: a triangular band attached anterior to the pubic symphysis.

- Make a distal cross section at the level of the navicular fossa of the **spongy urethra**. Note the erectile tissue surrounding the urethra.

- Make another more proximal cross section through the glans penis. Study the anatomical relations of **corona of glans, corpus cavernosum,** and **corpus spongiosum**.

Next, make another transverse section through the proximal part of the penis near its bulb.

- Observe the dark red cavernous structure of the erectile tissue of the corpus spongiosum and the two corpora cavernosa.

- Within the corpus cavernosum, identify the bilateral **deep artery of the penis** (artery of crus) that supplies the necessary blood to the erectile tissue. These arteries and also the artery to the bulb (i.e., to the corpus spongiosum) are **branches of the internal pudendal artery** (Fig. 3.13). This artery runs within the pudendal canal toward the symphysis pubis. Its branches include the artery to the bulb, the deep artery of the penis, and the dorsal artery of the penis. Store the detached penis in a plastic bag for future reference.

Examine the exposed **inferior fascia** of the deep perineal space (Fig. 3.13). Positively identify the sectioned urethra. Push a probe into the short **membranous portion** of the **urethra** that traverses the urogenital triangle close to the symphysis pubis.

Deep Perineal Space (Fig. 3.16)

Incise the inferior fascia of the urogenital diaphragm and remove it. You have now opened the **deep perineal space** or **pouch**. The contents of this space are:

- **Membranous Urethra.** It traverses the deep perineal pouch and extends from the inferior fascia inferiorly to the superior fascia of the deep perineal space superiorly. This is the shortest (about 1 cm), thinnest, narrowest, and least dilatable part of the urethra.

- **Sphincter Urethrae.** This important striated muscle surrounds the membranous urethra. When the muscle contracts, it compresses the urethra and stops the flow of urine.

⇦
GRANT'S 3.43B
ROHEN 319, 326
A.D.A.M. 4.44
NETTER 355
CLEMENTE 475-477

⇨
GRANT'S 3.37
ROHEN 331
A.D.A.M. 4.48
NETTER 357

⇦
ROHEN 326
NETTER 355
CLEMENTE 471, 473

⇦
GRANT'S 3.42
ROHEN 326
NETTER 355, 359
CLEMENTE 446, 473

⇦
GRANT'S 3.59B
ROHEN 328
A.D.A.M. 4.42, 4.44
NETTER 357
CLEMENTE 469, 470

⇦
GRANT'S 3.37
ROHEN 331
A.D.A.M. 4.48
NETTER 357
CLEMENTE 462

- **Deep Transverse Perineal Muscle.** This paired muscle originates at the pubic arch and meets the opposite muscle in a tendinous median raphe. The muscle and its raphe are attached to the perineal body.

- Other smaller structures include the **artery to the bulb,** the paired **bulbourethral glands** (Cowper's glands), and **branches** of the **pudendal nerve,** which supplies all muscles of the urogenital region.

Spread apart the muscle fibers of the deep perineal space and expose a small portion of the **superior fascia** of the deep perineal space. Realize that the **prostate gland** rests on the pelvic aspect of this superior fascia (Fig. 3.14). In addition, the superior fascia is related to the levator ani, particularly its anterior portion, the pubococcygeus or "puborectal sling."

> ***Note:*** The striated muscles stretching between the two sides of the pubic arch within the deep perineal space are also collectively known as the **urogenital diaphragm**. Although this term is part of the older anatomical nomenclature, you may still hear it; so, it is best to be familiar with it.
>
> Have all students in your group seen and studied the structures of the male urogenital triangle? If so, you may remove the wooden boards and/or ropes used to spread the lower limbs apart. Now return to the pelvic region.

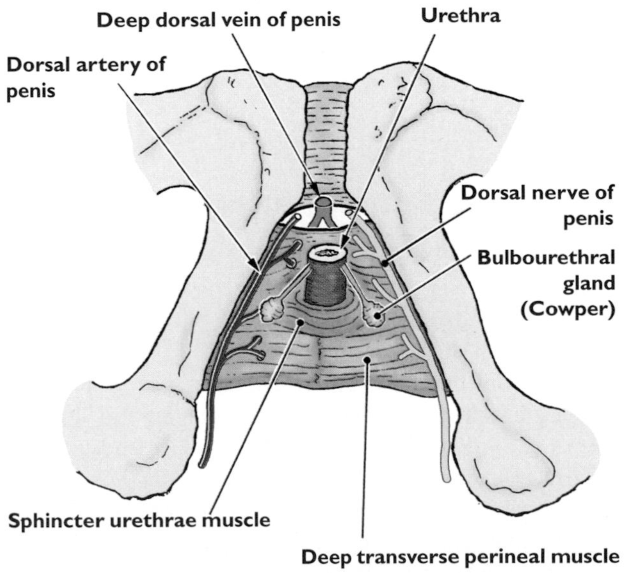

Figure 3. 16. Structures of the deep perineal space in the male.

Peritoneum in the Male Pelvis

Examine the **peritoneum** in the male pelvis (Fig. 3.17). The peritoneum passes from the anterior abdominal wall (**1**) to the level of the pubic bone (**2**) on to the superior surface of the urinary bladder (**3**). Next, it passes approximately 2 cm inferiorly along the posterior surface of the bladder (**4**) to cap the seminal vesicles which cannot be seen at this time (**5**). Posteriorly, the peritoneum lines the **rectovesical fossa** (**6**) to the middle part of the rectum. At this level, it covers only the anterior portion of the rectum. However, at higher levels it gradually envelops the sides of the rectum as well (**7**). Finally, at the third sacral vertebra, the peritoneum becomes the sigmoid mesocolon (**8**). The **paravesical fossa,** a peritoneal fossa, is apparent on each side of the bladder. The peritoneal recess on each side of the rectum is called the **pararectal fossa**.

Grant's 3.7
Rohen 316
A.D.A.M. 4.38
Netter 338
Clemente 439, 440
A.V.A. 3: 2.27.38

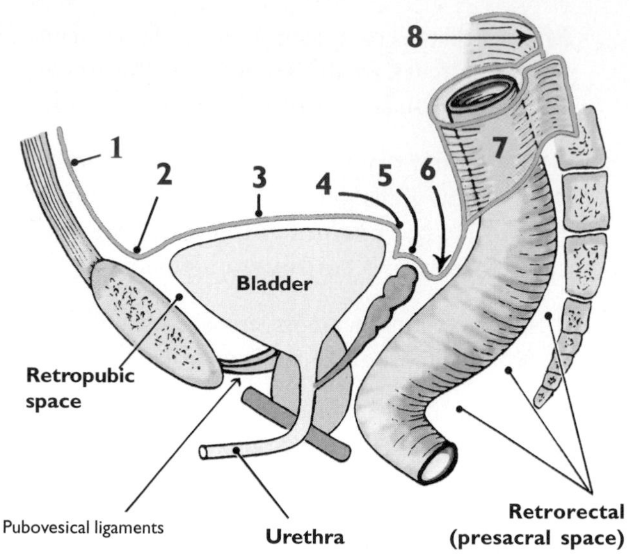

Figure 3.17. Peritoneum (green) in the male pelvis. The numbered portions of the peritoneum are explained in the text.

Structures Adhering to Peritoneum

With your fingers, detach the peritoneum from the pelvic wall and note the following structures that adhere to the peritoneum: **rectum**, **ureter**, **ductus deferens**, and **bladder**.

Grant's 3.6A
Rohen 316
A.D.A.M. 4.38
Netter 438, 440
Clemente 439, 440

Place your fingers between the symphysis pubis and anterior border of the bladder. Move the fingers to each side of the bladder. Inferiorly, the exploring finger is stopped by two cord-like thickenings of the pelvic fascia anchoring the neck of the bladder to the pubis; this is the **pubovesical ligament**.

> ***Clinical Correlation:*** As the bladder fills, the peritoneal reflection is elevated above the level of the pubic bones and raised from the anterior abdominal wall. Thus, a filled bladder can be surgically approached through an incision just above the pubic bones without entering the peritoneal cavity.

Retrorectal Space or Presacral Space
(Fig. 3.17)

Grant's 3.9A
Rohen 316, 317
A.D.A.M. 4.38
Netter 338
Clemente 445

The fused sacral vertebrae S3 to S5 and the coccyx are covered anteriorly with the rectum. Within the lesser pelvis, pass two fingers caudally behind the rectum and ease it off the sacrum and coccyx. Now, your fingers are in the deep **retrorectal space**. This space is limited inferiorly by a strong fascia investing the levator ani.

Push your fingers inferiorly and verify by palpation the inferior limit of the retrorectal (presacral) space.

Retropubic Space, Retrorectal Space, Nerves and Vessels

Retropubic Space (Fig. 3.17)

Grant's 3.7
Rohen 316, 317
A.D.A.M. 4.38
Netter 338
Clemente 440

The **retropubic space** (prevesical space, space of Retzius) is an extraperitoneal space that is U-shaped and lies between the symphysis pubis and the bladder and extends dorsally on each side of the bladder (Fig. 3.3). Posteriorly, the retropubic space is limited by the rectovesical fascia that contains arteries and veins of the bladder and of the internal genital organs. The retropubic space is filled with fat and loose areolar tissue that accommodates the expansion of the bladder.

Grant's 3.20
Rohen 325
A.D.A.M. 4.35
Netter 380
Clemente 456
A.V.A. 3: 2.34.18

Move your fingers laterally in the retrorectal space. Feel strands of **pelvic splanchnic nerves** (sacral parasympathetic outflow) on each side of the retrorectal space. These autonomic nerves branch off the ventral rami S2 through S4 after traversing the corresponding anterior sacral foramina (Fig. 3.18).

Clinical Correlation: Just as your fingers in the retrorectal space are limited inferiorly, so is the spread of an infection in this space. As a result of fascial arrangements, an infection, for example, a retrorectal abscess, cannot expand inferiorly. Instead, it is prone to rupture through the posterior wall of the rectum (which constitutes a lesser barrier) to drain into the rectum.

Since the pelvic splanchnic nerves (nervi erigentes; parasympathetic outflow of S2-S4; Fig. 3.18) are closely related to the lateral aspects of the rectum, they can also be easily injured during rectal surgery, for example, when the rectum must be entirely removed because of cancer. Injury to or loss of the pelvic splanchnic nerves results in impairment of bladder control and sexual function (loss of penile erection).

The process of well coordinated urination (micturition) is complex. It involves afferent pathways via the pelvic splanchnic nerves and the hypogastric nerves as well as micturition centers in the spinal cord and in the brain. Efferent pathways from the central nervous system to the bladder are mediated via sympathetic nerve fibers of the inferior hypogastric plexus and via parasympathetic fibers of the pelvic splanchnic nerves (Fig. 3.18). The pudendal nerve carries impulses to the striated and voluntary muscle fibers of the sphincter urethrae in the deep perineal space.

NETTER 368

GRANT'S TABLE 3.3
ROHEN 325
A.D.A.M. 413, 414
NETTER 374
CLEMENTE 410, 411
A.V.A. 3: 2.28.18

The common iliac artery divides into the external iliac artery and the internal iliac artery (Fig. 3.19). In the cadaver, follow the **internal iliac artery** and its branches to some extent. A complete dissection of these vessels will be done when the pelvic cavity is more accessible. Pay special attention to the obturator branch. With your finger, palpate the **obturator canal** that traverses the superior aspect of the obturator membrane. Once you have identified the obturator canal, you will also be able to find the **obturator artery** that runs together with the obturator nerve and vein. Follow the obturator artery proximally toward the internal iliac artery.

A.D.A.M. 4.22
NETTER 381
CLEMENTE 412

Clinical Correlation: Usually (in about 70% of cases), the obturator artery arises directly from the internal iliac artery. There is a slender anastomosis between obturator artery and inferior epigastric artery (a branch of the external iliac artery, Fig. 3.19). However, in about 25% of cases, the obturator artery may receive the bulk of its blood supply directly from the inferior epigastric artery. Which vascular arrangement can you identify in the cadaver? Surgeons must be aware of this vascular arrangement. The "anomalous" obturator artery is very vulnerable and can be easily injured during surgical repair of a femoral hernia. Uncontrolled bleeding from this vessel can be dangerous.

SCHEMATIC DIAGRAM OF NERVES TO THE BLADDER

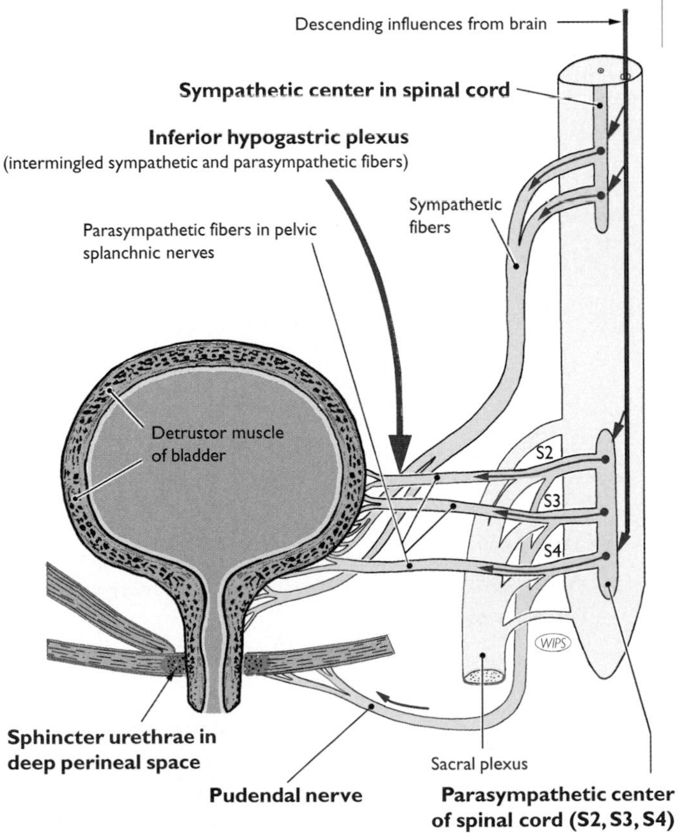

Figure 3.18. Schematic diagram of nerves to the bladder and the sphincter urethrae.

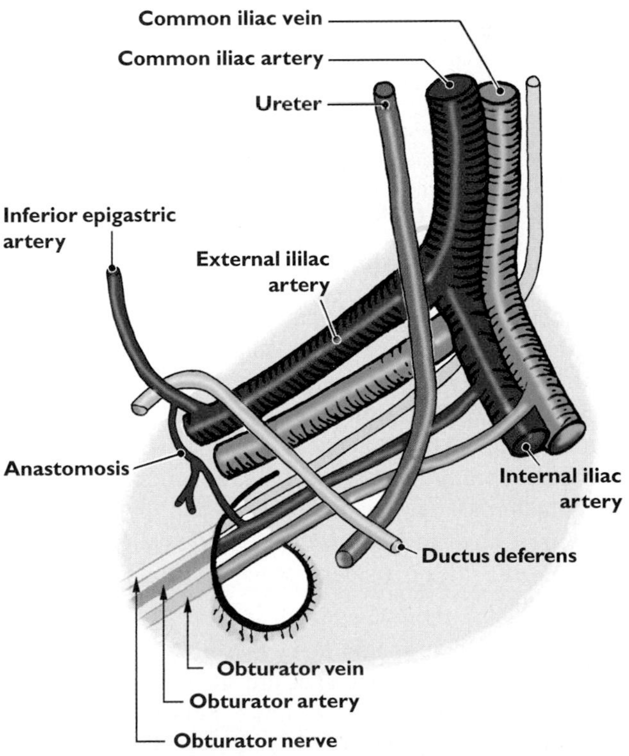

Figure 3.19. Structures on the lateral wall of the male pelvis. Note the medial position of the ureter and the ductus deferens.

Identify the **internal iliac vein** and some of its tributaries. Follow the vein to its junction with the **external iliac vein.** Here, the **common iliac vein** is formed. Note that the left common iliac vein lies directly posterior to the bifurcation of the aorta. This is of surgical importance, particularly in cases of abdominal aortic aneurysms.

GRANT'S 3.20
A.D.A.M. 4.15
NETTER 374
CLEMENTE 441
A.V.A. 3: 1.59.54

- On each side, identify the **ureter** as it crosses the external iliac vessels and the obturator vessels medially (Fig. 3.19). Follow it toward the urinary bladder as far as possible.

GRANT'S 3.13B, 3.20
ROHEN 316-319
A.D.A.M. 4.13
NETTER 338, 340, 372
CLEMENTE 439, 441

- Subsequently, identify the **ductus deferens** and follow it for some distance on its way to the prostate.
- Remove fat and areolar tissue surrounding vessels and ducts.
- Clean the accessible parts of the bladder wall, but do *not* destroy its blood supply.

Cleaning of the bladder wall will be facilitated by attaching a hemostat at its apex and pulling it taut. If in doubt whether or not the (collapsed) organ is really the bladder, make a small incision in the median plane and observe the lumen of this hollow organ. If the rectum interferes with the field of dissection, have your partner pull it to the left side. Frequently sponge the area to keep it clean. Moisten the dissecting field with mold-deterrent preservative fluid.

Pelvic Floor (Pelvic Diaphragm)

Lateral Wall of Pelvic Cavity

Identify the obturator foramen and the obturator nerve and vessels passing through the obturator canal. The obturator foramen (with its obturator membrane) is closed internally by the **obturator internus muscle.** Looking from within the lesser pelvis, only the most superior portion of the muscle can be seen at this time. Superiorly, the fascia of the obturator internus is thickened and forms a **tendinous arch** stretching from ischial spine to pubic bone. The **levator ani** arises, in part, from this tendinous arch (Figs.3.20B).

GRANT'S 3.13A
A.D.A.M. 4.10, 4.12
NETTER 335
CLEMENTE 457
A.V.A. 3: 2.16.54

The **pelvic diaphragm** is the fibromuscular floor that closes the inferior pelvic aperture. It is funnel-shaped. The rectum is anchored to it in the middle (Fig. 3.20A). The muscular components of the pelvic diaphragm can only be observed in part at this time, because of the intervening pelvic organs. The pelvic diaphragm will be com-

GRANT'S 3.5
A.D.A.M. 4.12
NETTER 335, 336
CLEMENTE 439, 455
A.V.A. 3: 2.18.54

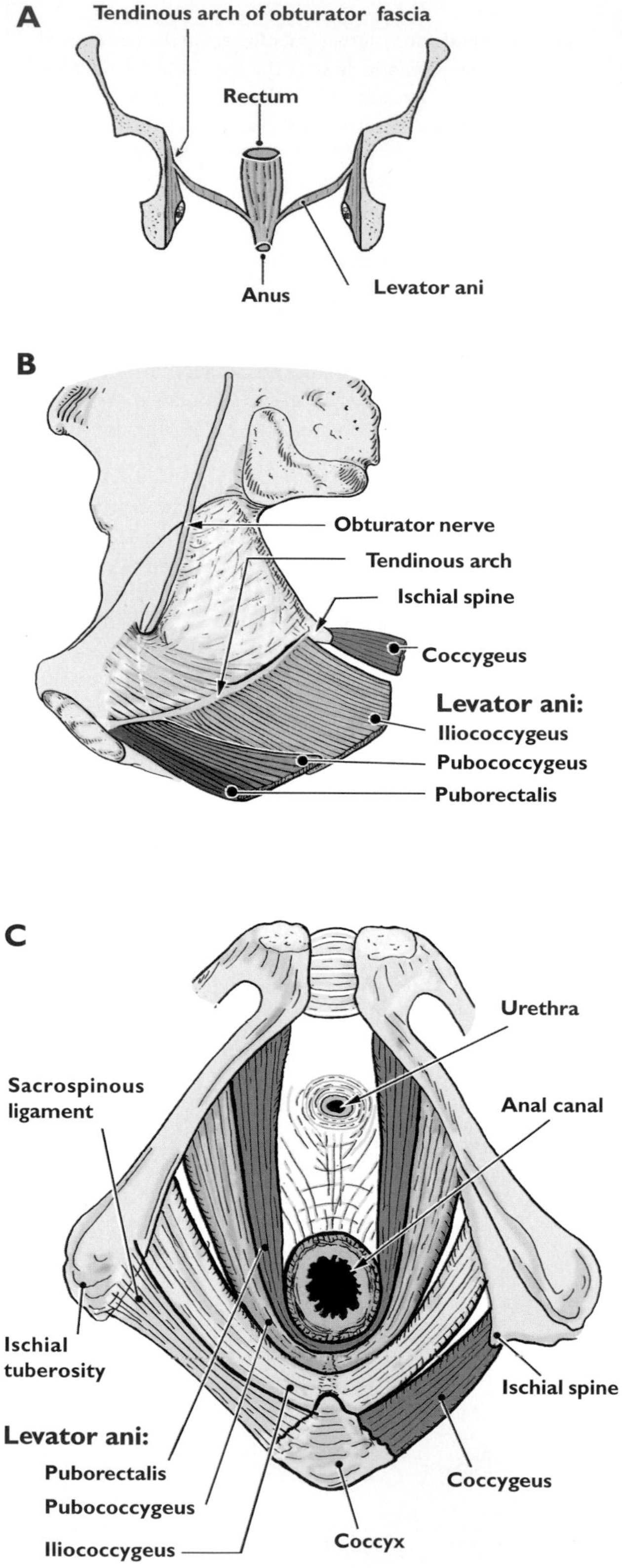

Figure 3.20. Levator ani in three different views. ***A,*** Funnel-shaped in coronal section. ***B,*** Originating from the tendinous arch medial to the obturator foramen. ***C,*** Forming the pelvic floor around the rectum in inferior view. Note two major components of the levator ani: the pubococcygeus and iliococcygeus. The third component, the coccygeus, lies deep to the sacrospinous ligament.

pletely dissected later after hemisection of the pelvis. However, it is important to have a conceptual understanding of these structures at this time.

The pelvic diaphragm is formed by the *two large levator ani muscles* and the *two smaller coccygeus muscles* (Fig. 3.20 B and C). The *external anal sphincter* may also be considered a part of the pelvic diaphragm. The funnel-shaped **levator ani** consists of three parts:

- **Puborectalis muscle**, the medial portion of the pubococcygeus muscle;
- **Pubococcygeus**, arising from the pubic bone;
- **Iliococcygeus**, arising from the tendinous arch.

The **pubococcygeus** is the thickened and most important part of the pelvic diaphragm. Fibers of the right and the left pubococcygeus unite *posterior* to the rectum. This union of fibers creates a U-shaped "puborectal sling" (Figs. 3.20C, 3.21). This sling is responsible for the curvature at the anorectal junction. During defecation, the puborectal sling relaxes, the anorectal junction is straightened, and the expulsion of fecal matter is facilitated. The **levator ani muscles** raise the pelvic floor and assist the anterior abdominal muscle in increasing the intra-abdominal pressure when necessary (e. g., during urination, straining, vomiting, forced expiration, and when lifting heavy objects).

The two **coccygeus muscles** arise from the ischial spine and form the posterior and smaller part of the pelvic diaphragm. Each coccygeus is essentially a triangular muscular sheet that lies posterior to the iliococcygeus muscle. The two coccygeus muscles assist the levator ani in supporting the pelvic organs.

Review all structures of the male pelvis and perineum that have been dissected and seen so far. Make sure your laboratory partners have also participated in the review process. Subsequently, the pelvis will be sectioned in the midsagittal plane to facilitate more detailed studies of pelvic structures.

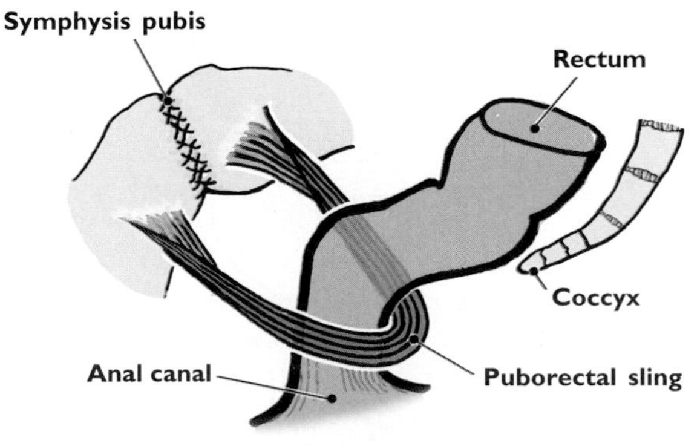

Figure 3.21. The *puborectal sling* is formed by the right and left puborectalis muscles which unite posterior to the rectum. The puborectalis is the thickened, medial portion of the pubococcygeus muscle.

GRANT'S 3.5
A.D.A.M. 4.50
NETTER 336
CLEMENTE 464
A.V.A. 3: 2.20.03

GRANT'S 3.10A, 3.22A
A.D.A.M. 4.50
NETTER 336
A.V.A. 3: 2.20.18

GRANT'S 3.6A
ROHEN 317
A.D.A.M. 4.35, 4.38
NETTER 338
CLEMENTE 445

Hemisection

Before you begin ...

Check with your instructor if you are allowed to proceed. The **goal** is to make a careful midsagittal split of all (soft and bony) structures from the perineum up to the level of vertebra L3. Subsequently, the body will be transected at the vertebral level of L3 to L4. One lower extremity (preferably the left one) remains attached to the rest of the body while the other side (preferably the right one) is mobilized. If this procedure is done with care, it will facilitate complete dissection and examination of the pelvis.

Section

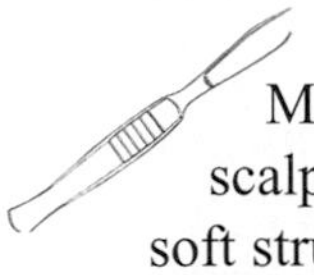

Make sure you are using a new and sharp scalpel. Use it to make a precise split of all soft structures in the midsagittal plane:

- Start posterior to the symphysis pubis in the midsagittal plane. Carry this midsagittal section through the entire bladder wall. Sponge the interior of the urinary bladder. Continue to cut inferior to the bladder and split the prostate gland.
- Subsequently, cut through the anterior and posterior walls of the rectum. Sponge it clean! Be careful *not* to cut into the sigmoid colon or any other loop of the GI tract! Now, the blade should have reached the anterior surface of the sacrum.
- Finally, push the knife inferior to the symphysis pubis with the cutting edge directed posteriorly. In the midsagittal plane, cut through the pelvic diaphragm from symphysis pubis to coccyx.

Obtain a suitable hand saw and make two cuts in the midsagittal plane:

- Cut through the symphysis pubis.
- Start at the coccyx and extend the midline cut through the sacrum up to the third lumbar vertebra. Be careful *not* to injure the nerves of the cauda equina. During sawing, pull these nerves laterally for protection.

If you have decided to mobilize the right lower extremity (which is preferred), proceed as follows:

- Cut horizontally through the right half of the intervertebral disc between L3 and L4 until this cut meets the superior extent of the midsagittal section of the vertebral column.

• Cautiously mobilize the right lower extremity to some extent. Cut nerves and blood vessels connecting the right lower limb with the rest of the body. Section the right ureter. Now, the right lower limb can be removed.

GRANT'S 3.37B
ROHEN 331
A.D.A.M. 4.10, 4.48
NETTER 343
CLEMENTE 462

Continue with your studies of the *male* pelvic structures using either half of the hemisectioned pelvis. The pelvic structures are now readily accessible. Examine and dissect these structures and note their topographical relations:

GRANT'S 3.16
ROHEN 318
A.D.A.M. 4.35
NETTER 358
CLEMENTE 442, 446

Urethra (Fig. 3.14)

The urethra is divided into **three portions: spongy or penile, membranous,** and **prostatic.** The **spongy portion** (penile urethra) has been studied already together with the anatomical components of the penis. The **membranous urethra** was seen earlier when the contents of the deep perineal space, or pouch, was explored. Now, in the bisected specimen, study the membranous urethra again. If the hemisection was done perfectly in the midsagittal plane, then the longitudinally opened halves of the membranous urethra should be present in each hemisectioned specimen. Otherwise, refer to the specimen that contains the membranous urethra. Note that it is only about 1 cm long and traverses the urogenital diaphragm.

GRANT'S 3.6
ROHEN 316, 317
A.D.A.M. 4.35, 4.38
NETTER 338
CLEMENTE 445
A.V.A. 3: 2.24.00

Within the deep perineal space, it is surrounded by a sphincter muscle, the **sphincter urethrae**. Be aware of the nerve supply to this important muscle (Fig. 3.18).

Prostate and Prostatic Urethra (Fig. 3.22)

In the bisected specimen, note that the prostate rests on the superior fascia of the urogenital diaphragm. Using a probe, identify the longitudinally sectioned **prostatic urethra.** Follow this structure proximally into the bladder.

Examine the **interior** of the **prostatic urethra**:

• Note its approximate length: 3 cm.

• On the posterior wall, observe a median ridge, the **urethral crest.** The ovoid enlargement of the crest is the **colliculus seminalis.**

• In the midline of the colliculus, find a small blind opening, the utricle.

• On each side of the utricle, find the minute **orifice** of the **ejaculatory duct.** You may have to use a magnifying glass.

GRANT'S 3.17
ROHEN 318
A.D.A.M. 4.10
NETTER 358
CLEMENTE 442, 446

• On each side of the urethral crest, observe a groove, the **prostatic sinus.** Here, the numerous ducts of the prostate open into the urethra.

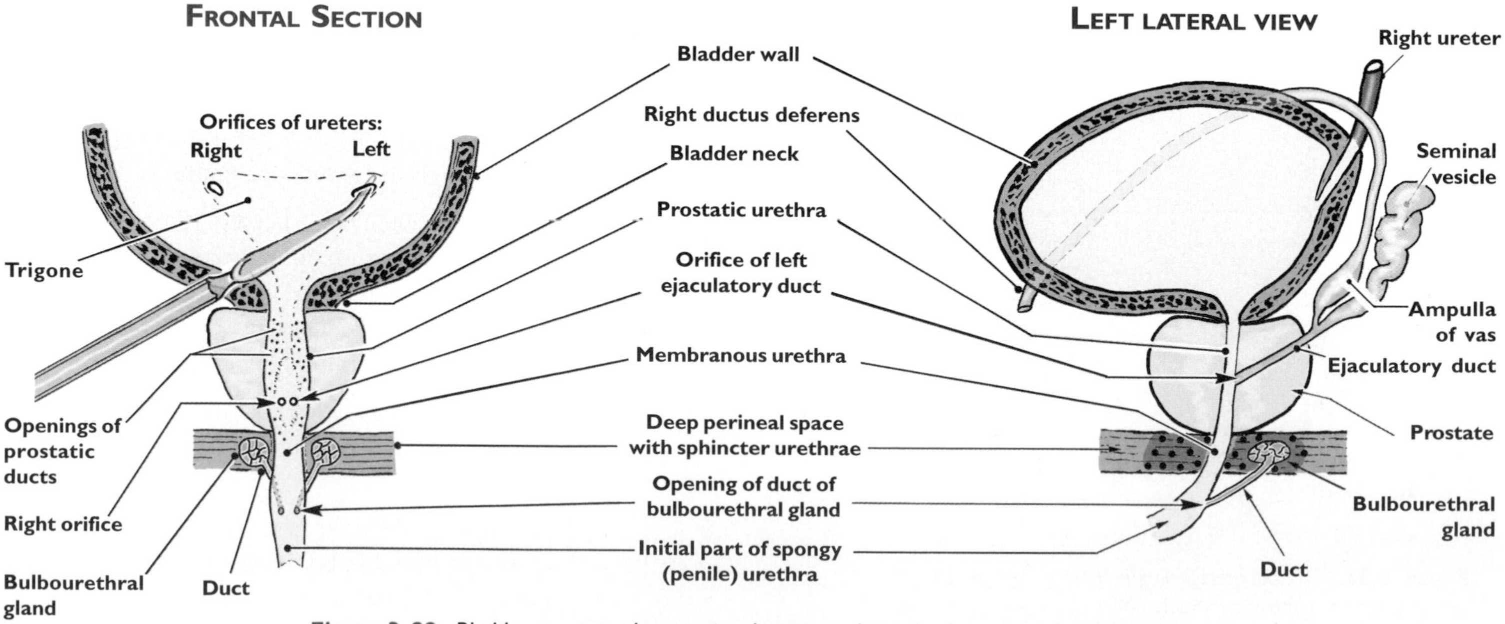

Figure 3.22. Bladder, prostate, deep perineal space, and proximal portion of male urethra on frontal section and in left lateral view. The probe is located at the left ureteric orifice.

Ductus (Vas) Deferens

Proceeed as follows (Fig. 3.23):

- Pick up the ductus deferens as it crosses the external iliac vessels medially. Note that the ductus is closely related to the inferior epigastric vessels.
- Follow the ductus deferens inferiorly and observe that is crosses the obturator nerve and vessels medially.
- Next, follow the ductus toward the bladder. Near the posterolateral angle of the bladder, it crosses anterior to the ureter (Fig. 3.23).
- Subsequently, follow the duct along the posterior aspect of the bladder. Here it expands to form the **ampulla**. Lateral to each ampulla lies a **seminal vesicle**. Each seminal vesicle is a convoluted tube.
- Using a probe, carefully expose the union of the ampulla and the **duct of the seminal vesicle**. This is the beginning of the **ejaculatory duct,** which traverses the posterior half of the prostate gland and terminates at the colliculus in the prostatic urethra (Fig. 3.22).

Urinary Bladder

During section of the pelvis, the urinary bladder was completely opened and divided into right and left halves. Examine the **muscular coat** of the organ. It consists of bundles of smooth muscle. This muscular coat is collectively called the detrusor urinae (L. *detrudere*, to thrust out).

Examine the **interior of the bladder**:

- The **trigone** (Fig. 3.22) is an equilateral triangle on the posterior wall (now divided). Its angles are formed by the **two orifices** of the **ureters** and the **internal urethral orifice.** The internal urethral orifice is situated at the lowest (most inferior) point of the bladder.
- Note that the mucous membrane over the trigone is smooth. Over the other parts of the bladder, it lies in folds when the bladder is empty.
- Pass a fine probe into the orifice of the ureter (Fig. 3.22). Verify that the ureter traverses the muscular wall of the bladder in an oblique fashion.

GRANT'S 3.14
ROHEN 316
A.D.A.M. 4.13, 4.24
NETTER 358
CLEMENTE 443
A.V.A. 3: 1.52.54

GRANT'S 3.15
ROHEN 3.16
A.D.A.M. 4.13, 4.24
NETTER 358
CLEMENTE 443, 449

GRANT'S 3.16
ROHEN 317
A.D.A.M. 4.13
NETTER 343, 358
CLEMENTE 442, 443

GRANT'S 3.17
ROHEN 318
A.D.A.M. 4.10
NETTER 358
CLEMENTE 442

A.D.A.M. 4.24
NETTER 338
CLEMENTE 443, 448

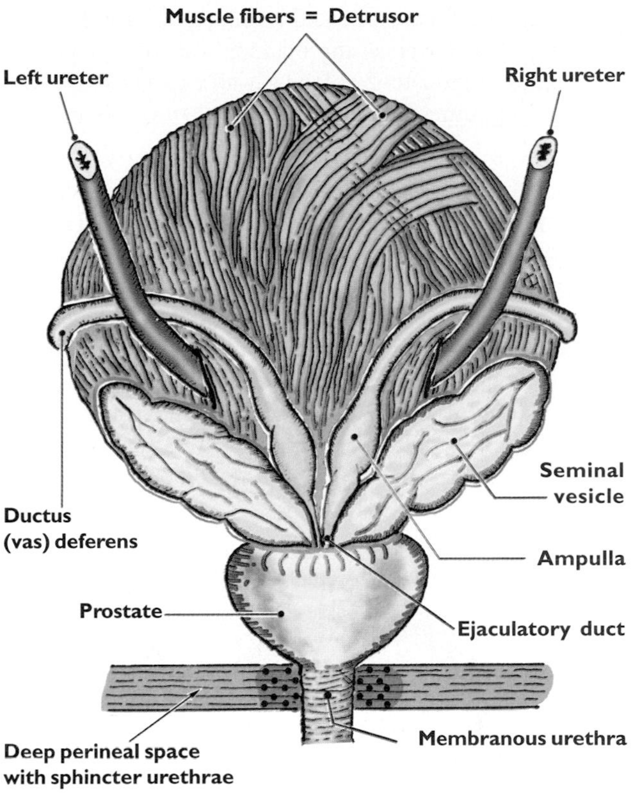

Figure 3. 23. Posterior view of urinary bladder, ureters, deferent ducts, seminal vesicles, and prostate.

Ureter (Fig. 3.23)

Pick up the ureter as it crosses the external iliac artery and follow it to the posterolateral portion of the urinary bladder. Here, at the ureterovesical junction, the ureter travels obliquely through the bladder wall.

> ***Clinical Correlation:*** What would happen if the ureters were just mere tubes, passively allowing the flow of urine? Imagine doing a hand stand or hanging by your feet; would the urine from a full bladder rush back into the kidneys? Fortunately and thanks to the ureteral peristaltic waves, this does not happen in a healthy person. However, in some persons the peristaltic movements are absent; and in these individuals the ureters are considerably dilated, a matter of significant clinical concern.
>
> The ureters are also involved in the often extremely painful passage of kidney stones. These stones have to pass through the ureters on their way from the kidney to the bladder. In the process, such stones may get stuck in the ureter.

Ureterovesical Junction

The junction between each ureter and the bladder (vesica) is appropriately called the ureterovesical junction. This area is of particular interest because it is clinically important. It is also ingeniously designed and constructed for maximal efficiency. Figure 3.24 and its enlarged inset illustrate that the ureter traverses the bladder wall obliquely. The ureter ends at the interior bladder wall as a slit-like opening, the **ostium**, through which the urine enters the bladder.

What then prevents the urine from flowing back (refluxing) into the ureters and toward the kidneys? The dynamics are twofold. To a certain extent, the slit-like opening acts as a valve, particularly when the bladder is only partially full (*Force A*). When the bladder contracts, muscles in the bladder wall compress the obliquely set portion of the ureter within the bladder wall (*Force B*). When the bladder is full (distended) with accumulated urine, the internal fluid pressure on the bladder wall flattens the ureter and thus effectively compresses it and blocks if off.

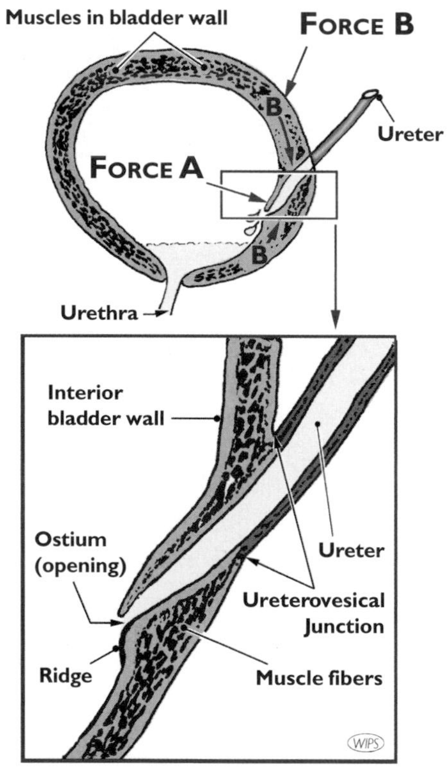

Figure 3.24. Ureterovesical junction and ostium (opening) of the ureter into the interior of the bladder.

> ***Clinical Correlation:*** The valve-like action at the **ureterovesical junction** (Fig. 3.24) works only if the bladder wall is of normal thickness. When the bladder wall is excessively thinned out (as in a chronically distended bladder with bladder outlet obstruction), the ureters cannot be adequately compressed within the bladder wall. As a result, urine will reflux into the ureters and toward the kidneys; and this leads to medically undesirable consequences for the kidneys.
>
> The ureterovesical junction is a relatively narrow passage; thus, a kidney stone can easily get trapped here. If this happens, the associated colicky pain can be severe. Once the stone has passed into the bladder, the pain stops suddenly.

GRANT'S TABLE 3.3
ROHEN 325
A.D.A.M. 4.13
NETTER 374
CLEMENTE 410
A.V.A. 3: 2.28.10

Internal Iliac Artery and Branches (Fig. 3.25)

You may not have time to dissect all 10 branches of the internal iliac artery. Demonstrate at least the following:

- Identify the **umbilical artery.** Note that it gives off 3 to 4 **superior vesical arteries** that supply the superior aspect of the bladder. The umbilical artery continues toward the anterior abdominal wall where it becomes the **medial umbilical ligament** (obliterated umbilical artery). Verify:

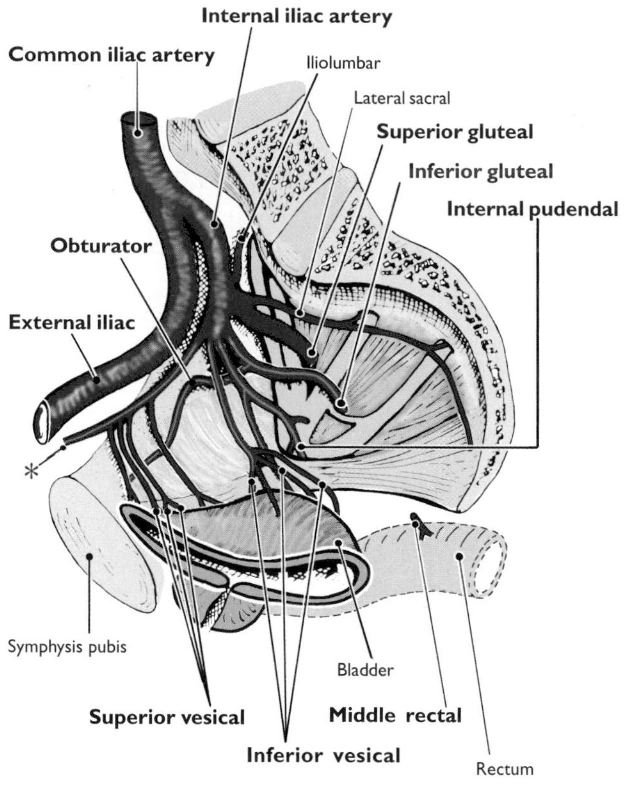

Figure 3.25. Internal iliac artery and its branches in the male pelvis. The asterick (*) denotes the obliterated umbilical artery.

- Trace the **obturator artery** from its point of origin toward the superior aspect of the obturator foramen.
- Follow a branch of the internal iliac artery to the posteroinferior part of the bladder and to the region of the prostate and seminal vesicles. This is the **inferior vesical artery** (not present in the female).
- The **middle rectal artery** is a small vessel to the lateral aspect of the rectum.
- Follow the important **internal pudendal artery** (which is larger in the male than in the female)

GRANT'S 3.12A
A.D.A.M. 4.53
NETTER 369
CLEMENTE 411, 453
A.V.A. 3: 2.29.23

to the inferior part of the greater sciatic foramen. This artery is closely related to the sacrospinous ligament. The internal pudendal artery has been encountered earlier in the pudendal canal where it gives off branches to the ischioanal fossa and where it divides into its terminal branches: the deep artery of the penis and the dorsal artery of the penis.

- The **inferior gluteal artery** also passes through the inferior part of the greater sciatic foramen. This vessel passes between the sacral nerves of the sacral plexus.
- The **superior gluteal artery** is relatively large and runs in close relationship to the lumbosacral trunk. This vessel leaves the pelvis through the superior part of the greater sciatic foramen.
- Identify some of the branches of the internal iliac artery in an iliac arteriogram.

Observe the **rectal venous plexus.** Note the numerous veins on the surface of the rectum. Observe the **vesical venous plexus** at the base of the bladder. It receives blood from the **prostatic venous plexus,** which lies ventral and lateral to the prostate. Pick up the **deep dorsal vein of the penis** just inferior to the symphysis pubis and verify that it empties into the prostatic venous plexus. Do not dissect these complex pelvic venous plexuses. Remove all tributaries to the internal iliac vein so that the arterial distribution can be clearly demonstrated.

Clinical Correlation: The venous plexuses in the pelvis intercommunicate. This is of considerable clinical importance (e.g., transportation of tumor cells along vascular channels).

The importance of the **rectal venous plexus** in cases of portal venous hypertension has been stressed earlier during dissection of the portal system. Remember that the superior rectal vein originates from the rectal venous plexus. The rectal venous plexus is also drained by the middle and inferior rectal veins that, in turn, empty into the caval system of veins. In portal venous hypertension, blood flow in the superior rectal vein may be reversed: portal blood may be carried to the rectal plexus and, from there, shunted into the caval system. The resulting increased blood flow and pressure in the rectal venous plexus leads to the development of hemorrhoids. Thus, in case of hemorrhoids, the physician must always evaluate the condition of the portal venous system. The portal venous system has no valves. This fact explains why the blood flow in the portal system can be easily reversed.

➪ *GRANT'S 3.11B*
A.D.A.M. 4.55
NETTER 365
CLEMENTE 450

⇦ *GRANT'S TABLE 3.3*
ROHEN 325
A.D.A.M. 4.13
NETTER 374
CLEMENTE 411
A.V.A. 3: 2.28.26

⇦ *GRANT'S 2.49*
NETTER 370
A.D.A.M. 4.15, 4.54
CLEMENTE 441

⇦ A.D.A.M. 4.15
NETTER 374
CLEMENTE 441

⇦ *GRANT'S 2.49, 2.50A*
ROHEN 282
A.D.A.M. 4.54
NETTER 370
CLEMENTE 455

Anal Canal (Fig. 3.26)

During bisection of the pelvis, the anal canal has been opened. Clean it thoroughly. Examine the interior features (this may be difficult to demonstrate in some cadavers):

- **Anal columns**. These are 5 to 10 longitudinal ridges of mucosa in the superior part of the anal canal. The terminal "branches" of the superior rectal vessels are contained in the anal columns. Here, the superior rectal veins of the portal system anastomose with middle and inferior rectal veins of the caval system. Abnormal increase in pressure in the valveless portal system leads to an enlargement of the veins contained in the anal columns, resulting in "internal hemorrhoids."
- **Anal valves,** semilunar folds uniting the lower ends of the anal columns. If these anal valves are torn by hard fecal material, an infection can occur and spread from the injured anal valves into the wall of the anal canal.
- In addition, examine the **sphincter muscles** of the **anus** and the puborectal sling on section.

Place a gloved finger into the split anal canal and proceed as follows:

- Palpate and visualize topographically related structures (as if performing a digital rectal examination).
- Palpate the muscular wall formed by the sphincter ani externus.

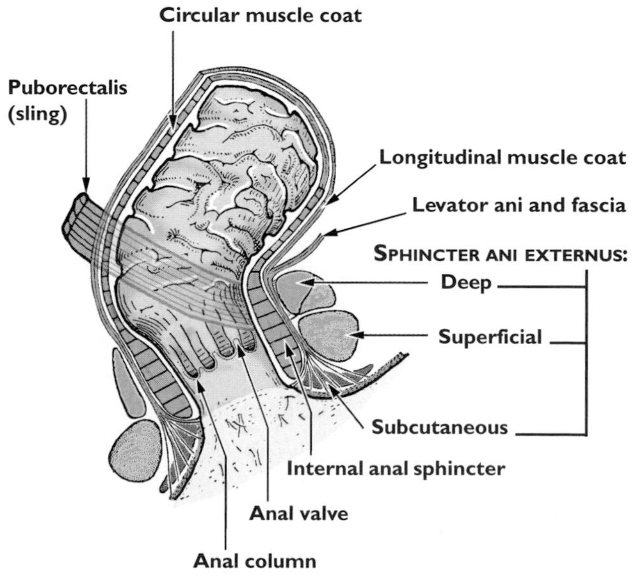

Figure 3.26. Rectum, anal canal, and anal sphincter.

- More superiorly, at the anorectal junction, feel the puborectalis (puborectal sling; part of levator ani).
- Verify that anterior to the finger (i.e., anterior to the rectum), the prostate and the seminal vesicles can be palpated.

Clinical Correlation: **Rectal examination** is an important part of every physical examination.The size and consistency of the prostate gland can be assessed. Normally, the wall of the rectum can be moved against the prostate because of the intervening areolar tissue. If this is not possible, one should suspect malignant tumor infiltration from prostate into rectum.

Posteriorly, the anterior surface of sacrum and coccyx can be palpated. Laterally, the ischioanal fossa can be examined. Thus, a pathological process (e.g., abscess) in these regions may be detected by digital examination. Appreciate this unique opportunity to combine digital palpation with visual observation.

Levator Ani

The levator ani is funnel-shaped (Fig. 3.20A). In the middle of this funnel, the prostate is supported anteriorly, and the rectum is positioned posteriorly (Fig. 3.17). Examine the **origins of the levator ani**: Identify the thickened fascia of the obturator internus stretching from pubic bone to ischial spine and forming a tendinous arch. From this **tendinous arch** the levator ani originates in part (Fig. 3.20B). Verify this. Identify the *three portions* of the **levator ani**:

- **Puborectalis muscle**, the medial portion of the pubococcygeus muscle; forming the puborectal sling;
- **Pubococcygeus**, arising from the pubic bone; it is the thickest and most important portion of the levator ani.
- **Iliococcygeus**, arising from the tendinous arch.

Identify the **coccygeus muscle** (Fig. 3.20 B and C). It stretches from the ischial spine to the coccyx and forms the posterior and smaller part of the pelvic diaphragm. The coccygeus is essentially a triangular muscular sheet that lies posterior to the iliococcygeus muscle. Note that the ischiococcygeus contributes to the sacrospinous ligament.

Piriformis Muscle

Observe its origin from the pelvic or ventral surface of the sacrum at segments S2, S3, and S4. Note that the muscle fibers converge and pass through the greater sciatic foramen. The ventral nerve rami S2 and S3 emerge between the digitations of the piriformis.

GRANT'S 3.21
ROHEN 446, 447
A.D.A.M. 5.26
NETTER 463-465
CLEMENTE 365-367
A.V.A. 3: 2.30.56

Sacral Plexus

The sacral nervous plexus is closely related to the anterior surface of the piriformis. In the cadaver, verify the following (Fig. 3.27):

- The **lumbosacral trunk** (L4, L5) contributes to the sacral plexus.
- The ventral rami of S2 and S3 emerge between the digitations of the piriformis.
- Ventral rami from L4 through S3 converge and form the large **sciatic nerve**. It passes through the greater sciatic foramen together with the piriformis.
- Usually, the **gluteal arteries** (branches of the internal iliac artery) pierce the sacral plexus: Often, the lumbosacral trunk and S1 are separated by the superior gluteal artery. Occasionally, the superior gluteal artery intervenes between L4 and L5. The inferior gluteal artery usually separates ramus S1 from S2.
- Ventral rami S2, S3, and S4 contribute to the **pudendal nerve** (Figs. 3.27 and 3.28). Remem-

GRANT'S 3.21B
ROHEN 447
NETTER 463
A.V.A. 2: 0.42.16

GRANT'S 3.13A
A.D.A.M. 4.10, 4.12
NETTER 335
CLEMENTE 457
A.V.A. 3: 2.17.53

GRANT'S 3.5
A.D.A.M. 4.12
NETTER 335, 336
CLEMENTE 439, 455
A.V.A. 3: 2.18.36

GRANT'S 3.4, 3.21A
ROHEN 325, 446
NETTER 465
CLEMENTE 410
A.V.A. 3: 2.16.37

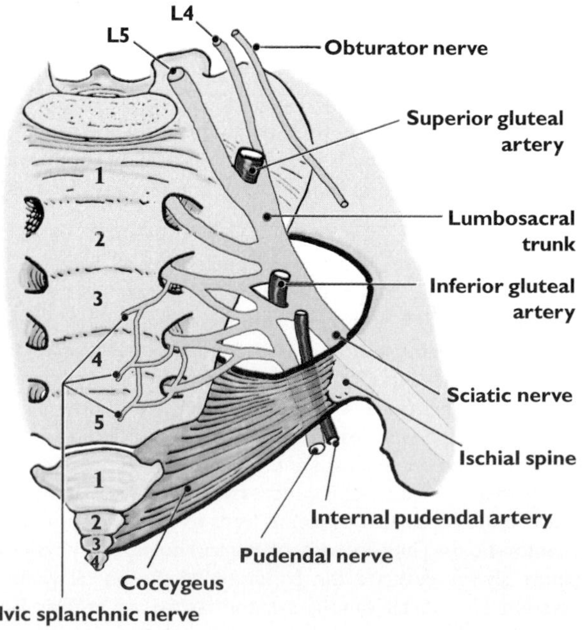

Figure 3.27. Sacral nerve plexus and related vessels.

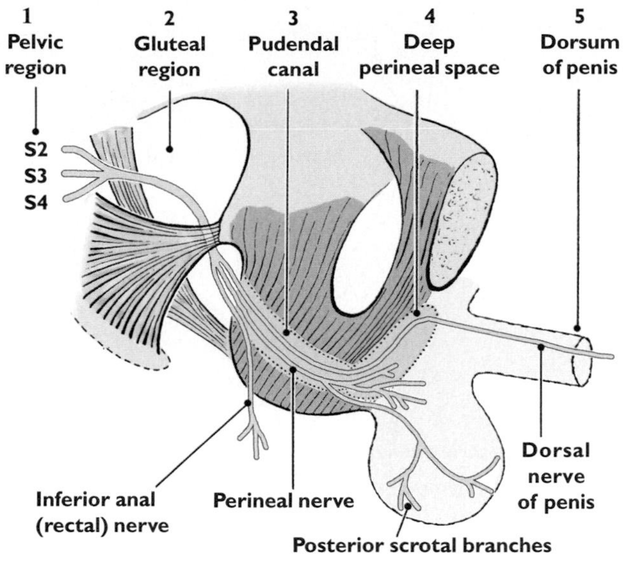

Figure 3.28. Diagram of the pudendal nerve. The nerve passes through 5 regions. It divides into 3 major branches.

ber, ventral rami S2, S3, and S4 contain preganglionic parasympathetic fibers (sacral parasympathetic outflow; pelvic splanchnic nerves). These autonomic nerves supply pelvic organs and the distal portion of the GI tract from left colic flexure to rectum.

- Note the sympathetic chain and its **ganglia** medial to the sacral foramina. These ganglia give off gray rami communicantes to the ventral sacral rami. Review the entire innervation of the *male* pelvis.

GRANT'S 3.23, 3.24
ROHEN 314
A.D.A.M. 4.19
NETTER 380, 381
CLEMENTE 456
A.V.A. 3: 2.34.00

Lymphatic Drainage of the Male Pelvis

GRANT'S 3.25
A.D.A.M. 4.21, 4.22
NETTER 379
CLEMENTE 369

Lymphatic channels are difficult to see unless injected with a dye. However, you may encounter lymph nodes in certain pelvic regions, particularly if there was a pelvic inflammatory or malignant process prior to death. Understand that the penis, scrotum, and spongy urethra have a different lymphatic drainage than the testes and prostate. This is of considerable clinical significance. Familiarize yourself with the lymphatic drainage of the rectum.

Female Pelvis and Perineum

General Arrangement

Study the general arrangement of the *soft parts* of the female pelvis (Fig. 3.29):

- The **perineum** is the area between the thighs.
- The perineal region is diamond-shaped and divided into two triangular areas, the **anal region** (or triangle) and the **urogenital region** (or triangle).

GRANT'S 3.26
ROHEN 332-335
A.D.A.M. 4.29
NETTER 337
CLEMENTE 394
A.V.A. 3: 2.23.50

- The **anal canal** is located in the anal triangle. It pierces the levator ani muscle.
- The **urinary bladder** is supported by the muscular pelvic floor.
- The **urethra** is short (3.5 to 4 cm). It pierces the anterior portion of the urogenital diaphragm.
- The **vagina** is about 7 to 8 cm long. The vagina also traverses the urogenital diaphragm.
- The posterior wall of the vagina is in contact with the rectum.

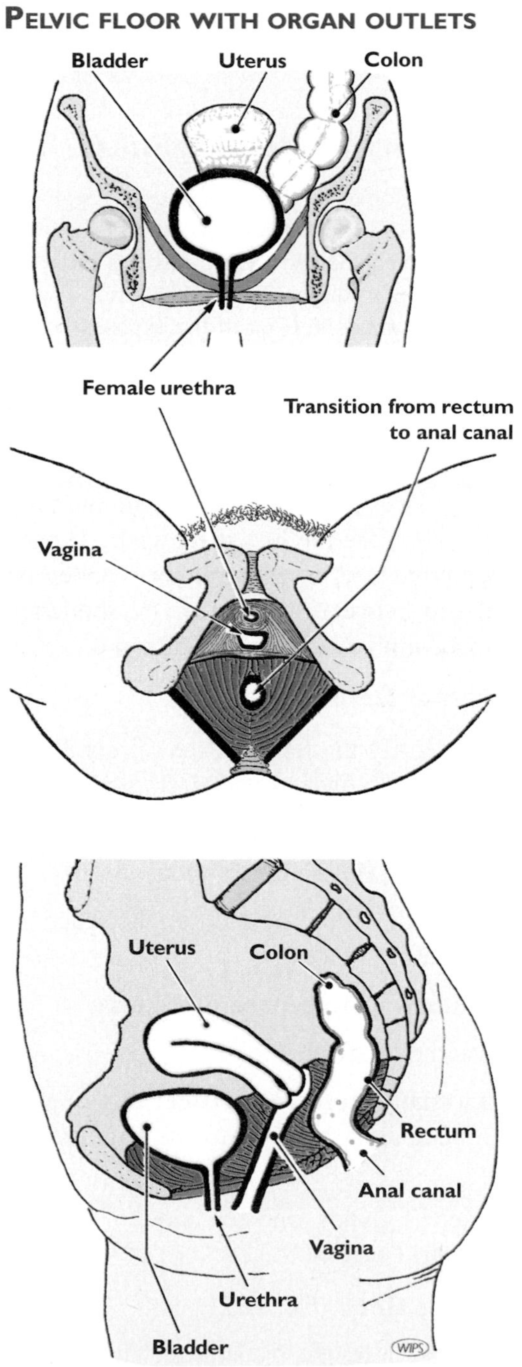

Figure 3.29. General arrangement of female pelvic organs, pelvic floor, and perineum.

- The middle portion of the anterior vaginal wall is in contact with the bladder.
- The **uterus** is about 7 cm long. It intervenes between bladder and rectum. The longitudinal axes of uterus and vagina are at almost a right angle.
- **Fornix of vagina** (L. *fornix*, arch). This circular gutter surrounds the intravaginal part of the cervix uteri. It is divisible into *anterior, posterior,* and *lateral parts*. Posteriorly, the fornix is larger than anteriorly.
- The **anal canal** and the **anus** are constructed as in the male.

The anal region has already been studied (see earlier part of this chapter). Now the urogenital region (triangle) must be dissected.

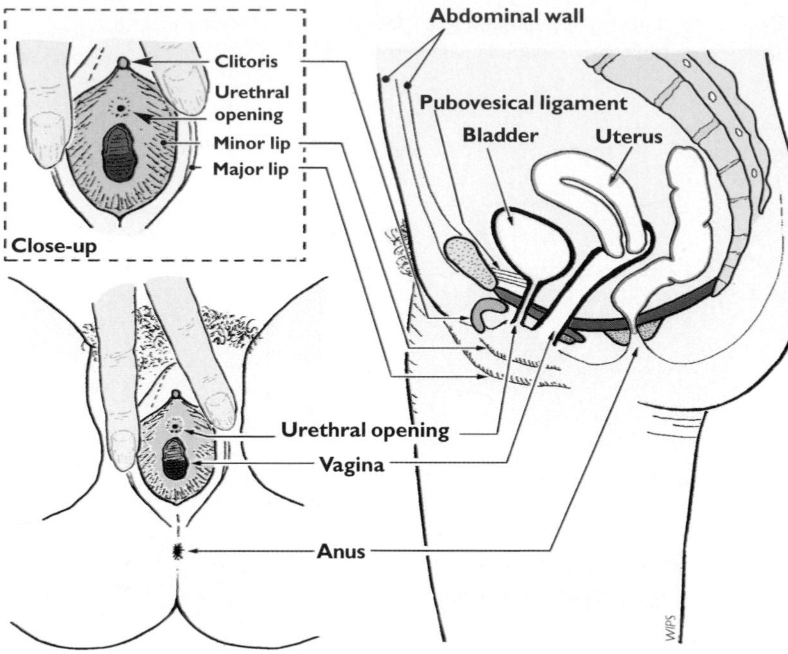

Figure 3.30. General arrangement of female external genitalia and pelvic organs.

Female Urogenital Region (Triangle)

The dissection of the female urogenital region will be done by using the so-called "traditional approach," which is preferred by many anatomists. The cadaver is in the supine position (face up). The thighs are widely stretched apart. The dissector sits or stands in front of the exposed perineal region (just as a gynecologist would). Usually, only one student can work on the region at a given time. The lighting must be excellent.

Place the cadaver in the supine position. Stretch the thighs widely apart. This can be accomplished by using either wooden boards placed between the feet or by abducting the lower limbs with the aid of ropes.

External Genitalia

Identify the female external genitalia, collectively known as *vulva* (Figs. 3.30, 3.31): Mons pubis;

Grant's 3.37F, 3.45
Rohen 340
A.D.A.M. 4.2
Netter 337, 350
Clemente 323, 324

- **Labia majora** and **minora**;
- Vestibule of the vagina (i.e., the space between the labia minora);
- **Clitoris** and **prepuce of clitoris**;
- Vaginal orifice;
- **External urethral orifice**; this opening lies immediately anterior to the vaginal orifice;
- Openings of the **paraurethral glands** or Skene's glands on each side of the external urethral orifice.

Netter 350

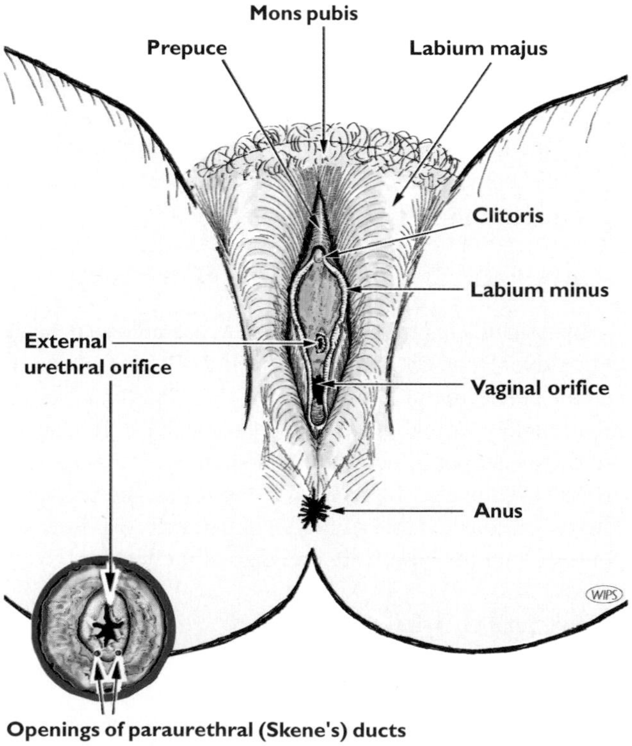

Figure 3.31. Female external genitalia.

Skin Incisions (Fig. 3.32)

Make a transverse skin incision that passes between both ischial tuberosities and crosses the midline between anal and vaginal orifices. Make a midline incision from the just established transverse incision toward the pubic symphysis, encircling the labia majora.

Proceed as follows:

- Reflect the skin flaps laterally and remove them.
- Raise the skin off the two labia majora, but leave the underlying mass of fat undisturbed.
- Place a finger into the ischioanal (ischiorectal) fossa and palpate the base of the urogenital triangle stretching between the ischial tuberosities via the perineal body. The **perineal body** is a fibromuscular node in the median plane where several perineal muscles converge and interlace.

GRANT'S 3.45, 3.46
ROHEN 342, 343
A.D.A.M. 4.39
NETTER 351
CLEMENTE 430

Study the mass of fat underlying each labium majus. Usually, it consists of a long finger-like process extending from the anterior abdominal wall and descending far into each labium majus. Closely related to this fat are the fascial bands of the distal part of the **round ligament** of the **uterus**. Lateral to the fat of the labium majus make a longitudinal cut.

GRANT'S 3.45
ROHEN 341
A.D.A.M. 4.23, 4.39
NETTER 351
CLEMENTE 397, 399

- Using a probe, find the **posterior labial nerves** and **vessels**, branches of the pudendal nerve and the internal pudendal artery, respectively.
- Next, on both sides of the symphysis pubis, cut horizontally down to the bone and scrape away the fatty tissue. This will leave exposed the prominent and tough **suspensory ligament of the clitoris.** This suspensory ligament extends from the symphysis to the fixed part of the clitoris.

Superficial Perineal Space (Fig. 3.33)

Remove the fatty tissue of the labia majora.

- Cut and discard the branches of the posterior labial nerves and vessels.
- Flush with the vaginal orifice, cut away the two labia minora. Note that they do not contain fat.
- Clean the dissection field as thoroughly as possible.
- Incise the **superficial perineal fascia** and insert your finger deep to it.

Your finger is now in the **superficial perineal space or pouch.** This space contains the greater vestibular glands and the superficial perineal muscles. These three paired muscles correspond to those in the male, but they are smaller.

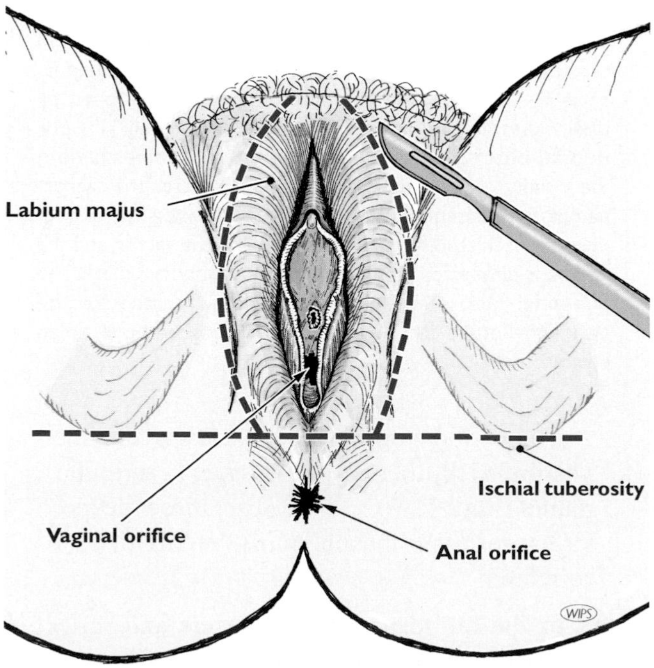

Figure 3.32. Skin incisions for the dissection of female external genitalia.

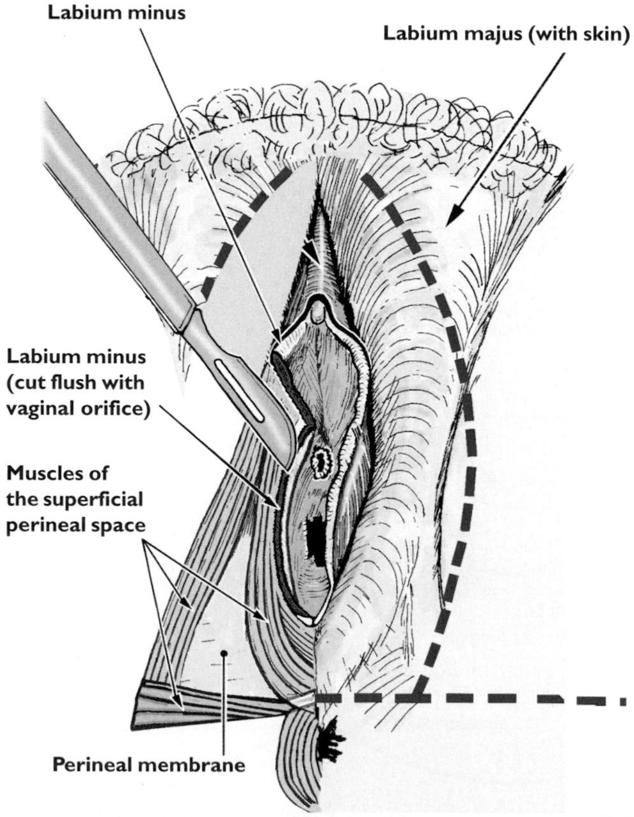

Figure 3.33. Removal of labia to expose the superficial perineal space.

Identify and clean the **three paired muscles** within the superficial perineal pouch (Fig. 3.34):

- **Transverse perinei superficialis** (superficial transverse perineal muscle), a slender muscular slip passing from the ischial tuberosity to the perineal body. Note that this **perineal body** (or central tendon) is a fibromuscular node in the median plane. At this point, several perineal muscles converge and interlace.
- **Ischiocavernosus**, arising from inner surface of ischial tuberosity and covering the unattached surface of the crus of the clitoris. *Function:* the muscle alters erection of the clitoris, once achieved, by forcing blood from the cavernous tissue of the crus of the clitoris into the distal corpus cavernosum of the clitoris.
- **Bulbospongiosus**, a broad muscular band surrounding the vaginal orifice like a sphincter. Posteriorly, it blends with the perineal body and muscle fibers of the sphincter ani externus. *Function:* the muscle forces blood from the spongy tissue of the bulb of the vestibule into the glans clitoris after erection is achieved. Identify the bulbospongiosus muscle and its relations to the other perineal muscles. When separating the three superficial perineal muscles from each other, note a small triangular area of exposed **perineal membrane**. This perineal membrane is the inferior fascia of the deep perineal space.

GRANT'S 3.37E, 346
ROHEN 342, 343
A.D.A.M. 4.41
NETTER 351
CLEMENTE 430

GRANT'S 346, 348
ROHEN 342
A.D.A.M. 4.41
NETTER 351, 352
CLEMENTE 430

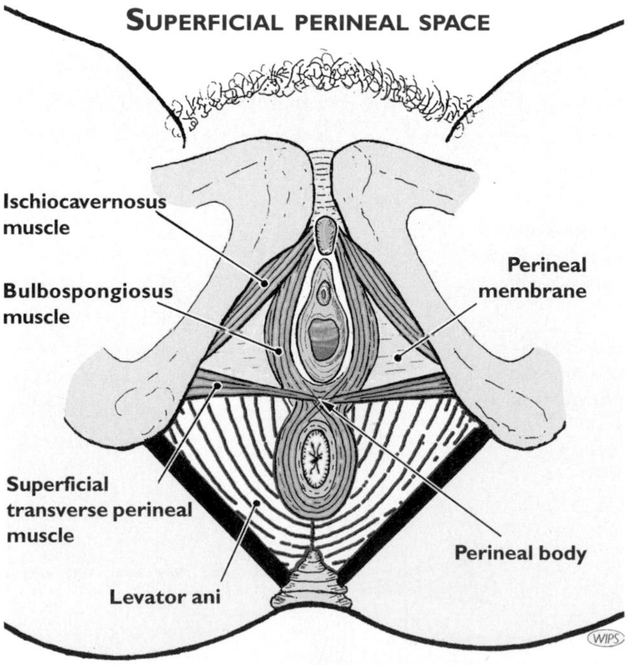

Figure 3.34. Superficial perineal space. Three paired muscles: superficial transverse perineal muscle, ischiocavernosus, and bulbocavernosus.

Clinical Correlation: The structures of the female pelvic floor are of great obstetric importance (Fig. 3.35). As the head of the baby pushes through the vagina, the vaginal wall is immensely stretched. Concomitantly, the structures surrounding the vaginal wall are also distended to a remarkable degree; this includes the muscles of the superficial and deep perineal spaces. The anus and the levator ani are forced posteriorly toward the sacrum and coccyx. The urethra is shifted anteriorly toward the pubic symphysis.

Perineal lacerations during childbirth are common. The superficial perineal muscles, notably the thick bulbospongiosus, may be torn as the child's head pushes through the perineum. To prevent tearing of perineal structures, it may be necessary to widen the external orifice of the birth canal by an episiotomy (surgical incision of perineum when laceration seems imminent during delivery). After complete delivery, this incision must be repaired with sutures. Intelligent repair of either lacerations or episiotomy wounds requires a good working knowledge of the female perineal region.

The perineal body is a fibromuscular node in the median plane where several perineal muscles converge and interlace (Fig. 3.34). The integrity of the perineal body in the female is of clinical importance. When the perineal body is injured during parturition (childbirth), it must be carefully repaired to avoid weakness of the pelvic floor with all its consequences (prolapse of bladder, uterus, or rectum). Thus, the anatomy of this region should be studied carefully.

The vulva is richly supplied with sensory nerve fibers. Thus, there is considerable pain when, during parturition, the head of the child is passing through the vulva and stretches its parts to the limit. The pain can be greatly diminished by locally anesthetizing the pudendal nerve bilaterally. This **pudendal block** is performed by injecting a local anesthetic in the vicinity of the pudendal nerve as it crosses the sacrospinous ligament near the ischial spine. During the procedure, the ischial spine is palpated through the vagina, and the needle is aimed toward this important bony landmark. The pudendal block is also performed to anesthetize the perineum locally for surgical repairs of lacerations or an episiotomy incision.

GRANT'S 3.48
ROHEN 343
A.D.A.M. 4.41
NETTER 352
CLEMENTE 430

The bulbospongiosus muscle covers the vestibular bulb and the greater vestibular gland (Fig. 3.36). To expose these deeper structures, the muscle must be divided or reflected.

- Cut the bulbospongiosus muscle and reflect it off the vaginal wall.

Now, the bulb of the vestibule and the greater vestibular gland adhering to the bulb

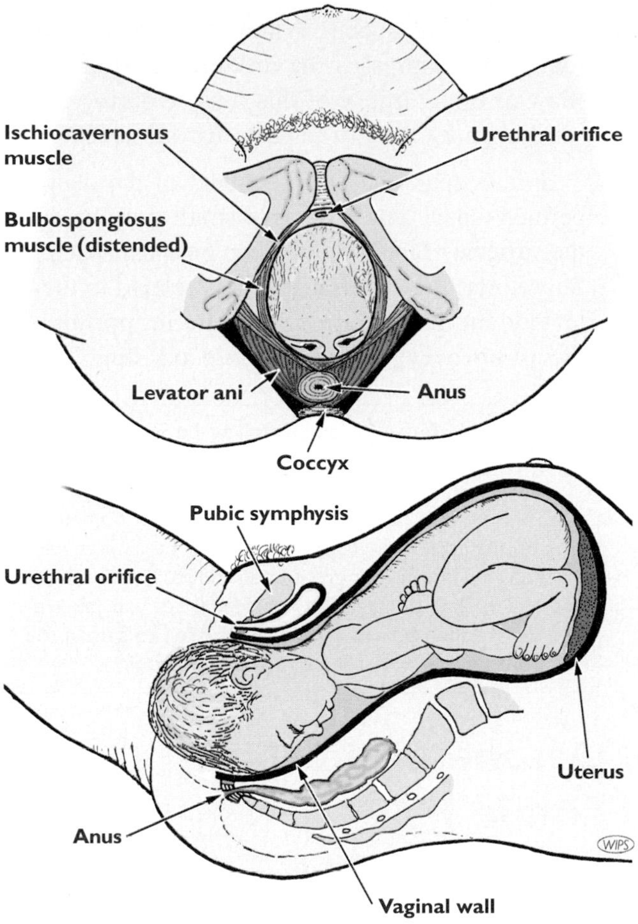

Figure 3.35. Pelvic floor during childbirth.

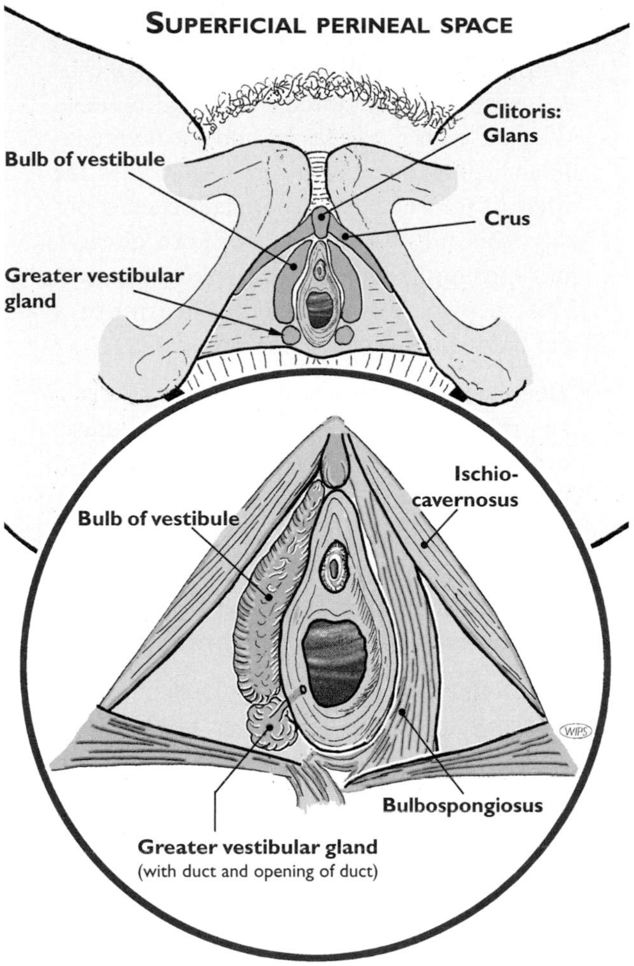

Figure 3.36. Superficial perineal space. Erectile tissue and glands.

can be examined (Fig. 3.36). The **bulbs of the vestibule** are two elongated (3 cm long) masses of erectile tissue on each side of the vaginal orifice. Anterior to the vaginal orifice, the two bulbs are united by a narrow band or commissure.

Attached to each posterior end of the bulb is the **greater vestibular gland** (vulvovaginal or Bartholin's glands). Attempt to find the duct of one of these small glands (Fig. 3.36). It opens into the vestibule in a groove between hymen and labium minus. The glands secrete lubricating mucus.

> *Clinical Correlation:* Acute inflammation of the greater vestibular gland (Bartholinitis) is of gynecological importance. As can be expected from the anatomical position of the gland, such inflammation (or abscess) will manifest itself by a substantial swelling of the lower (posterior) half of the labium, up to 5 cm in diameter. Enlarged and infected glands may also be palpated during rectal examination.

⇦
GRANT'S 3.37D, 3.48
ROHEN 341
A.D.A.M. 4.43
NETTER 352
CLEMENTE 431

⇦
GRANT'S 3.48
ROHEN 341
A.D.A.M. 4.43
NETTER 352
CLEMENTE 431

⇨
GRANT'S 3.47, 3.48
ROHEN 343
A.D.A.M. 4.41
NETTER 352
CLEMENTE 430, 431

With the handle of a scalpel, mobilize and free the **bulb of the vestibule**, thereby tearing the blood vessels that enter and leave the erectile tissue of the bulb. Reflect the bulb. Now the crura, body, and glans of the clitoris can be examined.

Clitoris (Fig. 3.36)

Identify the **glans,** which lies between two folds formed by labia minora. The anterior folds form the right and left sides of a hood over the glans, the **prepuce** of the clitoris (Fig. 3.31). The clitoris is homologous to the penis. It consists mainly of erectile tissue. Distinguish between its subdivisions: **glans, body,** and **crura.** Note that each crus is attached to the ischiopubic ramus. The clitoris has a rich blood and nerve supply (bilateral dorsal artery and nerve of clitoris).

Deep Perineal Space (Fig. 3.37)

Make sure that all structures of the superficial perineal space (three superficial perineal muscles, bulb of vestibule, and greater vestibular glands) have been removed. Incise the inferior fascia of the deep perineal space. Probably, this membrane has been torn already, thus opening the **deep perineal space or pouch.** This deep space is traversed by the **urethra** and the **vagina**. Identify the following:

⇦ *GRANT'S 3.37B* A.D.A.M. 4.45, 4.47 NETTER 352 CLEMENTE 428, 429

- **Deep transverse perineal muscle** (transversus perinei profundus). This paired muscle originates at the pubic arch and meets the opposite muscle in a tendinous raphe located just posterior to the vaginal wall. The muscle and its raphe are also attached to the perineal body. Examine the vagina in the deep perineal space together with the surrounding muscle.
- **Sphincter urethrae.** This important muscle partially surrounds the female urethra in the deep perineal space. When the muscle contracts, it compresses the urethra and stops the flow of urine. Injury of this muscle during parturition may lead to urinary incontinence.

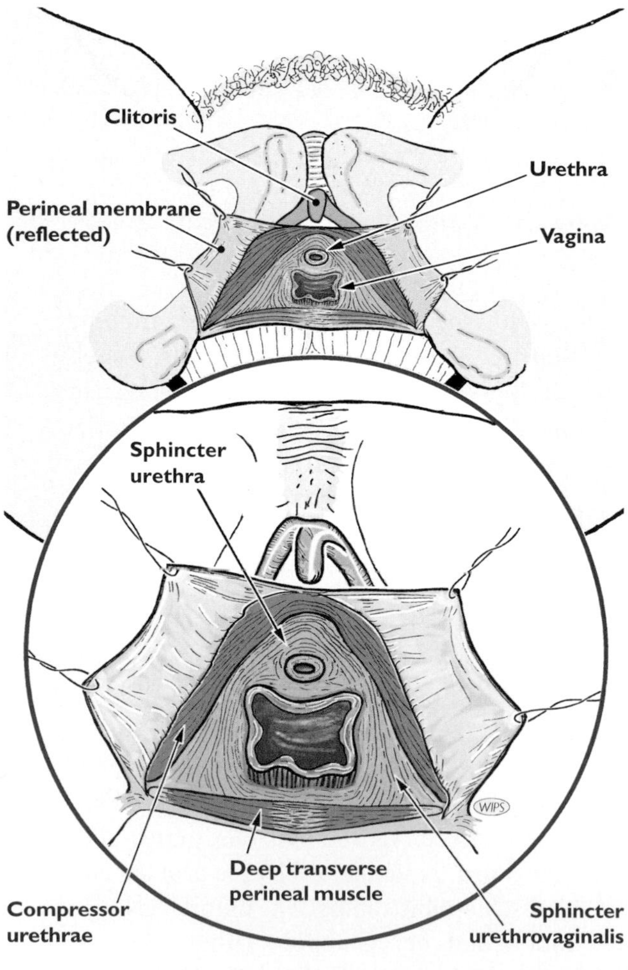

Figure 3.37. Deep perineal space exposed after reflection of perineal membrane.

⇦ *GRANT'S 3.49, 3.50* A.D.A.M. 4.45, 4.47 NETTER 352 CLEMENTE 428, 429

Spread apart the muscle fibers of the deep perineal space and expose a small portion of the **superior fascia** of the deep perineal space. Superiorly, the superior fascia is related to the levator ani, particularly to its anterior portion, the **pubococcygeus** or "puborectal sling."

> ***Note:*** The striated muscles stretching between the two sides of the pubic arch within the deep perineal space are also collectively known as the **urogenital diaphragm**. Although this term is part of the older anatomical nomenclature, you may still hear it; so, it is best to be familiar with it. Have all students in your group seen and studied the structures of the female urogenital triangle? If so, you may remove the wooden boards and/or ropes used to spread the lower limbs apart. Now return to the pelvic region.

Peritoneum in the Female Pelvis

> ***Dissection Note:*** It is possible that the female cadaver under dissection does not have a uterus. The removal of the uterus (hysterectomy), with or without the ovaries, is a common surgical procedure. Determine whether or not these organs are present in your specimen. If they have been surgically removed, examine these important organs in other cadavers.

⇨ *GRANT'S 3.26, 3.28* ROHEN 333 A.D.A.M. 4.37 NETTER 337, 339 CLEMENTE 394, 398

Examine the peritoneum in the female pelvis (Fig. 3.38). The peritoneum descends from the anterior abdominal wall (**1**) to the level of the pubic bone (**2**) on to the superior surface of the urinary bladder (**3**). Next, it passes from the bladder to the uterus (**4**). Here it forms the **vesicouterine pouch**. The peritoneum covers the fundus and body of the uterus. It extends over the posterior fornix and the wall of the vagina (**5**). Between the uterus and the rectum, the peritoneum forms the deep **rectouterine pouch** (**6**). From the bottom of the rectouterine pouch, the peritoneum passes on to the anterior surface and sides of the rectum (**7**). Finally, at the 3rd sacral vertebra, the peritoneum becomes the sigmoid mesocolon (**8**). The **paravesical fossa**, a peritoneal fossa, is apparent on each side of the bladder. The peritoneal recess on each side of the rectum is called the **pararectal fossa.**

Adnexa (L., *adnexum, adnexa,* connected parts).

This term is often used in a clinical context. It refers to the **uterine appendages:** the ovaries, uterine tubes, and ligaments of the uterus.

Broad Ligament of the Uterus (Fig. 3.39)

GRANT'S 3.27, 3.32A
ROHEN 333, 334
A.D.A.M. 4.25, 4.26
NETTER 344-346
CLEMENTE 399-405

At the sides of the uterus, two layers of peritoneum (from the posterior and anterior aspects of the uterus) come together to form a broad fold, the **broad ligament of the uterus**. This peritoneal fold extends to the lateral wall of the pelvis.

The **uterine tube** is contained within its free margin. The peritoneal fold that surrounds the uterine tube is called the **mesosalpinx** (Gr. *salpinx*, tube).

The **ovary** is attached to the posterior aspect of the broad ligament. The peritoneal fold that contains the ovary is the **mesovarium**. The broad ligament below the mesosalpinx is known as **mesometrium**. Mesovarium, mesosalpinx, and mesometrium are, of course, just portions of the broad ligament of the uterus. The loose fatty and areolar tissues enclosed between the two layers of the broad ligament are collectively called **parametrium** (Gr. *para*, beside; *metra*, womb, uterus).

Round Ligament of the Uterus

GRANT'S 3.26, 3.27
ROHEN 333, 334
A.D.A.M. 4.23, 4.25
NETTER 344, 345
CLEMENTE 399

It is visible through the anterior layer of the broad ligament. Observe its subperitoneal course over the pelvic brim toward the deep inguinal ring. It terminates in the labium majus.

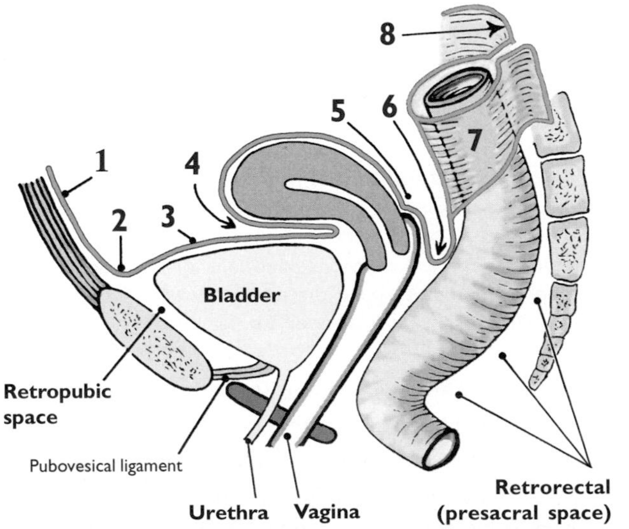

Figure 3.38. Peritoneum (green) in the female pelvis. The numbered portions of the peritoneum are explained in the text.

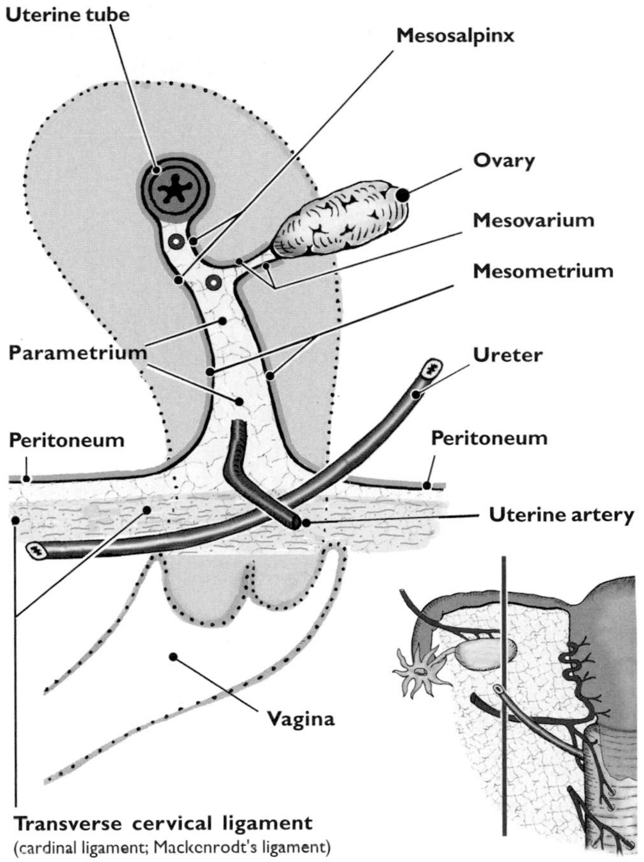

Figure 3.39. Broad ligament of uterus, its subdivisions and chief relations (paramedian section). Note the proximity of ureter and uterine artery. The **blue line** indicates the paramedian section through the broad ligament.

Other Ligaments

GRANT'S 3.27, 3.32A
ROHEN 333, 334
A.D.A.M. 4.23, 4.25
NETTER 344
CLEMENTE 401

The **ligament of the ovary** is a cord within the broad ligament connecting the ovary with the uterus at a point just below the uterine tube. The peritoneal fold covering the uterine tube extends laterally and posteriorly where it is continuous with the **suspensory ligament of the ovary**; this ligament contains the ovarian vessels. Once more, identify the **broad ligament of the uterus** as part of it stretches widely between the round ligament of the uterus anteriorly and the uterine tube posteriorly. Verify that the broad ligament separates the **vesicouterine pouch** from the **rectouterine pouch.**

Rectouterine Folds

GRANT'S 3.34
ROHEN 333, 334
A.D.A.M. 4.23, 4.25
NETTER 339, 344
CLEMENTE 419

These structures are sharp peritoneal folds containing true musculofascial ligaments, the **sacrouterine ligaments,** which anchor the uterus to the sacrum (Fig. 3.40). Observe that the rectouterine folds curve dorsally from the superior part of the cervix of the uterus past the sides of the rectum to the sacrum. Together, the right and left folds form the brim of the rectouterine pouch. The rectouterine folds with their underlying sacrouterine ligaments can be palpated by digital rectal examination.

In the female, the pelvic fascia is substantially thickened at the sides of the cervix and the vagina (Figs. 3.39, 3.40). This is the important **transverse cervical ligament** (lateral cardinal ligament; cardinal ligament; ligament of Mackenrodt). The ligament is triangular and holds the uterus in position by anchoring it to the lateral wall of the pelvis. Lateral to the uterus, push your finger inferiorly. Feel the stiff resistance and the firm support offered by the transverse cervical ligament.

⇦ *GRANT'S 3.34B* NETTER 341, 344 CLEMENTE 419

Structures Adhering to the Peritoneum

With your fingers, detach the peritoneum from the pelvic wall. Note the structures that adhere to the peritoneum:

⇦ *GRANT'S 3.26, 3.28* ROHEN 333 A.D.A.M. 4.27 NETTER 339, 342 CLEMENTE 394

- Rectum;
- Bladder;
- Ureter;
- Ovarian vessels;
- Round ligament of the uterus;
- Uterus.

Retropubic Space, Retrorectal Space, Nerves and Vessels

Retropubic Space (Fig. 3.38)

The retropubic space (prevesical space, space of Retzius) is an extraperitoneal space that is U-shaped and lies between the symphysis pubis and the bladder and extends dorsally on each side of the bladder. Posteriorly, the retropubic space contains arteries and veins of the bladder and of the internal genital organs. The retropubic space is filled with fat and loose areolar tissue, which accommodates the expansion of the bladder.

⇦ *GRANT'S 3.28* A.D.A.M. 4.27 NETTER 342 CLEMENTE 398, 419

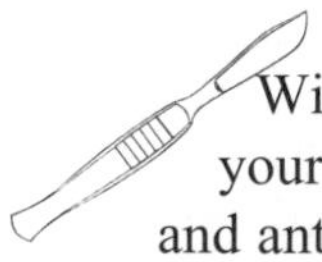

Within this extraperitoneal space, place your fingers between the symphysis pubis and anterior border of the bladder. Inferiorly, the exploring finger is stopped by cord-like thickenings of the pelvic fascia anchoring the neck of the bladder to the pubis. This is the **pubovesical ligament** (Fig. 3.38).

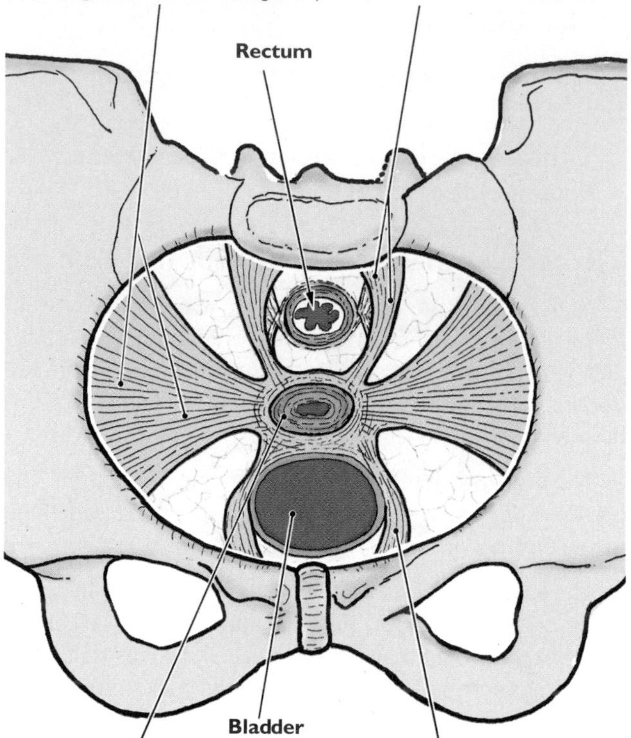

Figure 3.40. Transverse cervical ligament and other supportive ligaments of pelvic organs.

Retrorectal Space or Presacral Space

⇨ *GRANT'S 3.34* CLEMENTE 419

The fused sacral vertebrae S3 to S5 and the coccyx are covered anteriorly with the rectum. Pass two fingers caudally behind the rectum and ease it off the sacrum and coccyx. Now, your fingers are in the deep retrorectal space (Fig. 3.38). This space is limited inferiorly by a strong fascia investing the levator ani. Push your fingers inferiorly and verify by palpation the inferior limit of the retrorectal (presacral) space.

> ***Clinical Correlation:*** Just as your fingers are limited inferiorly, so is the spread of an infection in this space. As a result of this fascial arrangement, an infection, e.g., a retrorectal abscess, cannot expand inferiorly. Instead, it is prone to rupture through the posterior wall of the rectum (which constitutes a lesser barrier) into the rectum.

⇨ *GRANT'S 3.35A* A.D.A.M. 4.20 NETTER 383 CLEMENTE 365 A.V.A. 3: 2.34.20

Move your fingers laterally in the retrorectal space. Feel the strands of the **pelvic splanchnic nerves** (sacral parasympathetic outflow) on each side of the retrorectal space. These autonomic nerves branch off the ventral rami S2, S3, and S4 after traversing the corresponding anterior sacral foramina. Subsequently, the pelvic splanchnic nerves enter the **pelvic plexus** (or inferior hypogastric plexus), where parasympathetic and sympathetic fibers intermingle (structurally but not functionally). In the female, the pelvic plexus covers both sides of the rectum, uterus, vagina, and urinary bladder. Accordingly, clinicians often subdivide the pelvic plexus into a **rectal plexus, utero-vaginal plexus**, and **vesical plexus** (Fig. 3.41).

Clinical Correlation: Since the pelvic splanchnic nerves (parasympathetic outflow of S2, S3, S4) are closely related to the lateral aspects of the rectum, they can also be easily injured during rectal surgery; for example, when the rectum must be entirely removed because of cancer. Injury to or loss of the pelvic splanchnic nerves results in impairment of bladder control (see Figure 3.18).

Radical hysterectomy (for removal of cancer) involves the surgical removal of the uterus, the ovarian tubes, the ovaries and other adjacent structures, such as lymph nodes, connective tissue, and fatty tissue. Sometimes the adjacent nerve plexuses on both sides of the uterus cannot be spared. In that case, there is a certain interruption of nerve supply to the bladder, resulting in bladder dysfunction (see Figure 3.41).

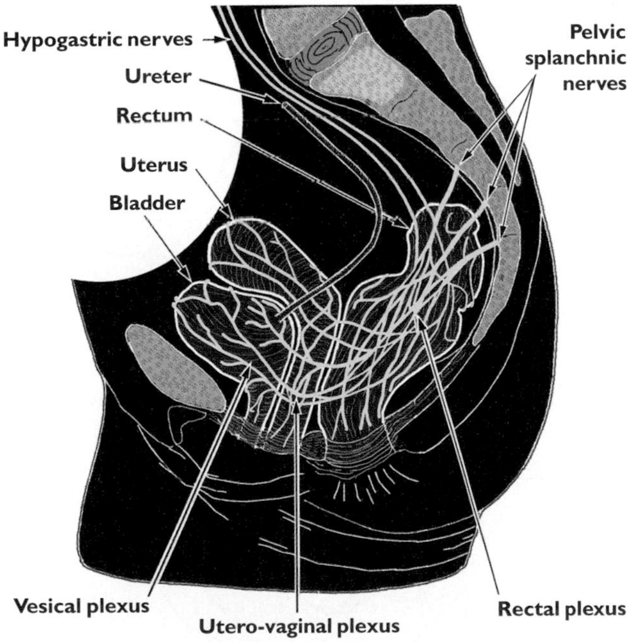

Figure 3.41. The female pelvic plexus (inferior hypogastric plexus).

The common iliac artery divides into the external iliac artery and the internal iliac artery. Follow the **internal iliac artery** and its branches to some extent (see Fig. 3.46).

GRANT'S 3.35
A.D.A.M. 4.20
NETTER 383
CLEMENTE 365
A.V.A. 3: 2.33.28

GRANT'S TABLE 3.3
ROHEN 325
A.D.A.M. 4.14, 4.31
NETTER 371, 373
CLEMENTE 410
A.V.A. 3: 2.28.40

A complete dissection of these vessels will be done when the pelvic cavity is more accessible. With your finger, palpate the **obturator canal** that traverses the superior aspect of the obturator membrane. Once you have identified the obturator canal, you will also be able to find the **obturator artery.** Follow this vessel proximally toward the internal iliac artery.

NETTER 373
CLEMENTE 410, 412

Clinical Correlation: Usually (in about 70% of cases), the obturator artery arises directly from the internal iliac artery. There is a slender anastomosis between the obturator artery and the inferior epigastric artery (a branch of the external iliac artery)(Fig. 3.19). However, in about 25% of cases, the obturator artery may receive the bulk of its blood supply directly from the inferior epigastric artery. Which vascular arrangement can you verify in the cadaver? Surgeons must be fully aware of this vascular arrangement. The "anomalous" obturator artery is very vulnerable and can be easily injured during surgical repair of a femoral hernia. Uncontrolled bleeding from this vessel can be dangerous. Study an iliac arteriogram.

A.D.A.M. 4.16, 4.31
NETTER 371
CLEMENTE 409, 410
A.V.A. 3: 1.59.54

Identify the **internal iliac vein** and some of its tributaries. Follow the vein to its junction with the **external iliac vein.** Here the **common iliac vein** is formed. Note that the left common iliac vein lies directly posterior to the bifurcation of the aorta. This is of surgical importance, particularly in cases of abdominal aortic aneurysms.

A.D.A.M. 4.23
NETTER 371
CLEMENTE 409, 418

On each side, identify the **ureter** as it crosses the external iliac vessels medially. Follow it inferiorly where it crosses the obturator vessels. Then trace it toward the urinary bladder as far as possible.

- Remove fat and areolar tissue surrounding vessels and ducts.
- Clean the accessible parts of the bladder wall, but do *not* destroy its blood supply.
- Cleaning of the bladder wall will be facilitated by attaching a hemostat at its apex and pulling it taut. If in doubt whether or not the (collapsed) organ is really the bladder, make a small incision in the median plane and observe the lumen of this hollow organ.
- If the rectum interferes with the field of dissection, have your partner pull it to the left side. Frequently sponge the area to keep it clean. Moisten the dissecting field with mold-deterrent preservative fluid.

Pelvic Diaphragm

Lateral Wall of Pelvic Cavity

Identify the obturator foramen and the obturator nerve and vessels passing through the obturator canal. The obturator foramen (with its obturator membrane) is closed internally by the **obturator internus muscle.** Looking from within the lesser pelvis, only the most superior portion of the muscle can be seen at this time. Superiorly, the fascia of the obturator internus is thickened and forms a **tendinous arch** stretching from ischial spine to pubic bone. The **levator ani** arises, in part, from this tendinous arch (Fig.3.42B).

GRANT'S 3.4
A.D.A.M. 4.11, 4.12
NETTER 334
CLEMENTE 457
A.V.A. 3: 2.16.54

The **pelvic diaphragm** is the fibromuscular floor that closes the inferior pelvic aperture. It is funnel-shaped. The rectum is anchored to it in the middle (Fig. 3.42A). The muscular components of the pelvic diaphragm can only be observed in part at this time, because of the intervening pelvic organs. The pelvic diaphragm will be completely dissected later after hemisection of the pelvis. However, it is important to have a conceptual understanding of these structures at this time.

GRANT'S 3.4
A.D.A.M. 4.11
NETTER 334
CLEMENTE 428
A.V.A. 3: 2.20.35

The pelvic diaphragm is formed by the *two large levator ani muscles* and the *two smaller coccygeus muscles* (Fig. 3.42 B and C). The *external anal sphincter* may also be considered a part of the pelvic diaphragm. The funnel-shaped **levator ani** consists of three parts:

- **Puborectalis muscle**, the medial portion of the pubococcygeus muscle;
- **Pubococcygeus**, arising from the pubic bone;
- **Iliococcygeus**, arising from the tendinous arch.

GRANT'S 3.4
A.D.A.M. 4.49
NETTER 333, 334
CLEMENTE 420, 426
A.V.A. 3: 2.18.52

The **pubococcygeus** is the thickened and most important part of the pelvic diaphragm. Fibers of the right and the left pubococcygeus unite *posterior* to the rectum. This union of fibers creates a U-shaped "puborectal sling" (Fig. 3.42 C and D). This sling is responsible for the curvature at the anorectal junction. During defecation, the puborectal sling relaxes, the anorectal junction is straightened, and the expulsion of fecal matter is facilitated. In the female, portions of the pubococcygeus muscle are inserted into the terminal portion of the vagina.

GRANT'S 3.21B, 3.22A
A.D.A.M. 4.49
NETTER 333, 334
CLEMENTE 420
A.V.A. 3: 2.19.55

The **levator ani muscles** raise the pelvic floor and assist the anterior abdominal muscle in increasing the intra-abdominal pressure when necessary (e. g., during urination, straining, vomiting, forced expiration, and when lifting heavy objects).

The two **coccygeus muscles** arise from the ischial spine and form the posterior and smaller part of the pelvic diaphragm. Each coccygeus is essentially a triangular muscular sheet that lies posterior to the iliococcygeus muscle. The two coccygeus muscles assist the levator ani in supporting the pelvic organs.

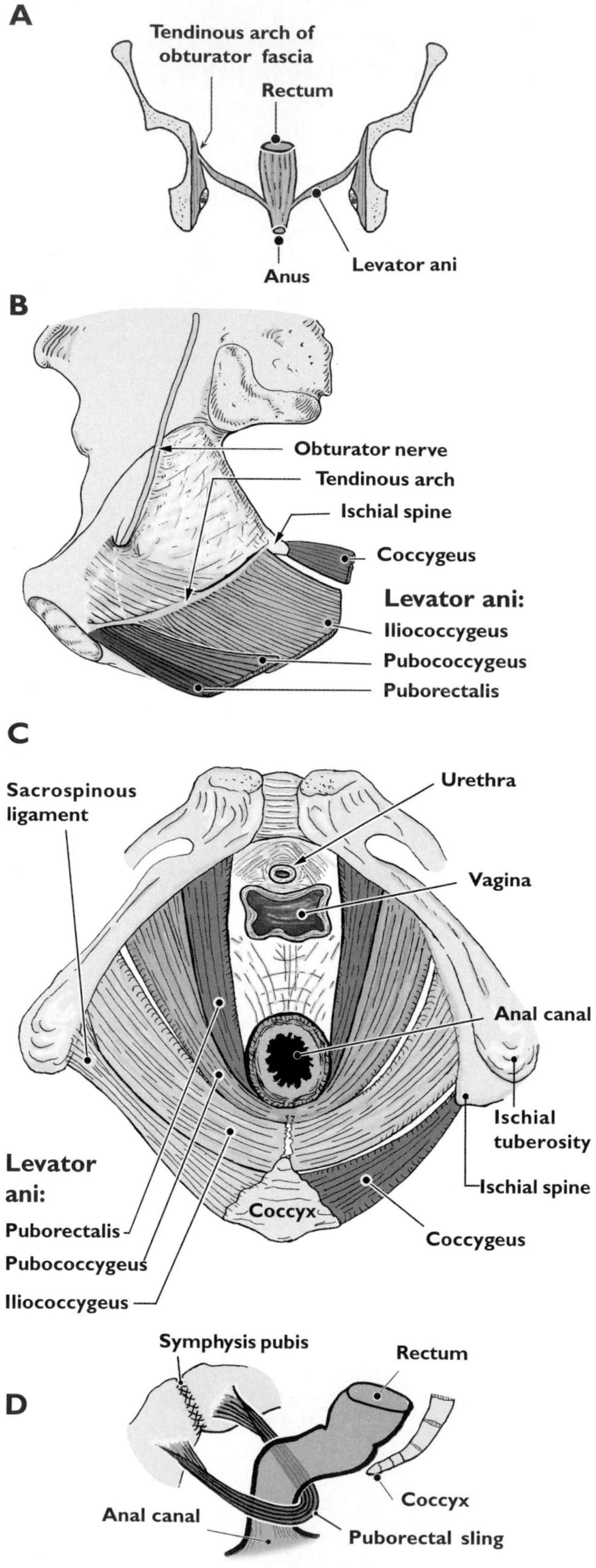

Figure 3.42. The pelvic diaphragm is formed by the levator ani and the coccygeus muscles. The levator ani is funnel-shaped in coronal section ***(A)***; originates from the tendinous arch ***(B)***; forms the pelvic floor around the rectum ***(C)***; and contributes to the *puborectal sling* ***(D)***.

> ***Clinical Correlation:*** The pubococcygeus, particularly the portions supporting the vagina and rectum, are frequently injured during childbirth. The supporting ligaments of the pelvic fascia (e.g., the cardinal ligament) may also be torn during parturition. As a consequence, the pelvic viscera are no longer adequately supported by the pelvic diaphragm. Pelvic organs may push downward and prolapse through the weakened vaginal wall (prolapse of bladder, cystocele; prolapse of rectum, rectocele), or the uterus may descend down the vaginal canal (prolapse of uterus).

Review all structures of the female pelvis and perineum that have been dissected and seen so far. Make sure your laboratory partners have also participated in the review process. Subsequently, the pelvis will be sectioned in the midsagittal plane to facilitate more detailed studies of pelvic structures.

Hemisection

Before you begin ...

Check with your instructor to determine if you are allowed to proceed. The **goal** is to make a careful midsagittal split of all (soft and bony) structures from the perineum up to the level of vertebra L3. Subsequently, the body will be transected at the vertebral level of L3 to L4. One lower extremity (preferably the left one) remains attached to the rest of the body while the other side (preferably the right one) is mobilized. If this procedure is done with care, it will facilitate complete dissection and examination of the pelvis.

Section

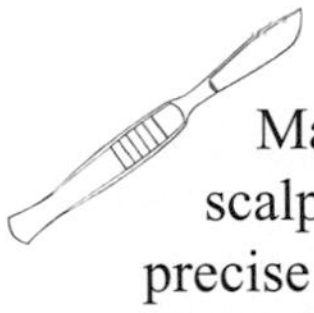

Make sure you are using a new and sharp scalpel. Use this instrument to make a very precise split of all soft structures in the midsagittal plane:

- Start posterior to the symphysis pubis in the midsagittal plane. Carry this midsagittal section through the entire bladder wall. Sponge the interior of the urinary bladder. Continue to cut inferior to the bladder until you have reached the urogenital diaphragm.
- Next, carry the midsagittal cut through the uterus. Include in this section the cervix of the uterus and the superior portion of the vagina.
- Subsequently, cut through the anterior and posterior walls of the rectum. Sponge it clean! Be careful *not* to cut into the sigmoid colon or any other loop of the GI tract! Now, the blade should have reached the anterior surface of the sacrum.

GRANT'S 3.26
ROHEN 335
A.D.A.M. 4.37
NETTER 337
CLEMENTE 394

- Finally, push the knife inferior to the symphysis pubis with the cutting edge directed posteriorly. In the midsagittal plane, cut through the pelvic diaphragm from symphysis pubis to coccyx.

Obtain a suitable hand saw and make two cuts in the midsagittal plane:

- Cut through the symphysis pubis.
- Start at the coccyx and extend the midline cut through the sacrum up to the 3rd lumbar vertebra. Be careful *not* to injure the nerves of the cauda equina. During sawing, pull these nerves laterally for protection.

GRANT'S 3.26
ROHEN 335
A.D.A.M. 4.37
NETTER 337
CLEMENTE 394

If you have decided to mobilize the right lower extremity (which is preferred), proceed as follows:

- Cut horizontally through the right half of the intervertebral disc between L3 and L4 until this cut meets the superior extent of the midsagittal section of the vertebral column.
- Cautiously mobilize the right lower extremity to some extent. Cut nerves and blood vessels connecting the right lower limb with the rest of the body. Section the ureter. Now the right lower limb can be removed.

Continue with your studies of the *female* pelvic structures using either half of the hemisectioned pelvis. The pelvic structures are now readily accessible. Examine and dissect these structures and note their topographical relations:

Urethra

GRANT'S 3.26
ROHEN 335
A.D.A.M. 4.39
NETTER 343, 353
CLEMENTE 394

If the hemisection was done perfectly in the midsagittal plane, then the longitudinally opened halves of the urethra should be present in each hemisectioned specimen. Otherwise, refer to the specimen that contains the urethra.

- Verify that the female urethra is a short muscular tube, about 5 to 6 mm in diameter and 3.5 to 4 cm in length.
- Trace the sectioned urethra anteroinferiorly from the urinary bladder to the **external urethral orifice**.
- Note that the urethra lies *anterior* to the vagina; therefore, the urethral orifice must also be located *anterior* to the vaginal orifice.

- Examine the portion of the urethra that passes through the **deep perineal space**. Note the solid **sphincter urethrae muscle**.

Close-up examination of the urethral mucosa with a magnifying glass will reveal numerous tiny orifices for the periurethral glands. The two largest of these glands open at the paraurethral orifice (orifice of Skene's duct), which lies just posterior to the urethral opening on either side of the midline (Fig. 3.31).

Ureter

Pick up the ureter as it crosses the external iliac artery. Verify that the ureter descends on the lateral wall of the true pelvis (pelvis minor) to a point close to the ischial spine. Here, the **uterine artery** crosses superior to the ureter.

Next, the ureter passes close to the lateral fornix of the vagina. At this point, the vaginal artery crosses inferior to the ureter. Trace the ureter to the posterosuperior angle of the bladder. Here, at the **ureterovesical junction**, the ureter travels obliquely through the bladder wall.

Anatomy and function of the ureter and the ureterovesical junction are identical in the female and male. For an account and an illustration of this important topic, please turn to pages 105-106).

⇦
GRANT'S 3.26
ROHEN 335
A.D.A.M. 4.39
NETTER 343, 353
CLEMENTE 394

⇨
ROHEN 333
A.D.A.M. 4.23
NETTER 343, 344
CLEMENTE 394, 397

⇦
A.D.A.M. 4.23
NETTER 342, 344

⇦
A.D.A.M. 4.23
NETTER 337
CLEMENTE 397

Urinary Bladder (Fig. 3.43)

During section of the pelvis, the urinary bladder was completely opened and divided into right and left halves. First, examine the bladder wall:

- With scissors and forceps, remove at least some portions of the peritoneum and the pelvic fascia that cover the bladder musculature.
- Identify the **muscular coat** of the bladder. It consists of complexly interwoven bundles of smooth muscle. This muscular coat is collectively called the detrusor urinae (L. *detrudere*, to thrust out).
- Define the area of the **bladder neck** and around the bladder outlet. Here, smooth muscle bundles form functional loop that acts like a sphincter, particularly in the female. This *internal sphincter* is involuntary and aids the more powerful, voluntary sphincter urethrae that is located in the deep perineal space.
- Verify that the bladder neck and the initial portion of the urethra are continuous and are positioned superior to (above) the pelvic floor.
- Using your fingers and a probe, explore the firm tissue that suspends the bladder neck and holds it in its appropriate location. These

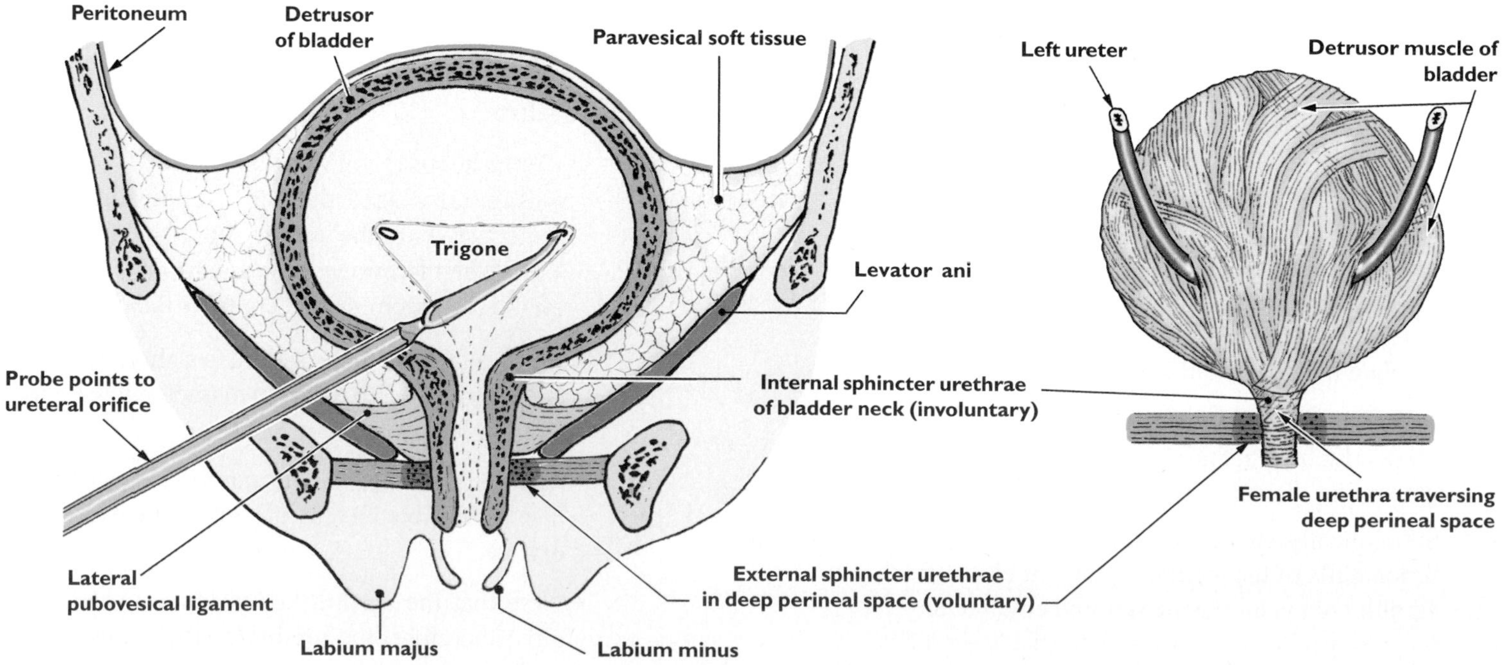

Figure 3.43. Urinary bladder and its support on the female pelvic floor.

fibrous strands are part of the pubovesical ligaments and their lateral extensions.

A.D.A.M. 4.39
NETTER 343

- Examine the lateral parts of the bladder wall and note that the bladder is surrounded by soft areolar tissue. This tissue can easily respond to and accommodate the extensive volume changes of an expanding or contracting bladder.

Clinical Correlation: The **anatomical suspension of the bladder neck** and of the initial portion of the female urethra above the pelvic floor is of considerable clinical importance. Only the well suspended bladder can maintain urinary continence during increased intraabdominal pressure.

When a person coughs, sneezes, laughs, or lifts heaviy objects, the pressure within the abdomen increases. This pressure increase has an effect on the bladder and puts it under "stress". The force of transmitted pressure from the abdomen (*arrows*) not only reaches the bladder but also the upper portion of the appropriately suspended urethra as well (Fig. 3.44).

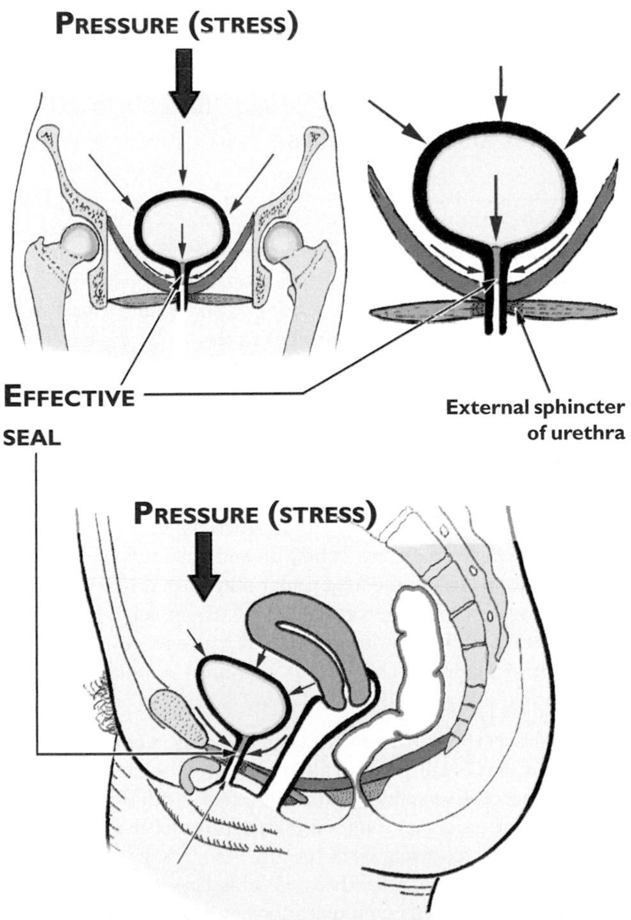

Figure 3.44. Healthy and well suspended bladder with good urinary stress tolerance. The ***blue arrows*** show the dynamics of transmitted pressure. The "effective seal" of the urethra is shown as a **green column**.

Thus, the same force that puts the urine in the bladder under pressure also compresses the urethra with equal pressure. No matter how high the abdominal "pressure stress" gets, the urethra is always equally tights. As a result, the bladder remains sealed. This phenomenon is known as **urinary stress tolerance**.

If the pelvic floor is weak and the bladder neck is no longer appropriately suspended (e.g., following several vaginal deliveries), the bladder and the upper portion of the urethra may descend onto the stretched and sagging pelvic floor. Now, the transmitted stress of abdominal pressure reaches the bladder and the urine in it; however, it can no longer reach and compress the upper portion of the urethra. Only the internal sphincter of the bladder neck and the possibly damaged external sphincter of the deep perineal space are left to keep the urethra sealed. This seal, however, is easily overcome by sudden abdominal pressure changes during coughing, sneezing, and straining activities. This important and common clinical phenomenon is known as **urinary stress incontinence**. [Excerpts from Sauerland, *The Well-Informed Patient Series*].

Examine the **interior of the bladder**, which is not different from the male urinary bladder:

GRANT'S 3.17
A.D.A.M. 4.39
NETTER 343, 353
CLEMENTE 442

- The **trigone** is an equilateral triangle on the posterior wall (now divided). Its angles are formed by the **two orifices of the ureters** and the **internal urethral orifice.** The internal urethral orifice is situated at the lowest (most inferior) point of the bladder.
- Note that the mucous membrane over the trigone is smooth. Over the other parts of the bladder, it lies in folds when the bladder is empty.
- Pass a fine probe into the orifice of the ureter. Verify that the ureter traverses the muscular wall of the bladder in an oblique fashion (Fig. 3.43).

Vagina (L. *vagina*, sheath)

GRANT'S 3.26, 3.32B
ROHEN 333, 336
A.D.A.M. 4.23, 4.27
NETTER 342, 345
CLEMENTE 394, 400

In the sectioned specimen, observe that the anterior vaginal wall is about 7.5 to 8 cm long. The posterior wall is slightly longer to accommodate the posterior vaginal fornix.

Once again, examine the relationship of the posterior fornix to the rectouterine pouch. Observe the close topographical relations of the lateral vaginal fornix and uterine artery. In the living, particularly in the pregnant woman the pulsations of the uterine artery may be felt through the lateral fornices. Realize that the vagina is so distensible that it can accommodate head and shoulders of a baby passing through the birth canal.

Uterus (Fig. 3.45)

Note its normal anteverted position. Observe that the longitudinal axes of the uterus and vagina are at an angle of approximately 90°. Realize that the position of the uterus must change when the bladder is full, or in pregnancy. Identify the following features of the uterus:

- **Cervix**, protruding into the vaginal canal. The **cervical canal** opens through the ostium uteri (external os) into the vagina. Review the strong ligamentous attachments that hold the cervix in place (sacrouterine ligament; transverse cervical or cardinal ligament).
- **Body of the uterus**. Identify the **vesical surface** facing the vesicouterine pouch, and the **superior surface** facing the rectouterine pouch. Note that the **lateral surfaces** are attached to the **broad ligament**. Structures to and from the uterus are contained in the loose areolar tissue between the two layers of the broad ligament. This tissue is the **parametrium**. Identify the **uterine cavity**. In a sagittal section, it is a mere slit. In a coronal section, it is triangular in shape (Fig. 3.45). Make a coronal section through the sectioned half of the uterus. Explore the uterine cavity and its continuation with the cervical canal and the uterine tube. The uterine mucosa is called **endometrium**. Observe the thick uterine wall composed of smooth musculature, the **myometrium**. Understand clinically important terms: *endometrium* (Gr. *endon*, within; *metra*, uterus); *myometrium* (Gr. *mys*, muscle); *parametrium* (Gr. *para*, beside). The **fundus** is the rounded part of the uterus that lies above the entrances to the tubes.

Uterine Tube (fallopian tube; oviduct).

With a pair of scissors, open one uterine tube longitudinally. Note the funnel-shaped **infundibulum** with its **fimbriae** (Fig. 3.45). Observe the narrow medial one-third of the uterine tube, the **isthmus**.

Clinical Correlation: The uterine tubes provide an open channel from the outside into the peritoneal cavity. With a probe, follow this channel from the vagina via the cervical canal, uterine cavity, and uterine tubes into the abdominal cavity. If available, study a hysterosalpingogram.

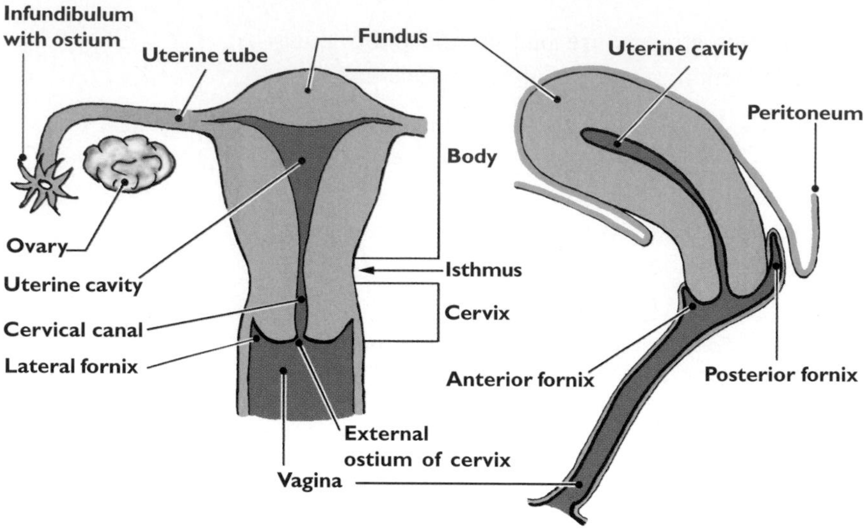

Figure 3.45. Uterus in coronal and midsagittal section.

GRANT'S 3.32A
ROHEN 336
A.D.A.M. 4.23, 4.25
NETTER 344-346
CLEMENTE 399, 401

Ovary (Fig. 3.45)

In nulliparous women, each ovary lies in a shallow depression bounded by ureter, external iliac vein, and uterine tube. If not already done, dissect the ovarian vessels throughout their course. Incise one ovary. The structure of the ovary varies with age. If the age of subject is less than 40 to 50 years, look for follicles.

GRANT'S 3.32B
ROHEN 337
NETTER 346
CLEMENTE 404

Clinical Correlation: In assessing certain pathological conditions, the topographic anatomical relations between lower urinary tract and vagina should always be remembered. The vagina lies posterior to the base of the bladder. Thus, a finger placed into the vagina can exert pressure on the posterior bladder wall.

The close relationship between vagina and posterior bladder wall has clinical implications: As a consequence of injuries sustained during labor and delivery, the bladder may be insufficiently supported by the muscular pelvic floor. In this condition and especially in the upright position, the full bladder may push downward and against the anterior vaginal wall. Eventually, a bulge appears in the anterior vaginal wall caused by the prolapsed bladder. This rather common condition is known as cystocele.

GRANT'S 3.31, 3.32
ROHEN 336, 337
A.D.A.M. 4.23, 4.25
NETTER 344-346
CLEMENTE 400, 401, 404

Similarly, the female urethra can prolapse, a condition known as urethrocele. The urethrocele, which is usually accompanied by a cystocele, occurs with weakening of the normal supporting structures of the pelvic floor; e.g., following birth trauma. As a result of post-surgical trauma, a urethrovaginal fistula can develop. This pathological communication between urethra and vagina allows urine to discharge constantly through the vagina, a most miserable although not life-threatening condition.

Internal Iliac Artery and Branches (Fig. 3.46)

The internal iliac artery supplies most of the blood to the pelvic viscera. You may not have time to dissect all branches of the internal iliac artery in the female cadaver. Demonstrate at least the following:

- Identify the **umbilical artery**. Note that it gives off 3 to 4 **superior vesical arteries** that supply the superior aspect of the bladder. The umbilical artery continues toward the anterior abdominal wall where it becomes the **medial umbilical ligament** (obliterated umbilical artery).
- Trace the **obturator artery** from its point of origin to the superior aspect of the obturator foramen.
- Next, identify the origin of the **uterine artery**. Usually, it arises directly from the internal iliac artery. Follow it to the inferior margin of the broad ligament and into the parametrium; i.e., into the areolar tissue between the two layers of the broad ligament. Subsequently, trace it to the lateral aspect of the uterus, specifically to the isthmus; i.e., the region between body and cervix of the uterus (Fig. 3.47).

⇨
GRANT'S 3.32B
ROHEN 338
NETTER 371, 373, 375
CLEMENTE 405-408

⇦
GRANT'S TABLE 3.3
A.D.A.M. 4.14
NETTER 371
CLEMENTE 410

⇦
GRANT'S 3.32B
ROHEN 338
A.D.A.M. 4.14
NETTER 371
CLEMENTE 405

- Note that the uterine artery divides into a large superior branch to the body and fundus of the uterus, and into a smaller branch to the cervix and vagina. Be aware of the **anastomosis between uterine** and **ovarian arteries.**
- Identify and trace the **vaginal artery** (Fig. 3.47). Follow some of its branches to the vagina and the posteroinferior parts of the urinary bladder. Note that the **ureter** is interposed between vaginal and uterine arteries.
- Pay particular attention to the relation between ureter and uterine artery (Fig. 3.47). Verify that the uterine artery crosses the ureter near the lateral fornix of the vagina.

> ***Clinical Correlation:*** The close proximity of ureter and uterine artery near the lateral fornix of the vagina is of considerable clinical importance. During hysterectomy, the uterine artery is tied off and cut. Inadvertently, the ureter may also be clamped, tied off, and severed. This will have serious consequences for the corresponding kidney.

Other Branches of the Internal Iliac Artery (Fig. 3.46):

- The **middle rectal artery** is a small vessel to the lateral aspect of the rectum.

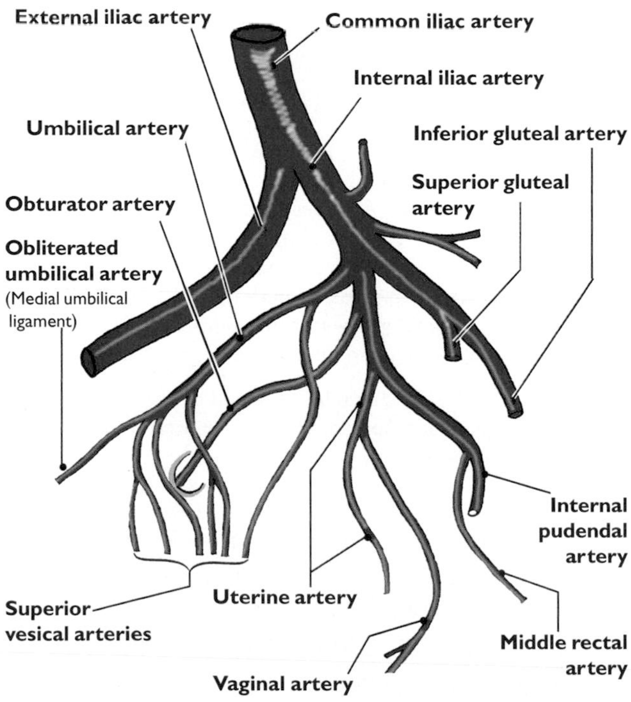

Figure 3.46. Internal iliac artery in the female pelvis.

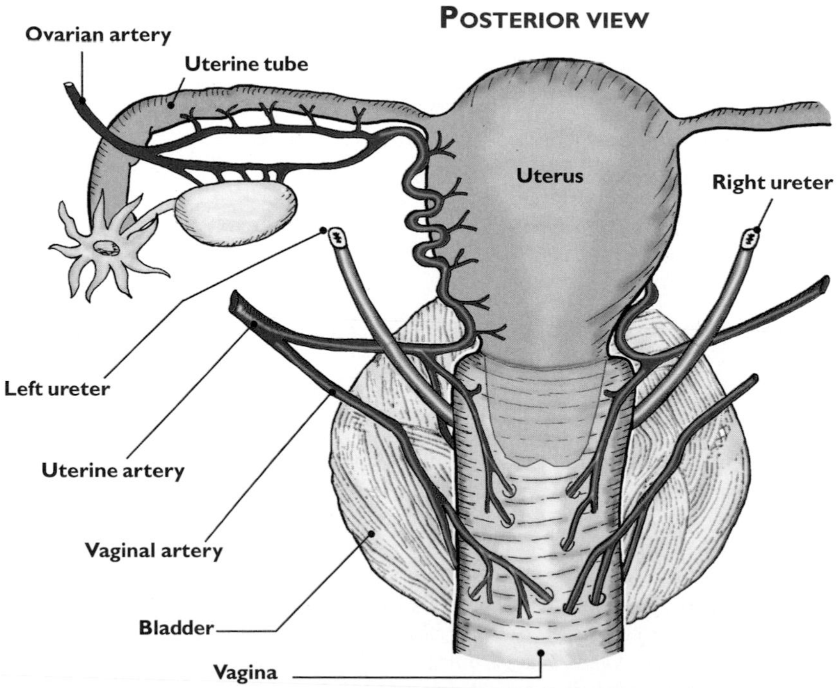

Figure 3.47. Arterial supply of uterus, vagina, and ovary. Note the crossing of ureter and uterine artery (posterior view).

- Follow the **internal pudendal artery** (which is smaller in the female than in the male) to the inferior part of the greater sciatic foramen. This artery is closely related to the sacrospinous ligament.

GRANT'S TABLE 3.3
A.D.A.M. 4.14
NETTER 373
CLEMENTE 410
A.V.A. 3: 2.29.23

- The internal pudendal artery has been encountered earlier in the pudendal canal where it gives off branches to the ischioanal fossa and where it divides into its terminal branches, supplying the muscles of the urogenital triangle and the erectile tissue of the clitoris.

GRANT'S 3.11B
A.D.A.M. 455
NETTER 365
CLEMENTE 450

- The **inferior gluteal artery** also passes through the inferior part of the greater sciatic foramen. This vessel passes between sacral nerves of the sacral plexus.

GRANT'S TABLE 3.3
A.D.A.M. 4.14
NETTER 373
CLEMENTE 410
A.V.A. 3: 2.28.27

- The **superior gluteal artery** is relatively large and runs in close relationship to the lumbosacral trunk. This vessel leaves the pelvis through the superior part of the greater sciatic foramen.

Pelvic Venous Plexuses

A.D.A.M. 4.16
NETTER 371
CLEMENTE 409

These plexuses are networks of veins that are located around the bladder, the uterus, and the rectum. The plexuses intercommunicate and eventually drain into the internal iliac vein. Do not dissect these complex pelvic venous plexuses. Remove all tributaries to the internal iliac vein so that the arterial distribution in the female pelvis can be clearly demonstrated.

> ***Clinical Correlation:*** The **venous plexuses in the pelvis** intercommunicate. This is of considerable clinical importance (e.g., transportation of tumor cells along vascular channels). The importance of the rectal venous plexus in cases of portal venous hypertension has been stressed earlier.
>
> The superior rectal vein originates from the rectal venous plexus. The rectal venous plexus is also drained by the middle and inferior rectal veins that, in turn, empty into the caval system of veins.
>
> In portal venous hypertension, blood flow in the superior rectal vein may be reversed: portal blood may be carried to the rectal plexus and, from there, shunted into the caval system. The resulting increased blood flow and pressure in the rectal venous plexus leads to the development of hemorrhoids. Thus, in case of hemorrhoids, the physician must always evaluate the condition of the portal venous system. The portal venous system has no valves. This fact explains why the blood flow in the portal system can be easily reversed.

Anal Canal

During bisection of the pelvis, the anal canal has been opened. Clean it thoroughly. Examine the interior features (this may be difficult to demonstrate in some cadavers):

- **Anal columns** (Fig. 3.48). These are 5 to 10 longitudinal ridges of mucosa in the superior part of the anal canal. The terminal branches of the superior rectal vessels are contained in the anal columns.

- **Anal valves.** These semilunar folds unite the lower ends of the anal columns (Fig. 3.48).

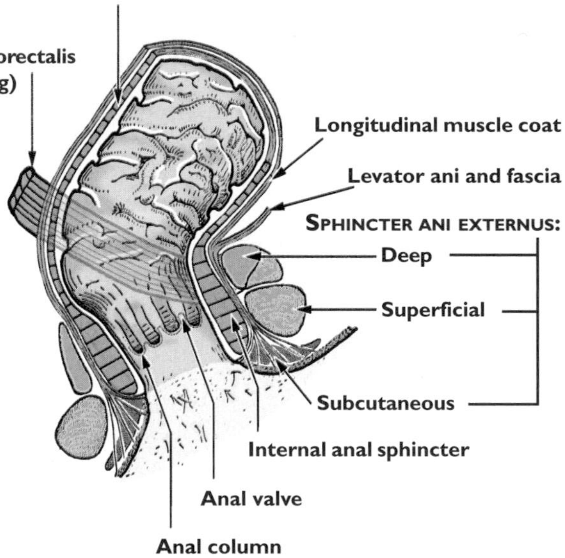

Figure 3.48. Rectum, anal canal, and anal sphincter.

> ***Clinical Correlation:*** At the level of the **anal columns**, the superior rectal veins of the *portal system* anastomose with middle and inferior rectal veins of the *caval system*. Abnormal increase in pressure in the valveless portal system leads to an enlargement of the veins contained in the anal columns, resulting in internal hemorrhoids.
>
> If the **anal valves** are torn by hard fecal material, an infection can occur and spread from the injured anal valves into the wall of the anal canal.

GRANT'S 3.12A
A.D.A.M. 4.55
NETTER 364-366
CLEMENTE 450-452
A.V.A. 3: 2.23.28

Examine the **sphincter muscles of the anus** (Fig. 3.48). At the inner aspect of the anal canal, identify the **internal anal sphincter**. Identify the **sphincter ani externus** that surrounds the anal canal. Note its three subdivisions (Fig. 3.48):

- Deep;
- Superficial;
- Subcutaneous.

Identify and examine the **puborectal sling** on the hemisectioned female cadaver. Verify that it is part of the levator ani.

Digital Examination of Rectum and Vagina (Fig. 3.49)

Perform digital examination of the female pelvic organs *per rectum*.

- Place a gloved finger into the split anal canal and palpate topographically related structures (as if performing a digital rectal examination).
- Palpate the muscular wall formed by the sphincter ani externus.
- More superiorly, at the anorectal junction, feel the puborectalis (puborectal sling; part of levator ani).
- Verify that anterior to the finger the posterior wall of the vagina and cervix of the uterus can be palpated.
- Place one finger of the other hand in the rectouterine fossa and note that the anterior wall of the rectum intervenes between the two fingers.

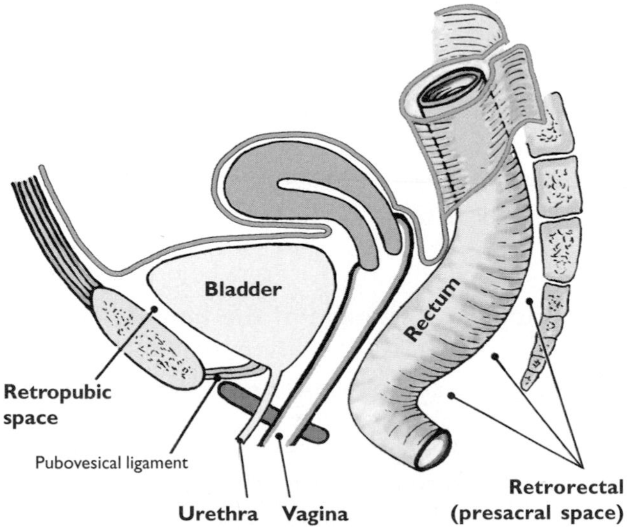

Figure 3.49. Structures that can be palpated by digital rectal and digital vaginal examination.

GRANT'S 3.26, 3.28
ROHEN 333
A.D.A.M. 4.37
NETTER 337
CLEMENTE 394

- Laterally, feel the sharp rectouterine fold.

Next, perform digital examination of the pelvic organs *per vaginam* (Fig. 3.49).

- Place one or two gloved fingers into the split vagina and palpate topographically related structures (as if performing a vaginal examination). Place the fingers of the other hand in the pelvis.
- Between the two hands, palpate and observe the following: urinary bladder, cervix of uterus, rectouterine pouch, and uterus.

Clinical Correlation: Digital rectal and vaginal examinations are very important procedures in assessing the disposition and condition of pelvic organs. Under pathological conditions, one can palpate the enlarged or displaced broad ligament, enlarged ovaries, and uterine tubes (inflammatory processes, tumors, cysts, ectopic pregnancies, etc.).

Note that only the posterior fornix of the vagina intervenes between the peritoneal cavity (rectouterine pouch of Douglas) and the outside (Fig. 3.49). Therefore, a needle can be pushed through the posterior vaginal fornix to aspirate pathological contents from the rectouterine pouch. Also, a culdoscope can be introduced through the posterior vaginal fornix into the abdominal cavity. The culdoscope allows visual observations of the uterine tubes, ovaries, posterior surface of the uterus, and anterior surface of the rectum.

GRANT'S 3.4
A.D.A.M. 4.49
NETTER 333, 334
CLEMENTE 420, 4.26
A.V.A. 3: 2.18.53

Levator Ani

The levator ani is funnel-shaped (Fig. 3.42). In the middle of this funnel, the vagina and uterus are supported anteriorly, and the rectum is positioned posteriorly (Fig. 3.49). Examine the **origins of the levator ani:** Identify the thickened fascia of the obturator internus stretching from pubic bone to ischial spine and forming a tendinous arch. From this **tendinous arch** the levator ani originates in part (Fig. 3.42B). Verify this. Identify the *three portions* of the **levator ani:**

- **Puborectalis muscle**, the medial portion of the pubococcygeus muscle; forming the puborectal sling;
- **Pubococcygeus**, arising from the pubic bone; it is the thickest and most important portion of the levator ani.

- **Iliococcygeus**, arising from the tendinous arch.

Identify the **coccygeus muscle** (Fig. 3.42 B and C). It stretches from the ischial spine to the coccyx and forms the posterior and smaller part of the pelvic diaphragm. The coccygeus is essentially a triangular muscular sheet that lies posterior to the iliococcygeus muscle. Note that the ischiococcygeus contributes to the sacrospinous ligament.

⇦ *GRANT'S 3.21B, 3.22A* A.D.A.M. 4.49 NETTER 333, 334 CLEMENTE 420 A.V.A. 3: 2.18.36

Piriformis Muscle

Observe its origin from the pelvic or ventral surface of the sacrum at segments S2, S3, and S4. Note that the muscle fibers converge and pass through the greater sciatic foramen. The ventral nerve rami S2 and S3 emerge between the digitations of the piriformis.

⇦ *GRANT'S 3.4, 3.21A* ROHEN 446 A.D.A.M. 4.12 NETTER 465 CLEMENTE 410

Sacral Plexus

The sacral nervous plexus is closely related to the anterior surface of the piriformis. In the cadaver, verify the following (Fig. 3.50):

⇦ ROHEN 446, 447 A.D.A.M. 5.26 NETTER 463-465 CLEMENTE 365-367 A.V.A. 3: 2.16.37

- The **lumbosacral trunk** (L4, L5) contributes to the sacral plexus.
- The ventral rami of S2 and S3 emerge between the digitations of the piriformis.
- Ventral rami from L4 through S3 converge and form the large **sciatic nerve**. It passes through the greater sciatic foramen together with the piriformis.
- Usually, the **gluteal arteries** (branches of the internal iliac artery) pierce the sacral plexus: Often, the lumbosacral trunk and S1 are separated by the superior gluteal artery. Occasionally, the superior gluteal artery intervenes between L4 and L5. The inferior gluteal artery usually separates ramus S1 from S2.
- Ventral rami S2, S3, and S4 contribute to the **pudendal nerve**. Note the proximity of the ischial spine and the pudendal nerve (Fig. 3.50). This fact is of obstetrical importance.

⇨ *GRANT'S 3.36* ROHEN 339 A.D.A.M. 4.21, 4.22 NETTER 377, 378 CLEMENTE 414 A.V.A. 3: 2.34.00

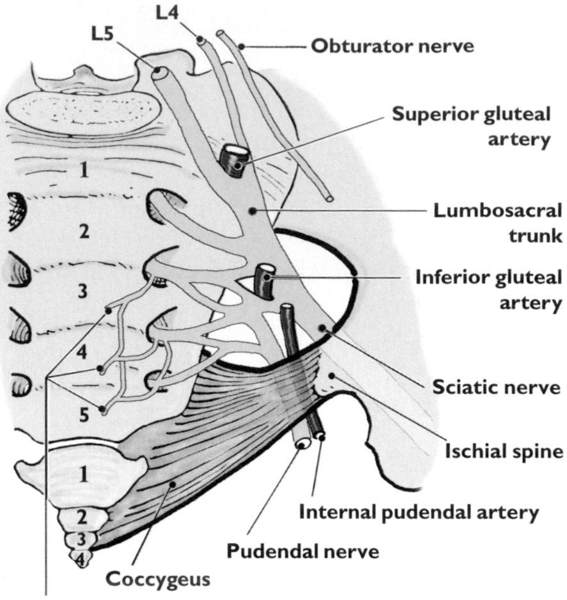

Figure 3.50. Sacral nerve plexus and related vessels. Note the proximity of the ischial spine to the pudendal nerve.

- **Pelvic splanchnic nerves.** The ventral rami S2, S3, and S4 contain preganglionic parasympathetic fibers (sacral parasympathetic outflow; pelvic splanchnic nerves). These autonomic nerves supply the female pelvic organs and the distal portion of the GI tract from left colic flexure to rectum.
- Note the sympathetic chain and its **ganglia** medial to the sacral foramina. These ganglia give off gray rami communicantes to the ventral sacral rami. Review the entire innervation of the *female* pelvis.

Lymphatic Drainage of the Female Pelvis

⇦ NETTER 384

⇦ *GRANT'S 3.23, 3.24* ROHEN 314 NETTER 383 A.V.A. 3: 2.32.02

Lymphatic channels are difficult to see unless they are injected with a dye. However, you may encounter lymph nodes in certain pelvic regions, particularly if there was a pelvic inflammatory or malignant process prior to death. Understand that the external genitalia have a different lymphatic drainage than the uterus and the ovaries. This is of considerable clinical significance. Be familiar with the lymphatic drainage of the rectum.

TEST 8

GAPP

GROSS ANATOMY PRACTICAL PRIMER

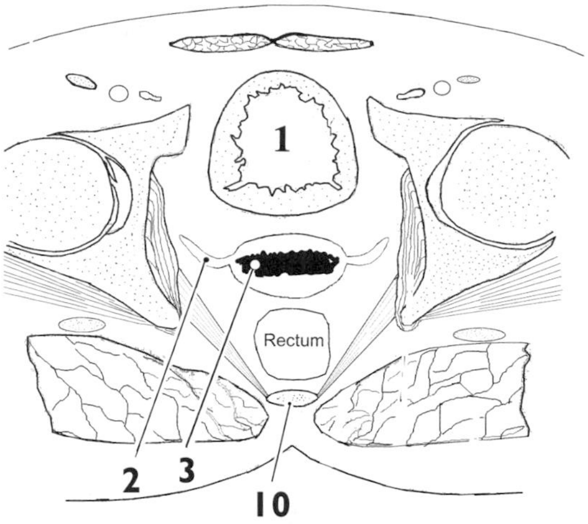

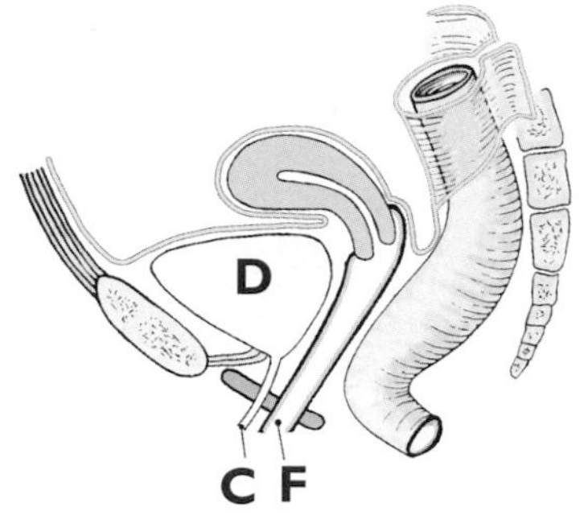

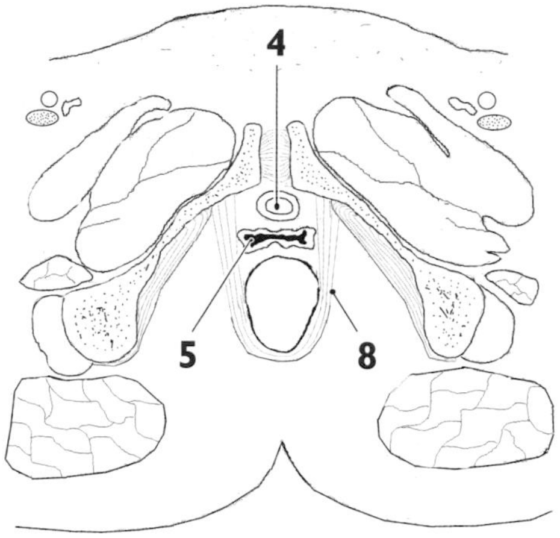

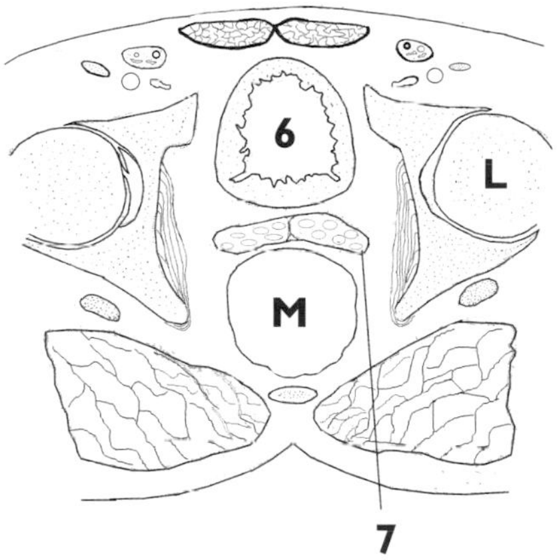

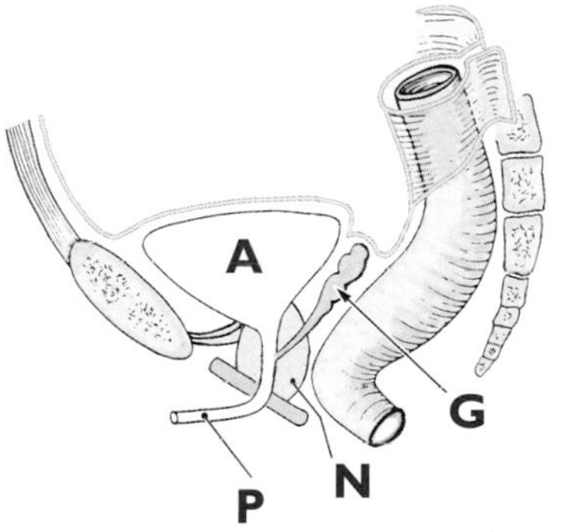

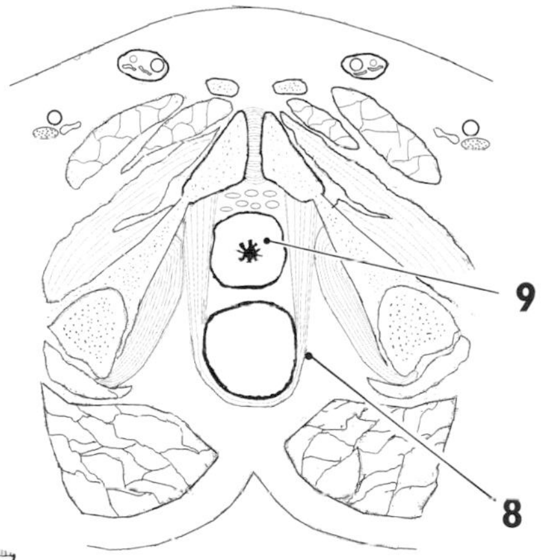

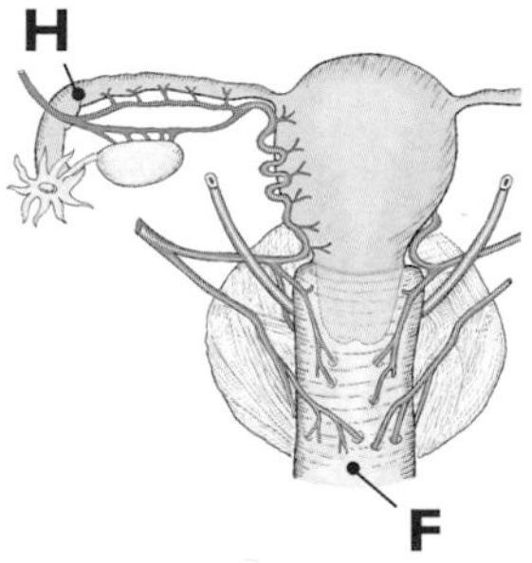

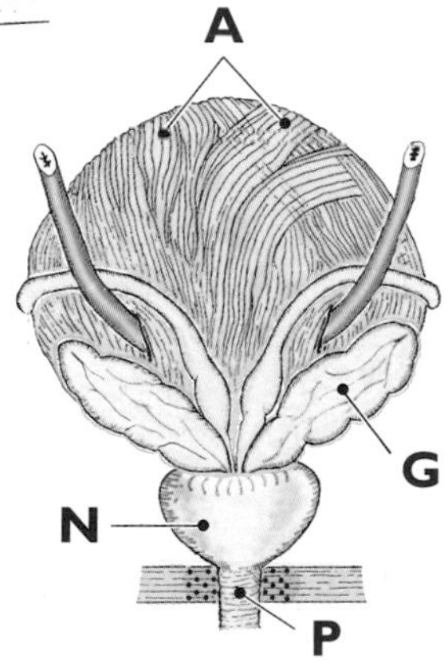

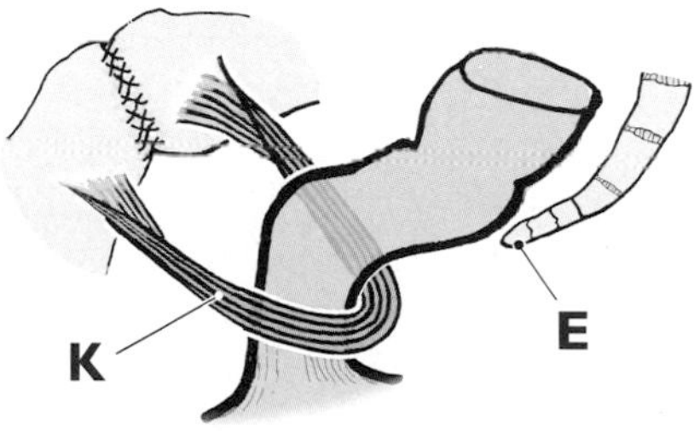

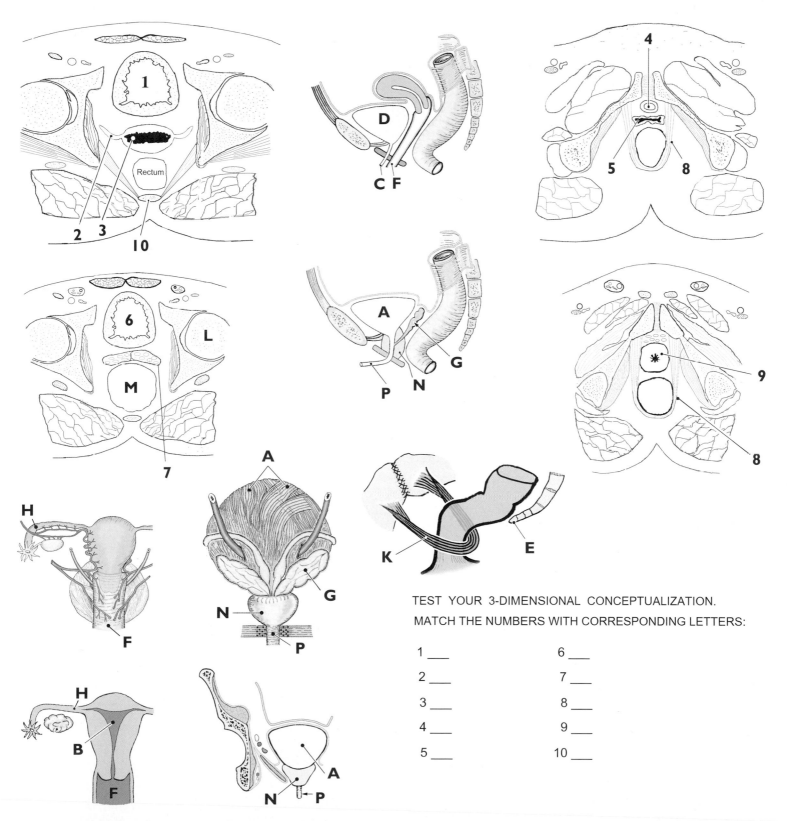

TEST YOUR 3-DIMENSIONAL CONCEPTUALIZATION.

MATCH THE NUMBERS WITH CORRESPONDING LETTERS:

1 ___	6 ___
2 ___	7 ___
3 ___	8 ___
4 ___	9 ___
5 ___	10 ___

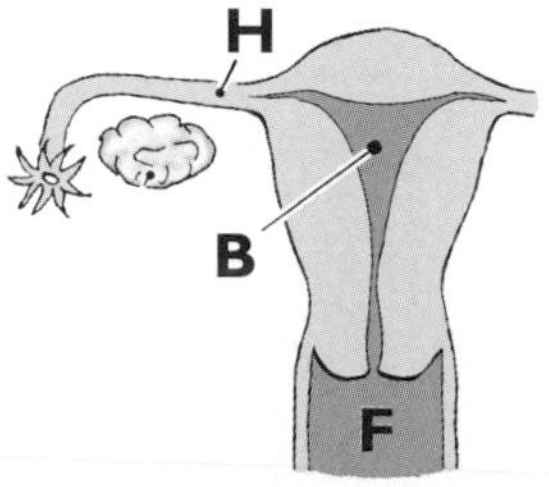

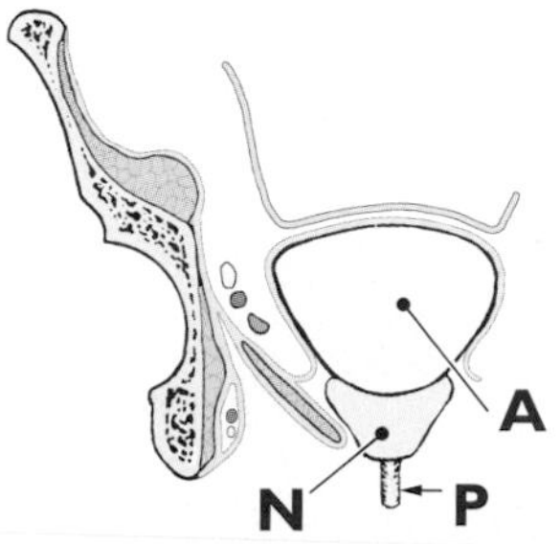

GAPP TEST: IF YOU MADE AN ERROR, REVIEW AND GAIN A BETTER UNDERSTANDING OF THE CONCERNED 3-DIMENSIONAL ANATOMICAL CONCEPT. GAPP KEY: 1-D, 2-H, 3-B, 4-C, 5-F, 6-A, 7-G, 8-K, 9-N, 10-E.

Notes:

CHAPTER 4

THE BACK

GRANT'S ATLAS OF ANATOMY, 10TH ED.:	
ROHEN, COLOR ATLAS OF ANATOMY, 4TH ED.:	ROHEN PAGE #
A.D.A.M. STUDENT ATLAS OF ANATOMY:	A.D.A.M. PLATE #
NETTER, ATLAS OF HUMAN ANATOMY, 2ND ED.:	NETTER PLATE #
CLEMENTE, ANATOMY, 4TH ED.:	CLEMENTE FIG. #
ACLAND'S VIDEO ATLAS OF HUMAN ANATOMY	A.V.A. Vol: hr:min:sec

Surface Anatomy

The back is the posterior aspect of the trunk to which the neck and the limbs are attached. Deep to the skin and superficial fascia are the muscles of the back. The surface anatomy of this region can be studied in a living subject or in the cadaver. Turn the cadaver in the prone position (face down).

⇦
GRANT'S 4.28
A.D.A.M. 1.2
CLEMENTE 623, 624

Palpate important bony reference points (Fig. 4.1): the iliac crest in the pelvic area and the spine and acromion of the scapula. Feel free to mark these areas with a grease pencil. Note the posterior median furrow between the bulges formed by the erector spinae muscles. These bulges are most notable in the lumbar region and are particularly pronounced in muscular specimens. Deep to the median furrow palpate the spinous processes of the vertebral column. The spinous processes of C7 and T1 are more prominent than the others, offering convenient reference points for counting the vertebrae up or down. Two superficial muscles, the trapezius and the latissimus dorsi, cover large areas of the back and are connected to the upper limb. In most cases, the superior border of the trapezius and its attachment to the scapula can be observed (Fig. 4.1).

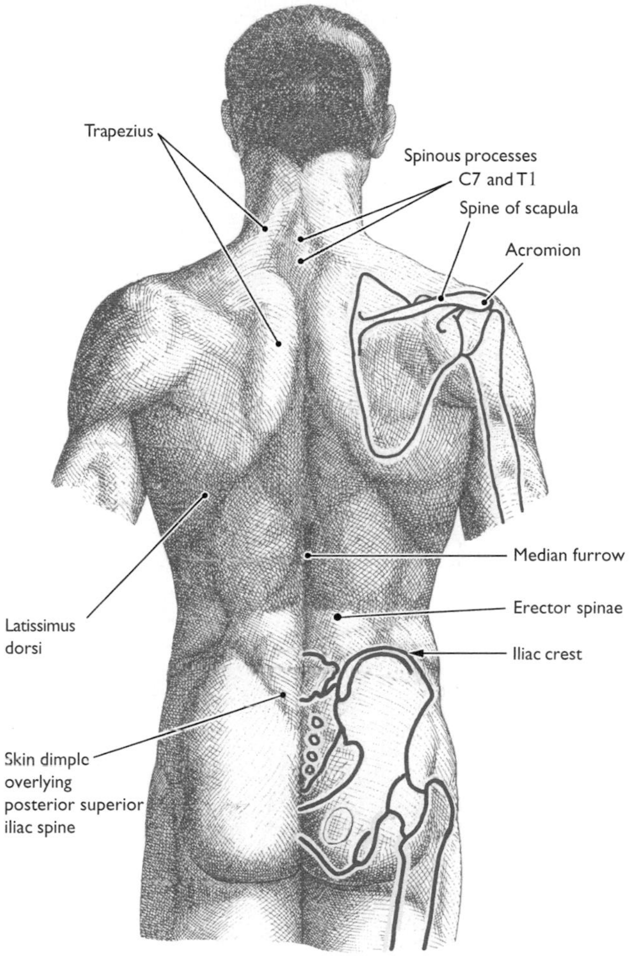

Figure 4.1. Surface anatomy of the back.

Vertebral Column

General Remarks

⇨
GRANT'S 4.1
ROHEN 182, 187
A.D.A.M. 1.7, 1.8
NETTER 142
CLEMENTE 655-657
A.V.A. 3: 0.02.16

The vertebral column (Fig. 4.2) constitutes the axis of the body. It consists of 33 vertebrae: 7 cervical (C), 12 thoracic (T), 5 lumbar (L), 5 sacral (S) that are fused as the sacrum, and 4 small coccygeal vertebrae (Co) that collectively form the coccyx , also known as the coccygeal bone or tail bone. The upper 24 movable vertebrae (cervical, thoracic, lumbar) allow flexibility and movement of the vertebral column. Each vertebra has a large vertebral foramen. In the articulated vertebral column, the vertebral foramina collectively form a bony tube, the vertebral canal. This canal encloses and protects part of the central nervous system, the spinal cord.

Bony Landmarks

Refer to a skeleton and to the cadaver, which must be in the prone position (face down). Identify the following bony landmarks:

- **Vertebral column** (Fig. 4.2)

⇨
GRANT'S 4.5, 4.6
ROHEN 189
NETTER 143
CLEMENTE 658
A.V.A. 3: 0.03.30

- Study a **thoracic vertebra** (Fig. 4.3). It consists of a weight-bearing body and a protective vertebral arch that is made up of two rounded **pedicles** (roots) and two flat plates or **laminae**. At the junction of pedicle and lamina,

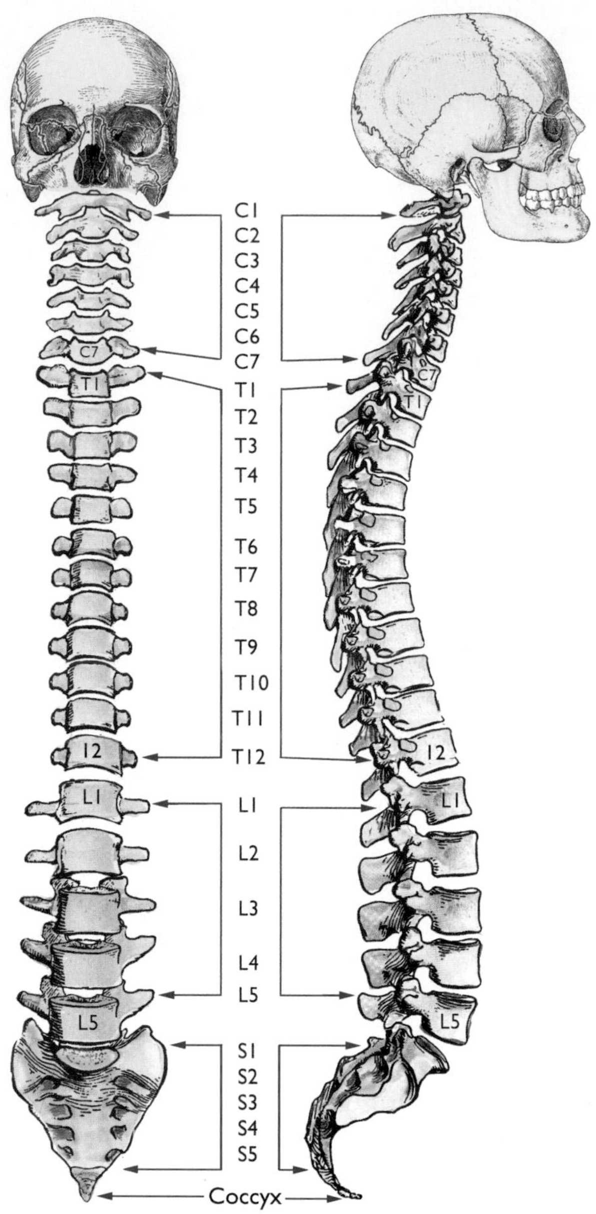

Figure 4.2. Vertebral column in anterior and lateral view.

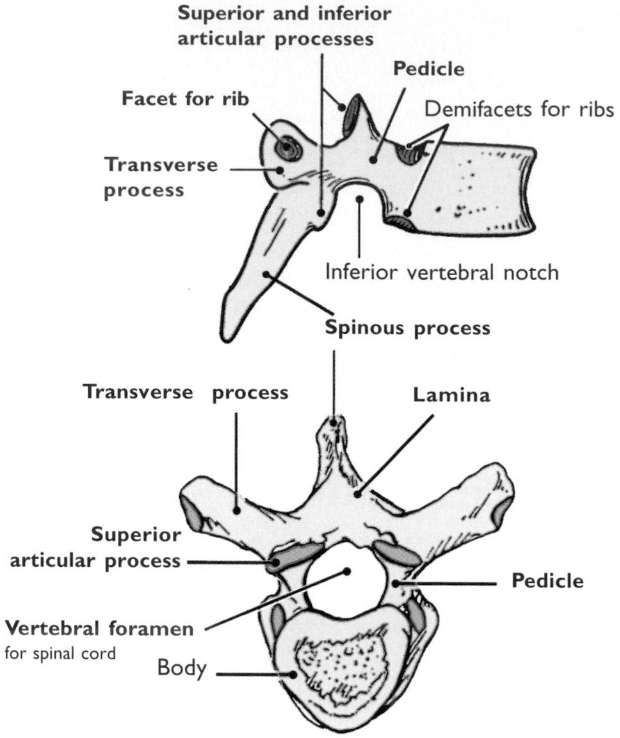

Figure 4.3. Typical thoracic vertebra in lateral and superior view.

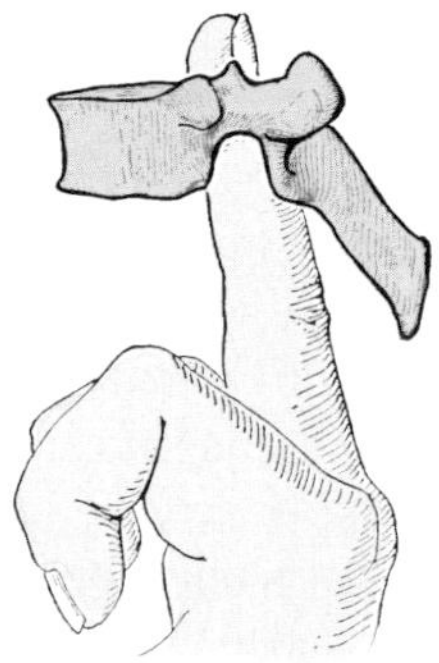

Figure 4.4. A vertebral foramen is not larger than a finger ring. In the articulated vertebral column, the vertebral foramina collectively form the bony vertebral canal.

a **transverse process** projects laterally, and **articular processes** project superiorly and inferiorly. At the junction of the two laminae, a **spinous process** projects posteriorly in the median plane. The bodies and transverse processes of the thoracic vertebrae have facets for the ribs (Fig. 4.3). Identify the large **vertebral foramen**.

- Place your index finger into the **vertebral foramen** of a vertebra. Observe that the size of the vertebral foramen is not larger than a finger ring and that the diameter of the vertebral foramina differs from vertebra to vertebra.
- In the articulated vertebral column, the vertebral foramina collectively form a bony tube, the **vertebral canal**. This canal encloses and protects the spinal cord.

⇨
GRANT'S 4.23, 4.24B
ROHEN 189
NETTER 144
CLEMENTE 657, 688
A.V.A. 3: 0.04.10

⇦
GRANT'S 4.9, 4.12B, 4.13
NETTER 143, 144
A.V.A. 3: 0.14.43

Understand that access to the contents of the spinal canal is possible by surgical removal of the laminae (laminectomy).

- Two adjacent vertebral bodies are united by a fibrocartilaginous **intervertebral disc**. This is a joint of the symphysis variety (Fig. 4.5).
- Two adjacent vertebral arches are united by their **articular processes**.
- An **intervertebral foramen** is completed between the pedicles of two adjacent vertebrae. It transmits the spinal nerve of the corresponding segment.
- The head of a rib articulates with two vertebral bodies and the intervening disc (Fig. 4.5). The tubercle of a

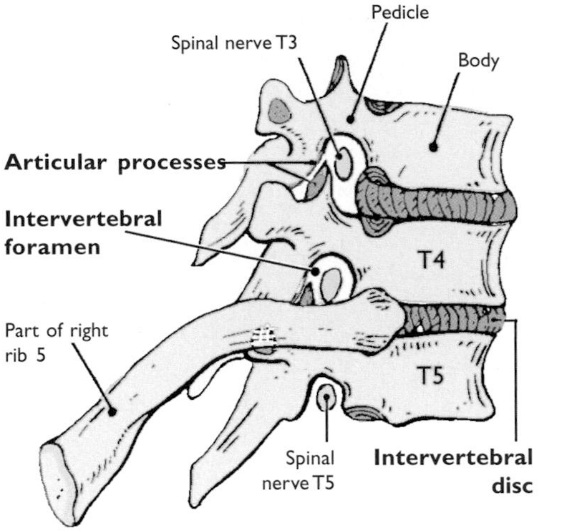

Figure 4.5. Part of vertebral column: intervertebral disc; intervertebral foramen with spinal nerve; portion of rib.

rib articulates with the transverse process of the vertebra with the same segmental number. The head of rib 5 articulates with vertebral bodies T4 and T5. The tubercle of rib 5 articulates with the transverse process of T5.

- Examine the **cervical vertebrae** (Fig. 4.6). Identify: the right and left **transverse processes**, each containing a characteristic opening, the **foramen transversarium**, that transmits the vertebral artery. Identify the **spinous processes** of all cervical vertebrae. Usually, the 7th cervical spine is the most prominent of the cervical spines. In the cadaver, run the finger down in the dorsal midline from external occipital protuberance, until it is arrested by the 7th cervical spine. Study radiographs of the cervical spine.
- The **atlas** (C1) does not have a spinous process but merely a **posterior tubercle** (Fig. 4.6). The **first thoracic spine** belongs to the **axis** (C2). It may be more prominent than the spine of C7.
- **Scapula** (Fig. 4.6). Identify its **spine.** Trace it from the medial border to the **acromion.** Palpate the **superior** and the **inferior angle** and the **medial or vertebral border** of the scapula.
- **Iliac crest** (Fig. 4.6). It terminates posteriorly in the **posterior superior iliac spine**. Here, the overlying skin often shows a dimple, since there are no fleshy muscle fibers.
- **Occipital bone** (Fig. 4.6). Note the **external occipital protuberance** or **inion** and the **nuchal lines.**
- **Mastoid process**

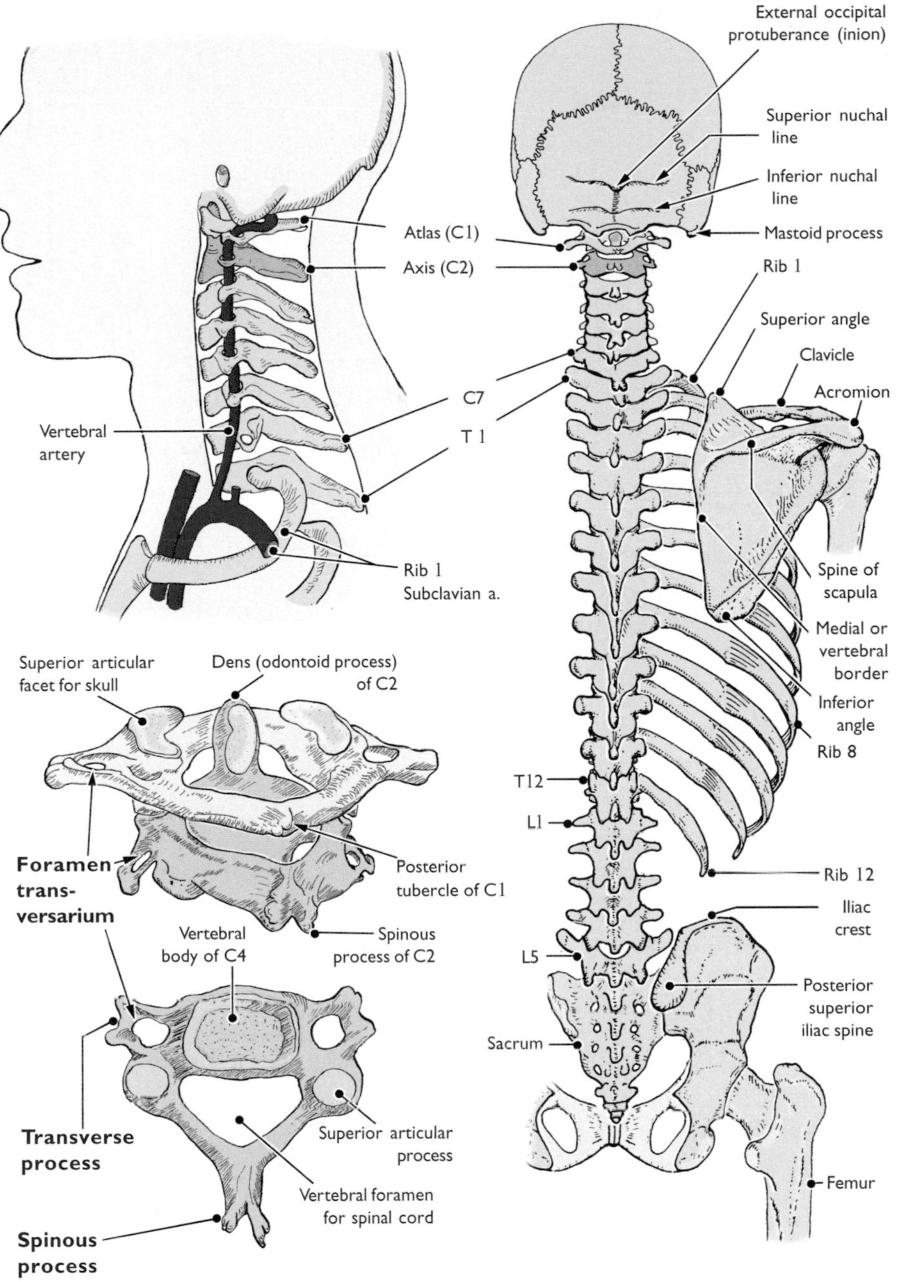

Figure 4.6. Bony landmarks of the back and vertebral column.

⇦
GRANT'S 4.1A
ROHEN 191
A.D.A.M. 1.9
NETTER 12
CLEMENTE 639-642
A.V.A. 1: 0.03.15

- There are **primary** and **secondary curvatures** of the spinal column. Identify these curvatures in a skeleton.

Clinical Correlation: With an imaginary line, connect the highest points of the left and right iliac crests. This line crosses the vertebral column at the 4th lumbar spine. The 3rd lumbar interspace is between the 3rd and 4th lumbar spines. A needle is usually introduced into the 3rd lumbar interspace to obtain cerebrospinal fluid (CSF) from the subarachnoid space (spinal tap or lumbar puncture) for diagnostic purposes.

Muscles of the Back

General Remarks

The muscles of the back are divided into three groups: superficial, intermediate, and deep. The **superficial group** anchors the upper limb to the axial skeleton. This anchorage extends from the skull to the pelvic girdle. The **intermediate group** functions in respiration. The **deep group** consists of intrinsic or "native" muscles of the back (dorsum). These are supplied by dorsal nerve rami (Fig. 4.7). Embryologically, the superficial and intermediate groups migrated from the ventrum and hence are supplied by ventral nerve rami.

GRANT'S 1.20
ROHEN 214
A.D.A.M. 1.35
NETTER 166
CLEMENTE 405

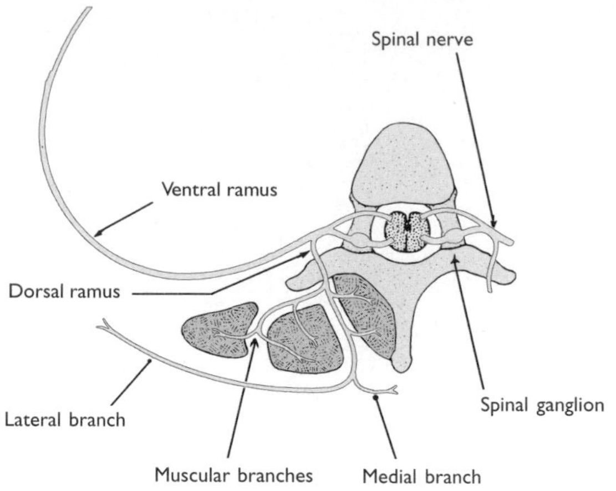

Figure 4.7. Schema of spinal nerve. Distribution of dorsal ramus to deep back muscles and skin of back.

Before you begin ...

To save time, skin and superficial fascia of the back will be removed together. The muscles of the superficial and intermediate groups will be reflected. Subsequently, the deep group will be studied. The dorsal aspect of the vertebral column will be exposed. The vertebral canal will be opened, and the spinal cord and its coverings will be studied. Finally, the muscles and nerves of the suboccipital region will be examined.

Skin Incisions

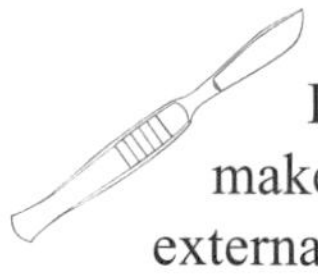

Refer to Figure 4.8. In the midline, make a vertical skin incision from the external occipital protuberance (*X*) to the level of the posterior superior iliac spines (*S*). Carry out the following transverse incisions:

- From *S* to *T*, along the iliac crest (if not already done for the dissection of the gluteal region);
- From *U* to *V*, at the level of the inferior scapular angle;
- From *R* to *B*, superior to the scapula and to the tip of the acromion, and on to point F. Here, make a complete circular skin incision at the root of the arm.
- From the external occipital protuberance (*X*) laterally to the base of the mastoid process (*M*).

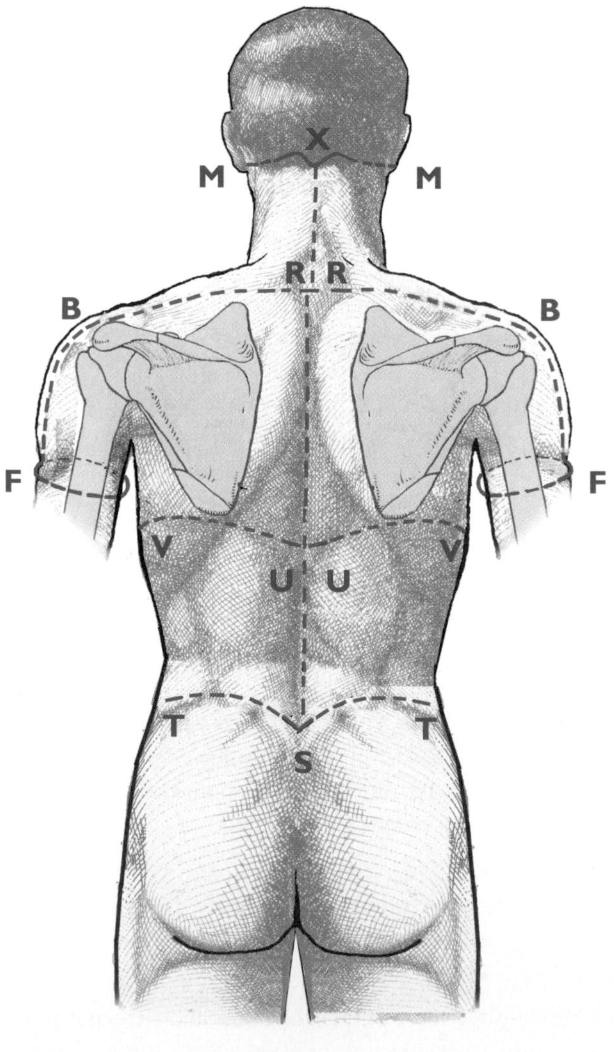

Figure 4.8. Skin incisions.

Skin Reflection and Special Attention in the Occipital Area. Reflect the skin in the area bounded by points *X*, *M*, and *R* (Fig. 4.8). In the underlying subcutaneous tissue, attempt

GRANT'S 4.29
A.D.A.M. 1.53
NETTER 163, 164
CLEMENTE 634

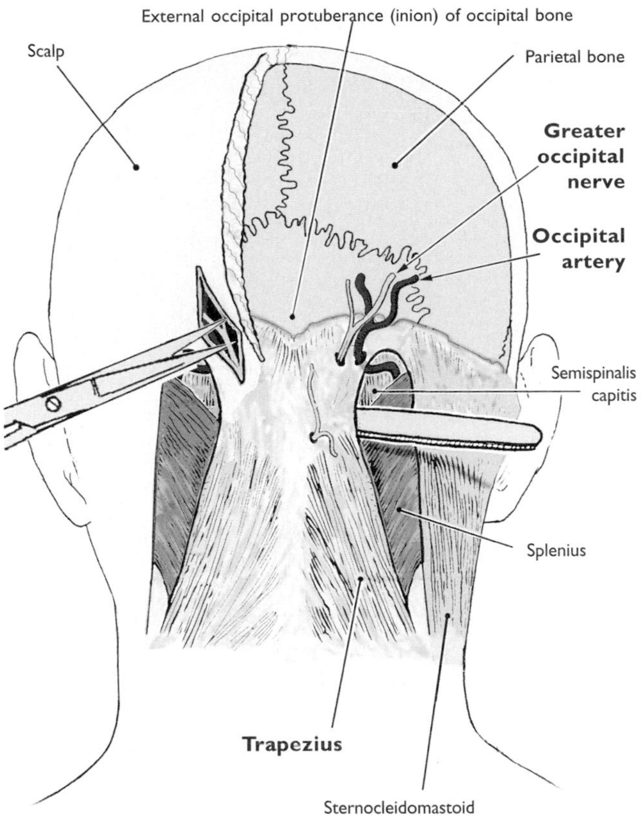

Figure 4.9. Greater occipital nerve and occipital artery.

to locate the **greater occipital nerve** and the accompanying **occipital artery** (Fig. 4.9). The nerve pierces the **trapezius muscle** about 3 cm inferolateral to the external occipital protuberance (inion). The artery lies lateral to the nerve. The deep fascia in this area is very dense and tough. Therefore, it may be difficult to find the nerve, even though it is large.

With scissors, split the deep fascia parallel to the expected course of the nerve (Fig. 4.9). If you find the occipital artery first, look for the nerve medial to it. Limit your time searching for the nerve. Check with your instructor. It is possible that you may have removed the distal portion of this cutaneous nerve with the skin.

Alternatively, with the handle of a scalpel or with a spatula, raise the free border of the superior portion of the trapezius muscle. The absence of fat in the area between the muscles makes it relatively easy to see the **greater occipital nerve** as it passes through the underlying semispinalis capitis muscle and then pierces the trapezius. You will later encounter the most proximal portion of the nerve as it emerges from the suboccipital triangle.

GRANT'S 1.20
ROHEN 214
A.D.A.M. 1.35
NETTER 166
CLEMENTE 13, 405
A.V.A. 3: 0.32.50

The greater occipital nerve is the dorsal ramus of C2. Read an account of the **dorsal primary divisions** or **dorsal rami** of the spinal nerves (Fig. 4.7). To save time, make no deliberate effort to display other cutaneous branches of the dorsal rami. However, several of these nerves may be seen piercing the trapezius or latissimus dorsi to enter the superficial fascia.

GRANT'S 4.29
ROHEN 214
A.D.A.M. 1.53
NETTER 163
CLEMENTE 625, 628

Reflect skin and superficial fascia of the back together. In doing this, you will also remove the medial and lateral cutaneous branches of the dorsal rami. These cutaneous branches course in the superficial fascia (or subcutaneous fat). Be careful **not** to incise the superficial fascia along the anterior border of the trapezius. Here, the spinal accessory nerve and other structures are in danger of being cut. The spinal accessory nerve and branches of ventral rami C2 to C4 supply the large trapezius muscle.

Superficial Muscle Group

GRANT'S 4.29
ROHEN 209
A.D.A.M. 1.53
NETTER 160
CLEMENTE 629
A.V.A. 1: 0.18.54

Clean two extensive muscles of the superficial group: **trapezius** and **latissimus dorsi** (Fig. 4.10). Notice that they cover almost the entire back. Observe two triangles associated with the latissimus dorsi: the triangle of auscultation, and the lumbar triangle.

GRANT'S 4.30
A.D.A.M. 1.53
NETTER 160
CLEMENTE 629
A.V.A. 1: 0.15.43

Clinical Correlation: The **triangle of auscultation** (Fig. 4.10) is bounded by the latissimus dorsi, trapezius, and rhomboid major together with the vertebral border of the scapula. Here, ribs 6 and 7 and the intercostal space 6 are free of overlying muscles. Thus, this area is particularly suited for auscultation (listening to sounds produced by thoracic organs, particularly the lungs).

The **lumbar triangle** (of Petit) is bounded by the latissimus dorsi, external oblique of the abdomen, and iliac crest (Fig. 4.10). Its floor is formed by the internal oblique of the abdomen. On rare occasions, this weak triangular space is the site of a "lumbar hernia."

Trapezius (Fig. 4.10). Observe the origin of this triangular muscle from the external occipital protuberance (inion), the ligamentum nuchae, and the spinous process of C7 and the spinous processes of T1 through T12.

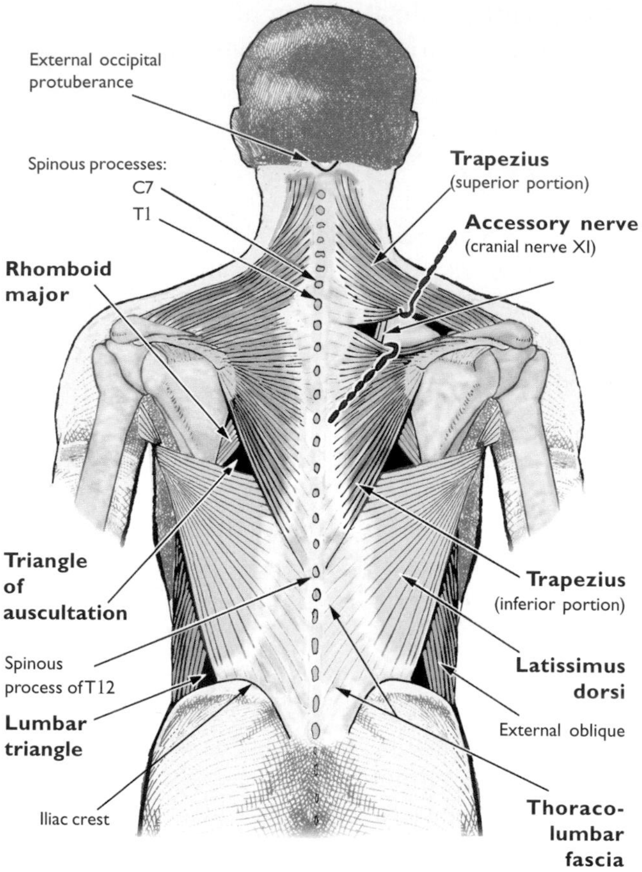

Figure 4.10. Exposure of dorsal scapular region.

The ligamentum nuchae is a strong, cord-like supraspinous ligament that extends from the external occipital protuberance to the spinous process of C7. Note that different parts of the **trapezius muscle** take different fiber courses:

- Fibers of the **superior portion** run inferolaterally and are inserted into the lateral third of the clavicle.
- Fibers of the **middle portion** run transversely. They are inserted into the acromion and spine of the scapula.
- Fibers of the **inferior portion** run superolaterally. These fibers converge into an aponeurosis near the medial end of the spine of the scapula.

The trapezius must be reflected in such a manner as (a) to allow complete access to underlying structures; and (b) to preserve its blood and nerve supply.

⇨
Grant's 4.29
Rohen 210
Netter 163
Clemente 634

⇦
Grant's 8.3, 8.4
Netter 395
Clemente 42
A.V.A. 1: 0.16.09

⇦
Grant's 4.29
Rohen 209
A.D.A.M. 1.53
Netter 395
Clemente 629
A.V.A. 3: 0.16.27

- Ask your partner to push the shoulder backward (posteriorly). This relaxes the trapezius.
- Pass your hand deep to the free lateral and inferior border of the muscle. Feel the loose fat and areolar tissue separating the trapezius from other muscles.
- With blunt dissection, using the handle of a scalpel and a finger, spread apart the muscle fibers at the level of the spine of the scapula (Fig. 4.10).
- Identify a portion of the **accessory nerve** (cranial nerve XI) that runs vertically on the undersurface of the trapezius muscle.
- Detach the muscle from its origin very close to the spinous processes. Start inferiorly. Carefully carry the detachment toward the external occipital protuberance. Frequently define and loosen the muscle with a finger before you proceed with the cutting.
- Finally, detach the trapezius from its insertion into the spine and acromion of the scapula. Do this with a scalpel, cutting very close to the bone. Now, the muscle is attached only to the clavicle.
- Reflect the muscle laterally.
- Study the **deep surface** of the reflected **trapezius muscle.** In the loose fatty tissue, find blood vessels and nerves.
- Using blunt dissection and a probe, identify the **accessory nerve**.
- Follow the accessory nerve inferiorly and note that it sends numerous twigs into the musculature of the trapezius muscle.

Dissection Note: The accessory nerve (cranial nerve XI) passes through the posterior triangle of the neck. However, do not follow the nerve into the triangle at this time. Keep the triangle undisturbed. This area will be dissected later with other head and neck structures.

If your dissection sequence was such that the posterior triangle of the neck has already been dissected, then establish the continuity of the accessory nerve in the triangle.

Latissimus Dorsi (Fig. 4.10). Verify the following:

- Its thin superior border extends laterally from the spinous processes of T6 and T7.
- Its most lateral fibers interdigitate with those of the external oblique inferior to the origin of the serratus anterior.
- The latissimus dorsi arises from the vast **thoracolumbar fascia** (lumbodorsal fascia) that covers the deep (intrinsic) musculature of the back.
- Superiorly, the muscle fibers of the latissimus dorsi converge. They form a broad tendon which is inserted into the humerus.
- Close to the tendon, the muscle receives its nerve supply. Do not explore either tendinous insertion or nerve supply at this time.
- Place your hand deep to the latissimus dorsi and lift it up slightly. With a scalpel, cut through its tendinous origin from the thoracolumbar fascia. Avoid cutting too close to the lumbar spinous processes.
- Reflect the muscle laterally.

Next, study the three remaining muscles of the superficial group: **rhomboideus major, rhomboideus minor,** and **levator scapulae**. They are inserted into the medial border of the scapula.

- Place your finger deep to the rhomboideus major and minor.
- Detach these muscles from the spinous processes. Reflect them laterally.
- On the deep surface of the muscles, look for nerves and blood vessels.
- Leave the levator scapulae undisturbed. However, observe three or four slips arising from the transverse processes of the upper four cervical vertebrae.
- At this point, all muscular attachments (with the exception of the levator scapulae) of the shoulder girdle to the vertebral column have been severed. As a result, the shoulder will easily fall forward (anteriorly).

GRANT'S 4.29
ROHEN 209, 210
A.D.A.M. 1.53, 1.55
NETTER 160
CLEMENTE 629
A.V.A. 1: 0.18.54

Intermediate Muscle Group

Following reflection of the superficial muscle group, the **intermediate muscle group** is readily accessible. Observe the thin sheets of the **serratus posterior superior** and **serratus posterior inferior.** These muscles are respiratory in action. Note their insertions into the ribs.

GRANT'S 4.30
ROHEN 209
A.D.A.M. 1.55
NETTER 161
CLEMENTE 630

Cut through the thin aponeuroses of both muscles at their origins from the spinous processes. Reflect the muscles laterally. Now, the muscles of the deep group are accessible.

Deep Muscle Group

The **muscles of the deep group** include (Fig. 4.11): **splenius capitis and cervicis, semispinalis capitis,** and the enormous mus-

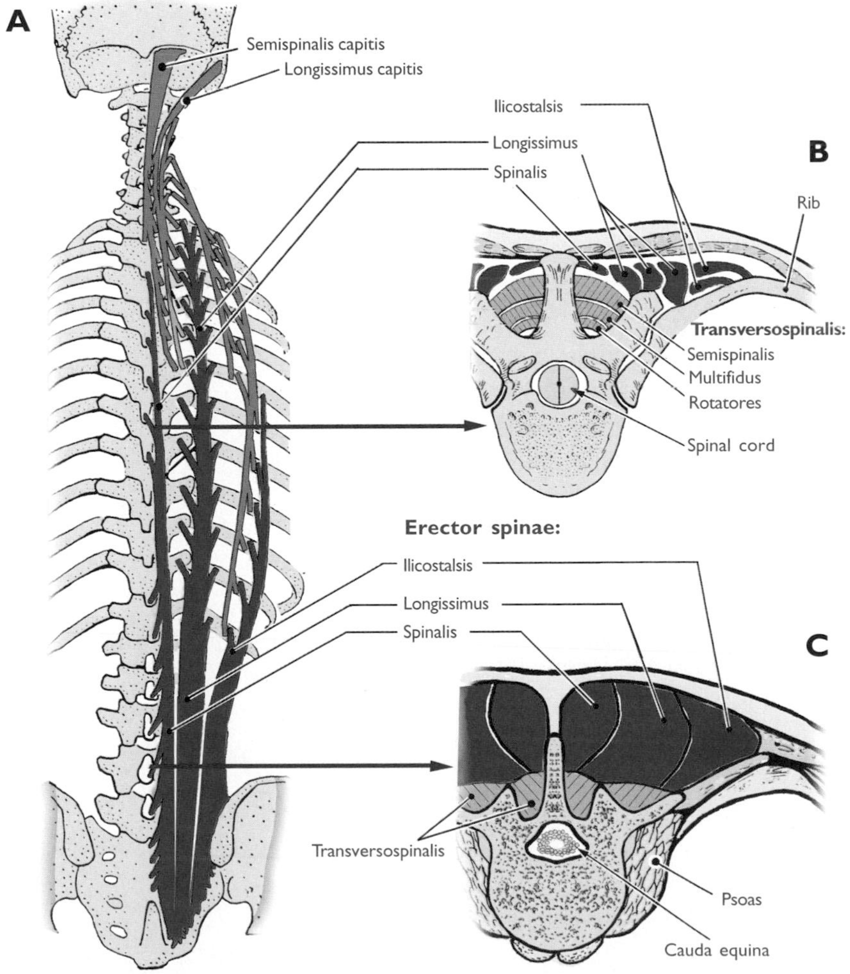

Figure 4.11. Deep muscles of the back: erector spinae and semispinalis capitis in schematic view **(*A*)** and schematic transverse sections at the thoracic level (*B*) and the lumbar level **(*C*)**.

culature collectively called the **erector spinae** and **transversospinalis.** Deep to the semispinalis capitis lie the small muscles of the suboccipital region.

Splenius Capitis and Cervicis (Gr. *splenion*, bandage; L., *caput*, head; *cervix*, neck).

- Identify the splenius capitis which is inserted into the occipital bone and the mastoid process.
- The splenius cervicis is inserted into the transverse processes of the upper cervical vertebrae.
- On one side only, detach the splenius where it arises from the ligamentum nuchae and spinous processes.
- Reflect the muscle laterally. Now, the semispinalis capitis is fully exposed.

The **semispinalis capitis** arises from the transverse processes of the upper thoracic vertebrae. It is inserted into the occipital bone between the nuchal lines. Note that it is traversed by the greater occipital nerve.

Erector Spinae or Sacrospinalis (Fig. 4.11). This bilateral structure is formed by long, vertically running muscle bundles on each side of the vertebral column. In the well developed specimen, it is a prominent and massive muscular bulge stretching from the pelvis to the skull. Distinguish **three columns** of the erector spinae: **iliocostalis, longissimus,** and **spinalis.**

The **iliocostalis** is the **lateral column of the erector spinae** (Fig. 4.11). As its name appropriately suggests, it arises from the ilium (iliac crest) and inserts into ribs (L. *costa*, rib). Identify the **three parts of the iliocostalis:**

- A lumbar part, arising from the iliac crest and inserting into the angles of the lower six ribs (Figs. 4.11 *A* and *B*);
- A thoracic part, arising from the six lower ribs and inserting into the six upper ribs (Figs. 4.11 *A* and *B*);
- A cervical part, arising from the upper six ribs and inserting into the transverse processes of

GRANT'S 4.31
ROHEN 210
A.D.A.M. 1.56
NETTER 161
CLEMENTE 630, 631
A.V.A. 3: 0.24.05

GRANT'S 4.32
ROHEN 210
NETTER 161
CLEMENTE 631
A.V.A. 3: 0.26.22

GRANT'S 4.36
ROHEN 211
A.D.A.M. 1.57
NETTER 161, 162
CLEMENTE 631
A.V.A. 3: 0.26.26

GRANT'S 4.33-4.35
ROHEN 211
A.D.A.M. 1.56
NETTER 162
CLEMENTE 6.32, 633
A.V.A. 3: 0.22.43

GRANT'S 4.31
ROHEN 210
A.D.A.M. 1.56
NETTER 161
CLEMENTE 630, 631
A.V.A. 3: 0.24.30

GRANT'S 4.36
ROHEN 192
NETTER 2, 5
CLEMENTE 757
A.V.A. 4: 0.06.02

the lower cervical vertebrae. Identify the general orientation of these muscular structures.

The **longissimus** (L., meaning the longest) is the **middle column of the erector spinae** (Fig. 4.11). It gives muscles slips to the transverse processes of the thoracic and cervical vertebrae. Identify the thoracic and cervical portions of the longissimus (Figs. 4.11 *A* and *B*). Note that its most superior portion, the **longissimus capitis**, inserts into the mastoid process of the skull.

Identify the **spinalis** which forms the **medial column of the erector spinae** (Fig. 4.11). It is relatively thin (about 2 cm). As the name implies, it is connected to the spinous processes of lumbar, thoracic and cervical vertebrae.

Function. Appreciate the fact that all three columns of the erector spinae extend the vertebral column if both sides work together. If only one side is active, the three columns bend the vertebral column laterally. Are you familiar with the nerve supply to the erector spinae (Fig. 4.7)?

Transversospinalis. On one side of the cadaver, remove the spinalis and the longissimus. This procedure will expose the space between spinous processes and transverse processes of the vertebrae. A number of short muscles (semispinalis, multifidus, rotatores) can be seen filling the groove between transverse and spinous processes (Figs. 4.11 *A* and *B*). These muscles are collectively called the **transversospinalis.** If required to define and dissect these short, obliquely running muscles, please refer to appropriate atlas illustrations.

Suboccipital Region

> ***Dissection Note:*** Students may or may not be required to dissect the suboccipital region. Check with your instructor. The following description will aid you in either dissecting this region or in understanding a prosected specimen.

Bony Landmarks

Refer to a skull and identify the following pertinent landmarks (Fig. 4.12):

- **Superior nuchal line**;
- **Inferior nuchal line**;

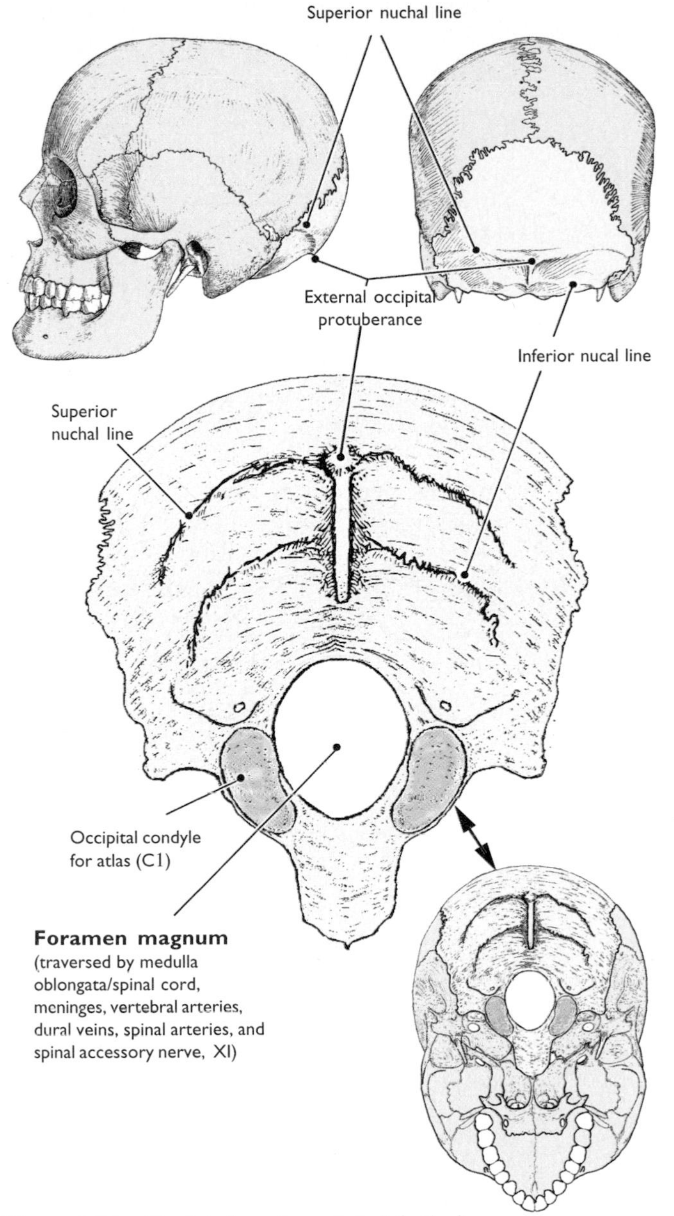

Figure 4.12. Occipital portion of skull (*yellow*).

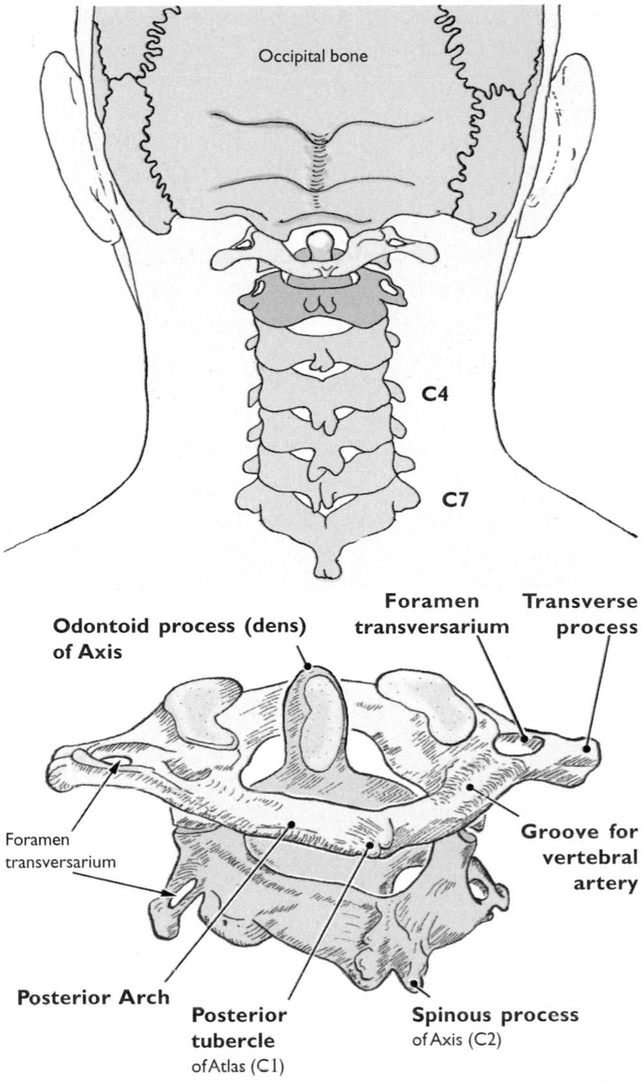

Figure 4.13. Essential bony landmarks of the cervical vertebral column. Atlas (C1) and Axis (C2) are articulated below.

- The area between the two nuchal lines;
- **External occipital protuberance** (or inion);
- **Foramen magnum**, which marks the boundary between brain stem and spinal cord.

Refer to a skeleton and examine the **cervical part of the vertebral column**. Identify the following pertinent landmarks (Fig. 4.13):

- On the **1st cervical vertebra or atlas,** identify the **posterior arch** with **posterior tubercle, transverse process**; **foramen transversarium** for the transmission of the vertebral artery, and **groove for the vertebral artery.**

⇨
GRANT'S 4.36, 4.37
ROHEN 211
NETTER 164
CLEMENTE 634, 635
A.V.A. 4: 0.29.51

⇦
GRANT'S 4.8-4.11
ROHEN 191
NETTER 12
CLEMENTE 639-646
A.V.A. 4: 0.12.09

- On the **2nd cervical vertebra** or **axis** identify the **spinous process, transverse process, foramen transversarium**, and the **vertebral foramen**.

Suboccipital Triangle

Identify the **semispinalis capitis** (Fig. 4.14). Detach the semispinalis capitis bilaterally close to its insertion into the occipital bone. Carefully reflect the muscle inferiorly. Take caution not to tear the **greater occipital nerve.** Trace this nerve through the substance of the semispinalis capitis. Deep to the muscle, follow the nerve to the lower border of the inferior oblique. The greater occipital nerve emerges between vertebrae C1 and C2. The bulk of this nerve is cutaneous to the posterior aspect of the scalp.

Identify and clean the **three muscles** bounding the **suboccipital triangle** (Fig. 4.14):

⇦
Grant's 4.37
Rohen 210, 211
A.D.A.M. 1.57, 1.58
Netter 164
Clemente 636
A.V.A. 4: 0.27.05

- **Obliquus capitis inferior** (inferior oblique). It bounds the triangle inferiorly. Verify that this muscle extends from the spinous process of the axis (C2) to the transverse process of the atlas (C1).
- **Rectus capitis posterior major** (rectus major). It bounds the suboccipital triangle medially. Follow it from the spinous process of the axis superolaterally to the inferior nuchal line. (The rectus minor lies medial to the rectus major. It originates from the posterior tubercle of the atlas.)
- **Obliquus capitis superior** (superior oblique). It bounds the triangle laterally. It lies deep. Follow it from the transverse process of the atlas to the occipital bone.

Demonstrate the **contents of the occipital triangle** (Fig. 4.14):

⇦
A.D.A.M. 1.57
Netter 164
Clemente 637, 638

- The **suboccipital nerve** (dorsal ramus of C1); note that the nerve emerges between the occipital bone and vertebra C1. The suboccipital nerve is a motor to muscles of the suboccipital region.
- The **vertebral artery**. On one side of the body, cut all dorsal musculature away from the transverse processes of C1 and C2. Identify the vertebral artery as it passes through the **foramina transversaria** of the axis and atlas. On the same side, scrape clean the **posterior arch of the atlas**. Note the thin **posterior atlanto-occipital membrane** that stretches from this arch to the posterior margin of the foramen magnum. Observe that the vertebral artery curves around the superior articular process of the atlas. Follow it in its groove on the arch of the atlas. Finally, the artery passes through a hiatus in the posterior atlanto-occipital membrane.

⇦
Grant's 4.38, 4.40A
Netter 14
A.V.A. 5: 1.32.10

Review the **articulated vertebral column.** Once more, examine all seven cervical vertebrae (Fig.4.13). Correlate your observations with corresponding radiographs. In a lateral radiograph of the cervical spine (also called lateral C-spine), identify the following:

⇦
Grant's 4.8
Rohen 192
Netter 12-14
Clemente 645
A.V.A. 3: 0.07.21

- **Posterior arch of atlas** (C1); note that there is only a **posterior tubercle** but no spinous process. The **posterior arch,** in part, surrounds the cervical spinal cord.
- **Anterior arch and anterior tubercle of atlas** (C1).
- **Dens (odontoid process) of axis** (C2). Note that the dens is closely related to the anterior arch of C1.
- **Spinous process of axis** (C2).

⇨
Grant's 4.11
Rohen 191
Netter 12-16
Clemente 645, 653
A.V.A. 4: 0.12.56

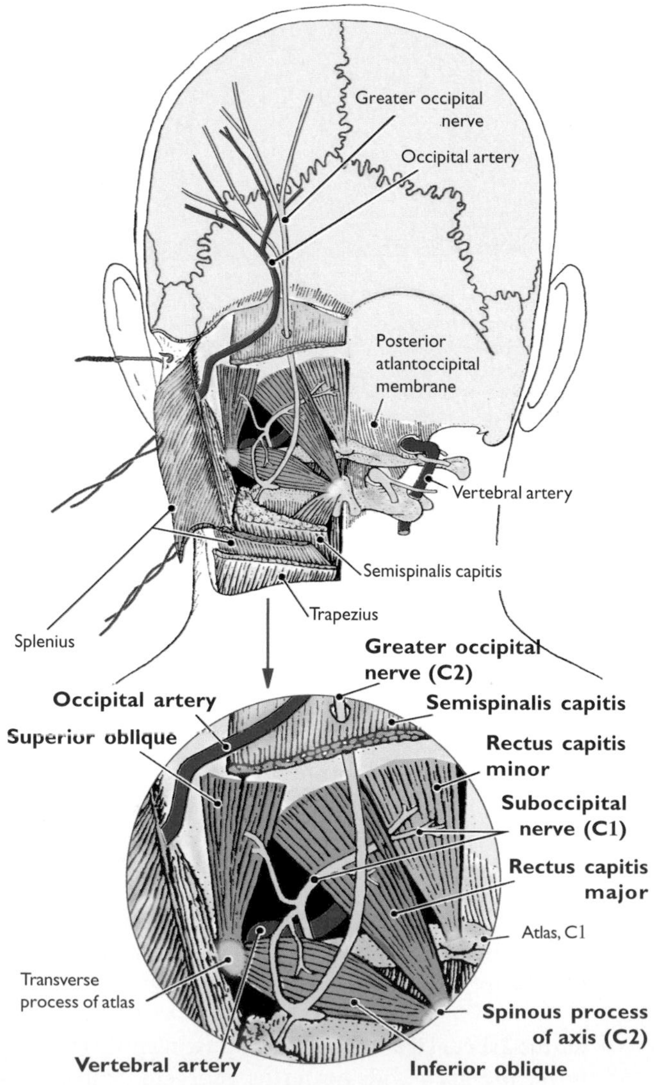

Figure 4.14. Suboccipital region.

Clinical Correlation: The radiographic evaluation of the C-spine is of enormous clinical importance, particularly in the evaluation of injuries sustained after falls or during automobile accidents. If a physician cannot competently recognize bony injuries of the C-spine (for example, a fractured dens), the cervical spinal cord may be compromised, the patient's life could be acutely endangered, or even death could be the tragic consequence.

GRANT'S 4.7, 4.8, 4.11
CLEMENTE 654

Vertebral Canal and Spinal Cord

General Remarks

Vertebral Canal (Fig. 4.15). The vertebral canal is a continuous hollow structure formed by the successive vertebral foramina of the cervical, thoracic, and lumbar vertebrae and, most inferiorly, by the sacral canal. This vertebral canal encloses and protects the spinal cord, its surrounding membranes (spinal meninges), and associated spinal blood vessels.

Spinal Cord (Fig. 4.15). The cylindrical spinal cord is part of the central nervous system. It is the (downward) continuation of the medulla oblongata of the brain. It begins at the foramen magnum of the occipital bone and usu-

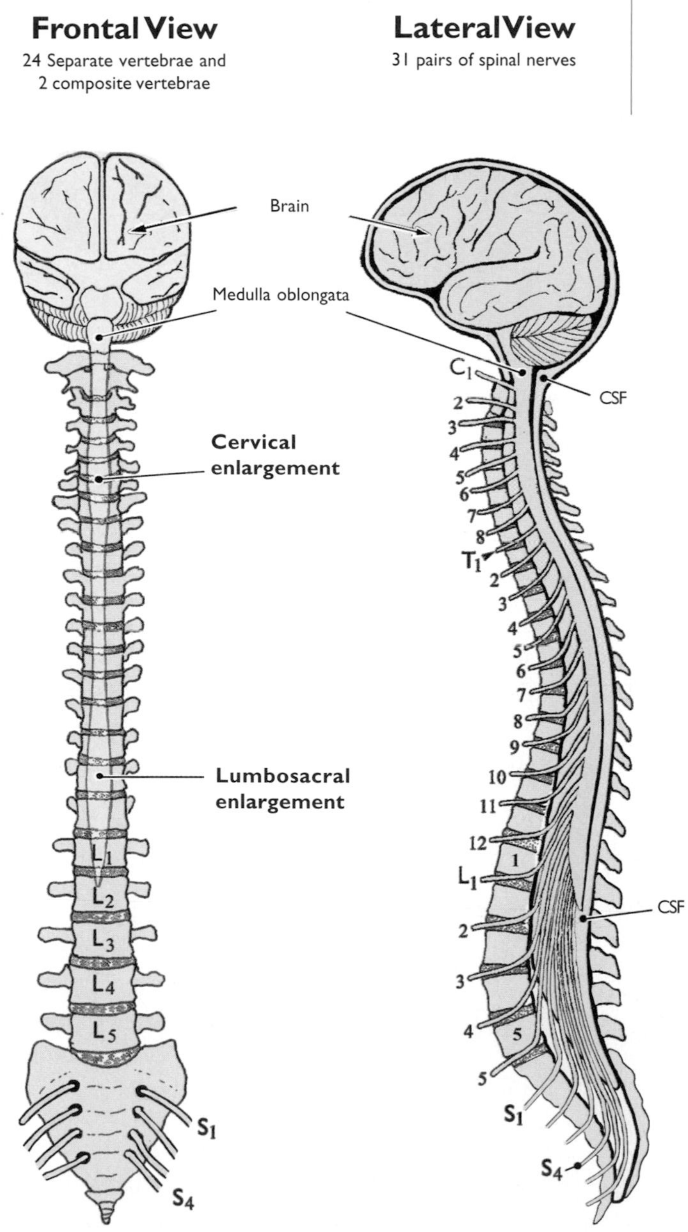

Figure 4.15. The spinal cord within the bony vertebral canal. Emergence of spinal nerves at various levels.

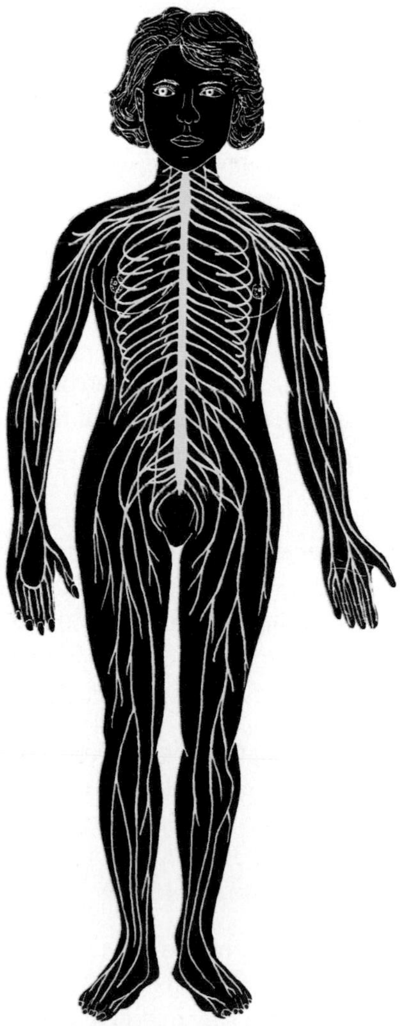

Figure 4.16. Schema of spinal cord with peripheral nerves. Note the cervical and lumbosacral enlargements that correspond to the large nerve supply of the upper limbs and lower limbs, respectively.

ally terminates at the level of the second lumbar vertebra (in the newborn infant the s pinal cord ends at a lower level, L3).

In the average adult, the spinal cord measures 42 to 45 cm (16 to 17 inches) in length. Corresponding to the large nerve supply necessary for the two upper limbs, the spinal cord has a **cervical enlargement** (Figs. 4.15, 4.16) that approximately extends from vertebral levels C3 to T2 (spinal cord segments C4 to T1). Similarly and corresponding to the large nerve supply necessary for the two lower limbs, there is a **lumbosacral enlargement** (Figs. 4.15, 4.16) of the spinal cord from vertebral levels T9 to T12 (spinal cord segments L2 to S3). Note the difference between *vertebral levels* and *spinal cord segments*. There are 31 pairs of spinal nerves (8 cervical; 12 thoracic; 5 lumbar; 5 sacral; 1 coccygeal).

Exposure of the Spinal Cord

Before the spinal cord and its surrounding membranes can be exposed, certain posterior structures must be removed. These include the dorsal musculature covering the vertebral canal and the posterior portion of the bony canal itself; i.e., the spinous processes and laminae of vertebrae.

Opening of the Vertebral Canal. Place a block under the pelvis to reduce the concavity of the lumbar region.

- Remove the dorsal musculature from T6 to L5. Scoop out the muscles that fill the groove between transverse and spinous processes (Fig. 4.11 B and C).

- In the lower thoracic (T6) region or in the lumbar (L1) region, remove several spinous processes with bone pliers. Note that the spines are attached to each other by **supraspinous ligaments** and **interspinous ligaments**.

- After removing the spinous processes, observe the strong and elastic **ligamenta flava**. These ligaments connect the laminae of adjacent vertebrae. They extend laterally to the intervertebral foramina and bound them posteriorly.

- Remove the **laminae** of several vertebrae (laminectomy). Do this about 1 cm from the midline, using a saw inclined to enter the vertebral canal. Remove individual pieces of bone with bone pliers. Protect your eyes from flying chips of bone. You have now entered the space of the vertebral canal.

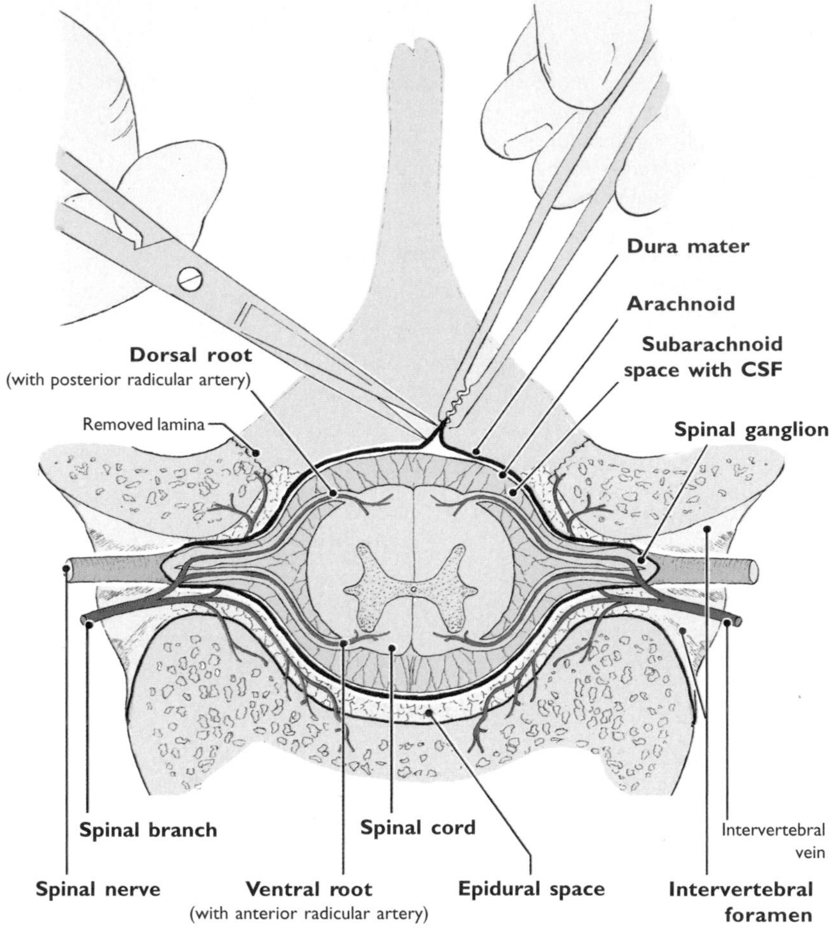

Figure 4.17. Membranes of the spinal cord.

GRANT'S 4.34, 4.35
ROHEN 211
A.D.A.M. 1.56
NETTER 162
CLEMENTE 633
A.V.A. 3: 0.22.35

GRANT'S 4.43 - 4.47
ROHEN 218
NETTER 148, 149, 155, 156
CLEMENTE 681, 682, 688
A.V.A. 3: 0.27.52

GRANT'S 4.26
CLEMENTE 674
A.V.A. 3: 0.17.00

Membranes of the Spinal Cord (Fig. 4.17):

- Identify the **epidural** or **extradural space.** Remove the fatty tissue (epidural fat) and veins (posterior internal vertebral venous plexus) from it.

- Expose and identify the **dural sac,** which terminates inferiorly at the level of S2.

- Next, carefully lift up a fold of dura mater with forceps (Fig. 4.17) and then create a small opening by cutting the fold with scissors. Extend the opening and incise the **dura mater** in the dorsal midline. Try to do this without damaging the underlying arachnoid mater.

- Identify the delicate **arachnoid mater** (membrane), incise it, and open the **subarachnoid space**. Using a probe, define and examine this space. In the living subject (but usually not in the embalmed cadaver), the subarachnoid space contains cerebrospinal fluid.

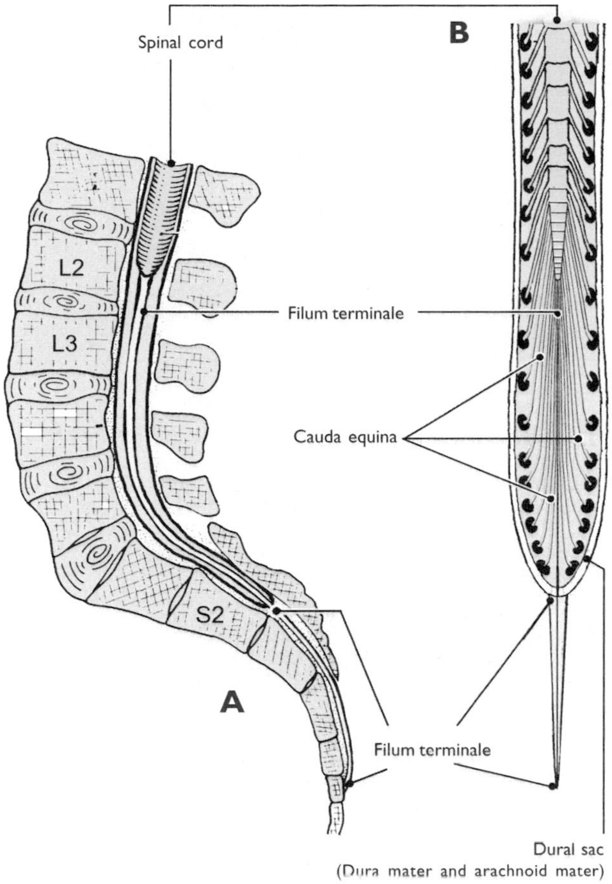

Figure 4.18. ***A***, Diagram of the lower portion of the vertebral canal and spinal cord. ***B***, Inferior portion of opened dural sac, spinal cord, and cauda equina.

Reflect the dura mater and the arachnoid mater. Note the following:

- **Spinal cord.** It is completely surrounded with delicate pia mater.
- On each side of the cord, the pia mater forms strong pointed prolongations. These are the **denticulate ligaments.** They secure the spinal cord to the dura mater. Usually, there are 21 points of attachment on each side.
- **Ventral and dorsal roots**. Using a probe, follow a ventral and a dorsal root to the point where they pierce the dura and enter the intervertebral foramen (Fig. 4.17).
- Look for small **blood vessels** that pass through the intervertebral foramina and course along the ventral and dorsal roots (Fig. 4.17). These are the **spinal branches** (of intercostal, lumbar or vertebral arteries, respectively) and their anterior radicular and posterior radicular branches. These vessels are vital for the proper neural functioning of the spinal cord. There are corresponding small *veins*. You may need to use a magnifying glass to inspect these small but important blood vessels.

GRANT'S 4.46, 4.48
ROHEN 214, 218
A.D.A.M. 1.36
NETTER 155, 156
CLEMENTE 688
A.V.A. 3: 0.15.28

- In the thoracic region, place a probe into an **intervertebral foramen** to protect the nerve within it. Using bone pliers, carefully remove the articular processes lying posterior to this foramen. Expose the **spinal ganglion** or dorsal root ganglion (Fig. 4.17). Identify the spinal nerve and follow it distally to the point where it divides into ventral and dorsal rami.

Dissection Note: It may be unnecessary to expose the entire spinal cord if demonstration or museum specimens are available. Consult with your instructor.

GRANT'S 4.41, 4.47
ROHEN 216, 217
A.D.A.M. 1.29, 1.36
NETTER 148, 149
CLEMENTE 682
A.V.A. 3: 0.30.35

In either the dissected or in a specially prepared museum specimen, study the following:

- **Cervical enlargement of the spinal cord**, corresponding to the large nerve supply of the upper limb, involving spinal cord segments C4 to T1.
- **Lumbar enlargement of the spinal cord**, corresponding to the large nerve supply of the lower limb, involving spinal cord segments L2 to S3. *Note:* These spinal cord segments do <u>not</u> correspond with the vertebral levels. The lumbar enlargement of the spinal cord extends approximately from vertebra T11 to vertebra L1.

GRANT'S 4.44, 4.47
ROHEN 216, 217
A.D.A.M. 1.30
NETTER 155
CLEMENTE 684, 688
A.V.A. 3: 0.29.05

- **Conus medullaris**, the end of the spinal cord, between vertebral levels L1 and L2. Of pediatric importance: at birth, the conus medullaris lies at the vertebral level of L3.
- **Cauda equina** (L., tail of horse). It is a collection of ventral and dorsal roots caudal to (inferior to) the termination of the spinal cord (Fig. 4.18).
- **Filum terminale** (Fig. 4.18). It is a delicate filament continuous with the pia mater. Its intradural portion ends at S2 where it is attached to the end of the dural sac. Its extradural prolongation ends at the coccyx.

GRANT'S 4.49
A.D.A.M. 1.30
NETTER 157-159
A.V.A. 3: 0.30.15

- **Spinal nerves**. Identify representative samples of spinal nerves (cervical, thoracic, lumbar, and sacral) and note that the spinal nerves are attached to the spinal cord via dorsal and ventral nerve roots.

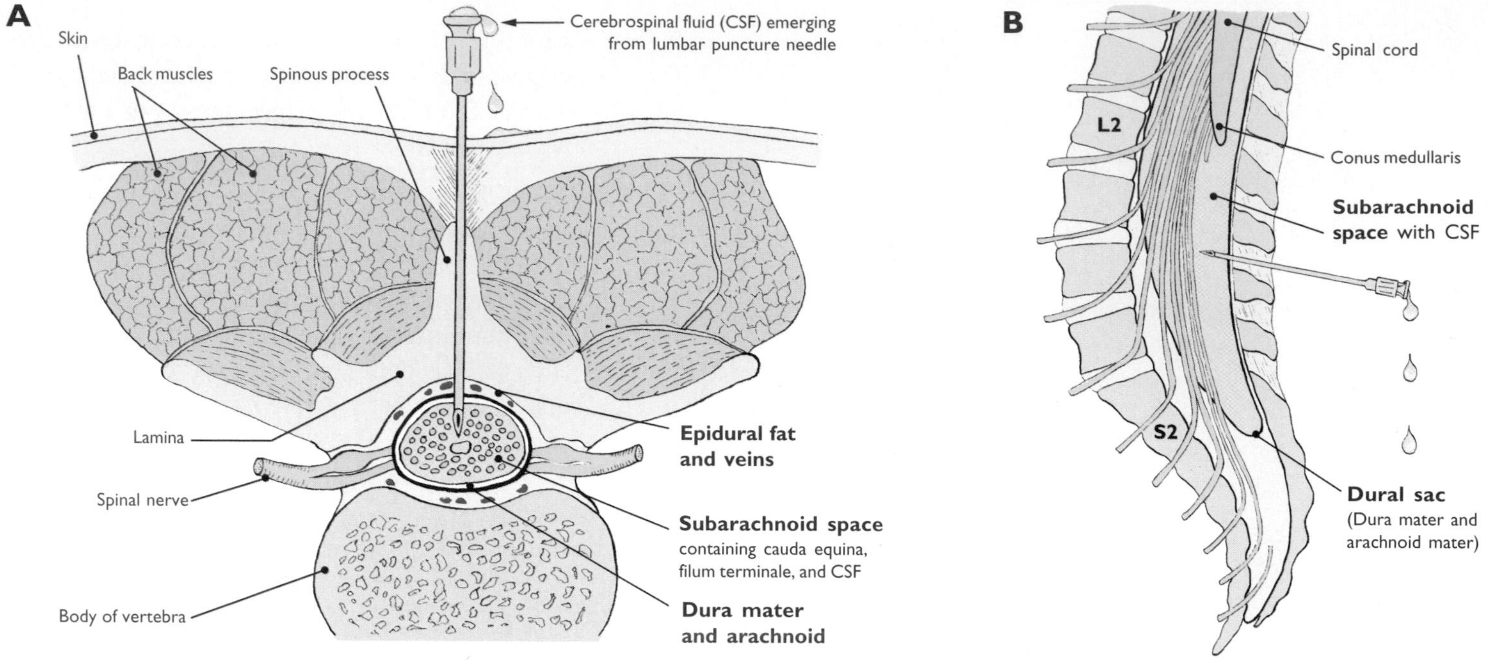

Figure 4.19. Lumbar puncture is best accomplished between vertebrae L3 and L4.

In relationship to the **spinal cord**, review the following:

- **Nerve plexuses.** ***(*1, see footnote)***
- Distribution of a **spinal nerve**. ***(*2)***
- **Dermatomes and myotomes**. ***(*3)***
- **Sympathetic chain** and its connections with spinal nerves. ***(*4)***
- **Blood supply** of the spinal cord. ***(*5)***

Clinical Correlation: **Lumbar Puncture** (Fig. 4.19). For diagnostic purposes, the cerebrospinal fluid (CSF) can be obtained from the subarachnoid space inferior to the conus medullaris. At this level, there is no danger of penetrating the central nervous system with the puncture needle. A special lumbar puncture needle with a stylus is inserted in the midline between the spinous processes L3/L4 or L4/L5. As the needle is advanced, it will pass through a layer of epidural fat that contains numerous small veins (of the posterior internal vertebral venous plexus). If the needle punctures one of these small veins, blood could emerge from the needle. After the needle passes through the dura mater and the arachnoid, it can tap the cerebrospinal fluid, which is normally under a positive pressure of less than 200 mm H_2O. If a deeply inserted needle encounters firm resistence, its tip has probably reached the vertebral body. The lumbar puncture needle may touch the nerve fibers of the cauda equina, causing a momentary sensation or muscle twitch in the innervated peripheral area. Great care must be taken to avoid infection of the subarachnoid space.

Regional Anesthesia. Following lumbar puncture, an anesthetic agent can be directly injected into the CSF (spinal block). The anesthetic effect on nerve roots of the cauda equina is very quick, resulting in regional anesthesia of the lower part of the body. The anesthetic agent can also be injected into the epidural (extraudal; peridural) space from where it diffuses gradually through the dura and arachnoid and eventually, over a period of 10 to 20 minutes, anesthetizes the nerve supply to the lower part of the body. This so-called epidural block is frequently used for pain control during child delivery.

Review the **lumbar vertebral column (*6)**. Correlate your findings with an anteroposterior (AP) and lateral radiograph of the lumbosacral spine. Pay special attention to **lumbar vertebrae L4 and L5** and the space between them. This is the location of the **intervertebral disc**. Intervertebral discs at L4/L5 are particularly prone to injuries (prolapsed nucleus pulposus with resulting compression of the cauda equina and corresponding neurological impairment).

(*1)	(*2)	(*3)	(*4)	(*5)	(*6)
GRANT'S 4.51	*GRANT'S 1.20*	*GRANT'S 4.52, 4.53*	*GRANT'S 4.48*	*GRANT'S 4.49*	*GRANT'S 4.13, 4.14*
NETTER 148	ROHEN 214	A.D.A.M. 1.31, 1.32	A.D.A.M. 1.35	A.D.A.M. 1.29, 1.30	A.D.A.M. 1.13
A.V.A. 1: 0.31.04	A.D.A.M. 1.35	NETTER 150	NETTER 153, 166	NETTER 157-159	NETTER 14
3: 2.30.55	NETTER 166	**CLEMENTE 625**	**CLEMENTE 690**	**CLEMENTE 683**	**A.V.A. 3: 0.14.44**
	CLEMENTE 13, 626		**A.V.A. 3: 1.19.05**		

TEST 9

GAPP

GROSS ANATOMY PRACTICAL PRIMER

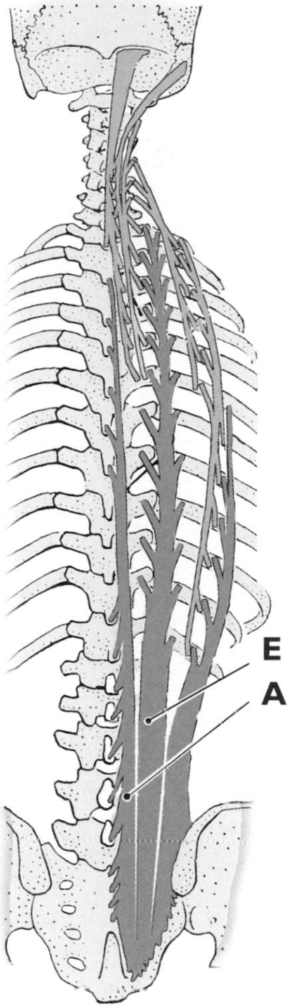

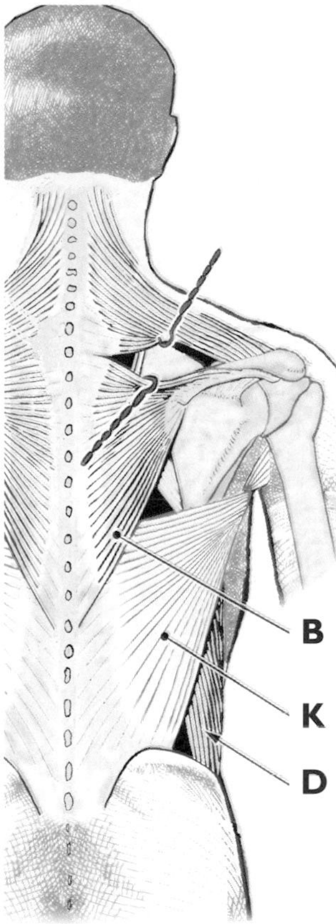

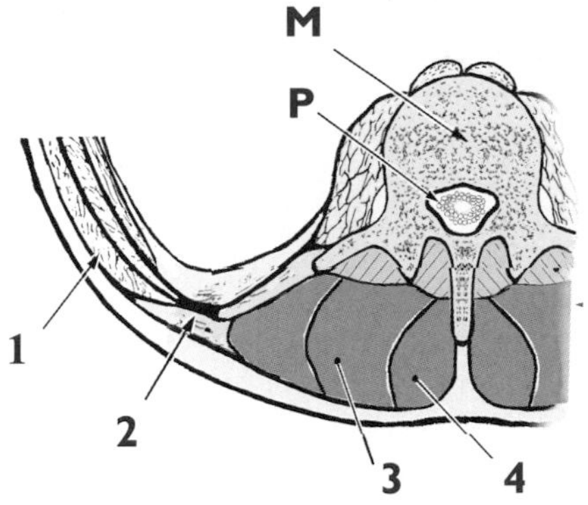

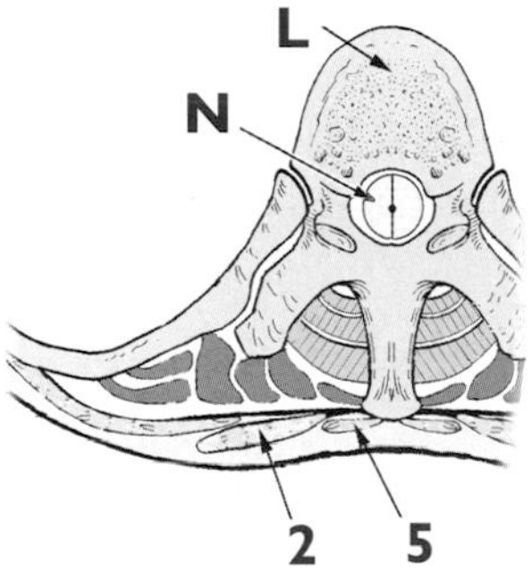

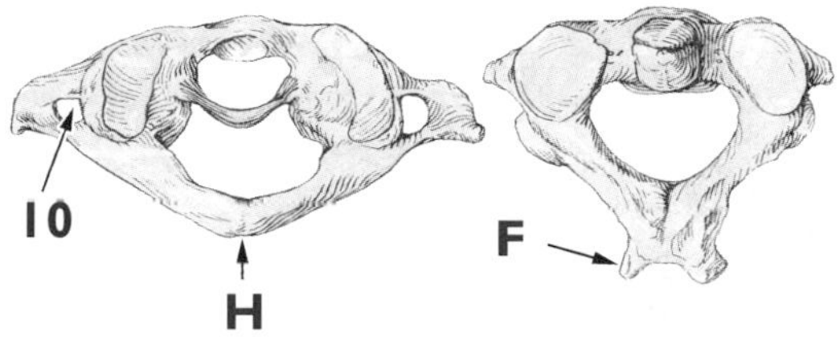

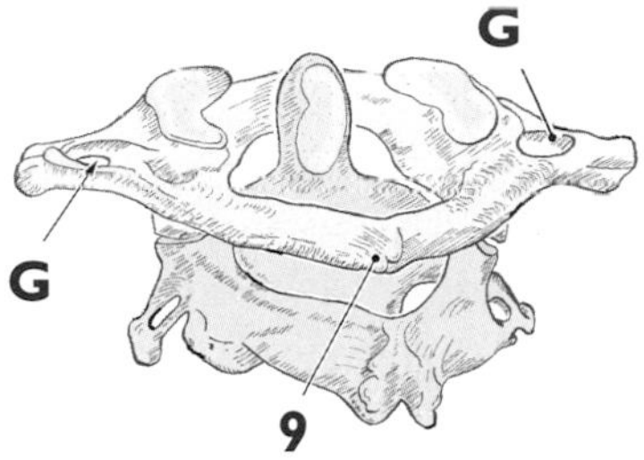

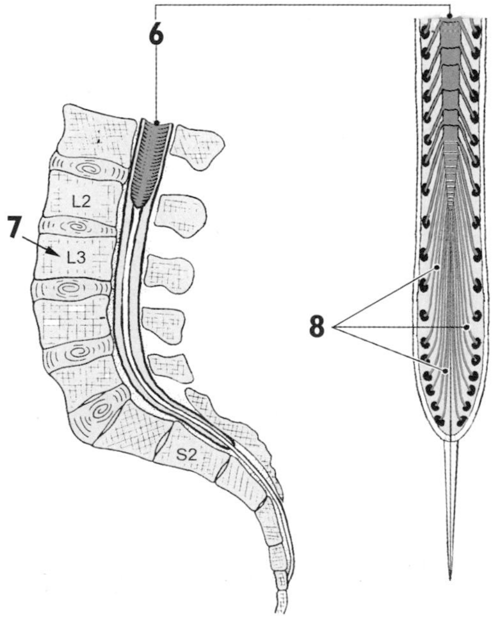

TEST YOUR 3-DIMENSIONAL CONCEPTUALIZATION.

MATCH THE NUMBERS WITH CORRESPONDING LETTERS:

1 ___	6 ___
2 ___	7 ___
3 ___	8 ___
4 ___	9 ___
5 ___	10 ___

GAPP TEST: IF YOU MADE AN ERROR, REVIEW AND GAIN A BETTER UNDERSTANDING OF THE CONCERNED 3-DIMENSIONAL ANATOMICAL CONCEPT. GAPP KEY: 1-D, 2-K, 3-E, 4-A, 5-B, 6-N, 7-M, 8-F, 9-H, 10-G

NOTES:

Chapter 5 The Lower Limb

Grant's Atlas of Anatomy, 10th Ed.:	*Grant's Fig. #*
Rohen, Color Atlas of Anatomy, 4th Ed.:	Rohen Page #
A.D.A.M. Student Atlas of Anatomy:	A.D.A.M. Plate #
Netter, Atlas of Human Anatomy, 2nd Ed.:	Netter Plate #
Clemente, Anatomy, 4th Ed.:	**Clemente Fig. #**
Acland's Video Atlas of Human Anatomy	**A.V.A. Vol: hr:min:sec**

Introductory Remarks

The essential functional requirements of the lower limb are weight bearing, locomotion, and maintenance of equilibrium. Anatomically, the lower limb is divided into three segments:

1. **Thigh,** the segment between hip and knee;
2. **Leg,** specifically the segment between knee and ankle;
3. **Foot.**

It is advantageous to dissect the lower limb in the following sequence: first, the superficial veins and nerves and the deep investing fascia of the entire lower limb will be examined. Next, the anterior and the medial regions of the thigh will be dissected. Subsequently, the gluteal region, back of thigh, and popliteal fossa will be explored. Finally, the three crural compartments of the leg will be dissected, and their contents will be followed onto the dorsum and into the sole of the foot.

Rohen 444
A.D.A.M. 5.15
Netter 510
Clemente 538
A.V.A. 2: 1.44.15

> **Note:** This manual is intended to guide you with the **dissection** of the human body. It is **not** the purpose of *Grant's Dissector* to provide you with a list of all muscles, their origins, insertions, and functions. However, you may find it advantageous to prepare or to copy such a list and to bring it to the laboratory for systematic review of all muscles of the lower limb you are held responsible for in your laboratory course.

Superficial Structures

Before you begin ...

Do *not* dissect at this time. Note that **superficial veins** and cutaneous nerves are contained in the **superficial fascia.** The first objective is to study these structures (superficial fascia; superficial veins; cutaneous nerves) of the entire lower limb as a whole. To accomplish this, the entire lower extremity will be skinned in an initial dissecting effort. The subcutaneous connective tissue and fat will be removed, leaving the more important superficial veins and nerves intact. Subsequently, the **deep fascia** will be demonstrated. The deep or investing fascia surrounds the various muscle compartments as well as the **deep system of veins.** Special attention will be paid to the clinically important **perforating veins,** which *perforate* the deep fascia and provide anastomoses between the deep and the superficial system of veins.

Grant's 5.4, 5.5
Rohen 445
Netter 508, 509
Clemente 489
A.V.A. 2: 1.43.00

Removal of Skin

Skin Incisions. With the cadaver in the supine position (face up), make skin incisions according to Figure 5.1. Be sure to cut only through the thickness of the skin. Do not cut into or remove the superficial fascia.

Make skin incisions as indicated by the *dotted lines* in Figure 5.1*A*: Anteriorly, vertically, and in the midline of the lower limb, starting inferior to the inguinal ligament, passing over the patella (knee cap), along the anterior portion of the leg and onto the dorsum of the foot. Make as many transverse skin incisions as needed to speed up the skinning process or to allow other students to participate. Cut transversely across the foot at the webs of the toes. Cut along the midline of each toe. Put traction on the skin as it is being removed, and keep the sharp knife directed against it to make the skinning process as efficient as possible. Leave the superficial fascia intact. Turn the skin flaps as far laterally as possible.

Subsequently, turn the cadaver into the prone position (face down) to remove the skin from the posterior aspect of the lower limb. As shown in Figure 5.1*B*, make a vertical cut, beginning inferior to the gluteal region, along the middle of the thigh and leg down to the heel. Extend the previously made transverse skin incisions posteriorly. If not already done (during the dissection of the pelvis), remove the skin from the gluteal region.

While the previously described skinning is under way, another student can remove the skin from the sole of the foot as indicated in Figure 5.1*C*.

Superficial Veins, Nerves, and Lymph Nodes

The next objective is to remove the superficial fascia while leaving intact the superficial veins and nerves. With the cadaver still in the prone position, examine the structures contained in the superficial fascia of the *posterior aspect* of the lower limb. Familiarize yourself with the expected course of **superficial veins** and **superficial nerves** (Fig. 5.2).

Grant's 5.4, 5.7
Rohen 445, 450
A.D.A.M. 5.16-520
Netter 508, 509
Clemente 489, 538
A.V.A. 2: 1.43.38

Pick up the **small saphenous vein** (Fig. 5.2) as it passes posterior to the lateral malleolus (ankle) and ascends toward the popliteal fossa (posterior to the knee). Note the numerous tributaries and communications with other superficial veins. Pay particular attention to the venous communications with the **great saphenous vein,** which runs at the medial aspect of the leg and knee.

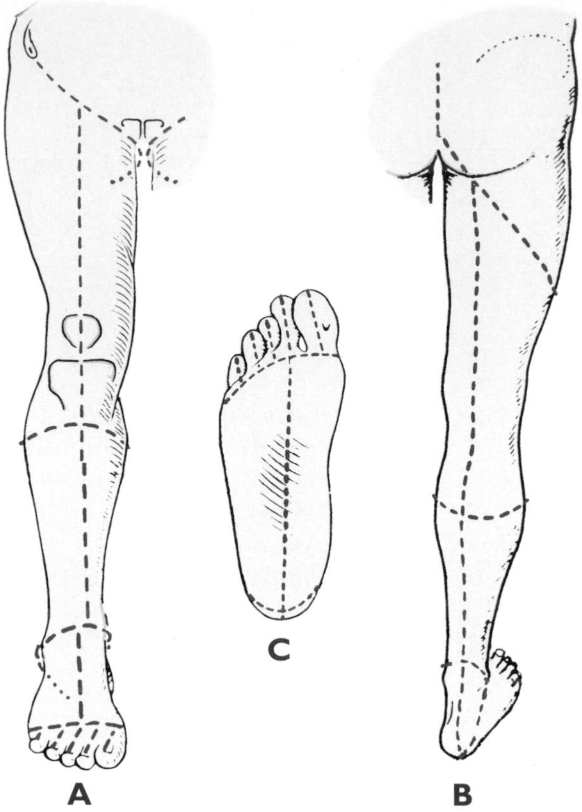

Figure 5.1. Skin incisions.

Grant's 5.7
Rohen 461, 464
A.D.A.M. 5.17, 5.19
Netter 509
Clemente 487
A.V.A. 2: 2.23.56

Observe that the **small saphenous vein** pierces the deep fascia in the popliteal fossa (at a deeper level, this vessel joins the popliteal vein). Identify **cutaneous nerves** related to the course of the small saphenous vein:

- The terminal branches of the **posterior cutaneous nerve of the thigh**. They emerge in the popliteal fossa. The more proximal portion of the posterior cutaneous nerve of the thigh runs deep to the investing fascia (Fig. 5.2, *dotted lines*); however, terminal cutaneous branches to the posterior aspect of the thigh pierce the fascia. Isolate at least one of the terminal twigs.

- The **sural nerve** (L. *sura*, calf of the leg). It pierces the deep fascia near the middle of the posterior aspect of the leg. Follow this nerve inferiorly as it courses together with the small saphenous vein posterior to the lateral malleolus toward the lateral aspect of the foot.

- Lateral to the sural nerve find the **lateral sural cutaneous nerve**.

Examine the **cutaneous nerves in the gluteal region**, also known as cluneal nerves (L. *clunis*, buttock). These nerves may have been removed earlier during the dissection of the perineum and pelvis. The cluneal nerves are derived from different sources (Fig. 5.2):

- Inferiorly, the **posterior cutaneous nerve of the thigh** sends cutaneous gluteal branches to the gluteal region around the inferior border of the gluteus maximus.
- Superiorly, the skin of the gluteal region is supplied by cutaneous branches of **dorsal rami L1, L2, and L3.**

Now, **remove** all connective tissue and fat of the **superficial fascia** from the posterior aspect of the leg, thigh, and gluteal region, leaving intact the deep fascia and the principal superficial nerves and veins. Be careful with tissue removal near the superficial veins. Demonstrate that the **superficial veins** are connected to **perforating veins,** which pierce the deep fascia and anastomose with the deep venous system.

Next, turn the cadaver over into the supine position (face up). First, examine the **superficial veins** of the anterior and medial aspects of the lower limb (Fig. 5.2).

- Start with the **great saphenous vein**, the longest vein in the body (Gr., *saphenous,* manifest; visible). Pick it up at the medial aspect of the knee, and follow it inferiorly along the medial side of the leg and anterior to the medial malleolus (medial ankle; same side as the great toe).
- Identify the veins on the dorsum of the foot and note that the **dorsal venous arch of the foot** is the main tributary to the great saphenous vein.
- Follow the great saphenous vein from the medial aspect of the knee superiorly to a point just inferior to the inguinal ligament. Here, the vein passes through an oval aperture in the deep fascia, the **saphenous opening or fossa ovalis,** to end in the femoral vein. This region will be dissected later following removal of the superficial fascia.

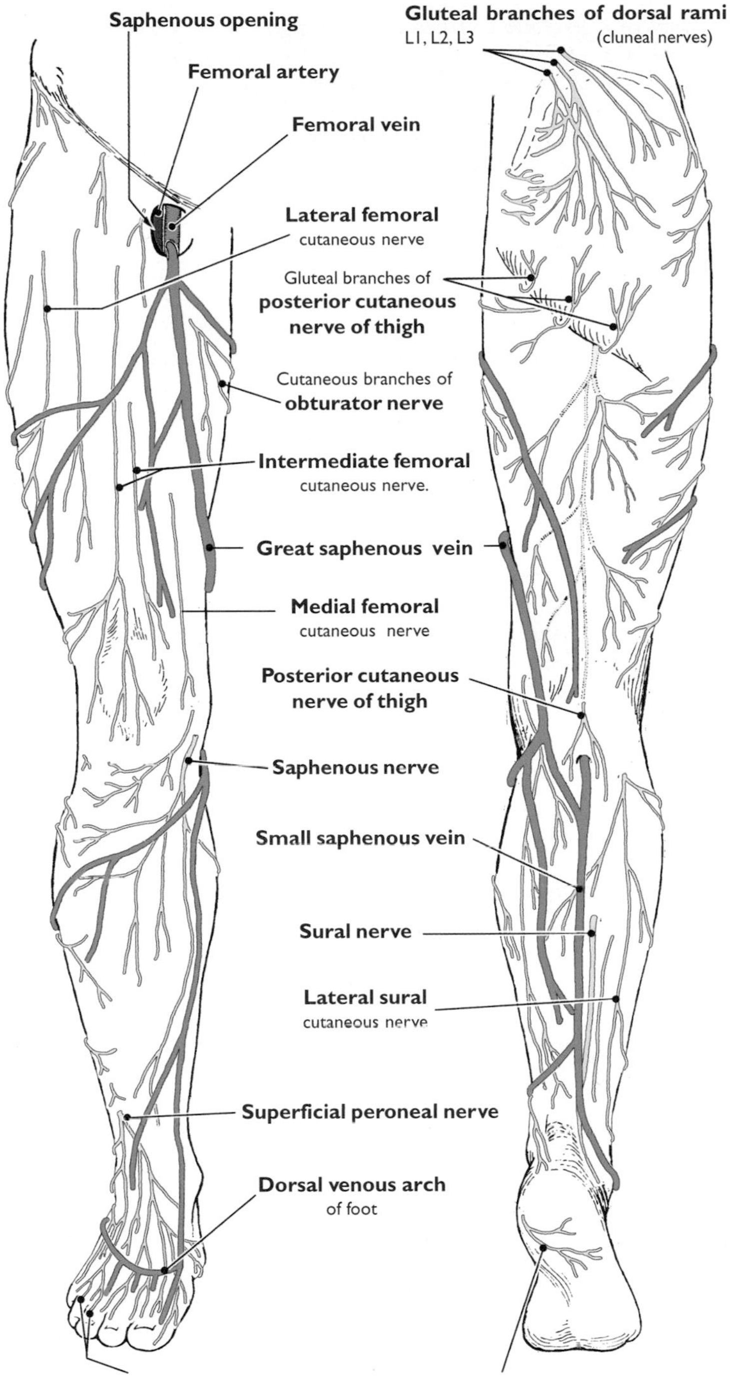

Figure 5.2. Superficial nerves and veins.

GRANT'S 5.14

GRANT'S 5.4B, 5.11
ROHEN 450, 451
A.D.A.M. 5.16
NETTER 508
CLEMENTE 489, 490
A.V.A. 2: 1.08.56

- Slit open the proximal portion of the great saphenous vein and observe one or two of its valves. There are 10 to 20 valves along the entire course of the vein.
- Gently remove the superficial fascia around the great saphenous vein, pull on the vein at various locations, and demonstrate again the existence of **perforating veins.**

> ***Clinical Correlation:*** Note that all superficial veins and even the perforating veins have valves that prevent the reflux of blood into lower regions and promote the venous blood flow in the direction toward the heart. If these valves become insufficient (i.e., "incompetent"), the veins become distended and tortuous, a condition known as **varicose veins.**
>
> For the purpose of coronary bypass surgery, portions of the great saphenous vein are removed and used as a graft vessel. When the great saphenous vein is tied off, blood from the original superficial drainage region of the vein must flow through the perforating veins into the deep venous system of the lower limb.
>
> The distal portion of the great saphenous vein is also used for a clinical procedure called "saphenous cutdown." If no veins can be located for emergent infusion purposes (e.g., in small infants, obese persons, or patients in shock with collapsed veins), the skin and superficial fascia is incised just anterior to the medial malleolus (side of the big toe), the vein is located, and a venous catheter is inserted for infusion purposes. In performing this procedure, the physician must be careful *not* to ligate the saphenous nerve (see below), or the patient will experience severe pain and later loss of sensation along the medial border of the foot.

Next, examine the **superficial nerves** of the anterior aspect of the lower limb (Fig. 5.2):

⇦ *GRANT'S 5.4, 5.7* ROHEN 450 A.D.A.M. 5.17. 5.18 NETTER 508 CLEMENTE 486, 520 A.V.A. 2: 2.24.26

- Identify the **saphenous nerve** as it pierces the deep fascia on the medial aspect of the knee. Verify that the nerve supplies the anterior and medial aspects of the leg and that it accompanies the great saphenous vein to supply the medial aspect of the foot.
- The lateral side of the foot, including the small (5th) toe, is supplied by terminal branches of the sural nerve. Verify this.
- Locate the **superficial fibular nerve** as it pierces the deep fascia in the lateral distal third of the leg. Follow it distally and note that it supplies the dorsum of the foot and sends **dorsal digital nerves** to most of the skin of thc toes. (It should be noted here that the skin between the 1st toe or big toe and the 2nd toe is innervated by a terminal branch of the deep fibular nerve, a matter of importance in the neurological assessment of nerve injuries in the leg).

⇦ *GRANT'S 5.7,* ROHEN 465 A.D.A.M. 5.17 NETTER 506, 508 CLEMENTE 531 A.V.A. 2: 2.21.17

Explore the nerve supply of the anterior and medial aspects of the thigh. Identify the **femoral cutaneous nerves: lateral, intermediate,** and **medial.** Inferior to the saphenous ring and medial to the great saphenous vein, attempt to find the **cutaneous branch of the obturator nerve.**

⇦ *GRANT'S 5.7* A.D.A.M. 5.17 NETTER 508 CLEMENTE 486, 489

⇨ *GRANT'S 5.9B* ROHEN 451 A.D.A.M. 5.27 NETTER 510 CLEMENTE 490, 491

Inguinal Lymph Nodes. Lymph vessels from the lower limb, lower anterior abdominal wall, gluteal region, perineum, and external genitalia drain into the **superficial inguinal lymph nodes** (Fig. 5.3). Identify **two groups of superficial nodes:**

- A horizontal group lies about 2 cm below the inguinal ligament.
- A vertical group is applied to both sides of the great saphenous vein.

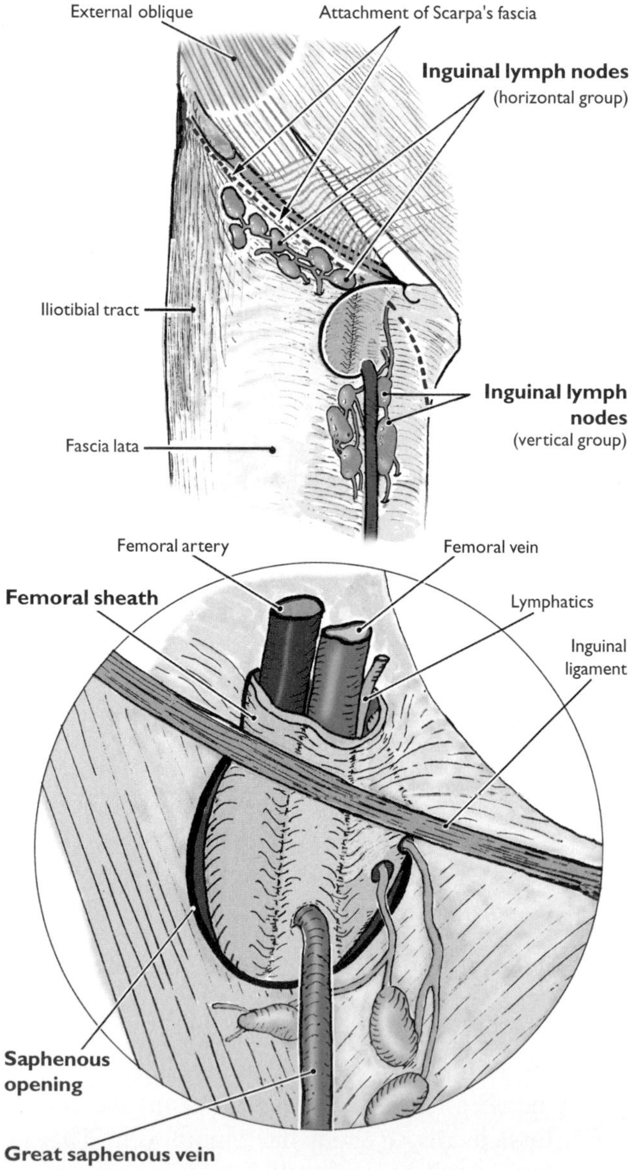

Figure 5.3. Fascia lata with saphenous opening, femoral sheath, and superficial inguinal nodes.

Realize that the superficial nodes are connected with one to three **deep inguinal nodes** that lie at a deeper level on the medial side of the femoral vein (they cannot be seen at this time). Correlate your anatomical observations and knowledge with the radiographic image of a lymphangiogram.

GRANT'S 5.9A

Finally, remove all superficial fascia, leaving intact the superficial inguinal lymph nodes, the deep fascia, and the principal superficial nerves and veins.

Deep Fascia and Saphenous Opening

Deep Fascia. With the superficial fascia removed, the full extent of the **deep fascia** of the lower limb can be appreciated. The deep fascia is a strong, dense layer of connective tissue that keeps the muscles in their various compartments much like a firm stocking. In the thigh (Fig. 5.3), the deep fascia is referred to as **fascia lata** (L., *latus*, broad). The lateral portion of the fascia lata is particularly strong and known as the **iliotibial tract.** Inferiorly, the deep fascia of the thigh is continuous with the deep fascia of the leg (area between knee and ankle). The thick and strong deep fascia of the leg is also known as the **crural fascia.** Underlying muscles may originate from the deep fascia (e.g., the tibialis anterior). The deep fascia may also form strong bands that hold muscles or tendons in place (e.g., extensor retinacula). There are areas where the deep fascia is absent because it is not needed (e.g., over the subcutaneous part of the medial surface of the tibia). Obviously, the deep fascia will have to be incised and removed to explore the deep structures of the lower limb.

GRANT'S 5.14
ROHEN 450
NETTER 508-510
CLEMENTE 492
A.V.A. 2: 1.19.45

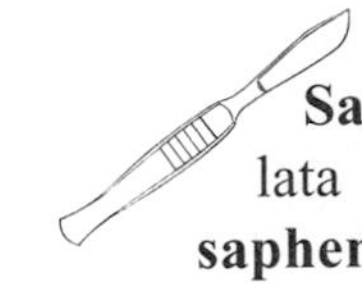

Saphenous opening. Clean the fascia lata (deep fascia) in the vicinity of the **saphenous opening** or fossa ovalis (Fig. 5.3). Proceed as follows:

- Note the femoral sheath that envelops the femoral vein, femoral artery, and deep lymph nodes.
- Insert a probe into the opening (Fig. 5.4) and ease back the underlying femoral sheath without injuring it. Define the round margin of the saphenous opening.
- Trace the **great saphenous vein** proximally to the femoral vein. Clean the vessels at their junction.
- Observe that the great saphenous vein hooks over the free inferior margin of the saphenous opening. Occasionally, the two vessels join slightly higher.

GRANT'S 5.11, 5.12A
ROHEN 451
A.D.A.M. 5.31, 5.32
NETTER 508, 510
CLEMENTE 495
A.V.A. 2: 0.34.26

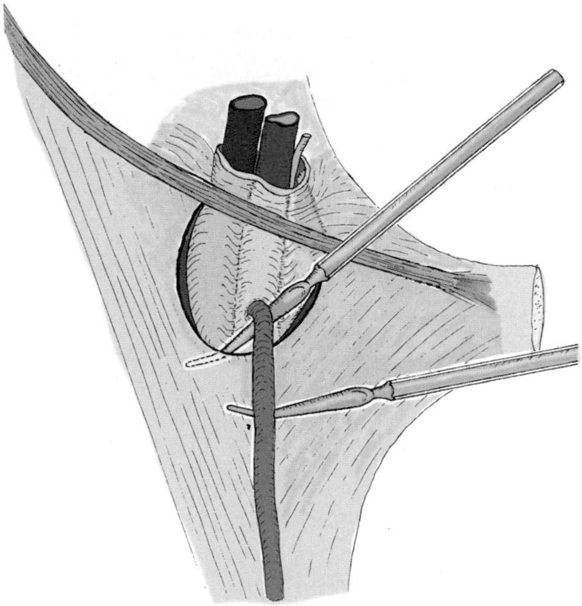

Figure 5.4. Use a probe to find and to define the margin of the saphenous opening.

- After you and your partners have studied the area, you may enlarge the saphenous opening by freely removing the deep fascia in its vicinity. This will widely expose the **femoral sheath.**

GRANT'S 5.12
A.D.A.M. 5.32
NETTER 244, 510
CLEMENTE 495

Femoral Sheath and Contents (Fig.5.5). This delicate sheath envelops the femoral artery, femoral vein, and some deep lymph vessels or nodes. Note that the femoral sheath is shaped like a short cone. The sheath is subdivided by two delicate vertical partitions into three compartments.

Dissect the three compartments as follows:

- In the midline of each compartment, make a vertical cut (Fig. 5.5).
- In the **lateral compartment** observe the femoral artery. Realize that this vessel is separated from the hip joint by the tough tendon of the psoas muscle (Fig. 5.5; *upper part*).

GRANT'S 5.12
CLEMENTE 496
A.V.A. 2: 0.36.36

- In the **middle compartment** identify the femoral vein.
- The **medial compartment** of the femoral sheath is the **femoral canal**.

The femoral canal, the short, conical medial compartment, contains lymphatics and loose areolar tissue (to allow for volume changes of the femoral vessels). The femoral ring is the small superior end (or mouth) of the femoral canal.

Pass a probe into the femoral canal (Fig. 5.5). Study the topographical relations of its mouth, the **femoral ring.** These relations are:

- Anteriorly, the inguinal ligament;
- Posteriorly, the pectineus muscle and its fascia;
- Medially, the sharp lateral edge of the lacunar ligament;
- Laterally, the femoral vein.

GRANT'S 5.12
CLEMENTE 496
A.V.A. 2: 0.36.36

Clinical Correlation: The femoral ring is a potentially weak area in the lower portion of the anterior abdominal wall. Knowledge of the femoral ring and canal is important in understanding the mechanism of **femoral hernia.** A femoral hernia is a protrusion of parts of abdominal viscera through the femoral ring into the femoral canal. Study Figure 5.5 and understand the following facts: by necessity, a femoral hernia must be relatively small since it is contained in the limited femoral canal, which is only about 1 cm in width. The hernia can usually be palpated below the inguinal ligament; it is frequently strangulated due to the rigid boundaries of the femoral ring and the tightness of the closely related inguinal and lacunar ligaments. Strangulation implies that the blood supply of the herniated bowel is impaired, and that tissue death (gangrene) is imminent. Femoral hernias are more common in women since the femoral ring in females is wider.

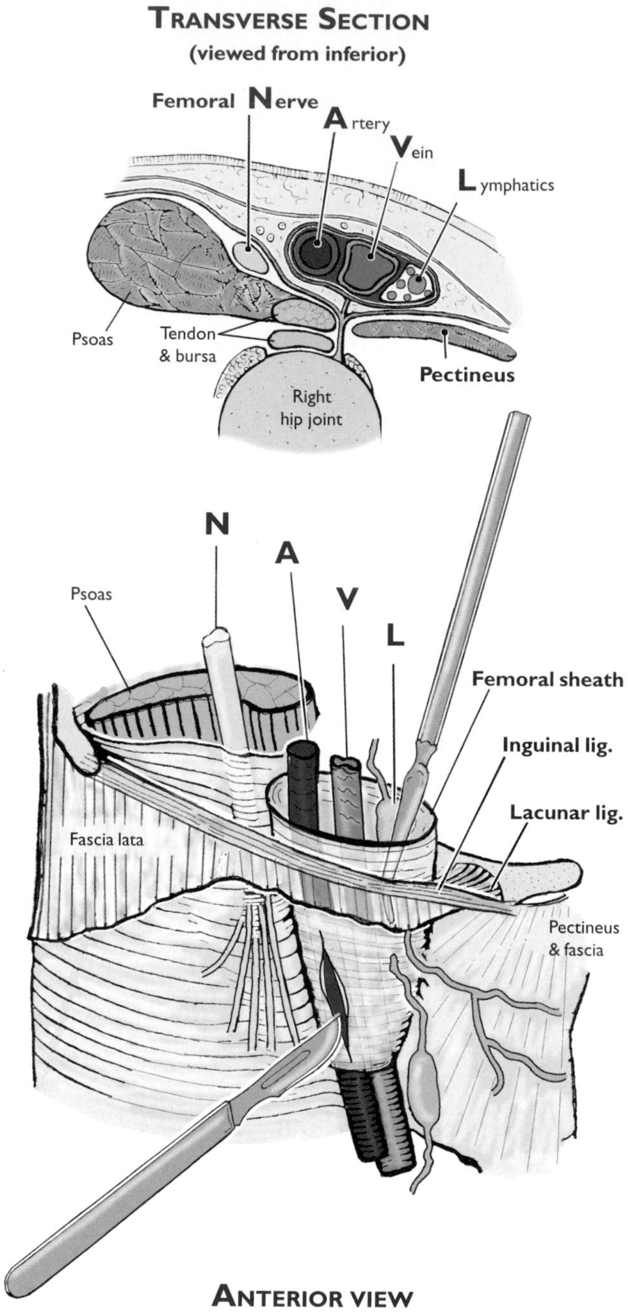

Figure 5.5. The femoral sheath and its three compartments. The lateral compartment has been incised to expose the femoral artery. The probe is located in the femoral canal. The femoral nerve **(*N*)** is located outside and lateral to the femoral sheath.

Anterior Region of Thigh

Bony Landmarks

Refer to a skeleton and study the following landmarks (Fig. 5.6):

GRANT'S 5.1
ROHEN 414, 415
A.D.A.M. 5.3, 5.4
NETTER 454, 455
CLEMENTE 559-562
A.V.A. 2: 0.01.40

- **Anterior superior iliac spine;**
- **Anterior inferior iliac spine;**
- **Pubic tubercle** (remember: the *inguinal ligament* stretches from the anterior superior iliac spine to the pubic tubercle);
- **Greater trochanter of femur;**
- **Lesser trochanter of femur;**
- **Lateral condyle** and **epicondyle** of femur;
- **Medial condyle** and **epicondyle** of femur;
- **Adductor tubercle** located on the medial epicondyle;
- **Linea aspera;**
- **Patella;**
- **Tuberosity** (tubercle) **of tibia.**

Femoral Triangle

GRANT'S 5.15
ROHEN 428
NETTER 458, 466
CLEMENTE 494
A.V.A. 2: 0.32.50

The **femoral triangle** is bounded superiorly by the **inguinal ligament,** laterally by the medial border of the **sartorius,** and medially by the medial border of the **adductor longus** (Fig. 5.7).

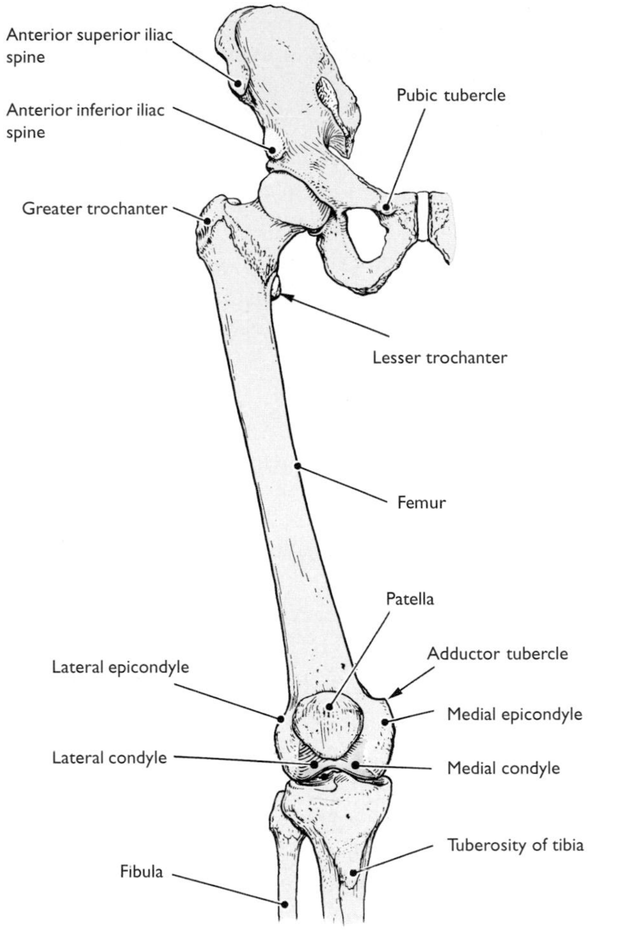

Figure 5.6. Bony landmarks pertaining to the anterior region of the thigh.

GRANT'S 5.12A, 5.15A
ROHEN 428
A.D.A.M. 5.29
NETTER 466
CLEMENTE 494
A.V.A. 2: 0.36.36

> ***Clinical Corelation:*** The femoral triangle contains the clinically important femoral vessels. The pulse of the femoral artery can be easily palpated about 3 cm inferior to the midpoint of the inguinal ligament.
>
> Within the triangle, the femoral vessels are also frequently used for diagnostic radiographic purposes. A special catheter can be inserted into either the femoral artery or the femoral vein. Catheters in the femoral artery can be advanced proximally into the aorta or selectively into aortic branches, such as the renal arteries or the mesenteric arteries. The catheter can be pushed via the aortic arch into the coronary arteries to obtain a coronary angiogram. In a similar fashion, a catheter in the femoral vein can be pushed through the inferior vena cava into the right atrium of the heart.

GRANT'S 5.15A
ROHEN 442
A.D.A.M. 5.13, 5.14
NETTER 466
CLEMENTE 494, 498
A.V.A. 2: 0.34.53

Clean the **femoral artery** and **vein** within the limits of the femoral triangle. Just inferior to the inguinal ligament, the artery gives rise to superficial branches of the abdominal wall and scrotum or labium majus. Pull the femoral artery and vein laterally and/or medially to observe branches and tributaries, respectively. Pay particular attention to the following three substantial arteries; these may arise from a large common stem, or they may arise independently from the femoral artery (Fig. 5.7):

GRANT'S 5.6, 5.21
ROHEN 442
A.D.A.M. 5.13, 5.14
NETTER 466, 477
CLEMENTE 498, 501
A.V.A. 2: 0.37.17

- **Profunda femoris artery** (deep artery of thigh). It pursues the same general direction

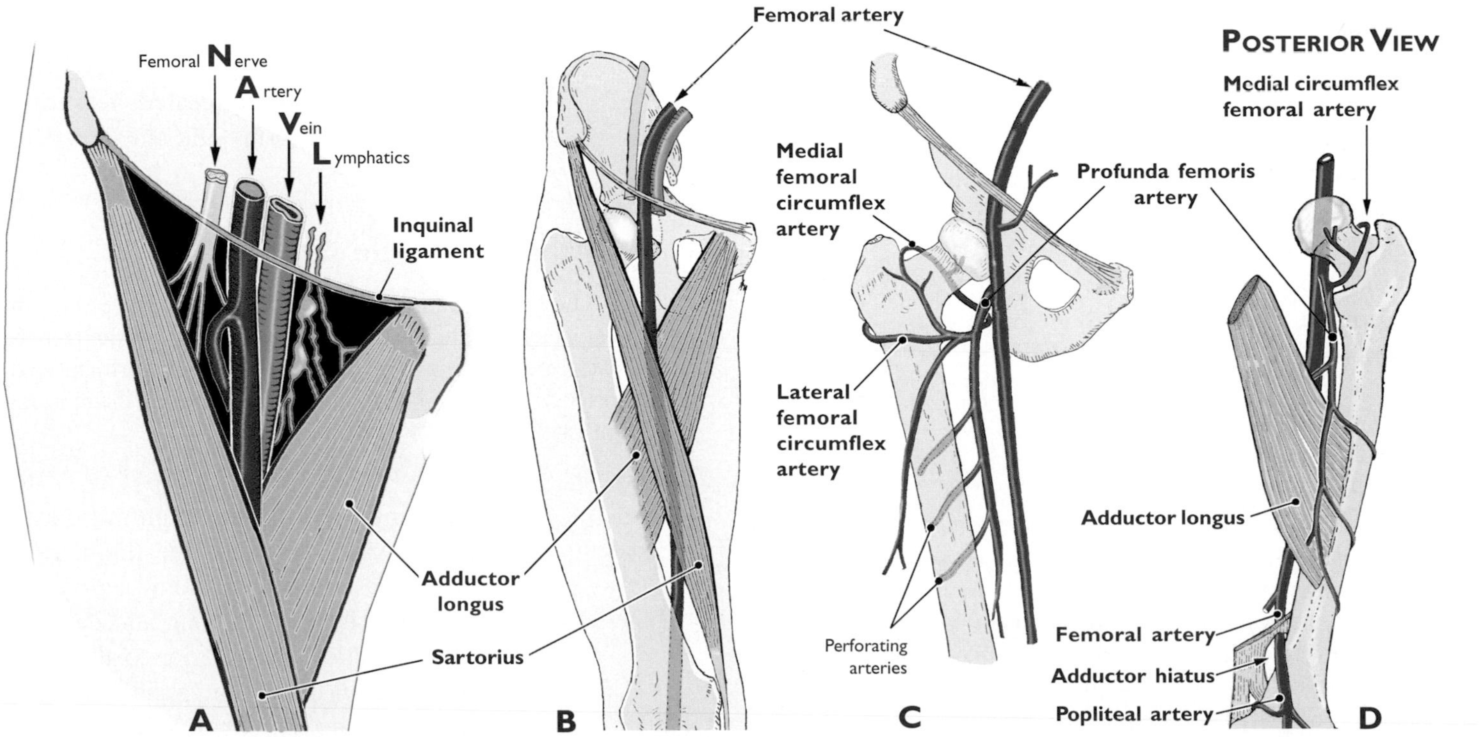

Figure 5.7. Femoral triangle and contents. Note that the femoral artery lies anterior to the hip joint.

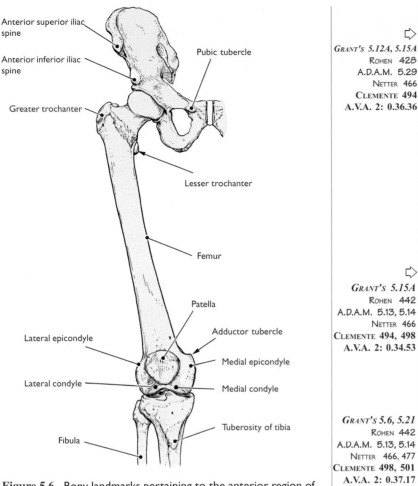

as the femoral artery, but on a plane posterior to the adductor longus muscle. It is accompanied by the profunda femoris vein.

Grant's 5.6, 5.21
Rohen 442
A.D.A.M. 5.13, 5.14
Netter 466, 477
Clemente 498, 501
A.V.A. 2: 0.37.17

- **Lateral circumflex femoral artery**.
- **Medial circumflex femoral artery**. This artery is clinically important since it supplies the bulk of blood to the head and neck of the femur.

Note that these three arteries are accompanied by corresponding veins. The largest of the veins is the **profunda femoris vein,** which drains into the femoral vein within the limits of the femoral triangle. Verify this fact.

- Preserve the principal veins (femoral; profunda femoris; great saphenous).
- In order to clarify the dissection field, remove all other smaller veins.
- Display the **floor of the femoral triangle** by removing fat and fascia, particularly from the **pectineus** and **adductor longus**.
- Open the interval between the contiguous borders of the **iliopsoas** and **pectineus.** Observe that the **medial circumflex femoral vessels** pass dorsally between these two muscles.

Grant's 5.16
Rohen 442
Netter 467
Clemente 498
A.V.A. 2: 0.37.31

Just lateral to the femoral artery, make a vertical cut through the fascia iliaca and expose the **femoral nerve** (Fig. 5.7). Follow the nerve inferiorly and observe numerous branches. Identify the **intermediate** and the **medial cutaneous nerve of the thigh** (Fig. 5.2). These nerves follow the medial border of the sartorius. The femoral nerve supplies the anterior muscle group of the thigh. Its muscular branches will be identified later.

Grant's 5.15A
Rohen 442
A.D.A.M. 5.29
Netter 466, 467
Clemente 498
A.V.A. 2: 0.40.43

Adductor Canal

In the middle third of the thigh, the femoral vessels and the saphenous nerve are contained in the **adductor canal** (Hunter's canal). The adductor canal is a narrow fascial tunnel that begins at the **apex of the femoral triangle**. It ends at the **adductor hiatus**, which is a slit-like opening or hiatus in the tendon of the **adductor magnus** (Fig. 5.7D). The femoral vessels pass through the adductor canal to reach the popliteal fossa (posterior to the knee). The adductor canal lies deep to the **sartorius muscle.**

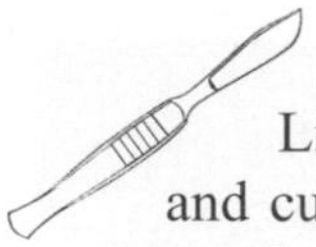

Lift the sartorius muscle out of its bed and cut it transversely near the apex of the femoral triangle. Reflect the inferior part of the sartorius inferiorly. Now the **adductor canal** is exposed and can be studied. Beginning at the apex of the femoral triangle, pass a probe into the canal and gently push it inferiorly. Slit open the fascial roof of the adductor canal. Study the **walls of the canal** and its boundaries:

Grant's 5.16, 5.21
Rohen 442
A.D.A.M. 5.29
Netter 4.66, 467
Clemente 498
A.V.A. 2: 1.03.10

- Laterally it is bounded by the **vastus medialis**;
- Posteromedially by the **adductor longus and magnus**;
- Anteriorly by the **sartorius**.
- Verify these relations on transverse section (Fig. 5.8).

Examine the whole length of the femoral vessels within the adductor canal. The **femoral vein** lies posterior to the **femoral artery.** Trace the femoral artery to the point where it passes through the **adductor hiatus** (Fig. 5.7 D). Here, the artery changes its name to **popliteal artery.** Note that the **saphenous nerve** accompanies the femoral vessels; however, it does *not* pass through the adductor hiatus. Instead, it runs anterior to the adductor magnus tendon toward the medial aspect of the knee. Follow the saphenous nerve inferiorly to the point where it pierces the deep fascia. This area is usually located between the tendons of the sartorius and the gracilis muscles.

Anterior Muscle Group

The powerful muscles of the thigh are divided into three main muscle groups: anterior, medial, and posterior (Fig. 5.8). Each muscle group has its own fascial compartment and its own nerve supply. The femoral nerve supplies the muscles of the anterior group (Fig. 5.9).

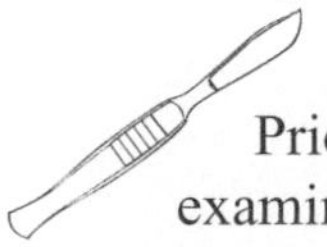

Prior to dissection of the thigh muscles, examine the deep fascia of the thigh, referred to as **fascia lata.** In the lateral region of the thigh, the **fascia lata** is strong and dense. Immediately posterior and inferior to the anterior superior iliac spine, the fascia lata encases a muscle, the **tensor fasciae latae**. Identify it (see Fig. 5.14). This muscle pulls

Grant's 5.16
A.D.A.M. 5.29
Netter 466
Clemente 492-494
A.V.A. 2: 0.19.44

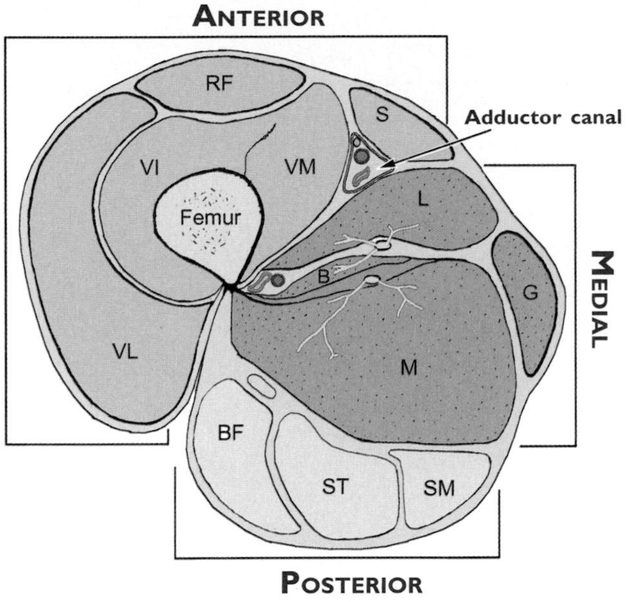

Figure 5.8. Transverse section of the right thigh, including the adductor canal and its contents. The three muscle groups of the thigh are *anterior*, *medial*, and *posterior*. *B*, adductor brevis; *BF*, biceps femoris; *G*, gracilis; *L*, adductor longus; *M*, adductor magnus; *RF*, rectus femoris; *S*, sartorious; *SM*, semimembranosus; *ST*, semitendinosus; *VI*, vastus intermedius; *VL*, vastus lateralis; *VM*, vastus medialis.

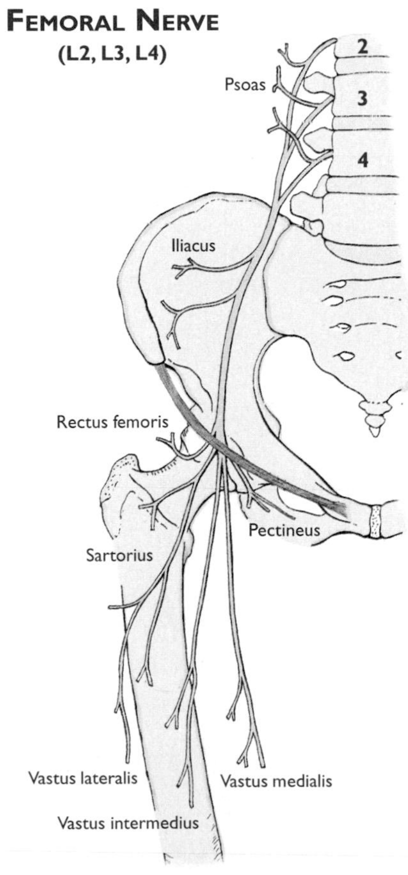

Figure 5.9. Scheme of motor distribution of the femoral nerve to the anterior muscle group of the thigh.

A.D.A.M. 5.29, 5.38
NETTER 471
CLEMENTE 493, 614
A.V.A. 2: 0.19.53

on a strap-like, longitudinal thickening of the fascia lata, the **iliotibial tract**. Split the fascia lata longitudinally between rectus femoris and vastus lateralis. Retract the iliotibial tract from the underlying vastus lateralis. With your fingers and the handle of the knife, follow the fascia lata posteriorly. Here, it is continuous with a very strong **intermuscular septum**, which is attached to the **linea aspera** on the posterior aspect of the femur.

GRANT'S 5.17B
ROHEN 452
A.D.A.M. 5.29
NETTER 4.58
CLEMENTE 493
A.V.A. 2: 0.23.40; 0.55.38

The **four muscles** of the anterior thigh (vastus lateralis, medialis, intermedius, and rectus femoris) are collectively known as the **quadriceps femoris.** The tendons of all four heads of the quadriceps unite to form a strong tendon. This tendon is inserted into the patella, and it continues inferiorly to the tibial tuberosity as the **ligamentum patellae** or **patellar liagment** (tendon) (Fig. 5.10).

Clinical Correlation: Tapping the **patellar liagment** (inferior to the patella) normally leads to the elicitation of the **quadriceps reflex** (patellar reflex; knee jerk). The tapping activates muscle spindles in the quadriceps. Afferent impulses from these muscle spindles travel in the femoral nerve to spinal segments L2, L3, and L4 (Fig. 5.9). From here, efferent impulses are mediated in motor fibers of the femoral nerve to the quadriceps, resulting in a jerk-like contraction of this muscle group. Obviously, intelligent clinical evaluation of the quadriceps reflex depends on thorough knowledge of the underlying anatomical substrate.

Identify the four muscles of the quadriceps femoris (Fig. 5.10):

GRANT'S 5.19A
ROHEN 451-453
A.D.A.M. 5.29
NETTER 458
CLEMENTE 497, 499
A.V.A. 2: 0.24.10

- Define the **rectus femoris** in the middle of the anterior thigh. Observe that the flattened inferior tendon of the muscle is inserted into the patella.
- Identify the **vastus lateralis**; it lies on the lateral side of the thigh.
- The **vastus medialis** covers the medial aspect of the thigh.
- Positioned between the vastus medialis and lateralis is the **vastus intermedius.** Expose the vastus intermedius by pulling the overlying rectus femoris either laterally or medially.

GRANT'S 5.21
ROHEN 453
A.D.A.M. 5.23, 5.29
NETTER 466, 467
CLEMENTE 498, 501
A.V.A. 2: 0.40.43

Identify motor branches of the femoral nerve to the following muscles (Figs. 5.9, 5.10):

- **Sartorius;**
- **Rectus femoris;**

- The **three vasti muscles** (vastus lateralis, medialis, intermedius);
- **Pectineus**. Usually, the pectineus is supplied by the femoral nerve. Find the small motor branch. Occasionally, the pectineus may have dual nerve supply by receiving an additional branch from the obturator nerve.

GRANT'S 5.21
ROHEN 453
A.D.A.M. 5.23, 5.29
NETTER 466, 467
CLEMENTE 498, 501

Pull on both the sartorius and rectus femoris muscles and verify that they span two joints, the hip joint and the knee joint. Thus, motion in these two joints is likely to occur during contraction of the sartorius and rectus femoris muscles. Examine each muscle individually and determine its action. The three remaining muscles of the quadriceps group (vastus medialis, vastus intermedius, vastus lateralis) act only on one joint, the knee joint. Verify this fact by determining the origins and insertions of these respective muscles. Examine the insertion of the ligamentum patellae into the tuberosity of the tibia. Palpate the patella (kneecap). It is a sesamoid bone, developed and contained within the ligamentum patellae.

GRANT'S TABLE 5.1
A.D.A.M. 5.7
NETTER 458
CLEMENTE 493, 497
A.V.A. 2: 0.24.37

Study the vasti muscles on transverse section (Fig. 5.8). Note that their attachments include large parts of the shaft of the femur.

GRANT'S 5.17B, 5.19A
ROHEN 451
A.D.A.M. 5.7
NETTER 458
CLEMENTE 497
A.V.A. 2: 0.48.33

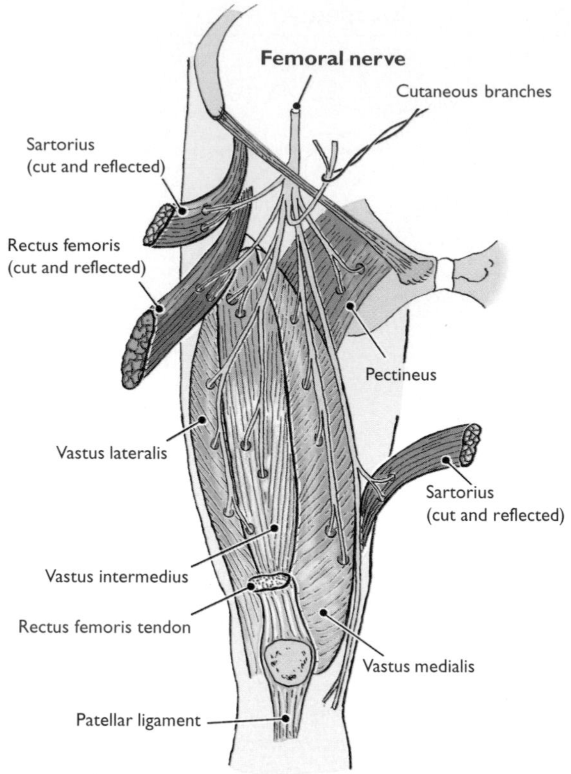

Figure 5.10. Muscular branches of the femoral nerve to the anterior muscle group of the thigh.

Medial Region of Thigh

The medial thigh muscles, also known as the adductor group, comprise the adductor magnus, adductor longus, adductor brevis, gracilis, obturator externus, and pectineus. This muscle group is supplied by the obturator nerve (Fig. 5.11). The pectineus, however, is mainly supplied by the femoral nerve (Fig. 5.9); sometimes it has a dual nerve supply from both the femoral and the obturator nerves. Similarly, the adductor magnus receives a dual nerve supply. Its hamstring portion is supplied by the sciatic nerve.

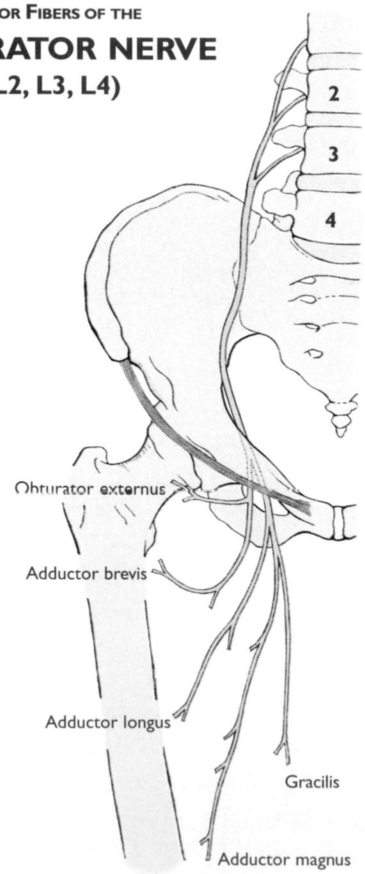

Figure 5.11. Scheme of motor distribution of the obturator nerve to the medial muscle group of the thigh.

Remove any remaining deep fascia from the medial side of the thigh to display the **adductors.** Proceed as follows:

- On the medial aspect of the thigh, follow the slender, strap-like **gracilis** inferiorly to its insertion into the tibia.
- Observe that **pectineus, adductor longus,** and **gracilis** originate from a curved line on the pubic bone.

GRANT'S TABLE 5.2
ROHEN 452, 453
A.D.A.M. 5.9
NETTER 458, 459
CLEMENTE 499, 500
A.V.A. 2: 0.17.27

- Trace the **pectineus** and **adductor longus** muscles as they fan out to their insertions along the linea aspera on the posterior aspect of the femur. Note that the **profunda femoris vessels** pass between the two muscles.

GRANT'S TABLE 5.2
ROHEN 452, 453
A.D.A.M. 5.9
NETTER 458, 459
CLEMENTE 499, 500
A.V.A. 2: 0.17.13

- Now, separate the adjacent borders of pectineus and adductor longus. Cut the adductor longus 5 cm inferior from its origin and reflect it (Fig. 5.12).

- The **adductor brevis** can now be seen at a deeper plane. On transverse section, verify that the adductor brevis lies posterior to the adductor longus (Fig. 5.8). Examine the adductor brevis. Note that part of it is covered by the pectineus.

- To expose the adductor brevis more fully, reflect the pectineus close to its origin (Fig. 5.12). Clean the adductor brevis. Do *not* damage nerves and vessels anterior to the muscle.

- Identify the nerve branches of the **obturator nerve**. Gently pull on the obturator nerve within the pelvis, or pass a probe along the nerve from the pelvis through the obturator foramen. The obturator nerve supplies motor fibers to the adductor muscles (Figs. 5.11, 5.12).

ROHEN 453
A.D.A.M. 5.23, 5.30
NETTER 467
CLEMENTE 501
A.V.A. 2: 0.41.10

Examine a transverse section of the thigh (Fig. 5.8) and note that some branches of the obturator nerve run anterior to the adductor brevis; others run posterior to the adductor brevis. Examine the *anterior* nerve branches in your cadaver specimen (Fig. 5.12). Next, verify that the *posterior* nerve branches pass between the **adductor brevis** and **adductor magnus.** Separate the two muscles with your fingers.

GRANT'S 5.33A
A.D.A.M. TABLE 5.3
NETTER 459, 467
CLEMENTE 500
A.V.A. 2: 0.12.43

NETTER 467, 471

Study the **profunda femoris artery** and its distribution (Fig. 5.7). To clarify the dissecting field, sacrifice the accompanying veins. Usually, the profunda femoris artery arises from the femoral artery 2 to 5 cm below the inguinal ligament. Clean the artery and some of its branches. Identify one or two of the **perforating arteries,** which encircle the femur and supply the adjacent musculature.

GRANT'S 5.20
ROHEN 453
NETTER 467
CLEMENTE 499, 500
A.V.A. 2: 0.16.14

GRANT'S 5.20, 521
ROHEN 453
NETTER 467, 477
CLEMENTE 498, 501
A.V.A. 2: 0.36.49

Cut the adductor brevis close to its origin and reflect it laterally to display the whole length of the **adductor magnus**. At this point, identify the **obturator externus** as it covers the external surface of the obturator membrane. Once more, note the anterior and posterior divisions of the obturator nerve. The accompanying arteries are branches of the obturator artery.

GRANT'S 5.18B
NETTER 457
CLEMENTE 516, 561
A.V.A. 2: 0.16.02

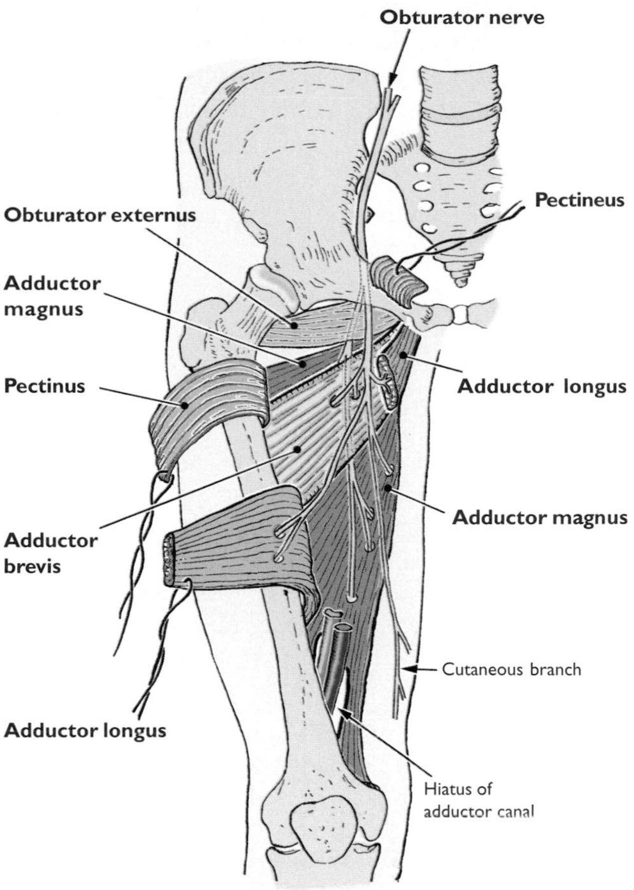

Figure 5.12. Medial region of thigh. The adductor group is supplied by the obturator nerve.

Examine the **adductor magnus**:

- Define the **hiatus** in the adductor magnus tendon through which the femoral vessels pass to become the popliteal vessels (Figs. 5.7, 5.12).

- Medial to the hiatus, trace the adductor tendon to its insertion into the **adductor tubercle** on the medial epicondyle.

- Note that the bulk of the adductor magnus is inserted by means of a broad aponeurosis into the **linea aspera** at the posterior aspect of the femur.

The adductors of the thigh (with exception of the slender gracilis muscle) span only one joint, the hip joint. The gracilis spans two joints by inserting into the medial surface of the tibia. Therefore, this muscle acts on the hip joint (adduction) and on the knee joint (flexion and medial rotation). Pull on the gracilis muscle and verify this fact.

Gluteal Region

General Remarks

The gluteal (buttock) region lies on the posterior aspect of the pelvis. It is formed by the large and prominent gluteus maximus and smaller gluteal muscles. The gluteal region was considered, in part, during the dissection of the perineum and pelvis (Chapter 3). The gluteus maximus was partially reflected so that the greater and lesser sciatic foramina could be defined, and the nerve and blood supply to the perineal region could be traced.

If the prescribed dissections of your gross anatomy course conform with the particular sequence of chapters in this manual, the previously mentioned procedures have been already performed. If you have not as yet dissected the perineum and pelvis, the gluteal region will be intact. At any rate, the area has already been skinned, the deep fascia has been demonstrated, and the cutaneous nerves of the region have been studied.

GRANT'S 5.23B, 5.25B
A.D.A.M. 5.1, 5.2
NETTER 509
CLEMENTE 483
A.V.A. 2: 0.20.43

GRANT'S 5.1B
ROHEN 414, 415
A.D.A.M. 5.4
NETTER 454, 455
CLEMENTE 561, 562
A.V.A. 2: 0.06.10

Important Landmarks

Refer to the skeleton and an articulated pelvis with intact ligaments. Identify the following landmarks (Fig. 5.13):

- **Greater sciatic notch**;
- **Lesser sciatic notch**;
- **Ischial spine** separating the greater and lesser sciatic notches;
- **Ischial tuberosity**;
- **Sacrotuberous ligament**;
- **Sacrospinous ligament**;
- The above mentioned two ligaments contribute to the formation of the **greater sciatic foramen** and the **lesser sciatic foramen**;
- **Greater trochanter of femur**;
- **Intertrochanteric crest**;
- **Trochanteric fossa,** a deep depression at the medial side of the greater trochanter.
- **Gluteal tuberosity** for the attachment of part of the gluteus maximus muscle.

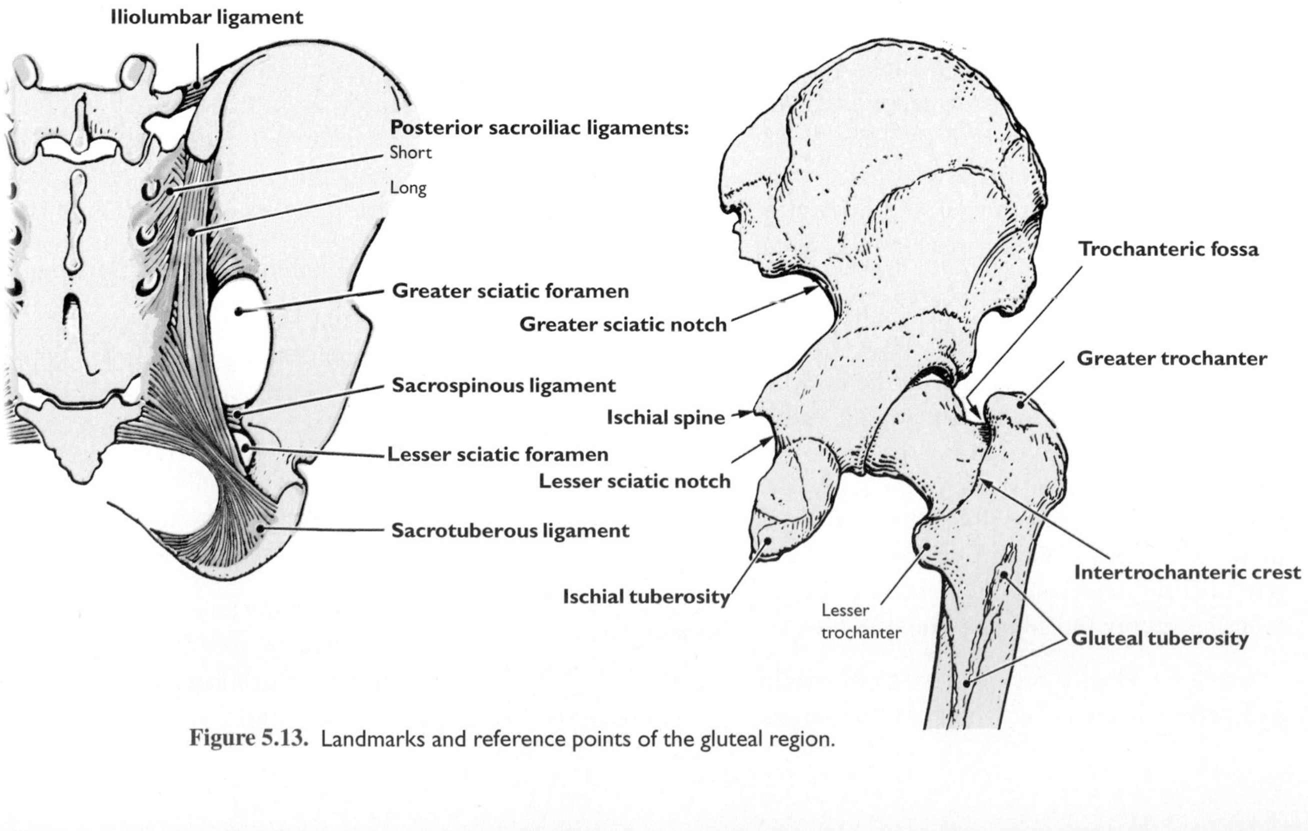

Figure 5.13. Landmarks and reference points of the gluteal region.

Gluteal Structures

Before you begin ...

The large gluteus maximus will be studied. The muscle will be reflected to allow access to the deeper plane of the gluteal region. The greater and lesser sciatic foramina are key areas. These foramina are traversed by important nerves, vessels, and muscles.

The **gluteus maximus** (Fig. 5.14) is a large, thick, quadrilateral muscle. Proximally, it is attached to the dorsal surfaces of the ilium, sacrum and coccyx as well as to the stout sacrotuberous ligament. Distally, its bulk is inserted into the iliotibial tract; a smaller portion is attached to the gluteal tuberosity of the femur. The muscle is a powerful extensor of the thigh.

GRANT'S 5.24B
ROHEN 430
NETTER 461
CLEMENTE 505
A.V.A. 2: 0.19.06

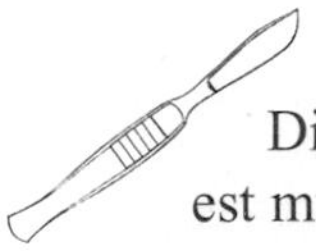

Dissect the **gluteus maximus**, the largest muscle in the body (Fig. 5.14):

GRANT'S 5.24B
ROHEN 430
A.D.A.M. 5.7, 5.8
NETTER 461
CLEMENTE 503, 504
A.V.A. 2: 0.20.43

- Define the superior and inferior borders of the vast, rhomboidal muscle.
- Carefully clean and define the inferior border of the muscle. Do not cut too deep, or you may sever the posterior cutaneous nerve of the thigh.
- Find and preserve the **posterior cutaneous nerve of the thigh** in the following manner:

GRANT'S 5.7B
ROHEN 454
A.D.A.M. 5.19
NETTER 509
CLEMENTE 504, 505

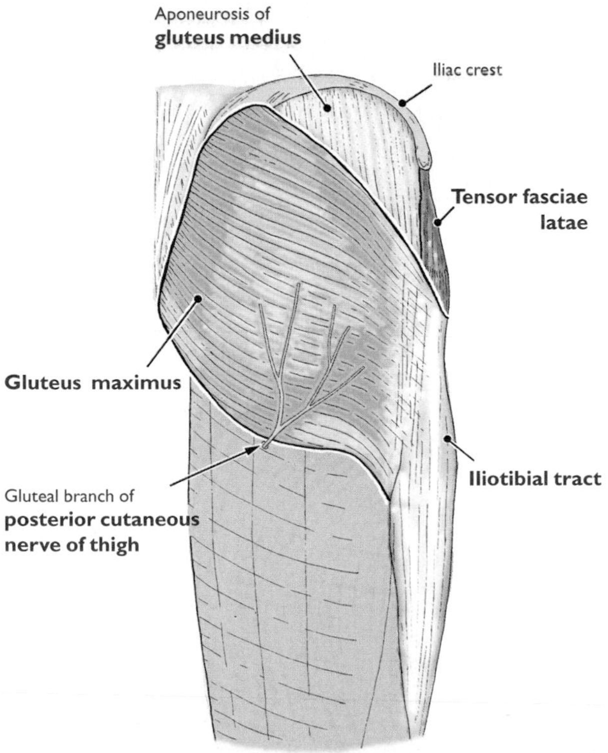

Figure 5.14. Muscles of the gluteal region; superficial dissection.

Midway between ischial tuberosity and greater trochanter, make a 5 cm longitudinal incision through the deep fascia of the posterior aspect of the thigh, just inferior to the inferior border of the gluteus maximus. Use a probe to locate the nerve just below the inferior border of the gluteus maximus.

- Now, remove the deep fascia from the entire gluteal region.
- Demonstrate the coarse muscle fibers of the gluteus maximus and their oblique direction.

A portion of the **gluteus medius** can be seen superior to the gluteus maximus (Fig. 5.14). Identify it. Push your fingers into the space between gluteus medius and maximus. *Note*: If the pelvis and perineum have been dissected previously, you will find the gluteus maximus reflected from its origin. If no prior dissection has been done in this area, proceed as follows:

- Refer to a bony pelvis and familiarize yourself with the sites of origin of the gluteus maximus from the iliac crest and the external surface of the ilium, the dorsal surfaces of the sacrum and coccyx, and from the sacrotuberous ligament.
- Detach the superior and medial portions of the muscle by cutting through its fibers very close to the posterior surfaces of the ilium, sacrum, and coccyx.
- Place your fingers deep to the inferior portion of the muscle. Note its attachment to the sacrotuberous ligament. Using a pair of scissors or a scalpel, carefully detach the muscle from this ligament.

GRANT'S 5.25A, 5.29
ROHEN 455
A.D.A.M. 5.33
NETTER 468
CLEMENTE 506, 507
A.V.A. 2: 0.43.04

- Gently reflect the muscle laterally. Observe the inferior gluteal nerve and vessels entering the muscle near its center. Cut the nerve and vessels close to the muscle, but leave a small button of the muscle attached to the nerve (to serve as an identifying indicator). Now, completely reflect the muscle laterally.
- Observe the insertions of the gluteus maximus (Fig. 5.15): the lower deeper quarter of the muscle is attached to the **gluteal tuber-**

osity of the femur; the remaining three quarters of the muscle are inserted into the **iliotibial tract**.

- The gluteus maximus slides over the **greater trochanter of the femur.** To protect the muscle from pressure and wear, it is separated from the greater trochanter by a bursa. Open this **trochanteric bursa,** which is the largest in the body. Observe another smaller bursa between the gluteus maximus and the ischial tuberosity.

Now, the deeper structures of the gluteal region are suitably exposed for examination (Fig. 5.15):

- Identify the **sciatic nerve,** the largest nerve in the body. Verify that the nerve is located midway between the ischial tuberosity and the greater trochanter.

GRANT'S 5.28
CLEMENTE 506
A.V.A. 2: 0.19.53

GRANT'S 5.25C

GRANT'S 5.28, 5.29
ROHEN 457
A.D.A.M. 5.33-5.35
NETTER 468, 469
CLEMENTE 506, 513
A.V.A. 2: 0.42.30

- Follow the sciatic nerve proximally to the point where it appears in the gluteal region inferior to the **piriformis muscle**.

- Be aware of possible variations. In the majority of cases, both the tibial and fibular (peroneal) divisions of the nerve pass together inferior to the piriformis. However, these nerve divisions may emerge separately at different levels of the piriformis muscle.

The **piriformis** occupies a key position in the gluteal region (Fig. 5.16). Verify that this muscle passes through the greater sciatic foramen and divides it. A number of vessels and nerves from the pelvis traverse the greater sciatic foramen to reach the gluteal region. Some of these structures enter the gluteal region superior to the piriformis; others enter inferior to the piriformis.

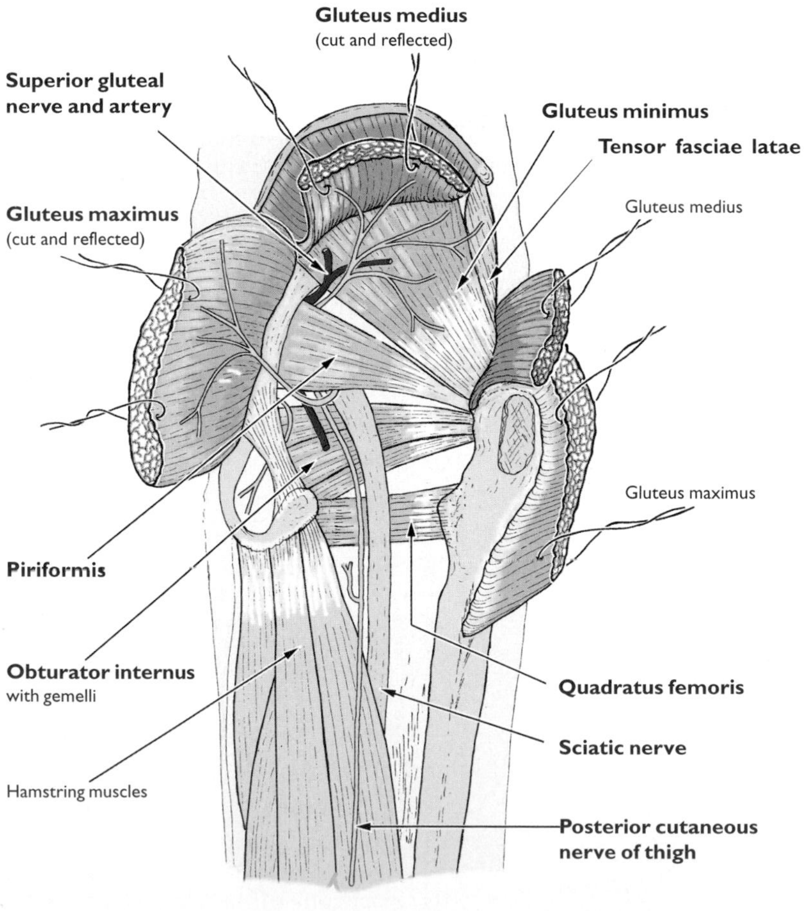

Figure 5.15. Muscles of the gluteal region; deep dissection. The gluteus maximus and medius are reflected to allow access to deeper layers.

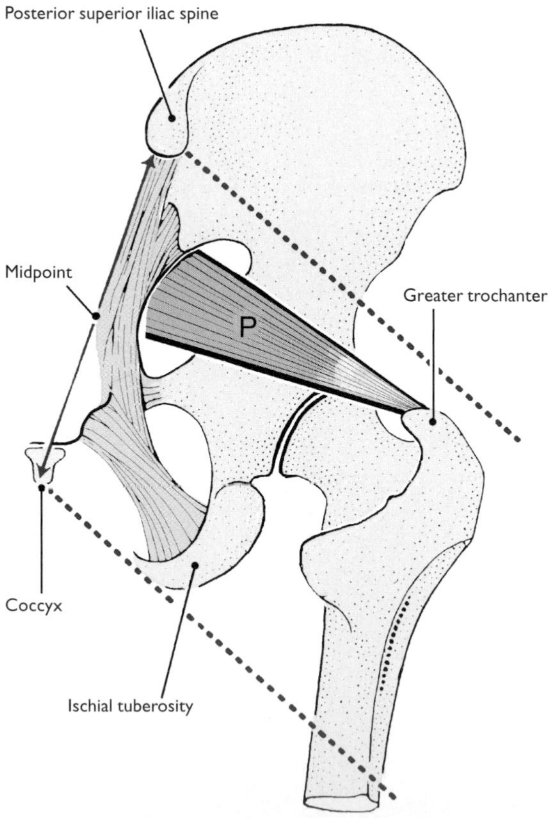

Figure 5.16. The reference line in the gluteal region is the readily defined inferior border of the piriformis muscle (*P*). The position of the gluteus maximus is indicated by *dotted lines*.

At the *superior border* of the piriformis (Fig. 5.17), identify the *stems* of the **superior gluteal nerve and vessels.** The more peripheral parts of these structures are covered by the **gluteus medius**.

GRANT'S 5.29
ROHEN 457
NETTER 468
CLEMENTE 506, 507
A.V.A. 2: 0.43.08

At the *inferior border* of the piriformis (Fig. 5.17), identify the following structures:

GRANT'S 5.29
ROHEN 457
A.D.A.M. 5.35
NETTER 468
CLEMENTE 410, 506
A.V.A. 3: 2.32.00

- **Inferior gluteal nerve and vessels** (which were cut during the reflection of the gluteus maximus).
- **Sciatic nerve,** the largest nerve in the body. Be aware that this important nerve has a rich blood supply via a continuous anastomotic chain of arteries.
- **Posterior cutaneous nerve of thigh,** running parallel to the sciatic nerve.

GRANT'S 5.31A
ROHEN 457
A.D.A.M. 5.35
NETTER 468
CLEMENTE 513
A.V.A. 2: 0.42.30

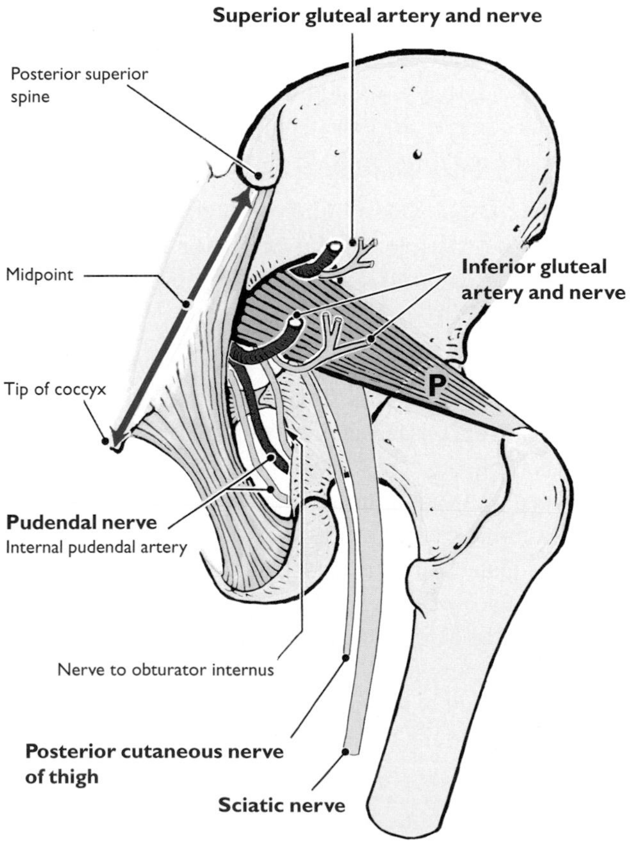

Figure 5.17. Structures passing through the greater sciatic foramen superior and inferior to the piriformis muscle (*P*).

- **Pudendal nerve** and **internal pudendal vessels.**

The **pudendal nerve and internal pudendal vessels** originate in the pelvis and appear only briefly in the gluteal region, entering through the **greater sciatic foramen.** They exit through the **lesser sciatic foramen** (Figs. 5.15, 5.17) to reach structures in the anal and urogenital regions. Push a probe along these structures through the lesser sciatic foramen into the **pudendal canal.**

Clinical Correlation: **Injury.** The large sciatic nerve and its branches supply with motor fibers numerous muscles in the lower limb: the hamstring muscles of the thigh (which primarily act on the knee joint) and the muscles of the three crural compartments of the leg (which act on the foot). The sensory fibers of the sciatic nerve and its branches innervate a large area of the lower limb. Thus, when the nerve is injured or impaired, significant peripheral neurologic deficits may occur. Fortunately, the sciatic nerve is deeply positioned and relatively well protected against injury. However, a deep knife wound or gun shot wound in the buttock region may severely injure or even complete sever the sciatic nerve. The superior portion of the nerve may also be damaged by a traumatic dislocation of the hip joint during an accident. Severe cases of sciatic nerve injury may result in paralysis of the flexors of the knee and all muscles below the knee. In addition, widespread numbness of the skin of the posterior aspect of the lower limb may occur. Familiarize yourself with the motor distribution of the sciatic nerve in the thigh (see Fig. 5.22) and with the motor distribution of sciatic nerve branches, the fibular (peroneal) nerves (see Fig. 5.31) and the tibial nerve (see Fig. 5.32).

Sciatica. Sciatica is defined as pain in the lower back and hip radiating down the back of the thigh, along the course of the sciatic nerve, into the leg. Sciatica is probably the most common disorder of the sciatic nerve. Initially, it was attributed to sciatic nerve dysfunction (hence the term). It is due to a herniated lumbar disk compromising the L5 or S1 root in the spinal canal. In addition to the pain of sciatica, there is numbness, tingling, and tenderness along the course of the nerve, and eventually loss of sensation and muscle function.

GRANT'S 5.31A
ROHEN 457
A.D.A.M. 5.35
NETTER 468
CLEMENTE 513

Metabolic Disorders. Like any other peripheral nerve, the sciatic nerve receives a rich blood supply that ensures its proper functioning. If this blood supply becomes insufficient due to vascular disease, nerve impairment may occur (peripheral neuropathy). Diabetes mellitus is the leading cause for such neuropathies. The longer nerves (such as fibers in the sciatic nerve) are affected first so that symptoms usually begin in the toes. Symptoms include numbness, tingling, needling, burning, sensations of cold or pain, and muscle cramps.

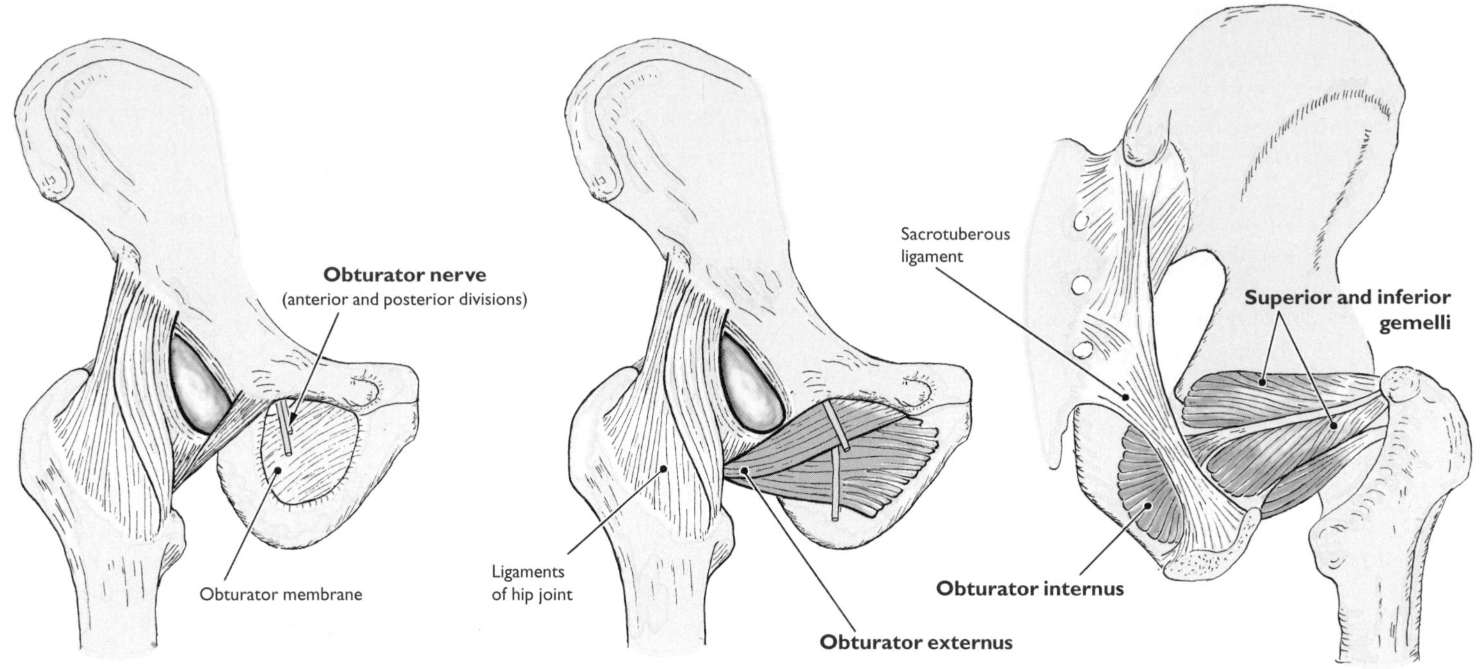

Figure 5.18. Structures related to the obturator foramen: obturator membrane, obturator nerve, obturator externus, and obturator internus with gemelli.

Identify the **obturator internus,** which traverses the lesser sciatic foramen (Fig. 5.18):

- Clean the tendon of the obturator internus as it inserts into the medial surface of the greater trochanter of the femur.
- Note that the tendon lies between the fleshy gemelli muscles. These two gemelli muscles are actually superior and inferior parts of the obturator internus and thus assist the obturator internus in its function.
- The fan-shaped obturator internus is attached to the pelvic surface of the obturator membrane.

GRANT'S 5.28, 5.29
ROHEN 457
A.D.A.M. 4.12
NETTER 4.68, 4.69
CLEMENTE 506, 507
A.V.A. 2: 0.13.10

Identify the **two gemelli muscles** (L. *gemellus*; twin) and related structures (Fig. 5.18):

- The **superior gemellus** arises from the ischial spine and surrounding area.
- The **inferior gemellus** arises from the ischial tuberosity.
- Inferior to the inferior gemellus, identify the **quadratus femoris** that stretches from ischial tuberosity to intertrochanteric crest of femur.
- Search with a probe near the greater trochanter and in the interval between the quadratus femoris and the inferior gemellus; there, locate the **obturator externus tendon**. It is inserted into the trochanteric fossa of the femur. Alternatively, detach and reflect the quadratus femoris to expose more widely the obturator externus muscle.
- The fan-shaped obturator externus is attached to the margins of the obturator foramen and to the external surface of the obturator membrane (Fig. 5.18).

GRANT'S 5.29, 5.32
ROHEN 457
A.D.A.M. 5.35
NETTER 468, 469
CLEMENTE 506, 511
A.V.A. 2: 0.13.51

GRANT'S 5.28
ROHEN 457
A.D.A.M. 5.36
NETTER 461
CLEMENTE 511
A.V.A. 2: 0.19.06

Identify the dense deep fascia covering the fan-shaped **gluteus medius**. Some of its fibers arise from this fascia. Verify this fact by vertically incising the deep fascia overlying the gluteus medius. In addition, a portion of the muscle arises from the external surface of the ilium.. Observe the gluteus medius tendon at its area of insertion into the lateral surface of the greater trochanter of the femur (Fig. 5.19). Understand that contraction of this muscle will lead to abduction of the thigh (abduction of hip joint). In walking and standing, the gluteus medius is the primary stabilizer of the hip joint.

GRANT'S 5.29
ROHEN 455, 457
A.D.A.M. 5.35
NETTER 468
CLEMENTE 506, 507
A.V.A. 2: 0.43.08

Once again, identify the **superior gluteal nerve and vessels** superior to the piriformis. Follow these vessels by sweeping your fingers deep to the gluteus medius. Your fingers

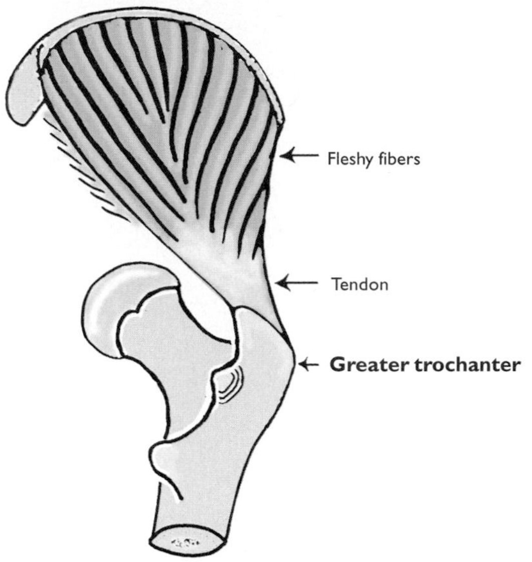

Figure 5.19. Fleshy and tendinous portions of the gluteus medius; insertion into the greater trochanter of the femur.

are now in the plane between gluteus medius and minimus. Sever the **gluteus medius** about 3 cm superior to its insertion into the **greater trochanter** of the femur. Gently reflect the proximal portion of the muscle superiorly and observe motor branches of the superior gluteal nerve entering the muscle (Fig. 5.15). Reflect the gluteus medius completely and identify the underlying **gluteus minimus.**

Occasionally, the gluteus medius and minimus are not well differentiated. The reason for this occasional fusion of the two muscles is the fact that they share a very similar fiber course and function. Observe the insertion of the gluteus minimus into the greater trochanter of the femur. Note branches of the superior gluteal nerve entering the muscle. Now, clean the entire **superior gluteal nerve** and follow a branch laterally to the **tensor fasciae latae** (Fig. 5.15).

Refer to a skeleton and the dissected specimen at the same time. **Study the functions of muscles in the gluteal region**. *Extend* the femur of the skeleton; in the living, this movement is accomplished by the gluteus maximus. *Abduct the femur;* this movement depends on the functional integrity of the three abductors of the hip joint: gluteus medius, gluteus minimus, and tensor fasciae latae.

GRANT'S 5.29
A.D.A.M. 5.35
NETTER 468
CLEMENTE 506
A.V.A. 2: 0.42.50

GRANT'S 3.22A, 5.32
ROHEN 325
A.D.A.M. 4.12
NETTER 333
CLEMENTE 410
A.V.A. 2: 0.13.20

GRANT'S 3.21
NETTER 373, 374
CLEMENTE 410, 411

GRANT'S 5.29
ROHEN 457
A.D.A.M. 5.35
NETTER 469
CLEMENTE 507

A.D.A.M. 5.21
CLEMENTE 502
A.V.A. 2: 0.21.06; 1.01.57

Intragluteal Injections. The gluteal region is commonly used for intramuscular injections of drugs. These injections should always be made superolaterally in the **superior lateral quadrant**. Why? Divide the gluteal region into four quadrants. Realize that injections into the two inferior quadrants will endanger and possibly paralyze the important sciatic nerve, or nerves and vessels entering the gluteal region inferior to the piriformis muscle. Injections into the superior medial quadrant may injure the stems of the superior gluteal nerve and vessels or an abnormally high peroneal division of the sciatic nerve. Intragluteal injections into the superior lateral quadrant are relatively safe since the superior gluteal nerve and vessels are well ramified in this region. Be sure the injection needle never deviates inferiorly or medially toward the greater sciatic foramen with its important structures.

Study the continuity of muscles, vessels, and nerves observed in the gluteal and pelvic regions.

- Within the pelvis minor, identify the fleshy part of the obturator internus covering the obturator foramen and membrane; then follow the muscle distally into the gluteal region.
- Within the pelvis, identify the piriformis muscle; then follow this muscle distally into the gluteal region and to the greater trochanter of the femur.
- Within the pelvis, study the gluteal vessels and their relationship to the piriformis muscle and the sacral plexus.
- Review the lumbosacral plexus and its contribution to the sciatic nerve.
- Note that the muscles of the gluteal region are supplied by branches of the lumbosacral nerve plexus.

Posterior Region of Thigh

Before you begin ...

The plan is to demonstrate the posterior muscle group of the thigh, the hamstring muscles, and the sciatic nerve. Subsequently, the dissection will be extended into the diamond-shaped popliteal fossa. The muscular boundaries of the fossa will be established, and the important contents of the popliteal fossa (nerves, vessels) will be identified. The proximal and distal continuity of these structures will be explored.

Important Landmarks

GRANT'S 5.1B
ROHEN 415-417
A.D.A.M. 5.4
NETTER 455, 478
CLEMENTE 561, 594
A.V.A. 2: 0.04.20; 2: 0.46.07

Refer to the skeleton and identify the following pertinent landmarks (Fig. 5.20):

- **Ischial tuberosity**;
- Lateral lip of **linea aspera**;
- **Lateral supracondylar line**;
- **Medial condyle** and **lateral condyle** of femur;
- **Apex**, **head**, and **neck of fibula**;
- **Medial condyle** of tibia;
- On the **posterior aspect of the tibia**: rough area for semimembranosus, popliteal area, and soleal line.

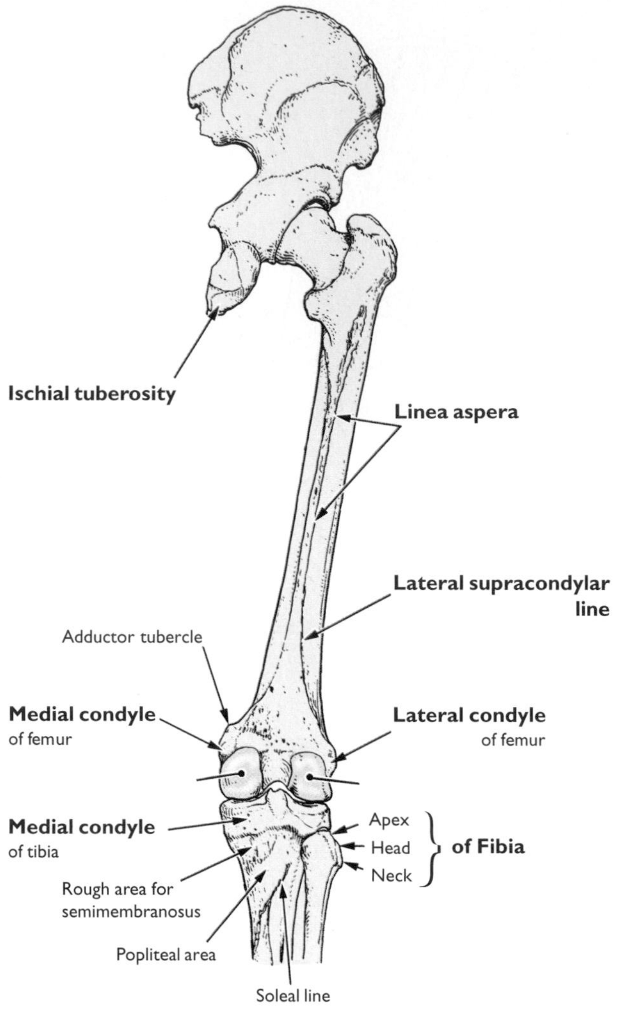

Figure 5.20. Bony landmarks of posterior aspect of thigh.

Posterior Muscle Group

GRANT'S 5.7B, 5.29
ROHEN 447, 456
A.D.A.M. 5.19, 5.20, 5.33
NETTER 504
CLEMENTE 504

Review the field of sensory innervation of the **posterior cutaneous nerve of the thigh**. Remove the deep fascia covering the posterior aspect of the thigh. Identify the posterior cutaneous nerve of the thigh; then reflect it superiorly. Clean the **sciatic nerve** and follow its branches to the posterior thigh muscles.

GRANT'S 5.25A
ROHEN 456
A.D.A.M. 5.8
NETTER 461
CLEMENTE 510
A.V.A. 2: 0.25.41

The posterior thigh muscles are also referred to as the **hamstring muscles**. This group is comprised of three large muscles (semitendinosus, semimembranosus, and biceps femoris). The hamstring muscles span two joints, the hip joint and the knee joint. The muscle group is supplied by the sciatic nerve.

> **Note:** The **hamstrings** are defined as the tendons of the semimembranosus, semitendinosus, and biceps femoris. In certain animals, such as pigs, these tendons are used to hang up hams for smoking. In quadrupeds the term refers to a tendon or tendons at the back of the joint between the knee and the fetlock of the hind leg. In the process of hamstringing, an animal is crippled and made inoperative by severing the hamstring tendons. Unfortunately, this procedure has also been used in humans to cripple rivals and adversaries.

Define and clean the hamstring muscles and separate them from one another (Fig. 5.21). These muscles are the **long head of the biceps femoris**, the **semitendinosus**, and the **semimembranosus**. Verify that these muscles have a **common site of origin**, the **ischial tuberosity.** Proceed as follows:

GRANT'S 5.24B, 5.25A
ROHEN 4.56, 457
A.D.A.M. 5.8
NETTER 461
CLEMENTE 511
A.V.A. 2: 0.26.50

- On the lateral side of the thigh, identify the long head of the biceps femoris (Fig. 5.21A). Pull the muscle laterally to demonstrate the sciatic nerve. Alternatively, sever the muscle at its superior third, reflect its ends, and thus expose the sciatic nerve and several of its muscular branches.

GRANT'S 5.25A
ROHEN 456, 457
A.D.A.M. 5.8
NETTER 461
CLEMENTE 511
A.V.A. 2: 0.26.17

- On the medial side of the thigh, identify the **semitendinosus** (meaning "half tendon") with its round and remarkably long tendon of insertion. Follow this tendon inferiorly to the medial surface of the superior part of the tibia.

GRANT'S 5.25A
ROHEN 456, 457
A.D.A.M. 5.8
NETTER 461
CLEMENTE 512
A.V.A. 2: 0.26.00

- Separate the semitendinosus from the **semimembranosus** (meaning "half membrane") with its substantial membranous tendon of origin (Fig. 5.21B). Follow the muscle inferiorly to a rough area of bone on the posterior part of the medial condyle of the tibia.

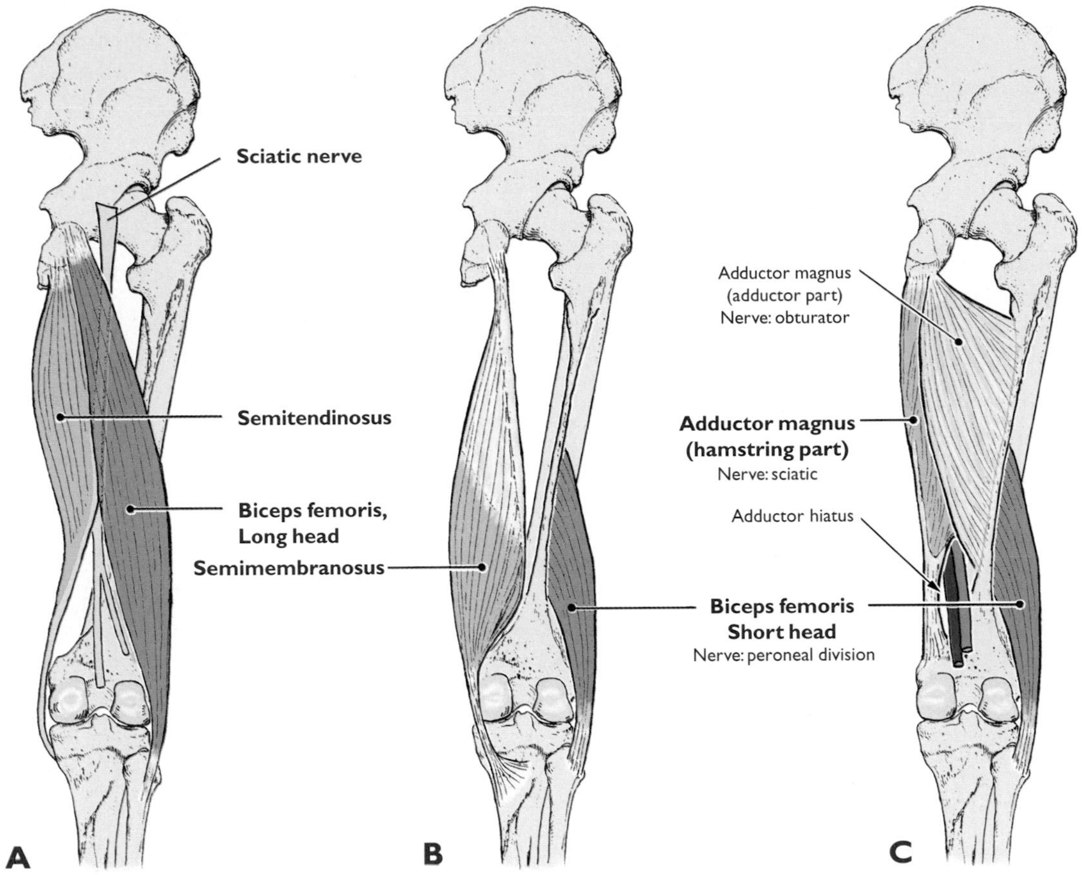

Figure 5.21. Muscles of the posterior thigh from superficial dissection ***(A)*** to deep dissection ***(C)***.

- On the lateral side of thigh, identify the **short head** of the biceps femoris (Fig. 5.21B). This muscle arises from the shaft of the femur. In contrast, the true hamstrings muscles arise from the ischial tuberosity. For this reason and the fact that the short head also has a different nerve supply, the short head of the biceps femoris does not belong to the hamstring muscles.

Verify that the most medial portion of the adductor magnus also arises from the ischial tuberosity (Fig. 5.21C). Identify the thick, fleshy mass of this medial portion that descends almost vertically.

Note that its rounded tendon is inserted into the adductor tubercle of the medial condyle of the femur. This is the **hamstring part of the adductor magnus**. It is innervated by the sciatic nerve, which also supplies the other hamstring muscles. In contrast, the larger remaining part of the adductor magnus is innervated by the obturator nerve.

⇦
GRANT'S 5.26
ROHEN 456, 457
A.D.A.M. 5.8
NETTER 461
CLEMENTE 512
A.V.A. 2: 0.27.02

⇨
GRANT'S 5.28, 5.29
ROHEN 457
A.D.A.M. 5.24, 5.34
NETTER 468
CLEMENTE 513
A.V.A. 2: 0.42.50

⇦
GRANT'S 5.20D
A.D.A.M. 5.9
NETTER 459
CLEMENTE 516
A.V.A. 2: 0.43.04

The hamstring muscles span two joints, the hip joint and the knee joint. Verify that the biceps femoris tendon is inserted into the head of the fibula. The semimembranosus has its insertion into the medial condyle of the tibia. The semitendinosus is inserted into the medial aspect of the tibia.

The principal actions of the hamstrings are flexion of the leg and extension of the thigh, especially during walking.

Once more, display the **sciatic nerve,** the largest nerve in the body. Review a scheme of its distribution (Fig. 5.22). Observe branches of the sciatic nerve as they enter the hamstring muscles.

Look for arteries supplying the hamstring muscles. Most of the blood is derived from the **perforating branches** of the profunda femoris artery, the chief artery of the thigh.

Popliteal Fossa

Define the superior angle of the diamond-shaped popliteal fossa (Fig. 5.23A): on the lateral side is the **biceps femoris.** On the medial side, identify the round **semitendinosus** and the fleshy **semimembranosus.** Define the lower angle of the popliteal fossa: here, the two bellies of the **gastrocnemius** are closely applied to each other. The gastrocnemius is the most superficial muscle in the posterior compartment of the leg; it is responsible for the prominence of the calf.

Dissect the **popliteal fossa** as follows:

- Place a block under the dorsum of the foot to relax the **gastrocnemius**.
- Incise the deep fascia at the medial and lateral borders of this muscle.
- At the lower angle of the popliteal fossa, insert your two index fingers between the contiguous bellies of the gastrocnemius, raise them, and pull them apart for a distance of about 5 to 10 cm (Fig. 5.23B).
- Now, the underlying parts of the **soleus, popliteus,** and **plantaris** muscles can be seen.
- Follow the **sciatic nerve** in the thigh distally toward the popliteal fossa.
- Note that it divides into two major branches, the **common peroneal nerve** and the **tibial nerve**. Identify these two nerves within the popliteal fossa.

⇦ *Grant's 5.41*
Rohen 457
A.D.A.M. 5.33
Netter 461
Clemente 515
A.V.A. 2: 1.12.00

⇨ *Grant's 5.42*
Rohen 457
A.D.A.M. 5.34
Netter 481-483
Clemente 515
A.V.A. 2: 1.12.23

⇦ *Grant's 5.8*
A.D.A.M. 5.22-5.26
Netter 4.63, 465

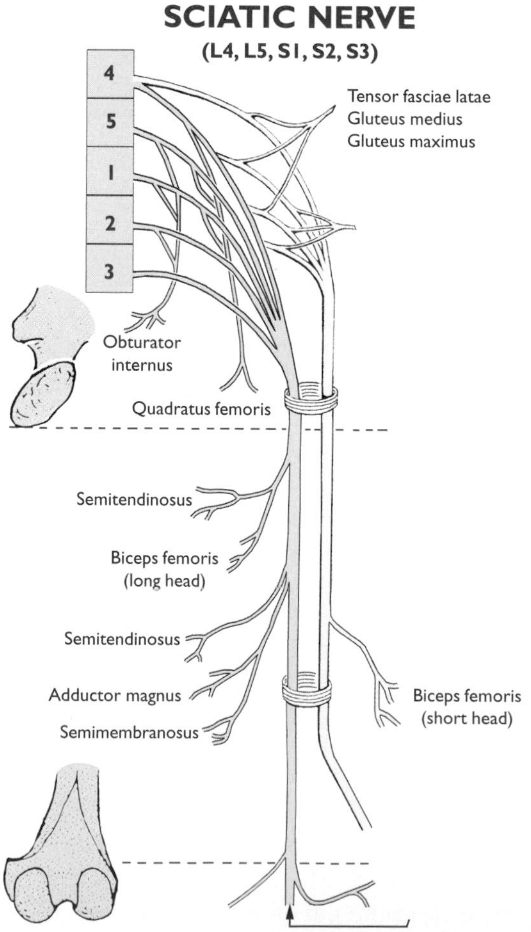

Figure 5.22. Contributions of the lumbosacral plexus to the gluteal nerves and to the sciatic nerve. Scheme of motor distribution of the sciatic nerve to the posterior muscle group of the thigh.

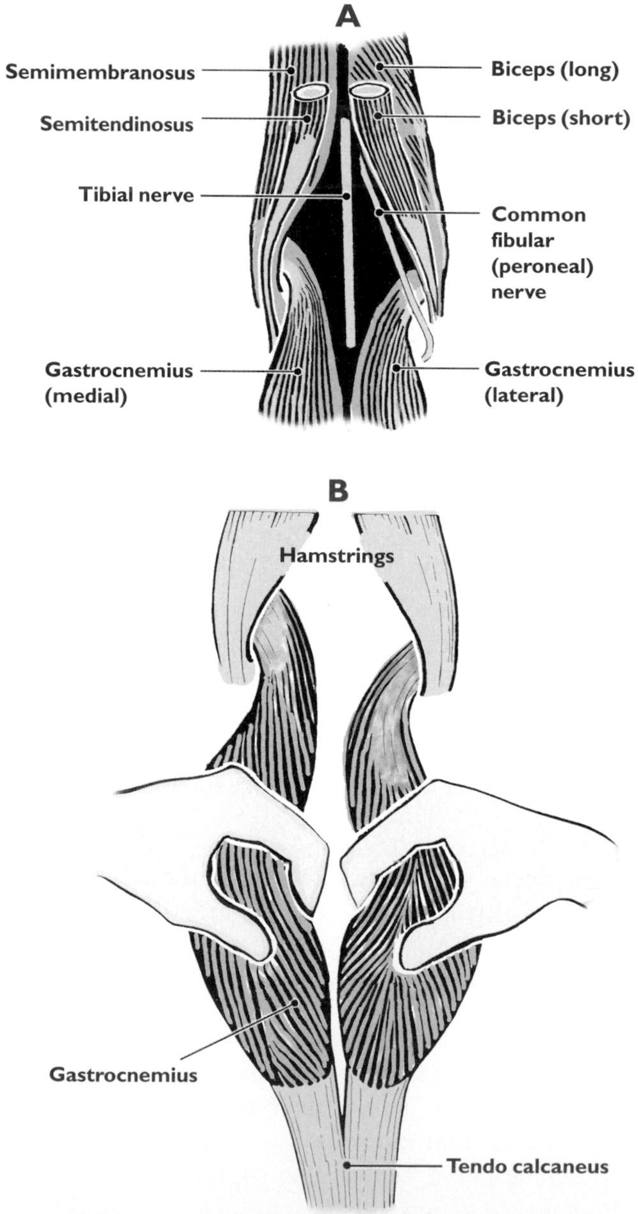

Figure 5.23. ***A,*** Boundaries of the diamond-shaped popliteal fossa. ***B,*** Pull the two bellies of the gastrocnemius forcefully apart to expose the underlying soleus muscle.

• Trace the **tibial nerve** to the lower limit of the fossa. Note that it passes through a gap in the origin of the soleus muscle. Display the nerve.

Observe the dense **vascular sheath** that envelops the **popliteal artery and popliteal vein**.

• Push a probe through the adductor hiatus, and establish the continuity of the femoral with the popliteal vessels (Fig. 5.24).

• Within the popliteal fossa, open the vascular sheath by incising it vertically. Extend the incision superiorly and inferiorly.

• Separate the popliteal artery from the popliteal vein. Cut away tributaries of the vein. This will clarify the dissection field.

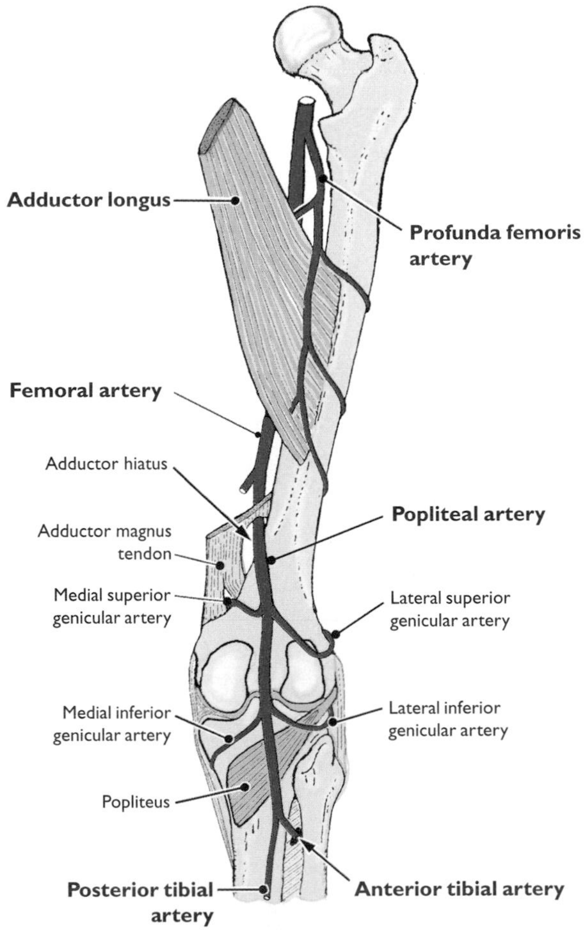

Figure 5.24. Posterior aspect of thigh and knee. At the adductor hiatus, the femoral artery is continuous with the popliteal artery. Note the genicular branches.

GRANT'S 5.42, 5.43
ROHEN 457
NETTER 482, 483
CLEMENTE 544
A.V.A. 2: 1.12.31

GRANT'S 5.45
ROHEN 460
NETTER 477
CLEMENTE 517
A.V.A. 2: 1.10.08

GRANT'S 5.6B, 5.31B
ROHEN 460
A.D.A.M. 5.34
NETTER 477
CLEMENTE 480, 543
A.V.A. 2: 1.09.36

GRANT'S 5.22B
A.V.A. 2: 1.05.34

ROHEN 470
CLEMENTE 620

• Retract the plantaris muscle laterally to expose fully the **popliteal artery** and some of its branches.

Spend a few minutes studying the elaborate arterial anastomoses around the knee joint (Fig. 5.24). Understand that these collateral vessels ensure adequate blood supply of the knee in case of injury. At this time, only the **superior lateral genicular artery** and the **superior medial genicular artery** can be seen. The inferior genicular arteries are still covered by the bellies of the gastrocnemius.

Verify that three slender muscles converge to an apex on the medial side of the proximal end of the tibia, essentially forming an inverted "tripod." These muscles are the **sartorius, gracilis, and semitendinosus.** Each muscle belongs to a different muscle group; thus each has a different nerve supply and a different site of origin on the hip bone. All three muscles span (i.e., act on) two joints, the hip joint and the knee joint.

Review the principal muscle groups of the thigh and their respective **nerve territories** (Fig. 5.25). The posteriorly located **hamstring muscles** are supplied by the **sciatic nerve.** The medially positioned **adductors** belong to the **obturator nerve** territory. The **femoral nerve** supplies the **sartorius and the quadriceps group** anteriorly and laterally to the femur. Correlate your anatomical observations with a transverse MRI of the thigh.

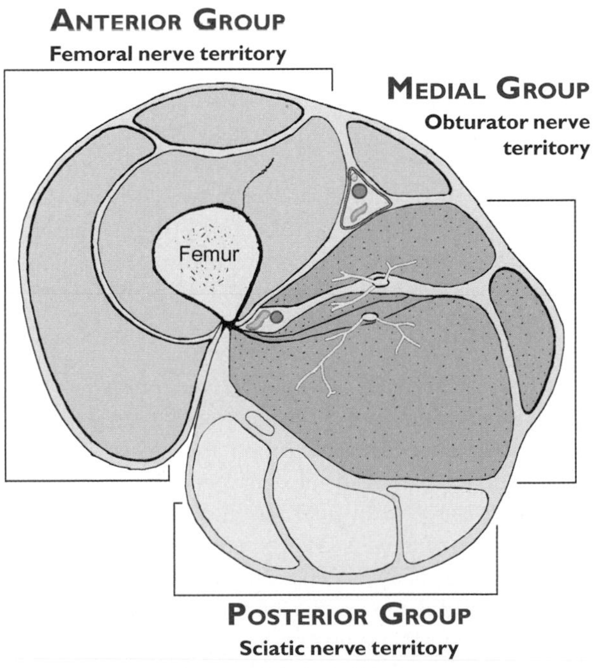

Figure 5.25. The three principal muscle groups of the thigh and their respective motor nerve territories.

Leg and Dorsum of Foot

General Remarks

The morphological organization and function of the leg will be best understood if a transverse section is studied and analyzed (Fig. 5.26). Before attempting dissection, understand the following facts:

⇦
Rohen 471
A.D.A.M. 5.46
Netter 487
Clemente 523, 616
A.V.A. 2: 1.33.40

- The two bones of the leg are unequal in size. The larger **tibia** lies medial; its medial surface is subcutaneous. The smaller **fibula** is deeply placed. Tibia and fibula are connected by an **interosseous membrane**.
- The investing deep fascia reaches the fibula by means of septa, the **anterior** and **posterior crural septa**.
- The two bones, their interosseous membrane, and the crural septa divide the leg into **three compartments: anterior, lateral** or **fibular** (peroneal), and **posterior**. Each compartment contains a synergistic muscle group. A nerve supplying these muscles runs in each compartment.
- The muscles in the **anterior crural compartment** are mainly concerned with **dorsiflexion of the foot** (turning of the foot upward) and with extension of the toes. The nerve within this compartment is the **deep fibular** (peroneal) **nerve** (Fig. 5.26). It is a branch of the common fibular nerve that passes around the lateral side of the neck of the fibula. The deep fibular nerve is accompanied by the **anterior tibial artery** that enters the anterior compartment through a gap superior to the proximal border of the interosseous membrane.
- The **lateral crural compartment** or **fibular** (peroneal) **compartment** contains two muscles for **plantar flexion** and **eversion of the foot**. The nerve within this compartment is the **superficial fibular** (peroneal) **nerve** (Fig. 5.26). It is a branch of the common fibular nerve that, in turn, is the smaller of the two terminal branches of the sciatic nerve.
- The **posterior crural compartment** contains several muscles whose principal function is **plantar flexion of the foot** and toes (turning foot downward). The muscles are divided into a **superficial group** and a **deep group** by an intermuscular septum. Note that the nerve of the posterior compartment runs between the superficial and deep groups (Fig. 5.26). This nerve is the **tibial nerve,** the larger of the two terminal branches of the sciatic nerve. The nerve is accompanied by the **posterior tibial artery**, a branch of the popliteal artery.

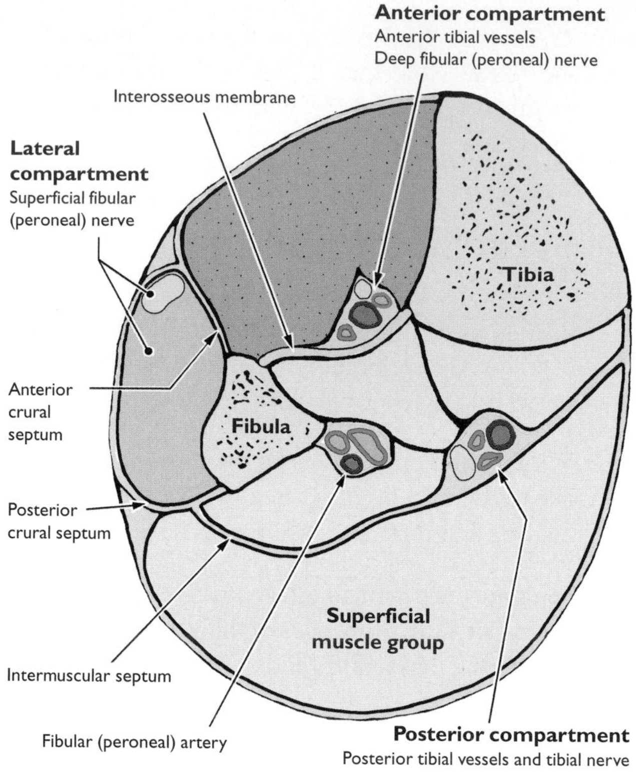

Figure 5.26. Schematic transverse section through the right leg. Note two bones, septa, and three crural compartments with contents.

Bony Landmarks

⇨
Grant's 5.68, 5.84
Rohen 416, 418
A.D.A.M. 5.5, 5.6
Netter 478-480, 488, 489
Clemente 589-598
A.V.A. 2: 1.15.55

Refer to an articulated lower limb of a skeleton. Identify the following landmarks (Fig. 5.27):

- **Medial condyle** and **lateral condyle of tibia**;
- **Anterior border of tibia**, descending from the tibial tuberosity; note that its proximal portion is sharp and prominent;
- **Head of fibula**;
- **Medial malleolus,** the large medial prominence at the ankle;
- **Lateral malleolus,** the lateral prominence at the ankle;

In the articulated foot, identify the **tarsus**, which consists of seven tarsal bones:

- **Talus** (L., ankle bone);
- **Calcaneus** (L. *calx,* heel);
- **Navicular** (L., little ship);
- **Cuboid** (Gr., cube-shaped);
- **Three cuneiformes** (L., wedge-shaped), 1st, 2nd, and 3rd.

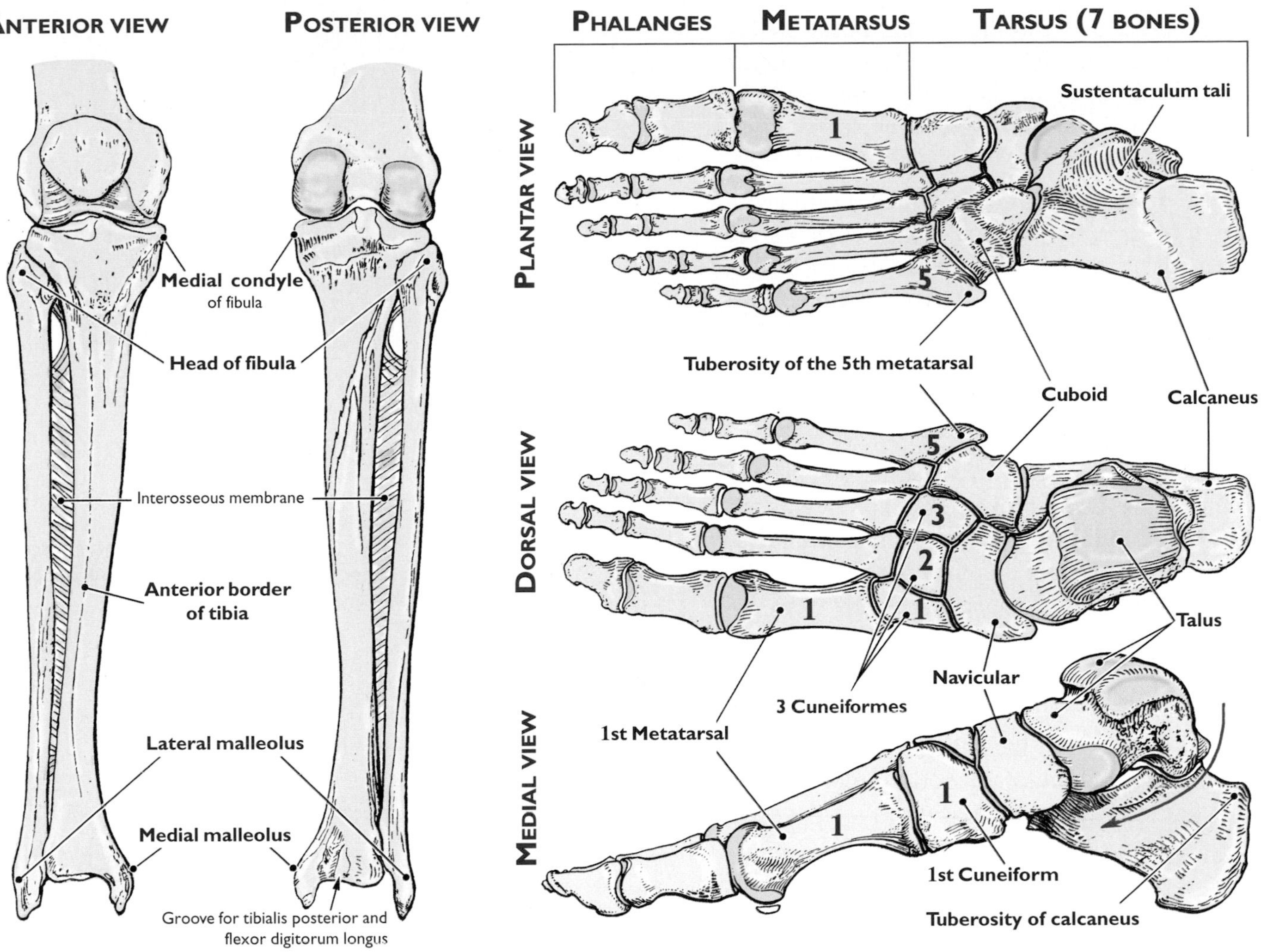

Figure 5.27. Bony landmarks of leg and foot.

On the calcaneus, identify:

- The **tuber calcanei** (tuberosity) for attachment of the tendo calcaneus or Achilles tendon;
- A groove below the **sustentaculum tali** (L., sustentaculum tali, support for talus) for the passage of the flexor hallucis longus tendon (blue arrow).

Examine the **metatarsus** and the **phalanges**:

- Identify the **five metatarsals** and the **tuberosity of the 5th metatarsal**.
- Note that the 1st toe has two phalanges, whereas the other toes have three.

Before you begin ...

After reflecting the skin, the crural compartments (anterior; lateral; posterior) will be dissected. The derivation and course of blood vessels and nerves will be explored, and their continuation onto the dorsum or into the sole of the foot will be demonstrated. The muscles of the crural compartments will be followed to their insertions in the foot.

GRANT'S 5.62
ROHEN 437, 4.38
A.D.A.M. TABLE 5.4
NETTER 484
CLEMENTE 522
A.V.A. 2: 1.29.30; 2.02.35

GRANT'S 5.62, 5.63
ROHEN 437, 438
A.D.A.M. 5.43, 5.44
NETTER 484, 485
CLEMENTE 521, 522
A.V.A. 2: 1.33.58

Anterior Crural Compartment and Dorsum of Foot

The **anterior compartment** (Fig. 5.26) is also known as the **extensor compartment** because its muscles extend (or dorsiflex) the foot. The four muscles of the anterior compartment are: tibialis anterior, extensor hallucis longus, extensor digitorum longus, and fibularis (peroneus) tertius. The deep fibular (peroneal) nerve supplies the muscles of the anterior compartment. The anterior tibial vessels provide the blood supply to the compartment. At the ankle joint, the anterior tibial artery becomes the clinically important dorsalis pedis artery. The superficial nerves and veins have already been dissected and demonstrated.

Place the cadaver in the supine position (face up). Review the **deep fascia.** Demonstrate that muscle fibers of the **tibialis anterior** arise from this deep fascia: make a vertical cut through the fascia just below the lateral tibial condyle, lift the edges of the deep fascia, and see the muscle fibers arising from the fascia (Fig. 5.28). Since the muscle takes origin from the fascia, this fascia must be strong and thick. Verify that the fascia is attached to the sharp anterior border of the tibia.

Grant's 5.62, 5.63
Rohen 437, 438
A.D.A.M. 5.43, 5.44
Netter 484, 485
Clemente 521, 522

The superior and inferior **extensor retinacula** are transversely directed thickenings of the deep fascia that hold tendons in place (Fig. 5.29). The **superior extensor retinaculum** extends across the tendons superior to the ankle joint. The **inferior extensor retinaculum** is Y-shaped. The stem of this Y is fixed to the calcaneus anterior to the lateral malleolus.

Grant's 5.65, 5.67
Rohen 437, 438
A.D.A.M. 5.43, 5.55
Netter 484, 493
Clemente 522, 532-534
A.V.A. 2 : 1.25.34

Laterally, the stem of the inferior extensor retinaculum is in broken continuity with the **inferior fibular** (peroneal) **retinaculum**. Define these retinacula and understand their function. What would happen if tendons were not held in place by these retinacula? Subsequently, cut vertically through the deep fascia overlying the anterior crural compartment.

The structures of the anterior crural compartment cross the ankle anteriorly. From the medial to the lateral side they are:

Grant's 5.62, 5.63
Rohen 437, 438
A.D.A.M. 5.43, 5.44
Netter 484
Clemente 522, 524
A.V.A. 2 : 2.03.42

- **Tibialis anterior**;
- **Extensor hallucis longus**;
- **Deep fibular** (peroneal) **nerve** together with **anterior tibial vessels**;
- **Extensor digitorum longus**. The lateral lower fleshy part of the extensor digitorum longus is the fibularis (peroneus) tertius.

Examine the components of the anterior crural compartment in greater detail. Begin with the muscles:

- Separate the muscles from each other and trace them to their origins.
- Trace the tendons of the muscles of the anterior crural compartment inferiorly to their insertions in the foot.
- Pull on the **tibialis anterior** tendon and confirm that the action of this muscle is dorsiflexion and inversion of the foot.
- Pull on the tendons of the **extensor hallucis longus** and the **extensor digitorum longus**. Observe that these muscles basically extend the digits and assist in dorsiflexion of the foot.

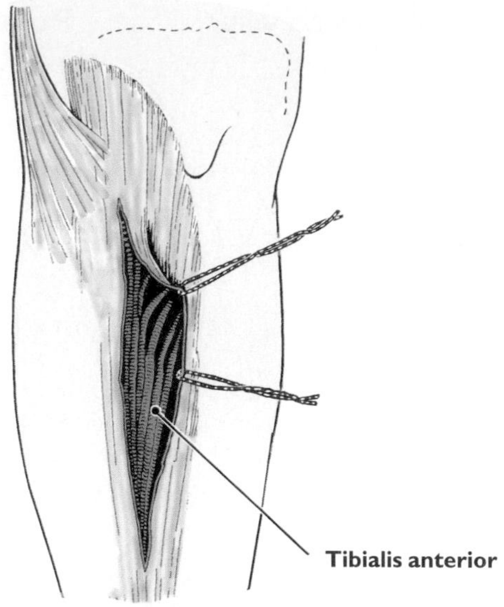

Figure 5.28. Deep fascia (incised) giving, in part, origin to the tibialis anterior muscle. Therefore, the fascia is aponeurotic, thick, and creates lines on the tibia.

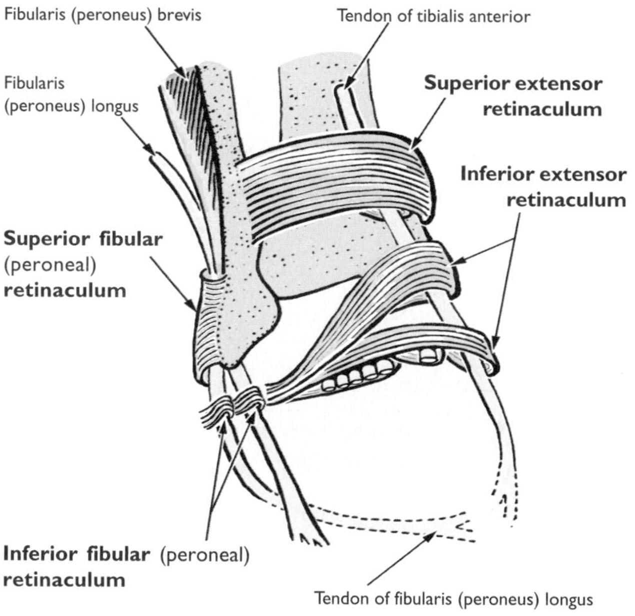

Figure 5.29. The retinacula hold tendons in place.

Grant's 5.64
Rohen 442, 466
A.D.A.M. 5.14, 5.43
Netter 485
Clemente 525
A.V.A. 2 : 1.47.05

Next, examine the vascular supply of the anterior crural compartment and the dorsum of the foot:

- Study the **anterior tibial artery** and the **deep fibular** (peroneal) **nerve**. Observe that artery and nerve occupy the median plane and have two tendons on each side of them. Trace the artery proximally to the point where it passes over the superior border of the interosseous membrane. Demonstrate the various branches of the anterior tibial artery.

- Note the **perforating branch** of the fibular artery that passes distal to the interosseous membrane. Occasionally, this perforating branch is large and may replace the dorsalis pedis artery.

GRANT'S 5.6B, 5.64A, 5.65D
ROHEN 469
NETTER 485, 495
CLEMENTE 525, 537
A.V.A. 2: 1.46.42

- Identify the **dorsalis pedis artery** (L. *pes, pedis,* foot). It is the continuation of the anterior tibial artery onto the dorsum of the foot. Note that the dorsalis pedis artery and its branches lie on the skeletal plane; there they remain intact even if all muscles are torn away. In the living, the pulse of the dorsalis pedis can be palpated.

GRANT'S 5.63, 5.64
ROHEN 468
A.D.A.M. 5.23
NETTER 485, 495
CLEMENTE 525, 537
A.V.A. 2: 1.49.37

- Demonstrate the **arcuate artery** across the base of the metatarsal bones. The **dorsal metatarsal arteries** originate from it.

- A deep plantar branch connects to the plantar arch in the sole of the foot.

- Note the **medial malleolar artery** to the medial ankle, the **lateral malleolar artery** to the lateral ankle, and **tarsal branches** to the tarsus. Usually, the lateral tarsal artery connects with the arcuate artery.

GRANT'S 5.65D
A.D.A.M. 5.13, 5.14
NETTER 495
CLEMENTE 537

Finally, examine the nerve supply of the anterior crural compartment and the dorsum of the foot:

- Demonstrate the **deep fibular** (peroneal) **nerve** (Fig. 5.30).

- Verify that this nerve is a branch of the common fibular (peroneal) nerve. Pull on the common fibular nerve posterior to the head of the fibula. Follow the nerve into the anterior crural compartment.

GRANT'S 5.8C
A.D.A.M. 5.23
NETTER 485
CLEMENTE 525
A.V.A. 2: 1.50.10

- Note and study the muscular branches (Fig. 5.31).

- Follow the deep fibular (peroneal) nerve onto the dorsum of the foot.

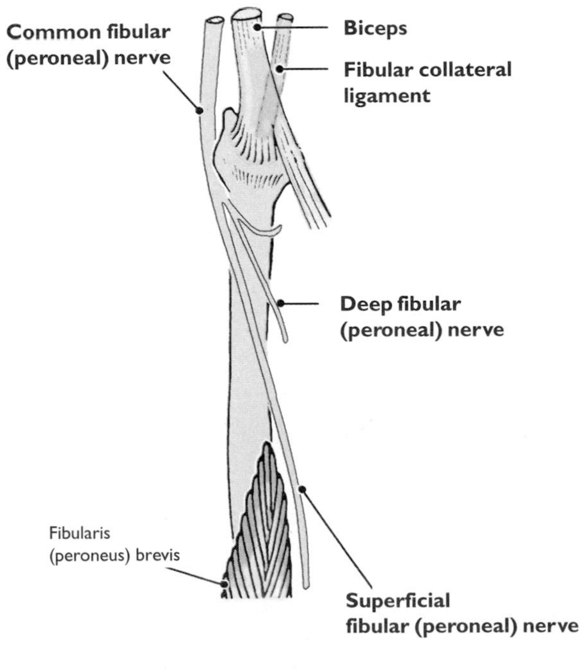

Figure 5.30. Common fibular (peroneal) nerve and its branches in contact with fibula.

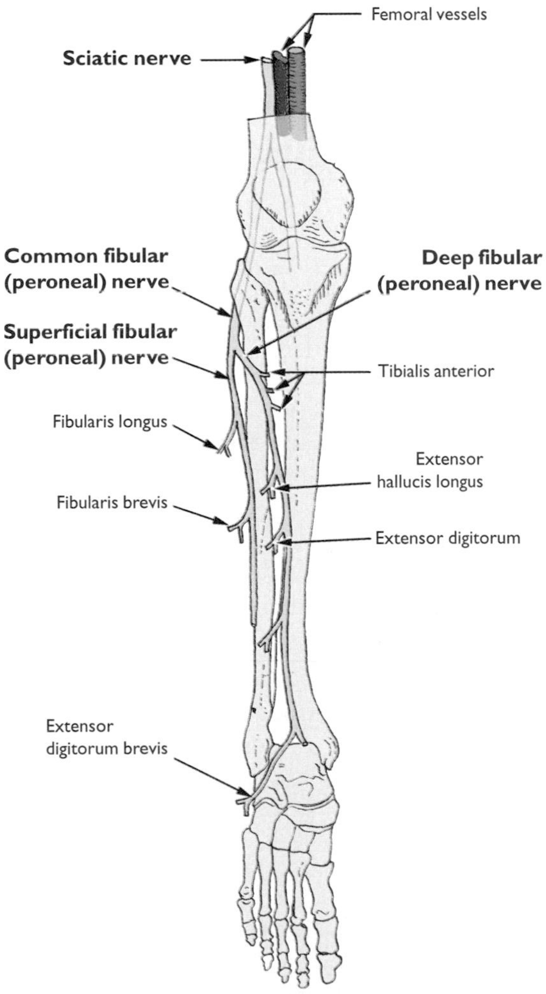

Figure 5.31. Scheme of motor distribution of the fibular (peroneal) nerve in the anterior and lateral crural compartments and the dorsum of the foot.

- Note the nerve branches to the two short extensors of the toes, **extensor digitorum brevis** and **extensor hallucis brevis**. Examine these muscles. They take origin from the calcaneus and are inserted into the extensor expansions of the toes.

GRANT'S 5.8C
A.D.A.M. 5.23
NETTER 485
CLEMENTE 525
A.V.A. 2: 2.05.05

Correlate your anatomical observations with a transverse section through the anterior crural compartment and a corresponding MRI.

Lateral Crural Compartment and Lateral Side of Ankle

The lateral crural compartment contains two muscles, the fibularis (peroneus) longus and the fibularis (peroneus) brevis. The nerve of this compartment is the superficial fibular (peroneal) nerve (Fig. 5.31); this nerve continues distally to supply the skin of the dorsum of the foot.

Dissect the structures within the lateral crural compartment:

- Open the **deep fascia** overlying the **lateral** (peroneal) **compartment**.
- In this compartment, identify its two muscles, the **fibularis (peroneus) longus** and the **fibularis (peroneus) brevis**. Distinguish these two muscles from each other.
- The fibularis brevis is inserted into the tuberosity of the 5th metatarsal bone.
- The fibularis longus hooks around the cuboid and travels medially in the sole of the foot. Its tendon in the sole of the foot will be dissected later. Realize (without dissection at this time) that this tendon is indeed long: it reaches as far as the inferior surface of the 1st metatarsal bone.

GRANT'S 5.61B, 5.62
ROHEN 435
A.D.A.M. 5.10
NETTER 486
CLEMENTE 522, 527
A.V.A. 2: 1.39.02

- Pull on the fibular (peroneal) muscles. Verify that they evert the foot.

Examine how the tendons of the fibularis longus and brevis are held in place (Fig. 5.29):

- The **superior fibular** (peroneal) **retinaculum** retains the tendons posterior to the **lateral malleolus**;
- The **inferior fibular retinaculum** holds them to the calcaneus. Follow the **fibularis longus tendon** to the point where it disappears into the sole of the foot.

GRANT'S 5.61C, 5.64A
ROHEN 466
A.D.A.M. 5.44
NETTER 485
CLEMENTE 525
A.V.A. 2: 2.21.17

Identify the nerve of the lateral crural compartment, the **superficial fibular** (peroneal) **nerve** (Fig. 5.31). It lies along the anterior border of the fibularis brevis. Follow the nerve distally. Its cutaneous branches to the dorsum of the foot have been examined earlier. Trace the nerve proximally and verify that it is a branch of the **common fibular nerve**. Push a probe parallel to the nerve as it passes between the fibula and fibularis longus. You may carefully divide this muscle over the probe to establish continuity of the common, superficial, and deep fibular nerves.

GRANT'S 5.60B, 5.62
ROHEN 466
A.D.A.M. 5.23, 5.24
NETTER 506
CLEMENTE 525
A.V.A. 2: 1.49.06

Clinical Correlation: Of all nerves in the body, the **common fibular** (peroneal) **nerve** is the most frequently injured. Once again, observe the superficial position of the nerve in relation to the head and neck of the fibula (Fig. 5.30 and 5.31). The nerve may be readily injured by superficial wounds, prolonged pressure by hard objects during sleep, anesthesia, and chronic illness, or by compression against the opposite patella while sitting with the knees crossed.

What are the neurological findings of common fibular nerve lesions? The nerves of the lateral and anterior crural compartments are affected. Consequently, eversion, extension (dorsiflexion) of the foot, and extension of the toes will be impaired. There is a "foot drop" resulting in a characteristic steppage gait. There may be some sensory loss on the dorsum of the foot and toes.

Sudden overuse of the anterior tibial muscles may lead to swelling and edema in the anterior crural compartment. This painful condition is known as "shin splints" in lay terminology.

Posterior Crural Compartment and Medial Side of Ankle

The **posterior crural compartment** lies posterior to the interosseous membrane that connects tibia and fibula (Fig. 5.26). The compartment contains the calf muscles that are divided into a superficial group (three muscles) and a deep group (four muscles). The tibial nerve supplies the superficial and deep muscle group (Fig. 5.32). The posterior tibial vessels are responsible for the blood supply.

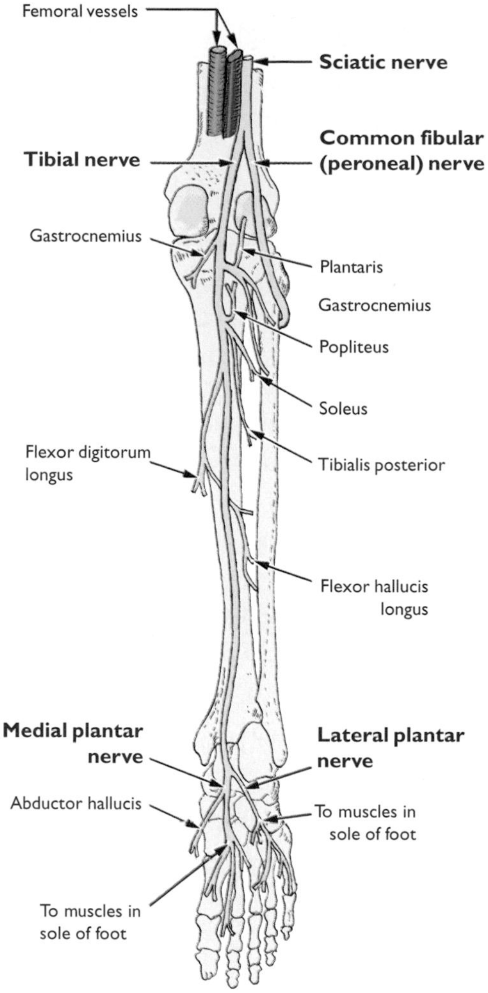

Figure 5.32. Scheme of motor distribution of the tibial nerve in the posterior crural compartment and in the sole of the foot.

Turn the cadaver into the prone position (face down). Identity the **deep fascia.** Cut it vertically from popliteal fossa to calcaneus, and reflect it laterally.

Dissect the **superficial muscle group** of the posterior crural compartment:

GRANT'S 5.70B, 5.70C
ROHEN 461
A.D.A.M. 5.45
NETTER 481
CLEMENTE 540, 541
A.V.A. 2: 1.30.54

- Identify the **gastrocnemius**. Pull the **two bellies (heads) of the gastrocnemius** apart. Follow them to the **tendo calcaneus** (Achilles tendon), the common tendon for the gastrocnemius and underlying **soleus**.
- Cut across the two bellies of the gastrocnemius well inferior to the entrance of their nerves.
- Reflect the proximal and distal portions of the bellies, and expose the underlying soleus. Verify that the two heads of the gastrocnemius originate from the medial and lateral condyles of the femur.

ROHEN 462
A.D.A.M. 5.45
NETTER 482
CLEMENTE 542
A.V.A. 2: 1.32.20

- Now, you can easily identify the **plantaris**. Occasionally, it is absent or doubled. This small muscle originates in the lateral supracondylar area of the femur and runs obliquely between gastrocnemius and soleus. Look for its long and thin tendon, located on the medial border of the tendo calcaneus. Although the plantaris muscle is of minor importance, its thin and long tendon is often used as tendon replacement in reconstructive surgery, notably in the forearm and hand.

GRANT'S 5.71
ROHEN 462, 463
A.D.A.M. 5.45
NETTER 483
CLEMENTE 544, 546
A.V.A. 2: 1.47.55

The **tibial nerve** and **posterior tibial vessels** are closely related to the intermuscular septum that separates the superficial from the deep muscles of the posterior compartment (Figs. 5.26, 5.33). To obtain access to the plane of this septum, the soleus must be reflected. Proceed as follows:

- Cut the **tendo calcaneus** (Achilles tendon) about 5 cm superior to its insertion into the tuberosity of the calcaneus.
- Reflect the tendon superiorly together with the fleshy parts of gastrocnemius and soleus.
- Pass two fingers superiorly between soleus and the loose intermuscular septum. Palpate the horseshoe-shaped origin of the soleus from tibia and fibula.
- Using a scalpel, detach the soleus from its tibial origin, but leave it attached to the fibula.
- Turn the muscle laterally. Now, the **intermuscular septum** is in full view.
- Slit the loose layer vertically to expose the **posterior tibial vessels** and the **tibial nerve** (Fig. 5.33). Free these structures from the surrounding connective tissue plane. Note that the artery is accompanied by two or more veins.

GRANT'S 5.71
ROHEN 462
A.D.A.M. 5.11, 5.45
NETTER 483
CLEMENTE 546, 548
A.V.A. 2: 1.35.16

Four muscles comprise the **deep group** of the posterior crural compartment. To aid in identification, it is useful to correlate a transverse section with a figure showing the origin of the muscles (Fig. 5.33). Note:

- The **flexor hallucis longus** lies lateral. It is closely attached to the fibula.

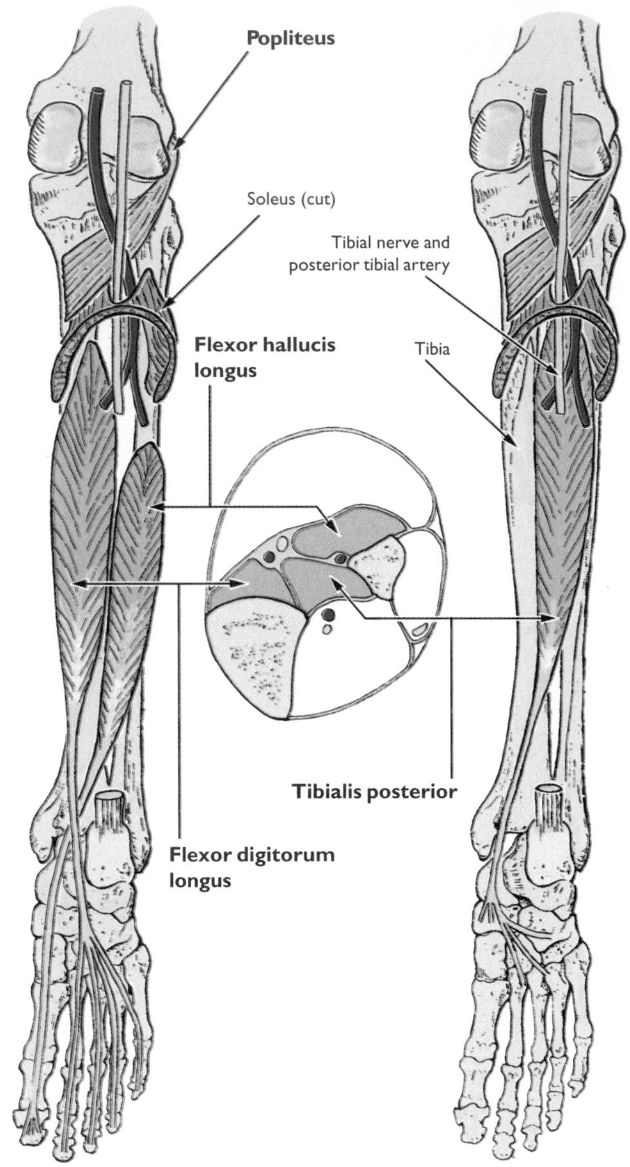

Figure 5.33. The deep muscle group of the posterior crural compartment.

Distally, its tendon is inserted into the most medial (1st) toe.

- The **flexor digitorum longus** lies medial. It is closely attached to the tibia. Distally, its tendons are inserted into the four toes. By necessity, the two longus tendons must cross each other.
- The **tibialis posterior** lies in the middle. It takes origin from the tibia, fibula, and the interosseous membrane. Distally, it is inserted into the inferior surfaces of various tarsal bones.

Identify and dissect the muscles of the **deep muscle group**. Their insertions will be demonstrated later during dissection of the sole of the foot.

⇨
Grant's 5.74, 5.78
Rohen 462
A.D.A.M. 5.11
Netter 483, 493
Clemente 534, 548
A.V.A. 2: 2.05.57

⇨
Grant's 5.43, 5.71B
Rohen 433
A.D.A.M. 5.11
Netter 483
Clemente 548
A.V.A. 2: 1.06.10

⇦
Grant's 5.71
Rohen 462
A.D.A.M. 5.11, 5.45
Netter 483
Clemente 546, 548
A.V.A. 2: 2.06.12

Proceed as follows (Fig. 5.33):

- Identify the **flexor hallucis longus** in the posterior compartment of the leg. Follow its tendon distally until it disappears in an **osseofibrous tunnel** (Fig. 5.34).
- Push a probe into the tunnel; then open it. Note that the tendon is surrounded by a synovial sheath.
- Temporarily lift out the tendon of the flexor hallucis longus. Verify that it runs in a **groove** below the **sustentaculum tali,** using the sustentaculum as a pulley.
- The **flexor digitorum longus tendon** passes along the medial border of the sustentaculum. Observe that the tendons of flexor digitorum longus and flexor hallucis longus cross each other (Figs. 5.33, 5.34).
- Identify the **tibialis posterior** and follow its tendon distally to the medial aspect of the foot.
- Turn to the popliteal fossa and identify the deeply positioned **popliteus** (Fig. 5.33). It is a flat, triangular muscle that is covered by the heads of the gastrocnemius. Note its close relationship with the popliteal artery.

Pulling on tendons and observing the resulting action is often informative. However, this maneuver may be difficult in cadavers with very stiff tissues.

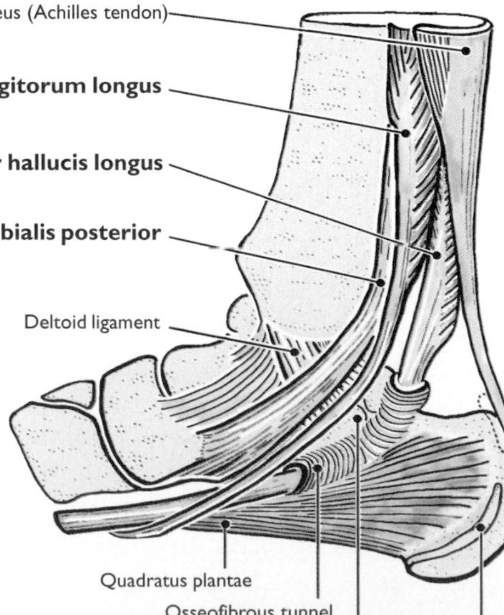

Figure 5.34. Deep structures on the medial side of the ankle.

• Pull on the flexor digitorum longus tendon. Observe that this muscle flexes the terminal phalanges of the four small toes (toes 2, 3, 4, 5) and also assists in plantar flexion and inversion of the foot.

• Pull on the tendon of the flexor hallucis longus. Observe flexion of the great toe (toe 1). The flexor hallucis longus also assists in plantar flexion and inversion of the foot.

• Verify that the **tibialis posterior** tendon passes superior to the sustentaculum tali. Pull on the tendon. Observe that the muscle inverts the foot and assists in plantar flexion.

Explore the vascular distribution in the back of the leg (Fig. 5.35). Clean the **posterior tibial artery** and the accompanying **tibial nerve**. Note that the artery is accompanied by two or more veins. The largest branch of the posterior tibial artery is the **fibular** (peroneal) **artery**. Identify the fibular vessels in the interval between tibialis posterior and flexor hallucis longus. At least two veins accompany the artery. Identify the fibular artery. Distally, search for its communicating branch and its perforating branch. Note the motor branches of the tibial nerve to the muscles of the posterior compartment (Fig. 5.32).

GRANT'S 5.74C
A.D.A.M. 5.45
A.V.A. 2: 1.46.33

GRANT'S 5.78, 5.79B
A.D.A.M. 5.11, 5.47
NETTER 483
CLEMENTE 541, 545
A.V.A. 2: 1.37.54

GRANT'S 5.71
ROHEN 443
A.D.A.M. 5.14
NETTER 483
CLEMENTE 546
A.V.A. 2: 1.45.52

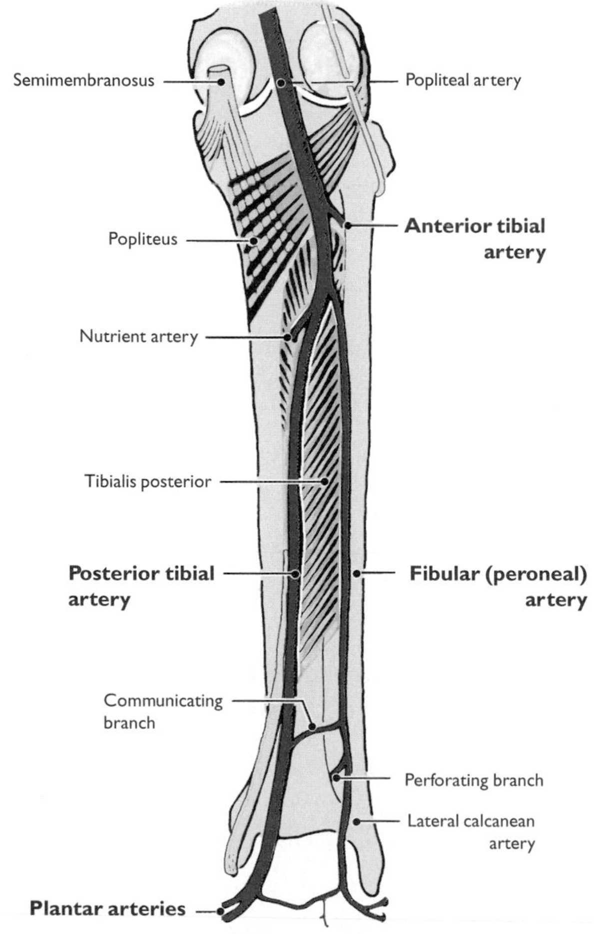

Figure 5.35. Arteries of the posterior aspect of the leg.

Now, review the **muscle groups** of the three crural compartments and their respective **nerve territories** (Fig. 5.36):

• The **muscles** in the **anterior compartment** (tibialis anterior, extensor hallucis longus, extensor digitorum longus, and fibularis tertius) are supplied by the **deep fibular** (peroneal) **nerve**.

• The two muscles in the **lateral compartment** (fibularis brevis, fibularis longus) belong to the territory of the **superficial fibular** (peroneal) **nerve**.

• All muscles of the **posterior compartment** (superficial: gastrocnemius, soleus, plantaris; deep: tibialis posterior, flexor digitorum longus, flexor hallucis longus, popliteus) are supplied by branches of the **tibial nerve.**

Review the compartmental organization of the leg by studying a transverse section. Correlate your anatomical observations with an appropriate MRI of the leg.

A.D.A.M. 5.46
NETTER 487
CLEMENTE 616, 617
A.V.A. 2: 1.33.45

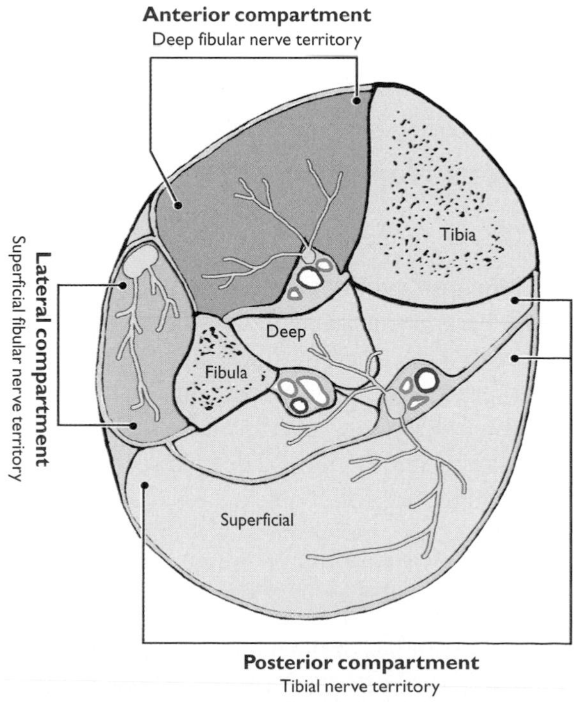

Figure 5.36. Three crural compartments and their respective motor nerve territories.

Sole of Foot (Planta)

General Remarks

Understand the following important facts:

- The **foot is arched longitudinally** (Fig. 5.37). Viewed from the medial side, the arch appears high. Viewed from the lateral side, the longitudinal arch is low. Can these facts be recognized in a footprint?

Grant's 5.82B, 5.84
A.V.A. 2: 1.53.45

- The **bearing points** of the foot are the calcaneus posteriorly, and the heads of the five metatarsal bones anteriorly. These bearing points are the ends of the longitudinal arches.

- The **plantar aponeurosis** (fascia) acts as a strong tie for the maintenance of the longitudinal arches. Therefore, it is logical that the plantar aponeurosis stretches from the calcaneus posteriorly to the five digits anteriorly. The plantar aponeurosis must be of considerable **strength** to perform its function. The aponeurosis is covered with thick skin. The toughness of the tissues in the sole of the foot often makes dissection difficult. Be aware of this fact in allotting your time.

Grant's 5.75
Rohen 439
A.D.A.M. 5.53
Netter 496
Clemente 549
A.V.A. 2: 1.56.14

- Deep to the plantar aponeurosis are **four layers of muscles.** These will be described later.

- The posterior tibial vessels are continuous with the **plantar vessels** in the sole of the foot .

- The tibial nerve sends two branches into the sole: The **medial plantar nerve** and the **lateral plantar nerve**.

Plantar Aponeurosis and Cutaneous Nerves

When dissecting the **plantar aponeurosis,** certain cutaneous nerves and vessels are easily cut. Therefore, attempt to secure these structures in the beginning. In a longitudinal direction, cut through the thick fatty fascia and a film of deep fascia (Fig. 5.38). Find the following nerves:

- **Medial calcanean nerve**, which supplies the skin of the heel.

- **Digital branches of the medial plantar nerve** (and artery); in part to the medial side of the great toe.

Grant's 5.75
Netter 496
Clemente 550

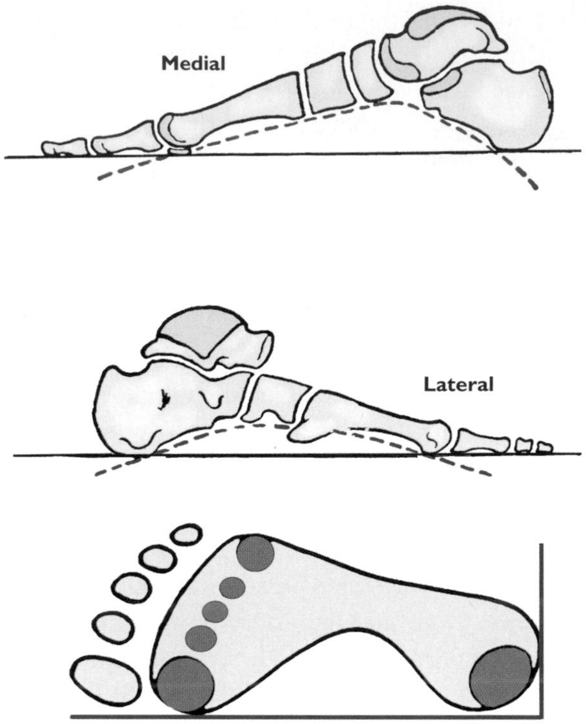

Figure 5.37. Medial and lateral longitudinal arches of the foot. Bearing points of the foot.

- **Digital branches of the lateral plantar nerve** (and artery); in part to the lateral side of the little toe.

- **Other digital nerves** may be traced now or later.

Plantar Aponeurosis. Proceed with the dissection as follows (Fig. 5.38):

Grant's 5.75
Rohen 439
A.D.A.M. 5.53
Netter 496
Clemente 549, 550
A.V.A. 2: 1.56.33

- Scrape the superficial fascia off the plantar aponeurosis. Note its proximal attachment to the calcaneus.

- Define the five diverging aponeurotic bands that pass to each toe.

- To expose the underlying muscles, split the plantar aponeurosis longitudinally throughout its length.

- Next, carefully cut it transversely close to the calcaneus and also in the anterior third of the foot.

- Reflect the flaps medially and laterally (Fig. 5.38).

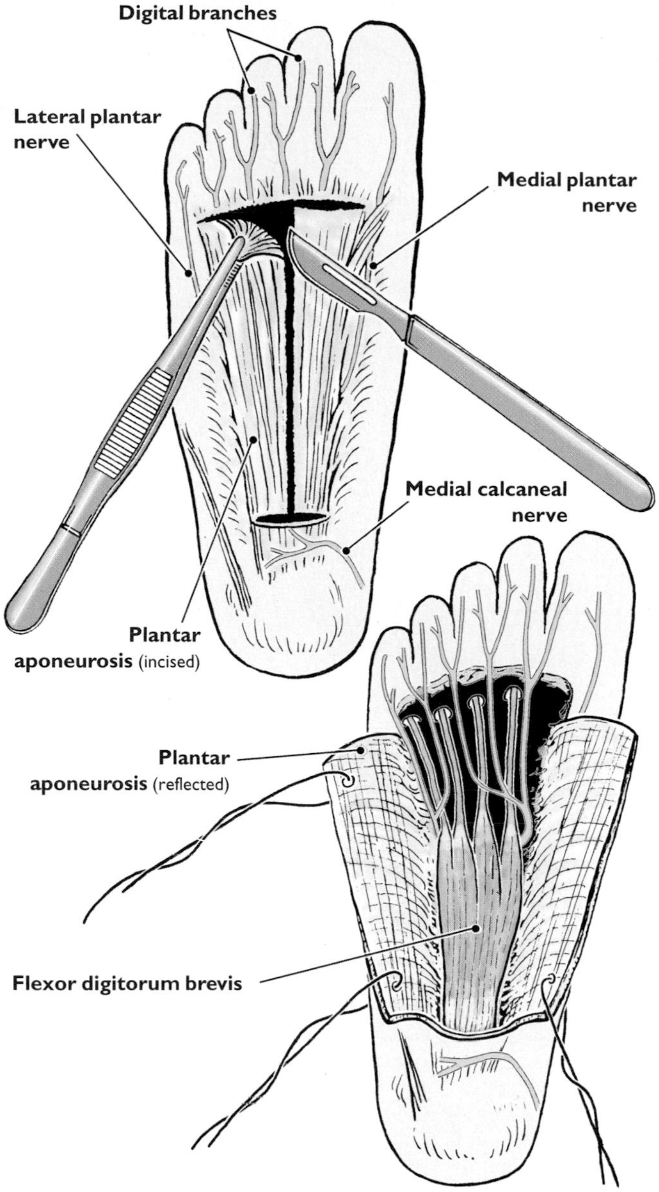

Figure 5.38. Incision in plantar aponeurosis, reflection of aponeurosis, and exposure of underlying flexor digitorum brevis. Cutaneous nerves of sole of foot.

GRANT'S 5.77
ROHEN 439
A.D.A.M. 5.12, 5.53
NETTER 497
CLEMENTE 551
A.V.A. 2: 2.13.12

- Separate the flaps from the **flexor digitorum brevis** that originates, in part, from the central portion of the plantar aponeurosis.

GRANT'S 5.77
ROHEN 439
A.D.A.M. 5.12, 5.53
NETTER 497
CLEMENTE 551
A.V.A. 2: 2.10.35

Muscle Layers

First Layer of Plantar Muscles. Proceed as follows (Fig. 5.39):

GRANT'S 5.6B, 5.8D
ROHEN 447
A.D.A.M. 5.14, 5.24
NETTER 483, 497
CLEMENTE 546, 550
A.V.A. 2: 2.19.55

- Medial to the plantar aponeurosis, expose the **abductor hallucis.** Note its origin from the calcaneus. What is its function? Be careful not to destroy the plantar digital nerve and artery to the medial side of the first (big) toe.

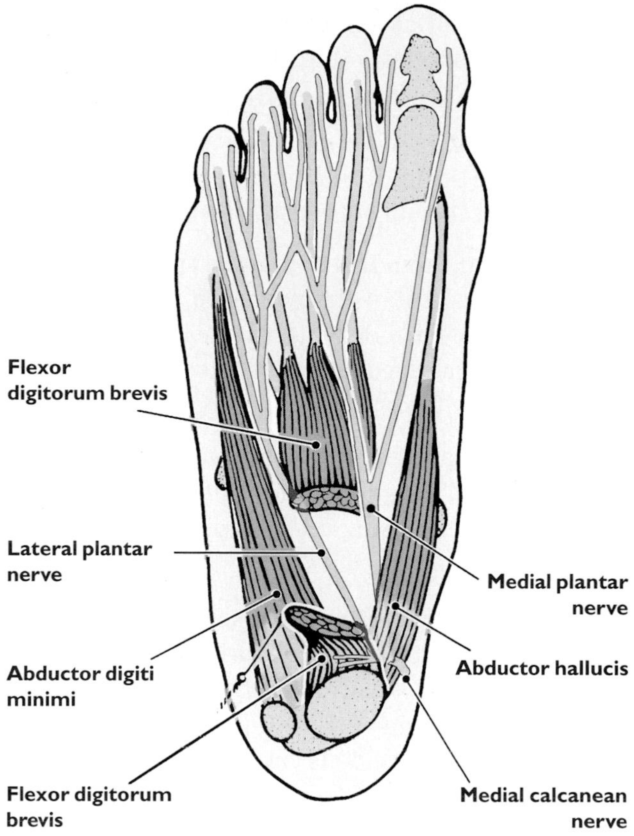

Figure 5.39. Sole of foot. First layer of muscles and plantar nerves.

- On the lateral side, expose and clean the **abductor digiti minimi**. Free the muscle and follow it to its origin and insertion. What is its function?
- In the middle between the two abductors, identify the **flexor digitorum brevis**. Trace its tendons anteriorly to digits 2, 3, 4 (and sometimes 5). In doing so, remove piecemeal the remaining and interfering distal part of the plantar aponeurosis. Subsequently, cut the flexor digitorum brevis close to the calcaneus and reflect it anteriorly.
- Establish the continuity of the posterior tibial artery and the tibial nerve with plantar structures. Follow nerve and artery into the sole by pushing a probe deep to the abductor hallucis. Carefully cut the muscle overlying the probe. Demonstrate the distribution of the **plantar nerves** and **arteries** (Fig. 5.39).

Second Layer of Plantar Muscles. Proceed as follows (Fig. 5.40):

- Reflect the flexor digitorum brevis as described previously. To make reflection easier, you may sacrifice some of the digital nerves and vessels (check with your instructor).
- Identify the **quadratus plantae** (flexor accessorius), a sheet of fleshy muscle in the posterior half of the foot. Note that the muscle arises from the calcaneus and is inserted into the tendon of the flexor digitorum longus.
- Now explore the distal portion of the **flexor digitorum longus tendon** in the sole of the foot. Note that it divides into four slips for toes 2, 3, 4, and 5.
- Four delicate **lumbricals** arise from the tendinous slips of the flexor digitorum longus. Note that these slips perforate the tendons of the flexor digitorum brevis. A similar arrangement of perforating tendons can be observed in the hand.

GRANT'S 5.78
ROHEN 440
A.D.A.M. 5.54
NETTER 498
CLEMENTE 552, 553
A.V.A. 2: 2.10.04

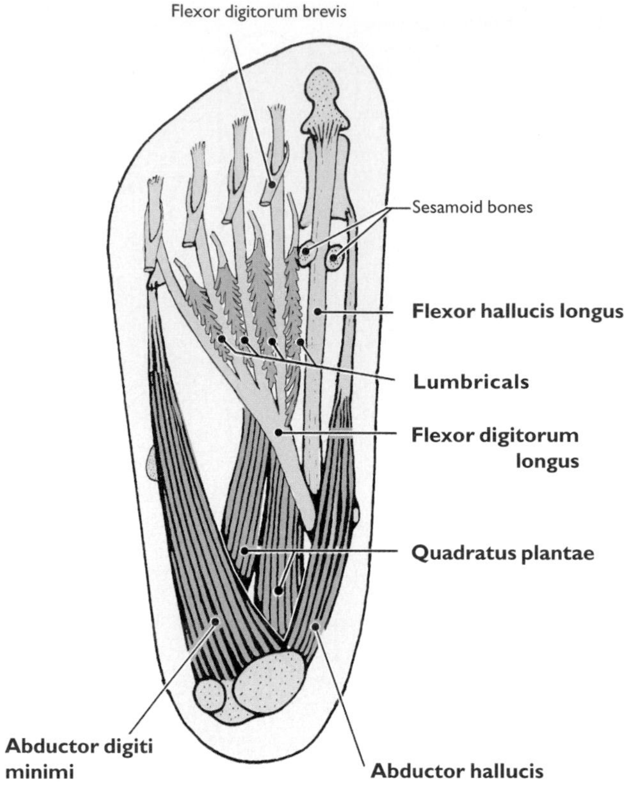

Figure 5.40. Sole of foot. Second layer of muscles displayed by removal of flexor digitorum brevis.

Third Layer of Plantar Muscles. Proceed as follows (Fig. 5.41):

- Cut through the flexor digitorum longus tendon where it is joined by the quadratus plantae. Reflect the distal part of the tendon anteriorly together with the lumbricals. Look for the small nerves supplying them.
- Now, the short muscles that occupy the anterior half of the foot are exposed. Identify the **flexor hallucis brevis**. This muscle covers the 1st metatarsal. It has two heads (medial and lateral) and two tendons. A **sesamoid bone** is attached to each of the tendons.
- Observe that the **tendon of the flexor hallucis longus** runs between the two sesamoid bones that form a guiding bony ridge for the tendon. Verify that the tendon of the flexor hallucis longus is inserted into the bases of the distal phalanx of the great toe.
- Follow the tendons of the flexor hallucis longus and flexor digitorum longus proximally toward the medial ankle. Once more, verify that the tendons cross each other.
- Identify the **adductor hallucis** for the big (1st) toe. It consists of a transverse head and an

GRANT'S 5.80
ROHEN 441
A.D.A.M. 5.54
NETTER 499
CLEMENTE 555
A.V.A. 2: 2.11.45

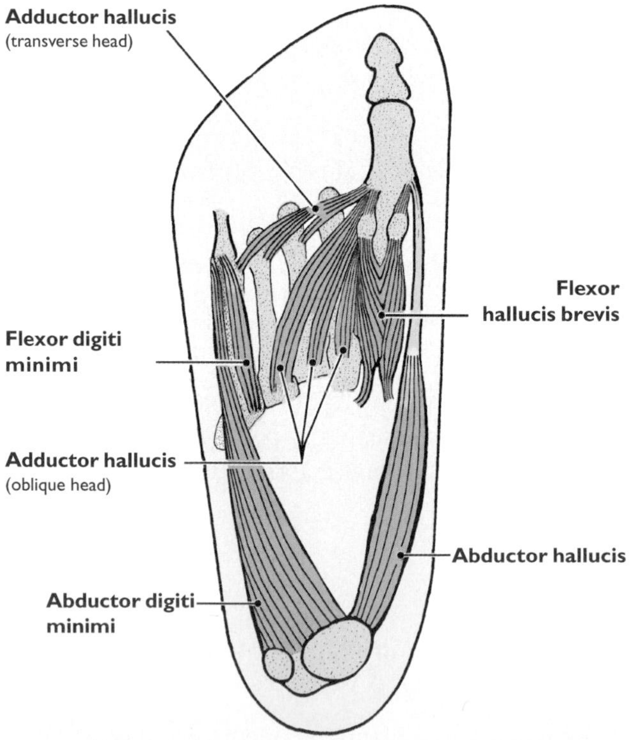

Figure 5.41. Sole of foot. Third layer of muscles displayed by reflection of flexor digitorum longus, quadratus plantae, and lumbricals.

oblique head. This muscle helps to maintain the transverse arch of the foot.

- Observe the **flexor digiti minimi** to the 5th digit.

GRANT'S 5.81
ROHEN 441
NETTER 500, 501
CLEMENTE 557, 558
A.V.A. 2: 2.09.00

Fourth Layer of Plantar Muscles. This layer consists of a compact muscular mass, the **interossei**. The four dorsal interossei are abductors, the three plantar interossei are adductors of the toes. The reference axis for abduction and adduction passes through the 2nd toe. The arrangement and action of the interossei is similar to that in the hand. Adduction and abduction of digits is more important in the hand than in the foot. Therefore, the interossei are more thoroughly discussed in the section for the hand.

- At this point, trace the **fibularis (peroneus) longus tendon** distally toward its insertion into the base of the 1st metatarsal and the medial cuneiform bone.

- Similarly, follow the tibialis posterior tendon distally and verify its multiple insertions into the navicular, cuneiforms, cuboid, and the bases of the 2nd, 3rd, and 4th metatarsals.

GRANT'S 5.76A
ROHEN 474
A.D.A.M. 5.14, 5.54
NETTER 500
CLEMENTE 554, 556

Identify the **plantar arterial arch**. Understand the essentials of the blood supply to the foot. Identify one or two of the **perforating branches** that connect the plantar arch with the dorsalis pedis artery. Find these branches in the intervals between the metatarsal bones.

GRANT'S 5.74, 5.96A
A.D.A.M. 5.56
NETTER 491
CLEMENTE 604, 606

Review the **medial side of the ankle** and its related tendons. Posterior to the medial malleolus, note the tibialis posterior, flexor digitorum longus, and flexor hallucis longus. Anterior to the medial malleolus observe the tibialis anterior. Finally, review the **lateral side of the ankle**. Posterior to the lateral malleolus, identify the fibularis (peroneus) brevis and fibularis (peroneus) longus.

Joints of the Lower Limb

General Remarks

It is advantageous to dissect the joints only in one lower limb. Keep the soft structures of the other limb intact for review purposes.

Refer to the articulated bones of the lower limb. Identify the following important joints that should be dissected:

1. **Hip joint**;
2. **Knee joint**;
3. **Ankle joint**;
4. **Joints of inversion and eversion**.

If time permits, you may dissect additional joints of the lower limb. Refer to Appendix II for a detailed text on the following joints:

- Tibiofibular joints;
- Various joints between the tarsal bones;
- Joints of the digits.

Hip Joint

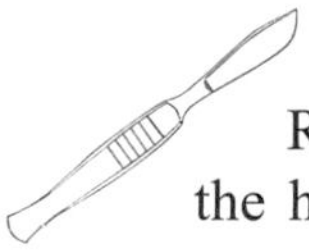

Review the essential bony features of the hip joint and its vicinity.

Anterior Relations of the Hip Joint. The **sartorius** projects across the neck of the femur. The **femoral artery** and the inguinal ligament project in relation to the head of the femur or the acetabulum.

Cut and reflect the sartorius, rectus femoris, pectineus, and the femoral nerve and vessels. Identify the **iliopsoas muscle**. Trace its tendon to the lesser trochanter, and sever it close to this bony landmark. Reflect it superiorly.

Study the anterior portion of the hip joint (Fig. 5.42):

- Moisten the strong and dense fibrous capsule of the hip joint to make it more pliable.

GRANT'S 5.33A
ROHEN 420
A.D.A.M. 5.41
NETTER 454
CLEMENTE 563
A.V.A. 2: 2.07.50

- Identify the ligaments that contribute to the formation of the **fibrous joint capsule**: the **iliofemoral ligament** and the **ischiofemoral ligament**.

- Examine the exceedingly strong **iliofemoral ligament.** Verify that the base of this triangular ligament is attached to the intertrochanteric line of the neck of the femur; its apex is attached to the anterior inferior iliac spine.

- Produce various motions of the femur and determine what movements render the exposed iliofemoral ligament taut and what movements make it flaccid. Extend the hip joint and observe that the iliofemoral ligament becomes taut. Thus, this ligament prevents overextension of the hip joint.

Open the **joint capsule** anteriorly by making a vertical incision along a line indicated by the former position of the psoas tendon (Fig. 5.42):

- Inside the capsule, observe the extensive **articular area of the head of the femur**.
- Abduct the femur so that the ischiofemoral ligament becomes relaxed. Define the **ligament of the head of the femur** by pushing a probe between it and the articular surface of the head.
- Rotate the limb laterally; note that you can see more of the articular surface.
- Rotate the limb medially; observe that the articular surface disappears in the acetabulum.
- At this stage, observe once more the **obturator externus**. Note the obturator nerve as it passes through its opening at the superior margin of the obturator membrane. Verify that the nerve is accompanied by the obturator vessels.

Posterior Relations of the Hip Joint: Turn the cadaver into the prone position (face down). Review the essential features of the gluteal region. Cut and remove all muscles that hold the femur close to the hip bone: piriformis, obturator internus with gemelli, quadratus femoris, gluteus medius and minimus, and obturator externus. Cut and reflect the obturator internus tendon to expose the posterior aspect of the hip joint fully.

Clean the posterior aspect of the **fibrous joint capsule** (Fig. 5.43):

- Identify the **ischiofemoral ligament** as it runs from acetabular rim to the neck of the femur.
- Note the **iliofemoral ligament**.

⇦ CLEMENTE 567
A.V.A. 2: 0.04.50

⇦ *GRANT'S 5.33A*
A.D.A.M. TABLE 5.3
NETTER 459
CLEMENTE 500
A.V.A. 2: 0.12.43

⇦ *GRANT'S 5.33B*
ROHEN 420
A.D.A.M. 5.41
NETTER 454
CLEMENTE 564
A.V.A. 2: 0.08.00

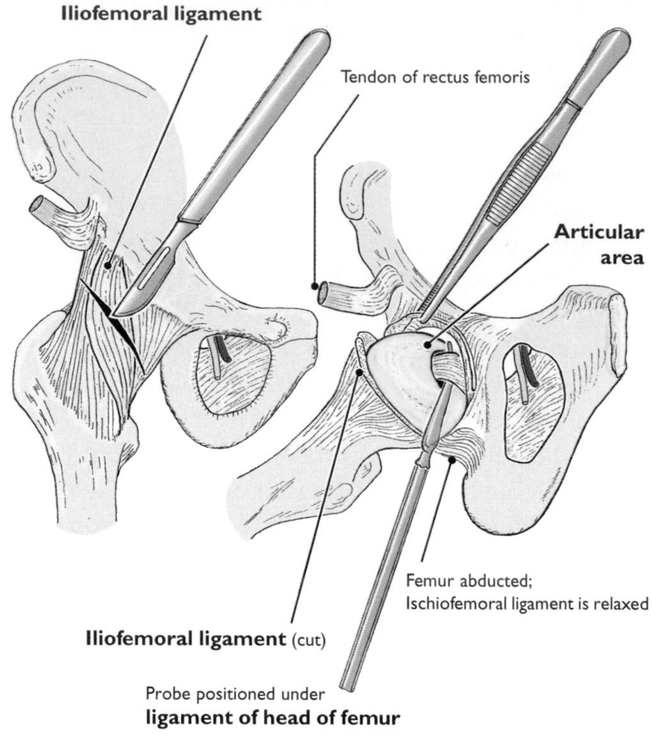

Figure 5.42. Anterior portion of hip joint.

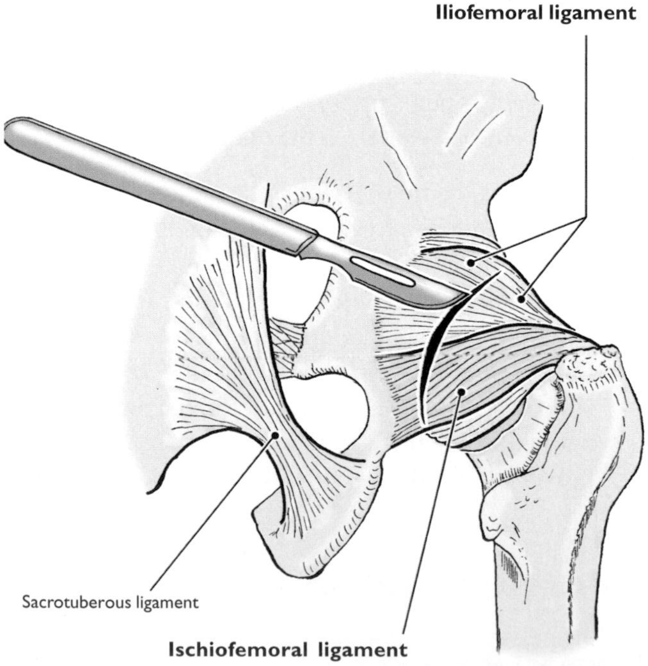

Figure 5.43. Posterior portion of hip joint.

- Relax the capsule by rotating the lower limb in the appropriate direction.
- Extend the hip joint and medially rotate the femur. Observe that the ischiofemoral ligament becomes taut, thus resisting hyperextension of the hip joint.
- Open the joint cavity by incising the capsule vertically (Fig. 5.43).
- Insert a probe, and explore the limits of the synovial cavity. Appreciate the thickness of the joint capsule.

The next objective is to dislocate the hip joint, i.e., to remove the head of the femur from its socket. Proceed as follows:

- Have the specimen in the prone position.
- Position the pelvis at the end of the table. Let the lower limb hang over the end of the table.
- Let your partner hold the pelvis steady.
- Simultaneously, flex the hip joint and forcibly rotate the femur medially. Persist in this maneuver until the **ligament of the head of the femur** ruptures. Subsequently, the head of the femur will pass out of the acetabulum onto the dorsum of the ilium.

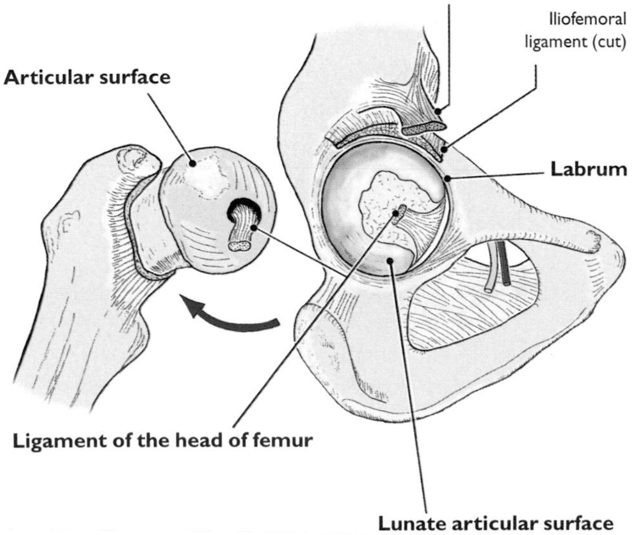

Figure 5.44. Head of femur removed from acetabular fossa.

GRANT'S 5.35, 5.37
ROHEN 421
NETTER 454, 470
CLEMENTE 565, 567
A.V.A. 2: 0.04.50

Examine the head and neck of the femur (Fig. 5.44):

- Observe the **articular surface** and the reflections of the synovial membrane.
- Note the pit for the **ligament of the head of the femur** or the stump of the torn ligament.

Socket for Head of Femur (or Acetabulum or acetabular fossa):

GRANT'S 5.36A
ROHEN 421
A.D.A.M. 4.4
NETTER 454, 470
CLEMENTE 568
A.V.A. 2: 0.07.07

- Identify the smooth **lunate articular surface** (Fig. 5.44).
- Note the torn **ligament of the head of the femur** (ligamentum teres).
- Observe that the **acetabular fossa** contains a fat pad that is lined with synovial membrane. With a probe, break through the synovial membrane and examine the underlying fat pad.

GRANT'S 5.34B

- Expose the blood vessels of the acetabular fossa; these are the acetabular branches of the obturator vessels. Note that a branch runs with the ligament of the head of the femur. This small branch contributes to the blood supply of the head of the femur.
- Reflect the ischiofemoral ligament from the femur.
- Attempt to find a small branch of the medial femoral circumflex artery.

GRANT'S 5.35

- Search for fine arterial twigs as they pass through tiny nutrient foramina to supply the neck and the head of the femur.
- In a similar fashion, a small branch of the lateral circumflex femoral artery supplies the more anterior portions of the head and neck of the femur. Study the clinically important blood supply to the head of the femur.

Clinical Correlation: A fracture of the femoral neck, particularly if it is close to the head, can disrupt the vital blood supply to the head. If the blood supply via the ligament of the head is minimal or also interrupted (as in a ruptured ligament), the head will become necrotic. Such necrosis is a common complication in femoral neck fractures of the elderly. The condition can be assessed radiologically. An injured or diseased hip joint may be surgically replaced by a hip prosthesis.

Study a radiograph of the hip and correlate it with a coronal section through the hip joint. In addition, study a transverse section of the hip joint.

Knee Joint

Review the bony landmarks related to the knee joint.

Medial Aspect of Knee Joint:

GRANT'S 5.46A
A.D.A.M. 5.48
NETTER 472
A.V.A. 2: 0.52.58

- Detach the tendons of the sartorius, gracilis, and semitendinosus from their insertions.
- Reflect the muscles and tendons. Remove the deep fascia.
- Deep to the tendons of the three muscles, identify the **tibial collateral ligament** of the knee.
- With a probe, explore the relations between the tibial collateral ligament and the **medial meniscus**. Verify that the deeper portion of the tibial collateral ligament is firmly attached to the medial meniscus.

Lateral Aspect of Knee Joint:

GRANT'S 5.47A
ROHEN 525
A.D.A.M. 5.48
NETTER 472
CLEMENTE 527
A.V.A. 2: 0.53.29

- Identify the **iliotibial tract**. It is about 2 to 3 cm wide. The tract is inserted into the anterior portion of the lateral tibial condyle.
- Cut the biceps tendon close to its insertion into the head of the fibula.
- Define the **fibular collateral ligament** of the knee. Notice that it does *not* blend with the underlying lateral meniscus. In fact, the space between fibular collateral ligament and lateral meniscus is wide enough so that the popliteus tendon can pass through it.

Anterior Aspect of Knee Joint:

GRANT'S 5.55
A.D.A.M. 5.48
NETTER 473, 476
CLEMENTE 569, 570, 574
A.V.A. 2: 0.54.49

- Identify the **expansions of the vasti muscles** and the **ligamentum patellae**.
- Palpate the patella. Verify the existence of the **prepatellar bursa** just anterior to the patella.
- Detach the quadriceps tendon from the patella. Be careful *not* to damage the underlying synovial capsule of the knee joint.
- Make a transverse cut immediately superior to the patella through the synovial capsule into the joint cavity. With a blunt instrument, carefully explore the extent of the capsule.
- Note the superior recess of the joint cavity. This sac-like recess is the **suprapatellar bursa** or **quadriceps bursa**.
- Just superior to the quadriceps bursa, make a wide horseshoe-shaped section through the quadriceps from epicondyle to epicondyle.
- Identify the quadriceps bursa. Note a layer of fat (fat pad) between bursa and femur.

Posterior Aspect of Knee Joint.

GRANT'S 5.57
A.D.A.M. 5.49
NETTER 476
CLEMENTE 575
A.V.A. 2: 0.56.28

- Remove the major vessels and nerves of the popliteal fossa.
- Cut the semimembranosus and other hamstring muscles well superior to the knee joint.
- Free the plantaris and both heads of the gastrocnemius from the joint capsule. Remove these muscles from their bony origins.
- Cut through the fleshly fibers of the popliteus and remove this muscle. During this procedure, the synovial capsule will be opened posteriorly.
- Observe that the capsule extends inferior to the lateral meniscus.
- Clear away the posterior aspect of the joint capsule. Remove any fat.
- Identify the **posterior cruciate ligament**.
- By means of transverse and vertical incisions, open the synovial cavity posterior to each femoral condyle.
- With a probe, explore the limits of the synovial cavity. Verify that the cruciate ligaments are located entirely *outside* the synovial capsule.

GRANT'S 5.49, 5.50A
ROHEN 422
NETTER 473
CLEMENTE 573-577
A.V.A. 2: 0.51.00

Interior of Knee Joint (Fig. 5.45). Turn to the anterior aspect of the knee joint and open the synovial capsule widely with a transverse incision. Carry the incision around the sides of the knee.

During development, the medial and lateral halves of the knee joint were originally two independent joint cavities separated by the membranes of the **intercondylar septum**. This septum partially breaks down anterior to the anterior cruciate ligament. Examine the anterior part of the septum, the **infrapatellar synovial fold**. Posterior to the infrapatellar fold, the septum is complete. Here, the synovial membranes are reflected across both sides of the cruciate ligaments. Therefore, the cruciate ligaments are situated outside the synovial cavity. However, they lie inside the fibrous joint capsule.

Snip through the infrapatellar fold. Verify that the femur and tibia remain attached to each other by four ligaments, the **two collateral ligaments** and the **two cruciate ligaments.** Rotate the femur medially. Note that the **fibular collateral ligament** becomes taut and stops the movement. Sever it. Note that medial rotation of the femur is now free and results in untwisting of the cruciate ligaments.

GRANT'S 5.50A, 5.52
ROHEN 422
NETTER 473, 475
CLEMENTE 576, 577
A.V.A. 2: 0.50.55

Verify that the strong cruciate ligaments cross each other (Fig. 5.45). The **anterior cruciate ligament** attaches the femur to the tibia *anteriorly*. The **posterior cruciate ligament** attaches the femur to the tibia *posteriorly*. Study the functions of the cruciate ligaments. Extend the leg (knee joint) maximally. In this position, observe:

GRANT'S 5.53, 5.54B
A.D.A.M. 5.51
NETTER 475
CLEMENTE 573
A.V.A. 2: 0.51.23

- The articular surfaces of femur and tibia are in maximal contact.
- The joint is "locked" in its most stable position.
- The anterior cruciate ligament is taut and prohibits further extension.

Flex the leg (knee joint). Observe:

- There is less contact between the articular surfaces.
- Some rotation occurs in the knee joint (at the expense of its stability).
- The posterior cruciate ligament prevents anterior displacement of the femur; i.e., it prevents the femur from sliding anteriorly off the "tibial plateau."
- With the leg (knee joint) flexed to a right angle, the tibia cannot be pulled anteriorly; it is held back by the anterior cruciate ligament.

Cut the anterior cruciate ligament (*not* the posterior one). Flex the leg to a right angle. Now, you will be able to pull the tibia anteriorly. This forward movement is an important clinical and diagnostic sign in cases of a ruptured anterior cruciate ligament.

GRANT'S 5.54
ROHEN 422
A.D.A.M. 5.50
NETTER 474
CLEMENTE 585-588
A.V.A. 2: 0.49.36

Study the menisci or semilunar cartilages (Fig. 5.45). Test the mobility of the menisci. The *C*-shaped **medial meniscus** is firmly attached to the tibia by the coronary ligament. Once again, examine its attachment to the tibial collateral ligament. The small

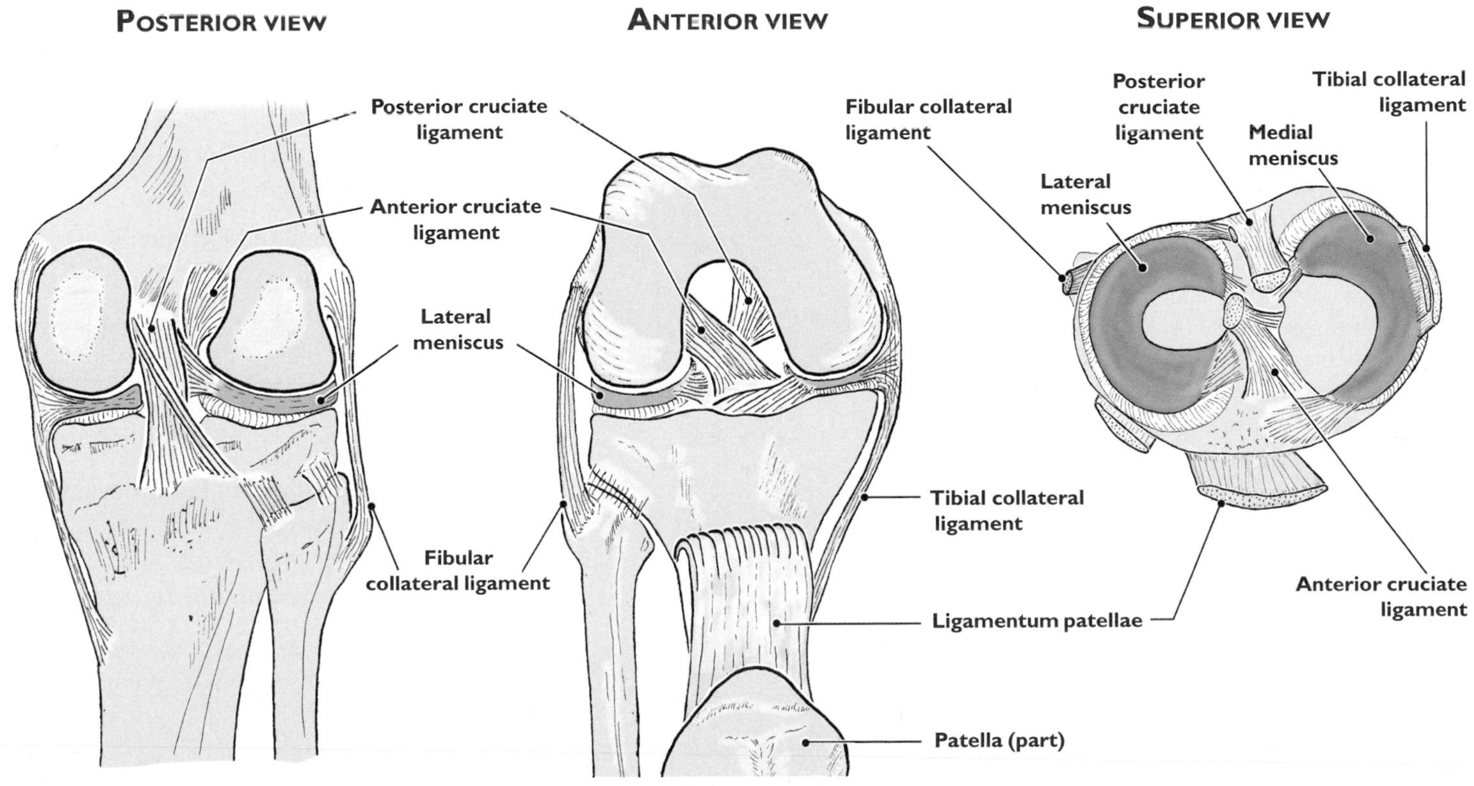

Figure 5.45. Right knee joint and associated structures.

O-shaped **lateral meniscus** is distinctly mobile. Remember, it has no attachments to the fibular collateral ligament.

Grant's 5.54
Rohen 422, 425
A.D.A.M. 5.50
Netter 474
Clemente 585-588
A.V.A. 2: 0.50.30

Clinical Correlation: The medial meniscus is injured about 6 to 7 times as often as the lateral meniscus. Why? The medial meniscus is firmly attached to the tibial collateral ligament and the underlying tibia. It is virtually immobile. During forceful abduction of the leg, the tension exerted by the tibial collateral ligament can result in tearing of the medial meniscus. In contrast, the slightly mobile lateral meniscus is *not* attached to the fibular collateral ligament and, therefore, less likely to be torn.

Forced abduction and lateral rotation of the leg may result in the simultaneous rupture or damage of three structures: (a) tibial collateral ligament; (b) anterior cruciate ligament; and (c) medial meniscus. This injury is typical for football players. It has been named the "unhappy triad."

When the anterior cruciate ligament is torn, the knee joint becomes very unstable. To test the stability of the knee, the examining physician will pull the tibia anteriorly. If such anterior displacement is present (so-called "anterior drawer sign"), a torn anterior cruciate ligament is diagnosed.

In patients, the cavity of the knee joint can be examined by inserting a fiberoptic arthroscope. Radiologists frequently perform arthrography, using injected contrast material and air to outline various soft structures of the knee joint. Usually, the interval between fibular collateral ligament and lateral meniscus can be well demonstrated, with the popliteus tendon intervening.

Grant's 5.45
Netter 477
Clemente 479, 480, 517, 519
A.V.A. 2: 1.10.10

Once more, review the extensive collateral blood supply around the knee joint. There are four named genicular branches (two superior branches and two inferior branches). In addition, there may be unnamed genicular branches that participate in the formation of the collateral vascular network around the knee. The vessels are closely applied to the skeletal plane. Note tiny nutrient foramina in the femur and in the tibia.

Grant's 5.48, 5.51B, 5.58, 5.59
Rohen 423
A.D.A.M. 5.52
Clemente 519, 571

Study radiographs of the knee region. In addition, correlate your anatomical observations with a sagittal and coronal MRI.

Ankle Joint

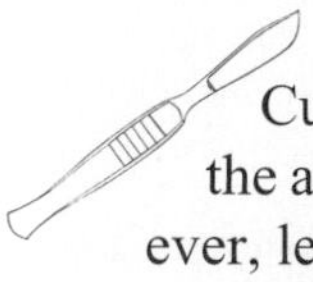

Cut and reflect the structures crossing the anterior aspect of the ankle joint. However, leave the tibialis anterior tendon intact.

Medial Side of Ankle Joint:

Grant's 5.86-588
Rohen 425, 426
A.D.A.M. 5.56
Netter 490, 491
Clemente 602, 606
A.V.A. 2: 1.23.26

- To display the medial aspect of the ankle joint, cut and reflect the flexor digitorum longus.
- Displace anteriorly (but do *not* cut) the tibialis posterior tendon.
- Now, clean and define the **medial or deltoid ligament**. It is a triangular ligament that attaches the medial malleolus to the tarsus.
- Note that the superficial fibers of this ligament are inserted into the whole length of the sustentaculum tali.
- The most anterior fibers radiate toward the navicular bone.
- The deep portion of the ligament anchors the medial malleolus to the talus. This fact is best appreciated on coronal (vertical) section.

Grant's 5.86, 5.87, 5.96
Rohen 426
A.D.A.M. 5.56
Netter 490, 491
Clemente 602, 604
A.V.A. 2: 1.39.50

Lateral Side of Ankle Joint:

- Identify the tendons of the fibularis (peroneus) longus and fibularis (peroneus) brevis. These tendons must be mobilized. Make sure that the superior and inferior fibular (peroneal) retinacula are slit open. Displace anteriorly (but do *not* cut) the fibularis longus and fibularis brevis tendons.
- Clean and define the ligaments that hold the lateral malleolus of the fibula to the tarsus: the **calcaneofibular ligament** and the **anterior talofibular ligament**.
- At this time, also identify the strong **anterior inferior tibiofibular ligament**, one of the structures that hold the tibia and fibular together.
- The **posterior talofibular ligament** can be best appreciated on coronal section.
- Correlate your anatomical observations with radiographs of the ankle joint.

Grant's 5.85, 592
Rohen 424
A.D.A.M. 5.58
Clemente 599

Plantarflex the foot and examine the joint capsule:

- Incise transversely the **articular capsule of the ankle joint**.
- Push the handle of the knife between body of talus and tibia.
- To display the **articular surfaces,** sever three ligaments that connect the fibula to the talus and calcaneus: calcaneofibular ligament, anterior talofibular ligament, and posterior talofibular ligament.
- Dislocate the foot by swinging it medially. The **deltoid ligament** or medial ligament of the ankle, which remains intact, acts as a hinge.
- Study the articular surfaces.

> ***Clinical Correlation:*** **Ankle injuries** are very common. Most often, the tripartite **lateral ligament** (calcaneofibular ligament; anterior and posterior talofibular ligaments) is involved by either being stretched or torn when the foot is forcefully inverted. The result is an **ankle sprain** with painful swelling of the lateral malleolus. In severe cases, the calcaneofibular and talofibular ligaments are torn, the lateral malleolus may be fractured, or its inferior tip may be avulsed. Such **fracture-dislocation** leads to a very unstable ankle joint. If the inversion of the foot is particularly violent, the tendon of the peroneus brevis muscle can be torn off the tuberosity of the 5th metatarsal bone, or the tuberosity itself may be avulsed. Radiologists routinely look for the tuberosity of the 5th metatarsal bone in cases of ankle injuries. Inversion injuries are more common than eversion injuries.

Joints of Inversion and Eversion

Study the movements of inversion and eversion of the foot in suitable bony specimens (wired laboratory skeletons can be damaged). With one hand, immobilize the ankle joint, i.e., hold the talus tightly between tibia and fibula. With the other hand, invert and evert the foot. Observe:

- The talus remains fixed in the ankle joint.
- The entire foot rotates about the inferior and anterior surfaces of the talus.
- This movement is augmented at the joint between calcaneus and cuboid.

Turn to the cadaver specimen. **Produce eversion** by pulling on the tendons of the peroneus longus and peroneus brevis. Follow the tendons to their insertions. **Produce inversion** by pulling on the tendons of the tibialis anterior and tibialis posterior. Follow the tendons clearly to their insertions.

GRANT'S 5.96
ROHEN 425
NETTER 490
CLEMENTE 607-609
A.V.A. 2: 1.29.38

Study the complex articular interactions between the talus on the one hand, and the calcaneus and navicular on the other. The objective is to disarticulate the talus from the rest of the tarsus. Proceed as follows:

- If not already done during dissection of the ankle, sever the ligaments that hold the lateral malleolus to the tarsus.
- Cut the interosseous talocalcaneal ligament. Cut the posterior part of the subtalar joint capsule.
- Force the handle of the knife between the talus and calcaneus.
- Swing the calcaneus and the foot medially. The deltoid ligament, which remains intact, acts as a hinge.

GRANT'S 5.93, 5.94
ROHEN 427
A.D.A.M. 5.56
NETTER 492
CLEMENTE 610, 611
A.V.A. 2: 1.22.08

Identify the posterior talar facet of the calcaneus for the subtalar joint (Fig. 5.46). Inspect the socket for the head of the talus. The articular components of this socket are formed by the **middle talar facet, anterior talar facet,** and **posterior articular surface of the navicular bone.** The floor of the socket is formed by the important **spring ligament**. Force a probe or needle through the floor of the socket. Next, approach the probe and ligament from the sole of the foot. Identify the **spring ligament or plantar calcaneonavicular ligament** (Fig. 5.47). This ligament and the tibialis posterior tendon are necessary for the support of the head of the talus. The socket for the head of the talus is of great importance to the integrity of the foot. The socket supports the "keystone" of the high medial arch.

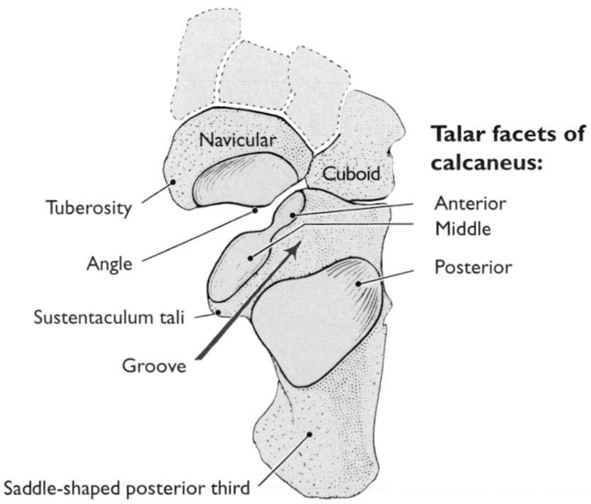

Figure 5.46. Bones of the foot on dorsal view. The talus has been removed to show where inversion and eversion take place.

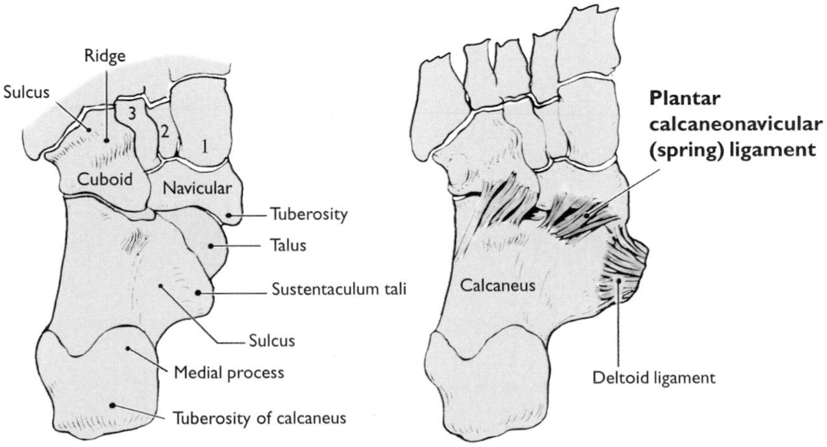

Figure 5.47. Bones of the foot on plantar view. Plantar ligaments of joints of inversion and eversion.

TEST 10

GAPP

GROSS ANATOMY PRACTICAL PRIMER

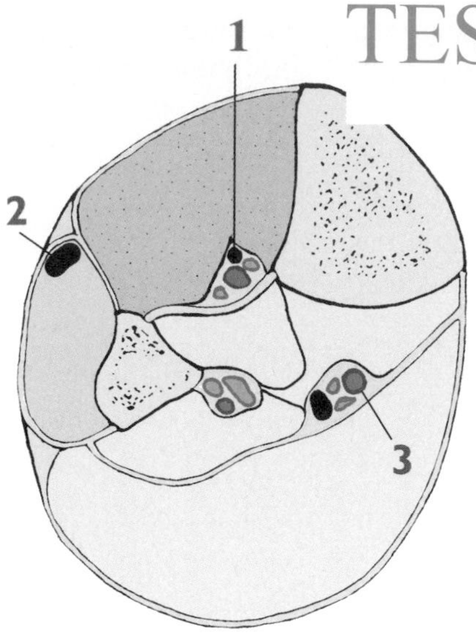

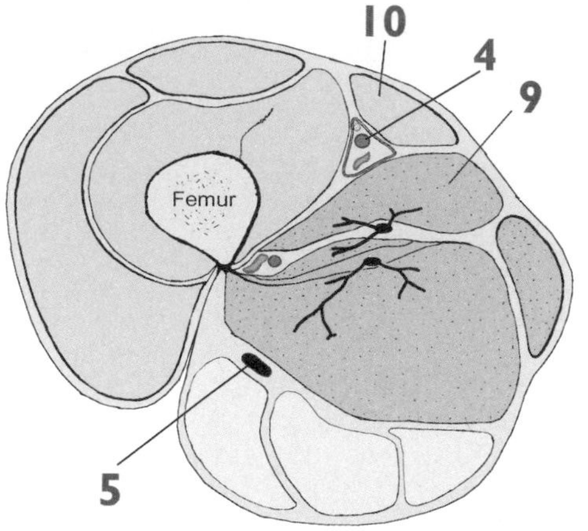

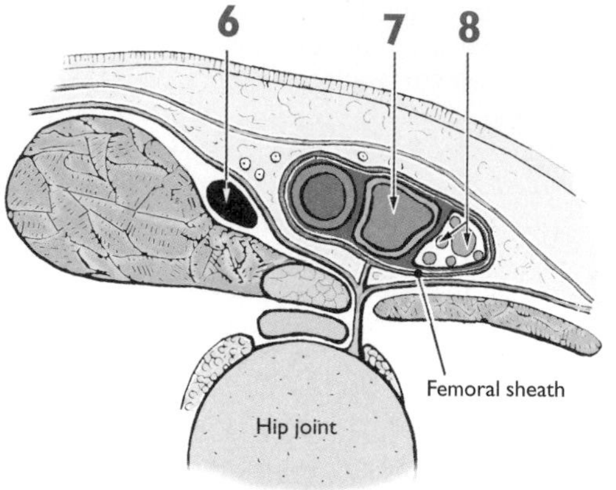

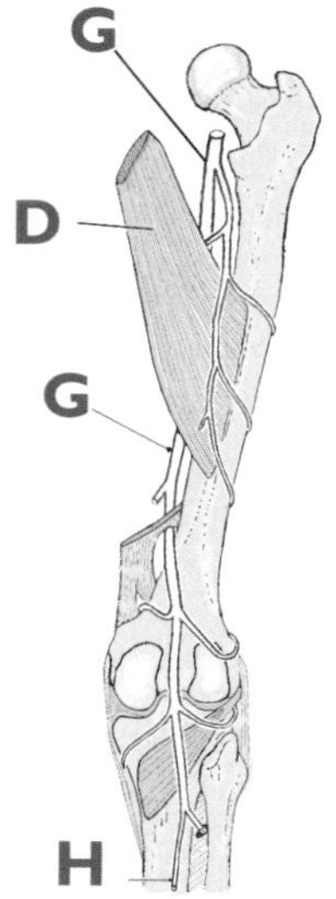

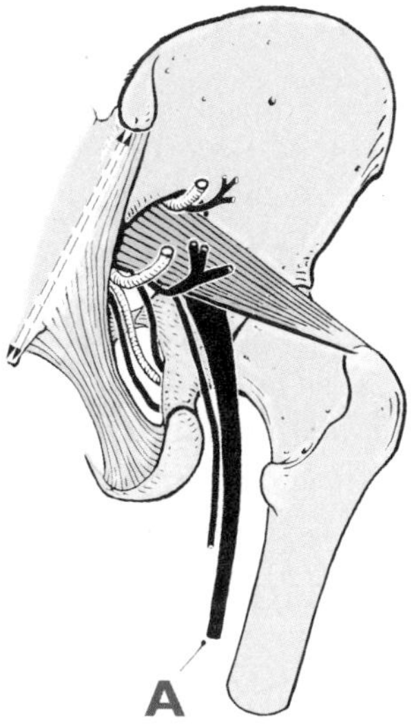

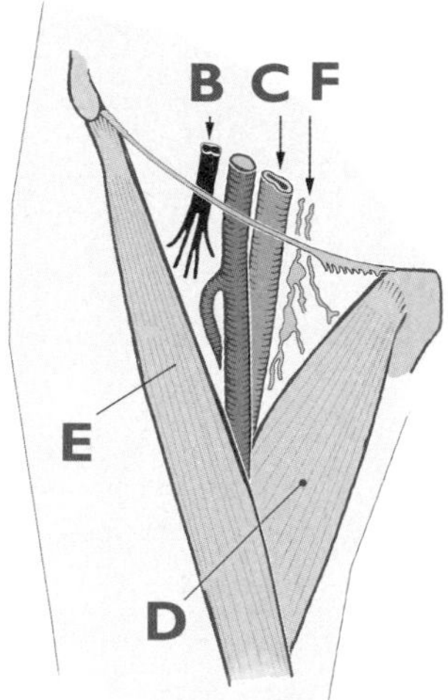

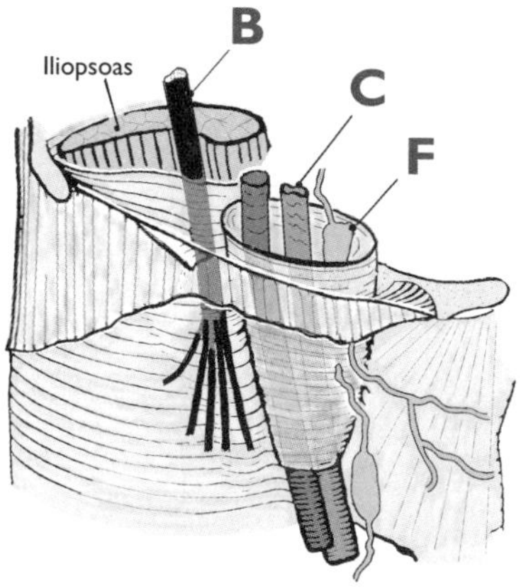

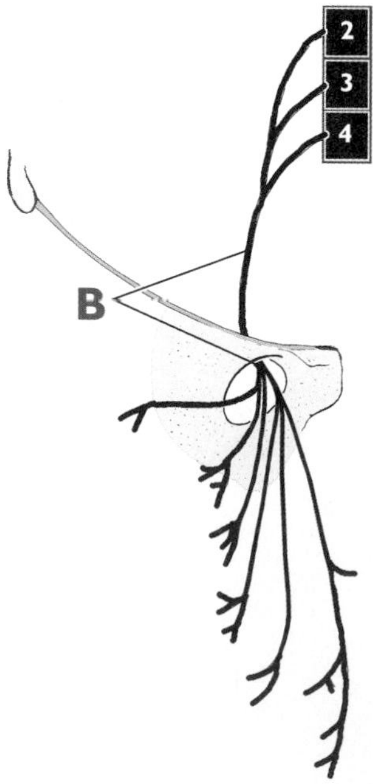

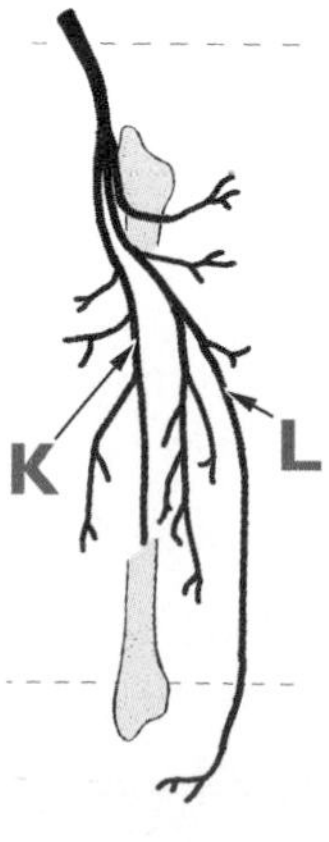

TEST YOUR 3-DIMENSIONAL CONCEPTUALIZATION.
MATCH THE NUMBERS WITH CORRESPONDING LETTERS:

1 ___	6 ___
2 ___	7 ___
3 ___	8 ___
4 ___	9 ___
5 ___	10 ___

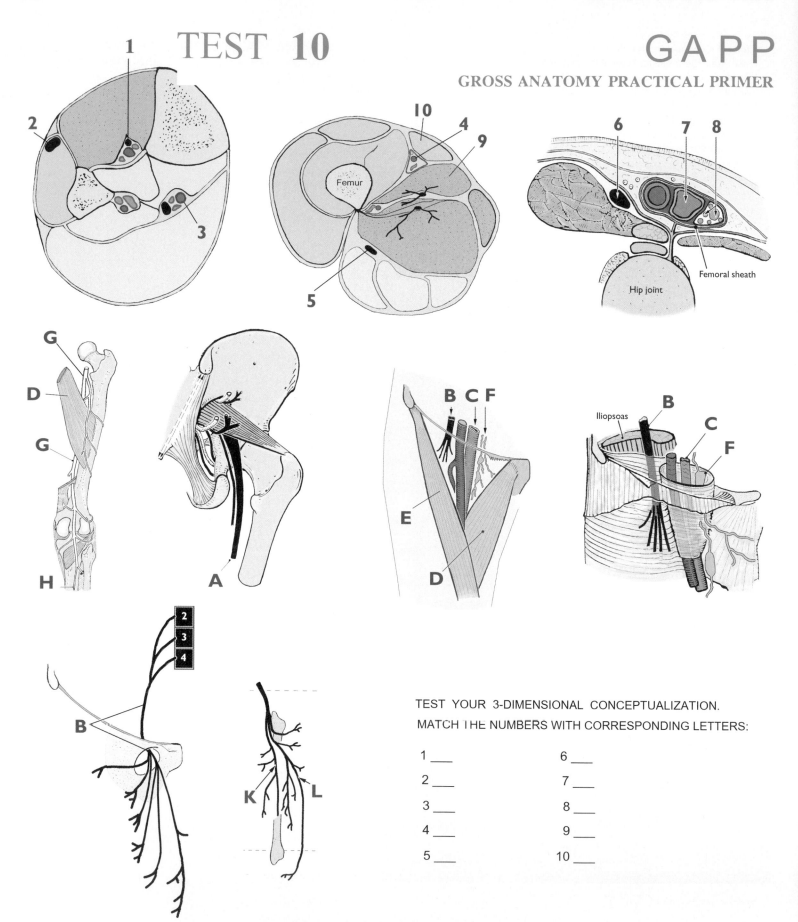

GAPP TEST: IF YOU MADE AN ERROR, REVIEW AND GAIN A BETTER UNDERSTANDING OF THE CONCERNED 3-DIMENSIONAL ANATOMICAL CONCEPT. GAPP KEY: 1-L, 2-K, 3-H, 4-G, 5-A, 6-B, 7-C, 8-F, 9-D, 10-E

Chapter 6 The Upper Limb

Grant's Atlas of Anatomy, 10th Ed.:	*Grant's* *Fig.* #
Rohen, Color Atlas of Anatomy, 4th Ed.:	Rohen Page #
A.D.A.M. Student Atlas of Anatomy:	A.D.A.M. Plate #
Netter, Atlas of Human Anatomy, 2nd Ed.:	Netter Plate #
Clemente, Anatomy, 4th Ed.:	Clemente Fig. #
Acland's Video Atlas of Human Anatomy	**A.V.A. Vol: hr.min.sec**

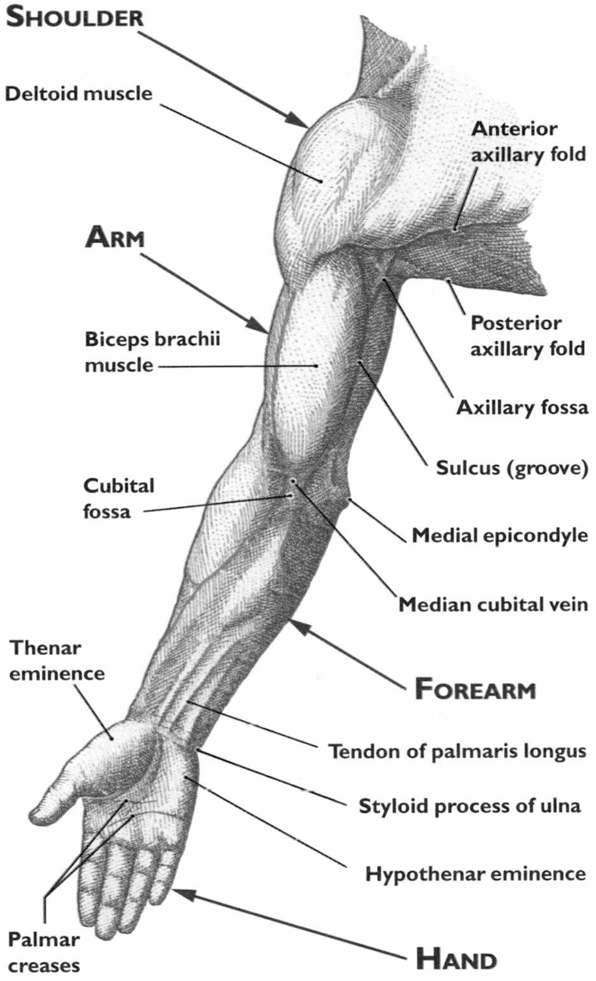

Figure 6.1. Surface anatomy of the right upper limb.

Introductory Remarks

The essential functional requirement of the upper limb is manual activity. Anatomically, the upper limb is divided into four segments (Fig. 6.1):

Grant's 6.9, 6.29A
A.D.A.M. 6.1, 6.2
Clemente 40, 623

- **Shoulder,** the junction of arm and trunk;
- **Arm** (brachium), the segment between shoulder and forearm;
- **Forearm** (antebrachium), the segment between arm and hand;
- **Hand** (manus).

Dissection Sequence. It is advantageous to dissect the upper limb in the following sequence: First, the superficial veins and nerves and the deep investing fascia of the entire upper limb will be explored. Next, the muscles acting on the shoulder joint will be studied. If ***The Thorax*** (Chapter 1) has been covered previously, the muscles of the pectoral region have already been identified during dissection of the anterior chest wall. If ***The Back*** (Chapter 4) has already been explored, the superficial group of back muscles connecting the upper limb to the vertebral column has already been studied. If you are assigned ***The Upper Limb*** before dissection of ***The Thorax*** and ***The Back***, the previously mentioned muscles of the shoulder region must as yet be dissected. Subsequently, the axilla and its contents as well as the brachial and anterior cubital regions will be explored. The flexor compartment of the forearm will be dissected and its contents will be followed into the palm of the hand. Finally, the extensor region of the forearm will be studied together with the dorsum of the hand.

Grant's 6.9, 6.29A
A.D.A.M. 6.1, 6.2
Clemente 40, 623

Surface Anatomy

The surface anatomy of the upper limb can be studied in a living subject or in the cadaver. In the supine position (face up), identify the following structures (Fig. 6.1):

- The **axillary fossa** (arm pit) between the **anterior axillary fold** and the **posterior axillary fold**;
- The rounded **shoulder region** with the **deltoid muscle**;
- In the **arm region**, a sulcus or groove on each side of the **biceps brachii muscle**;
- The **cubital fossa** with its prominent **veins**;

- The **forearm region** with its flexor muscles and the **tendon of the palmaris longus muscle**;
- On the **wrist region**, the **styloid processes** of the **radius** and the **ulna**;
- In the **hand**, the **palmar creases**, the **thenar eminence,** and the **hypothenar eminence**.

> ***Note:*** This manual is intended to guide you with the **dissection** of the human body. It is **not** the purpose of *Grant's Dissector* to provide you with a list of all muscles, their origins, insertions, and functions. However, you may find it advantageous to prepare or to copy such a list and to bring it to the laboratory for systematic review of all muscles of the upper limb you are held responsible for in your laboratory course.

Superficial Structures

Removal of Skin

Before You Begin ...

Do *not* dissect at this time. Note that **superficial veins** and **cutaneous nerves** are contained in the **superficial fascia.** The first objective is to study these structures (superficial fascia; superficial veins; cutaneous nerves) of the entire upper limb as a whole. To accomplish this, the entire upper extremity will be skinned in an initial dissecting effort. The subcutaneous connective tissue and fat will be removed, leaving the more important superficial veins and nerves intact. Subsequently, the **deep fascia** will be demonstrated. The deep or investing fascia surrounds the various muscle compartments.

Skin Incisions. Refer to Figure 6.2. If *The Thorax* has been dissected previously, all skin incisions and skin reflections, as outlined in Figure 6.2A, have already been made; if not, make the following skin incisions with the cadaver in the supine position:

- From the jugular notch *A* along the clavicle and across the acromion *B* to point *E*, about 10 cm distal to the acromion;
- From *A* to the xiphisternal junction *C*;
- From *C* superiorly and along the anterior axillary fold to point *E*; avoid the nipple;
- From *C* laterally until stopped by the table *D*.
- Refer to Figure 6.2C; at the root of the arm, make a complete circular incision from *E* to *E*;
- At the level of the wrist, make another circular incision from *G* to *G*;

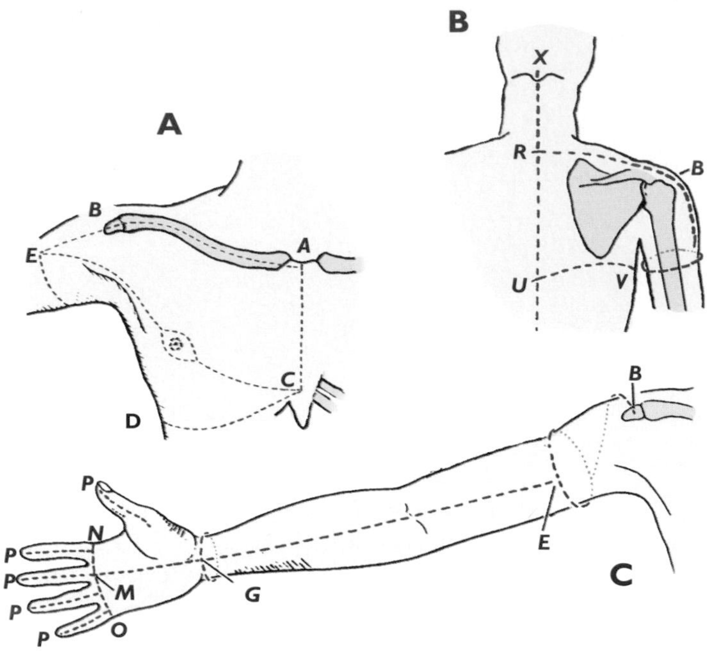

Figure 6.2. Skin incisions.

Grant's 6.4, 6.7
A.D.A.M. 6.15-6.20
Netter 448, 449
Clemente 44, 45, 58, 59, 76

- Join the two circular incisions with a longitudinal one on the anterior aspect of the upper limb from *E* to *G*; make additional transverse incisions as necessary to speed up the skinning process; reflect the skin of the arm and forearm medially and laterally; then, remove it completely; do not damage the superficial veins and cutaneous nerves in the superficial fascia;
- If the hand is tightly clenched, force it open and let your partner hold it open; make incisions in the middle of the palm from *G* to *M*, across the palm from *N* to *O*, and along the middle of all fingers to points *P*; remove the skin from the palmar and dorsal parts of the hand and finger; in peeling off the skin flaps from the fingers, proceed with intelligence and caution; note the thinness of the subcutaneous fat at the creases of the fingers; realize that there are digital nerves, vessels, and fibrous sheaths; these structures must not be destroyed.

If *The Back* has been dissected previously, all skin incisions and skin reflections as outlined in Figure 6.2B have already been made; if not, make the following skin incisions with the cadaver in prone position:

- In the midline, make a vertical skin incision from the external occipital protuberance *X* via *R* to a point at the approximate level of the inferior angle of the scapula *U*;

- Carry out a transverse incision from *U* to *V* at the level of the inferior scapular angle;
- Make a transverse incision from *R* to *B* (superior to the scapula and to the tip of the acromion) and on to the circular incision at the root of the arm; reflect the skin laterally and remove it; check with your instructor.

Superficial Fascia, Veins, and Nerves

In the living, the superficial veins are conspicuous through the skin. They are most frequently used for drawing blood and injecting medications. In the cadaver, the superficial veins are empty and are not conspicuous through the skin. However, they can be easily demonstrated in the superficial fascia. The brachial plexus supplies the upper limb with many cutaneous nerves. At various levels, these cutaneous nerves pierce the deep fascia and reach the superficial fascia and skin.

The next objective is to remove the **superficial fascia** while leaving intact the deep fascia and the principal superficial veins and nerves. With the cadaver in the prone position, examine the structures contained in the superficial fascia of the **posterior aspect of the upper limb** (Fig. 6.3).

On the dorsum of the hand, demonstrate a few tributaries to the **dorsal venous arch**. Note **superficial dorsal veins.**

GRANT'S 6.5
A.D.A.M. 6.15, 6.16
NETTER 449
CLEMENTE 76
A.V.A. 1: 1.55.21

The superficial veins of the hand drain into the **basilic vein** and the **cephalic vein.** These two structures will be followed proximally during dissection of the anterior aspect of the upper limb. The veins of the dorsum of the hand are often used for venipuncture and intravenous injection of fluids.

Investigate the structures contained in the superficial fascia of the **posterior aspect of the upper limb.** Familiarize yourself with the expected course of the **superficial nerves** and the cutaneous areas they innervate: cutaneous branch of the axillary nerve; intercostobrachial nerve; posterior brachial cutaneous nerve; posterior antebrachial cutaneous nerve; medial antebrachial cutaneous nerve; lateral antebrachial cutaneous nerve. Pay special attention to the cutaneous nerve branches that supply the dorsum of the hand.

GRANT'S 6.10
ROHEN 378
A.D.A.M. 6.19, 6.20
NETTER 449
CLEMENTE 59, 76
A.V.A. 1: 2.01.04

GRANT'S 6.4
ROHEN 376
A.D.A.M. 6.16
NETTER 448, 449
CLEMENTE 44, 58
A.V.A. 1: 1.55.52

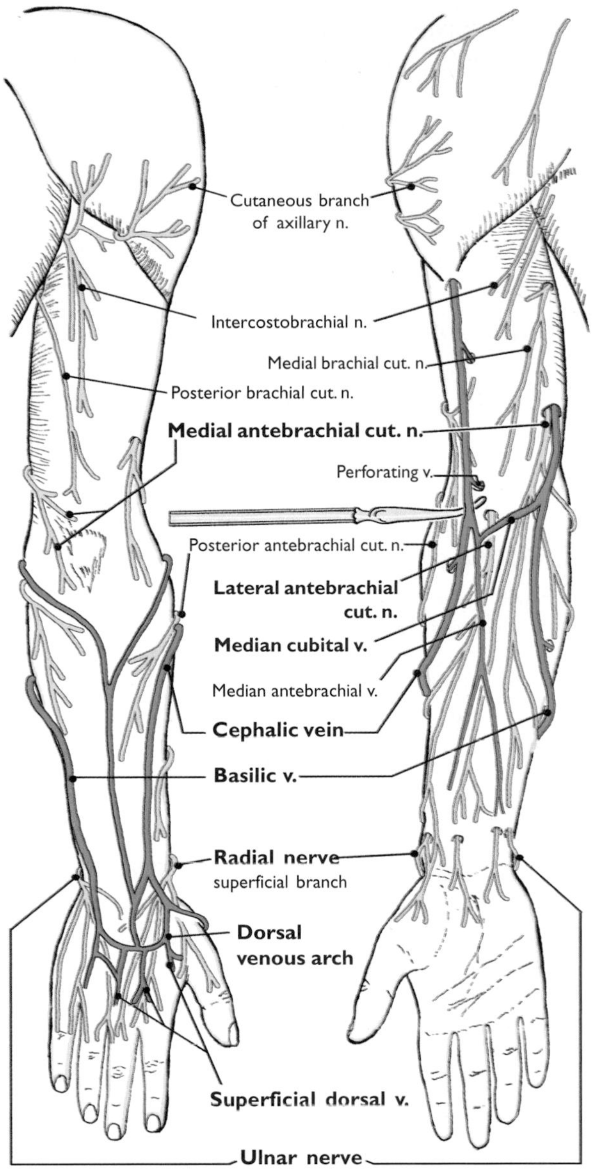

Figure 6.3. Superficial nerves and veins. With a probe, lift up superficial veins and note perforating veins.

Identify and trace to some extent the following two nerves:

- At the radial aspect of the wrist, use a probe and pick up the **superficial branch of the radial nerve;**
- At the ulnar aspect of the wrist, identify the **dorsal branch of the ulnar nerve.**

Next, turn the cadaver over into the supine position, and examine the structures contained in the **superficial fascia of the anterior aspect of the upper limb** (Fig. 6.3). Focus your attention on the **superfi-**

cial veins. On the radial side of the forearm, use a probe and pick up the **cephalic vein**. On the ulnar side of the forearm, identify the **basilic vein.** Follow these two main, superficial veins proximally. Verify the following:

- Superiorly, the **cephalic vein** passes into the interval between the deltoid and pectoralis major muscles.
- The **basilic vein** runs on the medial aspect of the forearm and arm. Before reaching the axilla superiorly, it pierces the deep fascia.
- In the cubital fossa, the cephalic vein and the basilic vein communicate by means of the **median cubital vein.** The veins in the region of the cubital fossa are prominent and easily accessible; therefore, they are commonly used for venipuncture.
- With a probe, lift up various portions of the principal superficial veins (Fig. 6.3). Note that they are connected to **perforating veins** that perforate the deep fascia and drain deeper structures.

Investigate the **superficial nerves** contained in the superficial fascia of the **anterior aspect of the upper limb** (Fig. 6.3). Familiarize yourself with the expected course of these **superficial nerves** and the cutaneous areas they innervate: intercostobrachial nerve; medial brachial cutaneous nerve; **medial antebrachial cutaneous nerve** with ulnar and anterior branches; **lateral antebrachial cutaneous nerve** with anterior and posterior branches; posterior antebrachial cutaneous nerve; and various palmar cutaneous branches. The nerves to the fingers will be explored later.

Deep Fascia

The **deep fascia of the arm** is known as the **brachial fascia.** It is connected with the humerus by two fascial intermuscular septa, thus creating an anterior and a posterior fascial compartment for the muscles of the arm (Fig. 6.4). Superiorly, the brachial fascia is continuous with the deep fascia covering the pectoralis, the deltoid, and the latissimus dorsi muscles. Inferiorly, the brachial fascia is continuous with the **deep fascia of the forearm, the antebrachial fascia.** In the cubital fossa, the antebrachial fascia is connected to the biceps brachii muscle via a strong triangular band. This is the **bicipital aponeurosis**, which protects deeper structures in the cubital fossa. At the level of the wrist, the antebrachial fascia is thickened posteriorly and anteriorly to create strong transverse bands. The posterior band, the **extensor retinaculum,** retains the extensor tendons in their position. The anterior band, the **flexor retinaculum**, forms part of a tunnel that contains the flexor tendons.

GRANT'S 6.4
ROHEN 376
A.D.A.M. 6.16
NETTER 448, 449
CLEMENTE 44, 58
A.V.A. 1: 1.55.56

GRANT'S 6.7A
ROHEN 378
A.D.A.M. 6.17
NETTER 448, 449
CLEMENTE 44, 58

GRANT'S 4.29
ROHEN 209
A.D.A.M. 1.53
NETTER 160
CLEMENTE 6.29
A.V.A. 1: 0.56.54

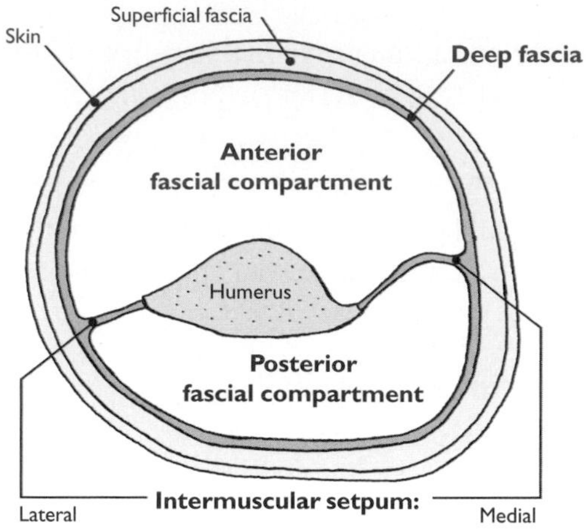

Figure 6.4. The brachial fascia and the fascial compartments of the arm.

Remove all superficial fascia, leaving intact the deep fascia, and the principal superficial nerves and veins. Examine the **deep fascia** of the upper limb. Positively palpate and identify the obliquely running **bicipital aponeurosis** in the cadaver and in your own cubital fossa (see Fig. 6.24). Obviously, the deep fascia will have to be incised and removed in order to explore the deep structures of the upper limb.

Back and Shoulder Region

General Remarks

If *The Back* (Chapter 4) has already been explored, the superficial group of back muscles connecting the upper limb to the vertebral column has already been studied. If you are assigned the upper limb before dissection of the back, the previously mentioned muscles of the shoulder region must, as yet, be dissected and studied. These muscles include the **trapezius, latissimus dorsi, the rhomboids, and the levator scapulae.** The latissimus dorsi acts directly on the arm, since it is inserted into the humerus. The trapezius, rhomboids, and levator scapulae act primarily on the scapula. Positional changes of the scapula are transferred to the humerus (since the scapula and the humerus articulate with each other. Review these previously dissected and mentioned muscles (Chapter 4).

Four muscles (supraspinatus, infraspinatus, teres major, and teres minor) arise from the dorsal surface of the scapula and insert into the upper portion of the humerus.

Bony Landmarks

Refer to a skeleton and study the following bony landmarks on the **scapula** (Fig. 6.5):

GRANT'S 6.1
ROHEN 349-351
A.D.A.M. 1.3, 1.4
NETTER 392, 393
CLEMENTE 92-95, 104
A.V.A. 1:0.03.15

- Identify the **acromion**.
- The **spine** separates the dorsal surface of the scapula into **supraspinous fossa** and **infraspinous fossa**.
- At the lateral scapular border, the two spinous fossae are connected by the spinoglenoid notch.
- Observe the **glenoid cavity** for the articulation with the head of the humerus. Above the glenoid cavity, note the **supraglenoid tubercle**; below it, observe the **infraglenoid tubercle.**
- Identify the **coracoid process.** Note the **scapular notch** incising the superior scapular border at the base of the coracoid process.

On the **humerus** identify the following features (Fig. 6.5):

- **Head**, articulating with the glenoid cavity of the scapula;
- **Greater tubercle,** located laterally;
- **Lesser tubercle,** located anteriorly;
- **Intertubercular sulcus or bicipital groove** between the two tubercles;
- **Deltoid tuberosity** for the insertion of the deltoid muscle;
- **Sulcus for radial nerve or spiral groove**.

Structures of Shoulder Region

Before You Begin ...

The deltoid muscle will be detached from its scapular origin and the course of its nerve and artery will be studied. Subsequently, the four muscles arising from the dorsal surface of the scapula (supraspinatus, infraspinatus, teres major, teres minor) will be dissected and their nerve and blood supplies will be demonstrated.

Dissection. Place the cadaver into the prone position. Dissection will be easier if the arm is abducted about 45° and the shoulder is allowed to fall forward. Use a wooden block if necessary.

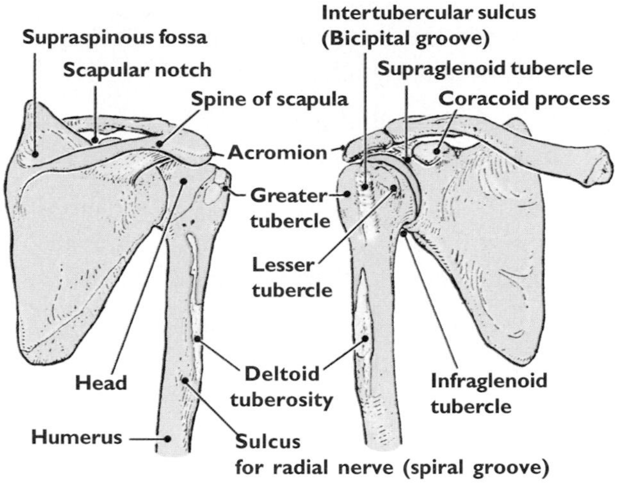

Figure 6.5. Bony landmarks of the shoulder region.

GRANT'S 6.31A
ROHEN 360-363
A.D.A.M. 6.8, 6.50
NETTER 403
CLEMENTE 54-57
A.V.A. 1: 0.19.53

Define the borders of the **deltoid muscle.** Verify its origin from the lateral third of the clavicle, spine, and acromion of scapula.

With a scalpel, detach the deltoid from the spine and the acromion of the scapula. Leave the muscle attached to the clavicle. Reflect the deltoid anteriorly. Observe the **axillary nerve** and the **posterior circumflex humeral artery** entering its deep surface. Dissect the nerve and vessels. Verify that the axillary nerve also supplies the **teres minor** (Fig. 6.6).

Push your fingers parallel to the axillary nerve and posterior circumflex humeral vessels into a space. This space is the **quadrangular space** (Fig. 6.6). Define the borders of the quadrangular space:

- Superiorly, the capsule of the shoulder joint;
- Laterally, the surgical neck of the humerus;
- Medially, the long head of the triceps brachii;
- Inferiorly, the upper border of the teres major.

GRANT'S 6.30
A.D.A.M. 6.34
NETTER 403
CLEMENTE 52
A.V.A. 1: 0.58.00

Note the **long head of the triceps brachii.** Verify that it passes between teres minor and teres major and attaches to the infraglenoid tubercle. With your fingers, separate the **long head** and the **lateral head** of the triceps. Define the **triangular interval** between the two heads of the muscle inferior to the teres major (Fig. 6.6). With a probe, explore the **floor** of the triangular interval:

- Identify the humerus, forming the bony floor of the triangle;
- Identify the **radial nerve** and the **profunda brachii artery** within the triangle;
- Observe that the nerve and artery lie in a broad groove directly on the humerus. This is the spiral groove or sulcus for the radial nerve.

Next, explore the **supraspinatus** and **infraspinatus muscles** in their respective fossae, the supraspinous fossa and the infraspinous fossa. To clear the area, reflect the trapezius anteriorly. If dissection of the superficial back muscles has been done properly, the trapezius will remain attached only to the clavicle. Its nerve and blood supply should still be intact. Remove deep fascia from the supraspinatus and infraspinatus muscles. Push your finger into the space bounded by the levator scapulae, superior border of the scapula, and anterior margin of reflected trapezius. Since this space is filled with loose fat, use scissors and forceps to remove it. Run your finger along the superior border of the scapula. Feel the ligament that bridges the scapular notch medial to the base of the coracoid process. This is the **suprascapular ligament** (Fig. 6.7).

⇦
Grant's 6.30, 6.31A
Rohen 361
A.D.A.M. 6.27, 6.34
Netter 396
Clemente 33, 52
A.V.A. 1: 0.11.31

The next objective is to demonstrate the nerve and blood supply to the muscles occupying the supraspinous and infraspinous fossae (Fig. 6.7):

⇦
Grant's 6.30
Rohen 382
A.D.A.M. 6.49, 6.50
Netter 397
Clemente 34
A.V.A. 1: 0.29.36

- Vertically, cut across the **supraspinatus muscle**, about 5 cm lateral to the superior angle of the scapula; that is, medial to the scapular notch and the suprascapular ligament.
- With the handle of the scalpel, free the lateral portion of the supraspinatus from its fossa. Reflect it laterally.
- Now, observe and clean the **suprascapular nerve and artery**. The nerve passes inferior to the suprascapular ligament whereas the artery passes superior to it.
- Next, cut vertically across the **infraspinatus muscle**, about 5 cm lateral to the vertebral border of the scapula.
- Peel loose the lateral portion of the muscle. Reflect it laterally.

⇨
Grant's 6.26B, 6.27B
Rohen 382, 383
A.D.A.M. 6.49, 6.50
Netter 397, 398
Clemente 34

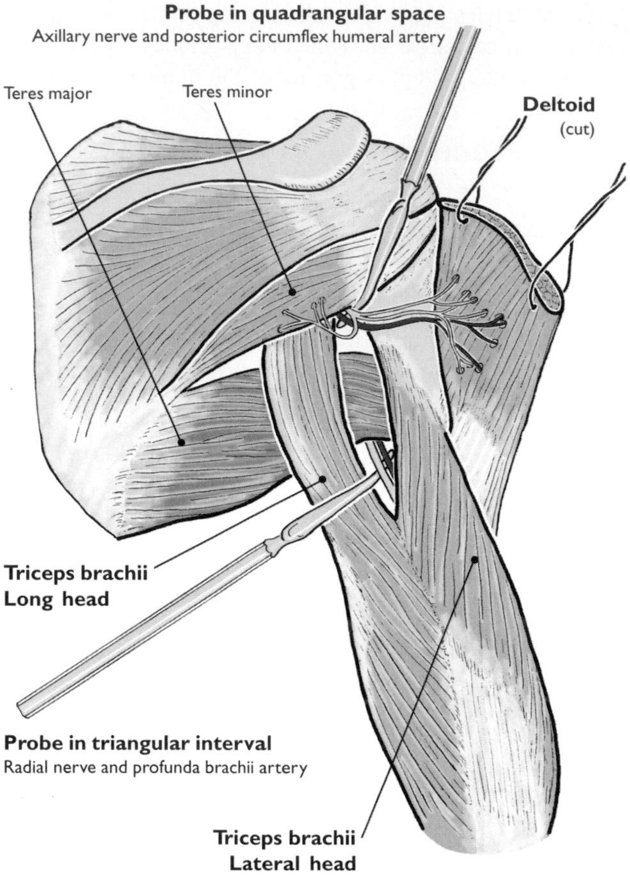

Figure 6.6. Dorsal scapular region. Quadrangular space and triangular interval.

- Note the **suprascapular artery and nerve** reaching the muscle via the spinoglenoid notch (Fig. 6.7).

Follow the **suprascapular artery and nerve** superiorly into the fossa bounded by the levator scapulae, the superior border of scapula, and the trapezius. Both nerve and artery are lateral to a small "rounded" muscle, the **posterior belly of the omohyoid**, which arises medial to the scapular notch. Deep within the fossa, find the **transverse cervical artery**. The transverse cervical artery is a branch of the thyrocervical trunk. It continues to the deep surface of the trapezius where it supplies the middle third of this muscle. The transverse cervical artery contributes also to the collateral blood supply of the scapular region (Figs. 6.7, 6.8). This collateral circulation is extensive and ensures blood supply to the upper limb if the blood flow through the axillary artery is insufficient.

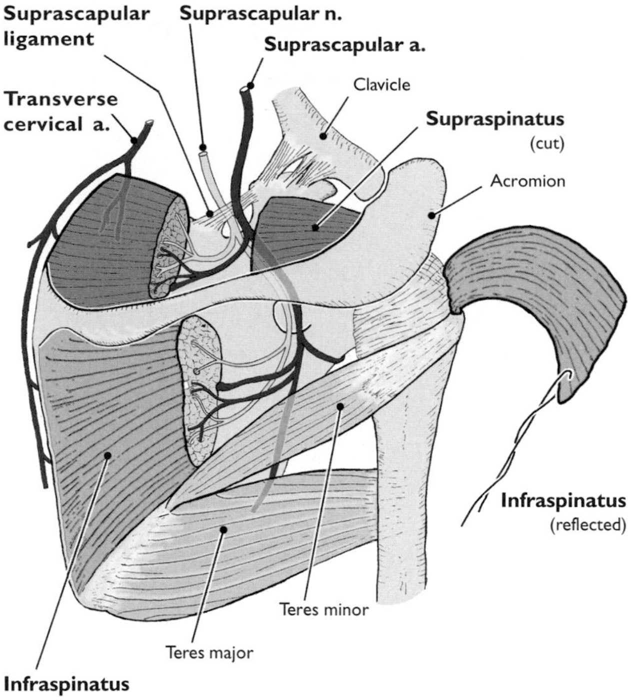

Figure 6.7. Blood and nerve supply to the supraspinatus and infraspinatus muscles.

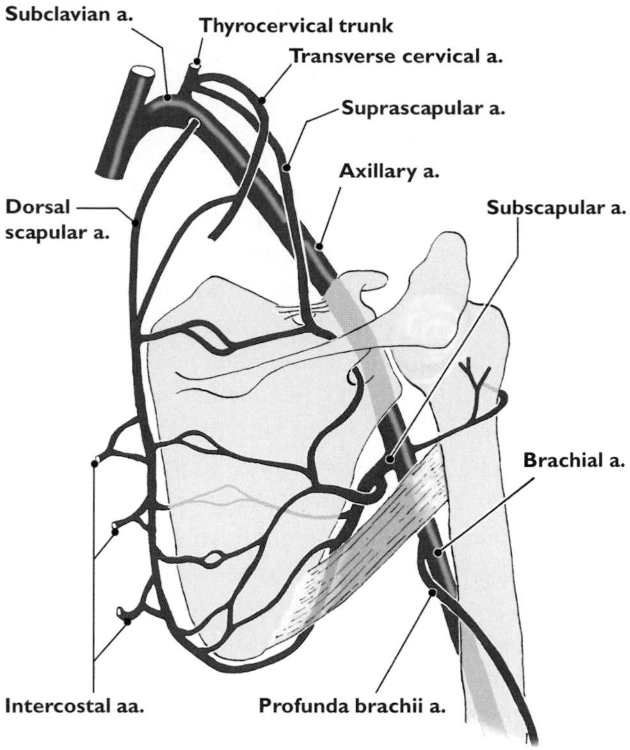

Figure 6.8. Extensive collateral blood supply of the scapular region.

Dissection Note: In 70% of the cases, there is a **dorsal scapular artery** that arises from the second or third part of the subclavian artery.The artery runs deep to the rhomboid layer of muscles to supply the rhomboids, the levator scapulae, and the serratus anterior. It also sends small branches to the dorsal and ventral surfaces of the scapula, providing anastomoses with the suprascapular and the subscapular arteries.When the dorsal scapular artery does *not* arise independently from the subclavian artery (in 30% of the cases), it is usually a branch of the transverse cervical artery. Regardless of its point of origin, the artery that runs deep to the rhomboid layer is called the **dorsal scapular artery.**

Clinical Correlation: The scapular region has an extensive collateral circulation (Fig. 6.8). Its surgical importance becomes apparent during ligation (placement of thread or clamp) of an injured axillary or subclavian artery. In an emergency, and particularly when a modern surgical facility is not available, the axillary artery may be ligated between the thyrocervical trunk and the subscapular artery. In this case, the direction of the blood flow in the subscapular artery becomes reversed, allowing arterial blood from anastomoses to reach the portion of the axillary artery distal to the ligature (*arrows* in Fig. 6.9). Note that, in case of ligature, the subscapular artery receives its blood via several anastomoses with the suprascapular artery, transverse cervical artery, dorsal scapular artery, and some intercostal arteries. Ligation of the axillary artery distal to the subscapular artery interrupts the blood supply to the arm entirely and is intolerable. In the modern and sophisticated surgical setting, ligation of a severly injured axillary artery may not be necessary; instead, a vascular graft may be used to reestablish regular blood flow.

⇦
GRANT'S 6.26B, 6.27B
ROHEN 3.82, 383
A.D.A.M. 6.49, 6,50
NETTER 397, 398
CLEMENTE 34

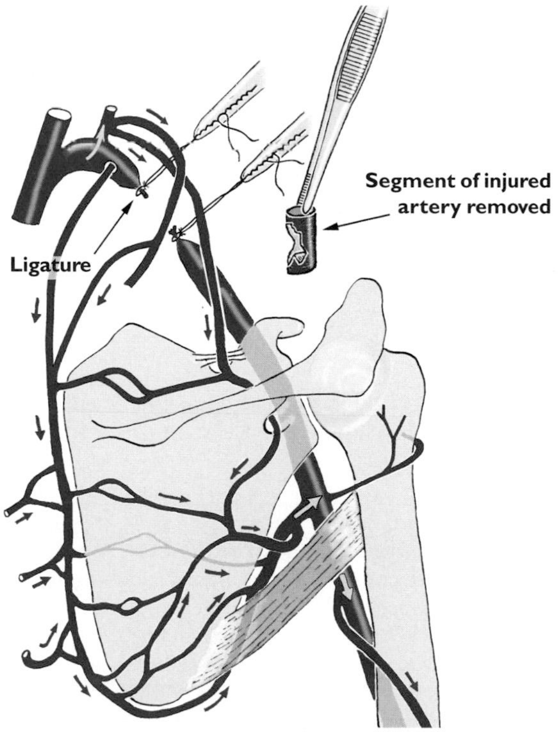

Figure 6.9. Collateral circulation to arm after ligation of the axillary artery. *Arrows* indicate dirrection of adjusted blood flow.

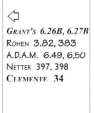

Study the insertion of the four muscles arising from the dorsal surface of the scapula (Fig. 6.10). Verify that the tendons of the **supraspinatus, infraspinatus,** and **teres minor muscles** fuse with the capsule of the shoulder joint to form the major portion of the "rotator cuff". These tendons insert into the **greater tubercle of the humerus.** Sometimes, the tendons of the infraspinatus and teres minor muscles are inseparable. The teres major is attached to the medial lip of the intertubercular sulcus of the humerus. Understand the principal actions of these four muscles. The supraspinatus abducts the arm, infraspinatus and teres minor rotate the arm laterally, and the teres major rotates the arm medially. Demonstrate that the supraspinatus tendon covers part of the capsule of the shoulder joint (Fig. 6.11A). Between the deltoid muscle and the acromion superiorly and the supraspinatus tendon inferiorly lies a bursa. This bursa (synovial sac) is the **subacromial bursa**. Identify the bursa and explore its extent with a probe.

Grant's 6.28
Rohen 380
A.D.A.M. 6.33, 6.34
Netter 396
Clemente 33, 34
A.V.A. 1: 0.12.45

Grant's 6.36A
A.D.A.M. 6.29, 6.35
Netter 394
Clemente 102

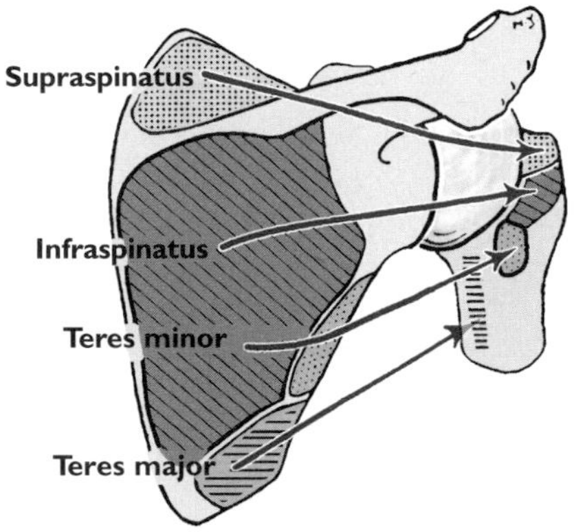

Figure 6.10. Proximal and distal attachment sites of four scapular muscles.

> ***Clinical Correlation:*** **Attrition of the supraspinatus tendon** is a common finding among middle-aged persons. As the supraspinatus tendon degenerates and wears away, the underlying joint capsule is thinned and eventually opened. This attrition of the supraspinatus tendon and the joint capsule ultimately leads to a wide-open communication between the shoulder joint and the subacromial bursa (*Inset*, Fig. 6.11B). The result is a "painful shoulder" (pathologically evidenced by a rupture of the rotator cuff of the shoulder joint with limitation of rotation of the arm).

Grant's 6.36B

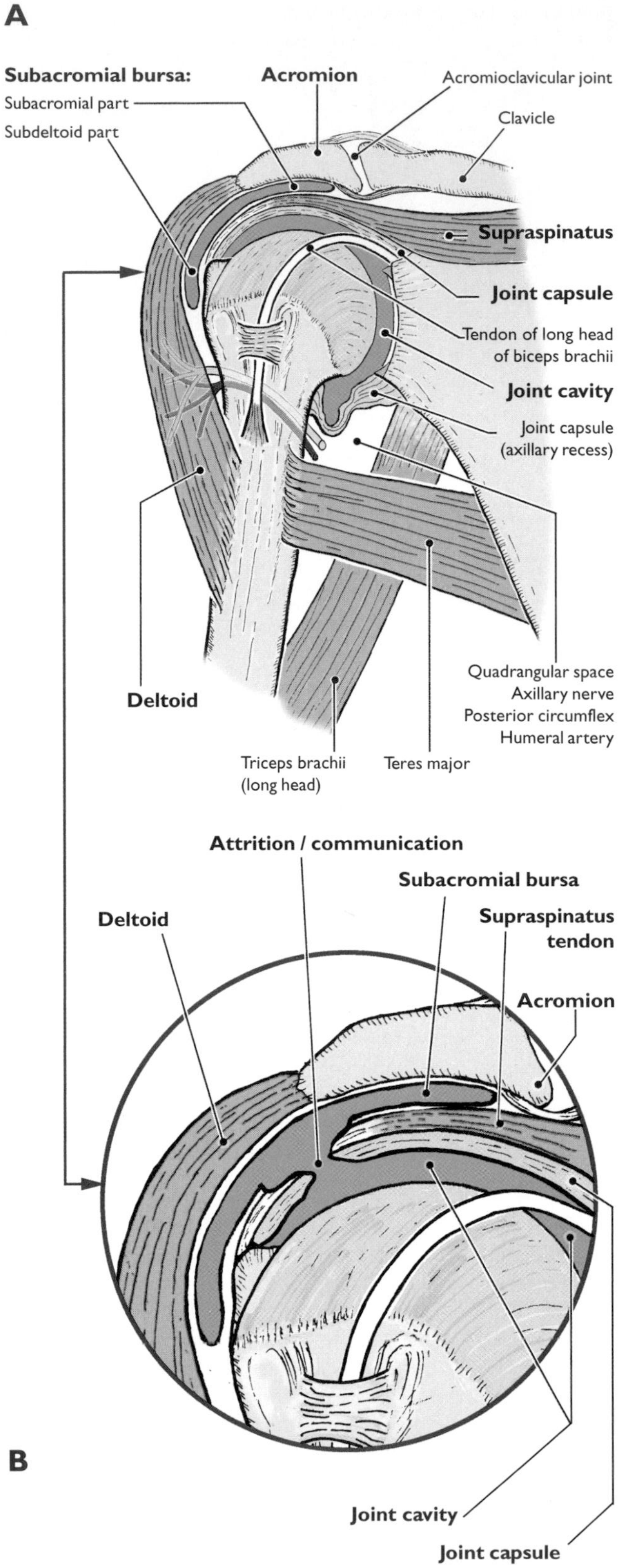

Figure 6.11. *A,* Subacromial bursa and its relationship to the acromion, the deltoid muscle, and the tendon of the supraspinatus muscle. Coronal section; anterior view. *B,* Attrition of supraspinatus tendon and underlying joint capsule leads to communication between shoulder joint and subacromial bursa.

Pectoral Region

The pectoral region (L., *pectus*, chest) covers the anterior and part of the lateral chest wall. The mammary gland is superficial. The muscles of the region comprise the pectoralis major, pectoralis minor, subclavius, and serratus anterior. The pectoralis major muscle is inserted into the humerus. The other muscles are inserted into the scapula and clavicle, which form part of the pectoral girdle. If ***The Thorax*** (Chapter 1) has been covered previously, the mammary gland and the muscles of the pectoral region have already been identified during dissection of the anterior chest wall. Please refer to the first part of Chapter 1, ***Thoracic Wall***.

Dissect or review the following structures:

- **Mammary gland** and its lymphatic drainage;
- **Pectoralis major** and related structures (deltopectoral triangle; clavipectoral fascia; cephalic vein; medial and lateral pectoral nerves);
- **Pectoralis minor** and **subclavius**.

At this point, identify and study the **serratus anterior muscle**. Note its extensive fleshy origin from the upper eight ribs. It is inserted into the whole length of the medial border of the scapula. Identify the serratus anterior on the surface (Fig. 6.12) and on a transverse section (Fig. 6.13). Review the components of the **pectoral girdle**. Finally, review the muscles acting on the scapula and study various **scapular movements**.

Axilla

General Remarks

The axilla is the region between the arm or brachium and the chest (Fig. 6.12). Palpate your own axillary fossa and verify that it is a pyramidal space. The axillary fossa possesses an apex, a base, and four walls. The apex is bounded by the clavicle ventrally, the upper border of the scapula dorsally, and the 1st rib medially. The base of the pyramidal space is the skin and fascia of the armpit. The **four walls of the axilla** are (Figs. 6.12, 6.13):

- **Anterior wall**, the muscular anterior axillary fold;
- **Posterior wall**; consisting of muscles covering the ventral surface of the scapula;

GRANT'S 1.3-1.5
ROHEN 245
NETTER 167-169
CLEMENTE 6-11
A.V.A. 1: 0.18.26

GRANT'S 1.2, 1.15, 6.10
ROHEN 245, 246
A.D.A.M. 1.37, 1.38, 6.28
NETTER 174, 175
CLEMENTE 16-24
A.V.A. 1: 0.17.07, 0.14.04

GRANT'S 6.9
A.D.A.M. 6.29-6.32
NETTER 400, 515
CLEMENTE 17-19
A.V.A. 1: 0.18.20

GRANT'S 6.13, 6.15
ROHEN 363
A.D.A.M. 6.30
NETTER 400
CLEMENTE 19, 21
A.V.A. 1: 0.18.55

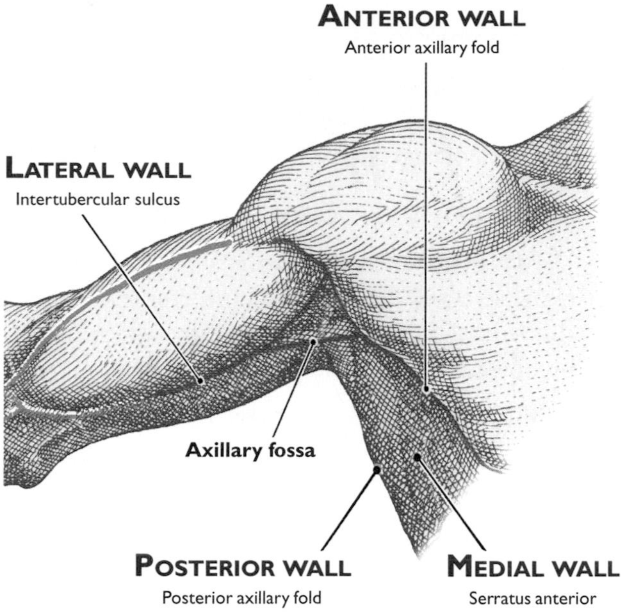

Figure 6.12. Surface anatomy of axilla.

- **Medial wall**; consisting of the upper portion of the thorax with overlying serratus anterior muscle;
- **Lateral wall**; the narrow vertical groove of the humerus intervening between the converging anterior and posterior walls, i.e., the intertubercular sulcus.

The **contents of the axilla** consist of the **axillary sheath**, **lymphatics**, portions of **muscles**, and intervening fat and connective tissue (Fig. 6.13).

Walls of Axilla

Anterior Wall of Axilla. Review the **pectoralis major** and **pectoralis minor** (Fig. 6.13). These muscles were discussed in detail with the dissection of the pectoral region (Chapter 1).

- Reflect the pectoralis minor superiorly.
- Reflect the pectoralis major toward the arm.
- Abduct the arm to a right angle. Have your partner hold the limb in this position with the elbow raised off the table. This procedure relaxes the structures within the axilla.

Posterior Wall of Axilla (Fig. 6.13). Identify and palpate the three muscles that form the posterior wall of the axilla:

- **Latissimus dorsi** (responsible for producing the posterior axillary fold);

- **Teres major**;
- **Subscapularis**. Do *not* clean these muscles at this time. This will be done after tracing nerves and blood vessel from the axillary contents.

GRANT'S 6.13, 6.15
ROHEN 363
A.D.A.M. 6.30
NETTER 400
CLEMENTE 19, 21
A.V.A. 1:0.19.30, 0.11.03

Medial Wall of Axilla (Fig. 6.13):

- Verify that the medial wall is formed by the expansive and flat **serratus anterior**. Note that this muscle covers the ribs and intercostal muscles.

GRANT'S 6.10
ROHEN 363
A.D.A.M. 6.33
NETTER 174, 175
CLEMENTE 21, 24, 29, 30
A.V.A. 1: 0.14.04

- With your fingertips, follow the muscle dorsally toward the medial margin of the scapula. Do *not* clean the muscle at this time so that its nerve and blood supply remain undisturbed.

Lateral Wall of Axilla (Fig. 6.13):

GRANT'S 6.15B, 6.16
NETTER 400
CLEMENTE 19
A.V.A. 1: 0.06.51

Identify the **intertubercular sulcus** of the humerus. The sulcus is also called the **bicipital groove** since the tendon of the long head of biceps brachii lodges in it; note the tendon in its specific location.

Contents of Axilla

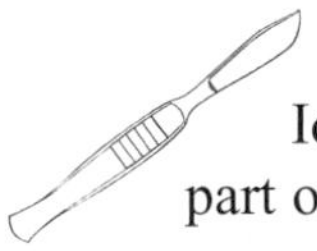

Identify the following three muscles as part of the contents of the axilla (Fig. 6.13):

GRANT'S 6.13-6.15
A.D.A.M. 6.29
NETTER 400
CLEMENTE 19
A.V.A. 1: 0.56.04

- Tendinous **long head of biceps brachii;** it lies within the intertubercular sulcus; it arises from the supraglenoid tubercle of the scapula;
- **Short head of biceps,** lying medial to the tendon of long head;
- **Coracobrachialis,** the most medial of the muscles; observe that the coracobrachialis and short head of biceps are attached to the coracoid process of the scapula.

GRANT'S 6.13, 6.14
ROHEN 374, 375
A.D.A.M. 6.29, 6.31
NETTER 400, 405
CLEMENTE 23
A.V.A. 1: 0.28.00

Axillary Sheath (Fig. 6.13). This sheath envelops the remaining contents of the axilla; i.e., the axillary artery, the axillary vein, and the cords of the brachial plexus. If the axillary vein and its tributaries have already been removed, the axillary sheath must have been opened. If the axillary vein is still present, remove it and its tributaries so that the dissection field of the axilla can be clarified.

GRANT'S 6.12, 6.15A
ROHEN 388
A.D.A.M. 6.29
NETTER 400
CLEMENTE 19

Axillary Artery (Fig. 6.14). This large artery begins at the lateral border of the 1st rib where it is continuous with the **subclavian**

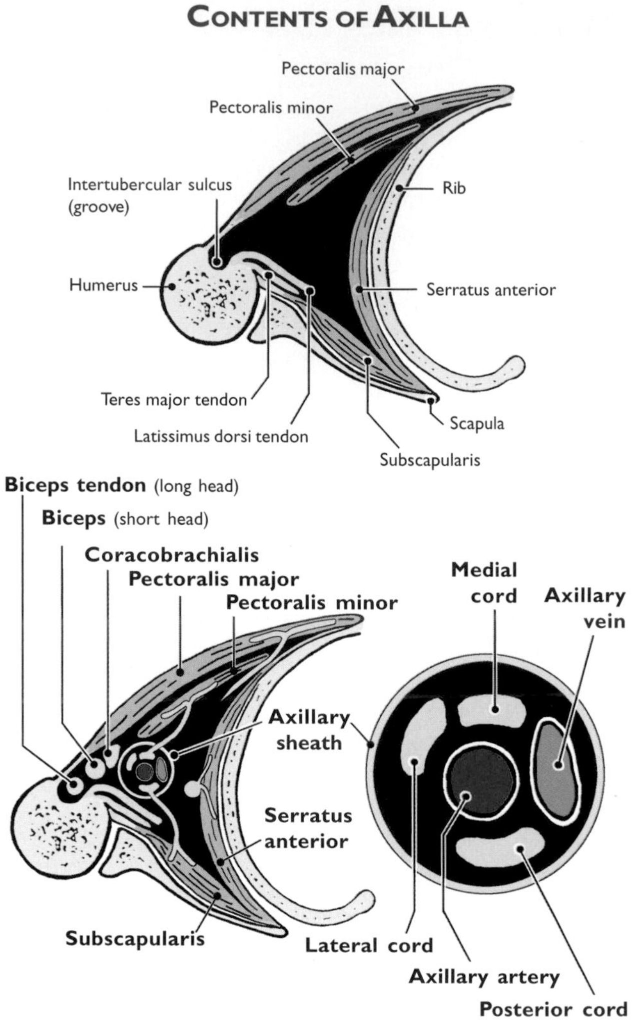

Figure 6.13. Walls and contents of axilla (schematic transverse section).

artery. The axillary artery ends at the inferior border of the teres major muscle. At this point, it continues distally as the **brachial artery.** Positively identify the three parts of the axillary artery:

- The first part is located between the lateral border of the 1st rib and the superior (medial) border of the pectoralis minor;
- The second part lies deep to the pectoralis minor;
- The third part extends between the inferior (lateral) border of the pectoralis minor and the inferior border of the teres major.

The three parts of the axillary artery give rise to various arterial branches. There is con-

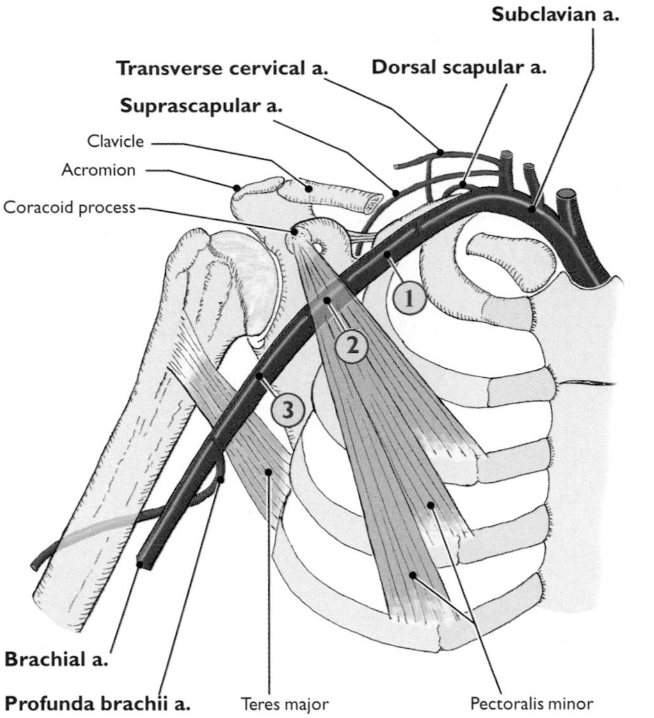

Figure 6.14. The three parts of the axillary artery: *1,* lateral border of first rib to medial border of pectoralis minor; *2,* posterior to pectoralis minor; *3,* lateral border of pectoralis minor to inferior border of teres major.

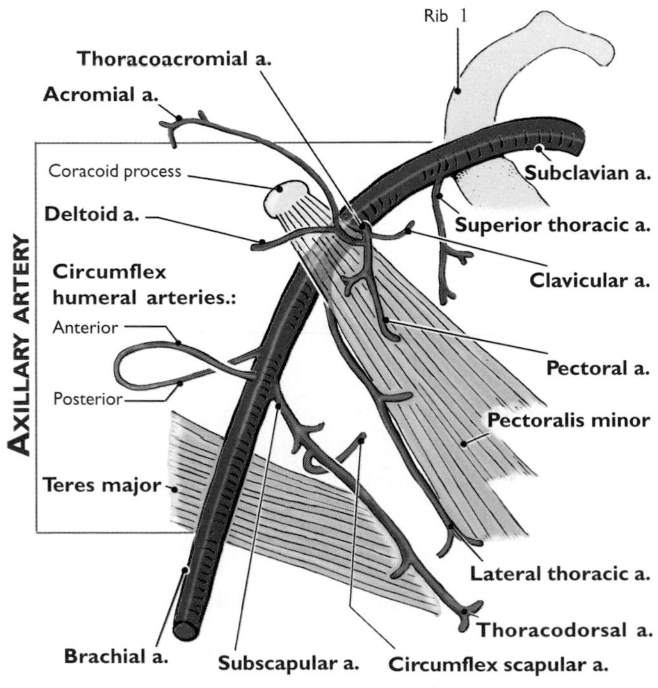

Figure 6.15. Branches of the axillary artery (schematic).

siderable variation in the branching pattern of the axillary artery. If the pattern is different in your specimen, note that the branches are named according to their distribution rather than their point of origin.

GRANT'S 6.13, 6.14
ROHEN 374, 375
A.D.A.M. 6.29, 6.31
NETTER 400, 405
CLEMENTE 23
A.V.A. 1: 0.28.25, 1.09.54

Axillary Artery and Its Branches (Fig. 6.15). The axillary artery is surrounded by the cords and branches of the brachial plexus. These nerves must *not* be destroyed. They should be retracted during dissection of the axillary artery and its branches. Using scissors and forceps, clean the following structures:

Branch of the **first part** of the **axillary artery**: This single, small vessel is the **superior (or supreme) thoracic artery** that supplies part of the 1st and 2nd intercostal spaces.

Branches of the **second part** of the **axillary artery** (Fig. 6.15). These are the **thoracoacromial artery** and the **lateral thoracic artery** that arise deep to the pectoralis minor muscle:

GRANT'S 6.13
ROHEN 374, 375
A.D.A.M. 6.13
NETTER 400, 405
CLEMENTE 20, 23, 30
A.V.A. 1: 0.29.53

- Identify the short wide **trunk of the thoracoacromial artery** at the superior border of the pectoralis minor muscle, and follow its branches (**acromial**; **deltoid**; **pectoral**; **clavicular**) to their respective fields of distribution.
- Next, identify the origin of the **lateral thoracic artery,** and follow it to the pectoral muscles. (In females of reproductive age, this vessel is relatively large since it also supplies the lateral portion of the mammary gland).

Branches of the **third part** of the **axillary artery** (Fig. 6.15):

GRANT'S 6.14
ROHEN 374, 375, 388
A.D.A.M. 6.13
NETTER 400, 405
CLEMENTE 23, 32
A.V.A. 1: 0.30.04

- First, identify the largest branch of the axillary artery, the **subscapular artery.** Trace it along the lateral border of the subscapularis muscle. The vessel continues inferiorly as the **thoracodorsal artery**, which supplies the latissimus dorsi muscle. Note another branch of the subscapular artery, the **circumflex scapular artery**, which contributes to the rich anastomotic arterial network around the scapula. Follow other branches of the subscapular artery to the various muscles, the subscapularis, latissimus dorsi, and serratus anterior.
- Next, search for the two circumflex humeral arteries. Note that the larger vessel, the **poste-**

rior circumflex humeral artery, passes through the quadrangular space together with the axillary nerve. Establish continuity of the vessel. With one finger, approach the quadrangular space from the axilla; with another finger, approach the quadrangular space from dorsally. Positively identify the posterior circumflex humeral artery as it passes through the quadrangular space.

- Look for the smaller **anterior circumflex humeral artery**.

Brachial Plexus (Fig. 6.16). *Note:* Only the infraclavicular part of the plexus will be dissected at this time. The supraclavicular part will be dissected with the neck. The axillary artery is surrounded by the **three cords** of the brachial plexus: lateral, medial, and posterior. First, identify the **lateral** and **medial cords** and their branches. Proceed in the following manner:

- Identify the **musculocutaneous nerve.** It is the most lateral nerve of the plexus and enters the substance of coracobrachialis.
- Trace the musculocutaneous nerve proximally to the **lateral cord** (Figs. 6.16, 6.17).
- Identify the other terminal branch of the lateral cord: this is the lateral root of the median nerve. Follow it distally and identify the **median nerve.**
- Trace the medial root of the median nerve proximally to the **medial cord**.
- Identify the other terminal branch of the medial cord, the **ulnar nerve**.

Note that the three nerves (musculocutaneous; median; ulnar) describe the letter *M* anterior to the axillary artery (Fig. 6.17). The medial cord has a large collateral branch: the **medial cutaneous nerve** of the **forearm**. Follow this nerve distally to the point where it pierces the deep fascia. With tape or a string, retract the axillary vessels and the M-shaped anterior nerves. This procedure exposes the **posterior cord** of the brachial plexus. Clean and dissect its branches (Fig. 6.18):

- The **axillary nerve,** passing through the quadrangular space with the posterior circumflex humeral artery;

◁
GRANT'S 6.14
ROHEN 374, 375
A.D.A.M. 6.33, 6.34, 6.40
NETTER 400-403
CLEMENTE 23
A.V.A. 1: 0.30.07

◁
GRANT'S 6.20
ROHEN 390
A.D.A.M. 6.22
NETTER 400, 401
CLEMENTE 26-28
A.V.A. 1: 0.31.05

▷
GRANT'S 6.21
NETTER 400
CLEMENTE 24
A.V.A. 1: 0.34.46

◁
GRANT'S 6.13
ROHEN 391
A.D.A.M. 6.22
NETTER 400
CLEMENTE 24
A.V.A. 1: 0.32.15

◁
GRANT'S 6.14, 6.21
ROHEN 390
A.D.A.M. 6.22, 6.23
NETTER 400
CLEMENTE 27, 32
A.V.A. 1: 0.32.56

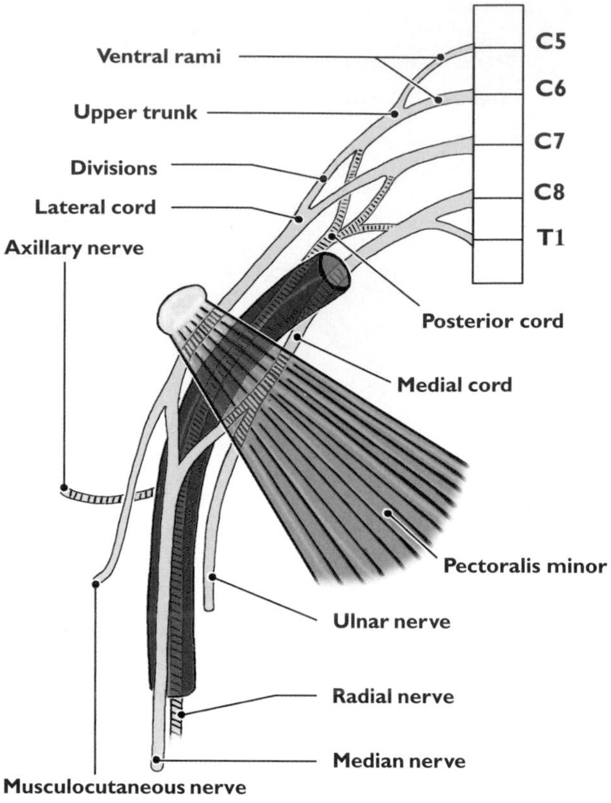

Figure 6.16. Brachial plexus.

- **Subscapular nerves** to the **subscapularis muscle**;
- The **nerve** to the **teres major** and **deltoid**;
- The **nerve** to the **latissimus dorsi**, the **thoracodorsal nerve**.
- Verify that these nerves run in the loose areolar or fatty tissue anterior to the subscapularis muscle; use probe and scissors to clean these nerves.
- Trace the pectoral nerves of the reflected pectoral muscles to their origins from lateral and medial cords (Fig. 6.13).
- Follow the **subscapular artery** and its branches. Note its largest branch, the **circumflex scapular artery**.
- Review the motor nerve supply to the scapular and shoulder regions (Fig. 6.19). Identify each muscle and the nerve that supplies it.

Examine the **contents** of the **axilla** with special reference to an important bony landmark: the **tip** of the **coracoid process.** Palpate this landmark. Verify:

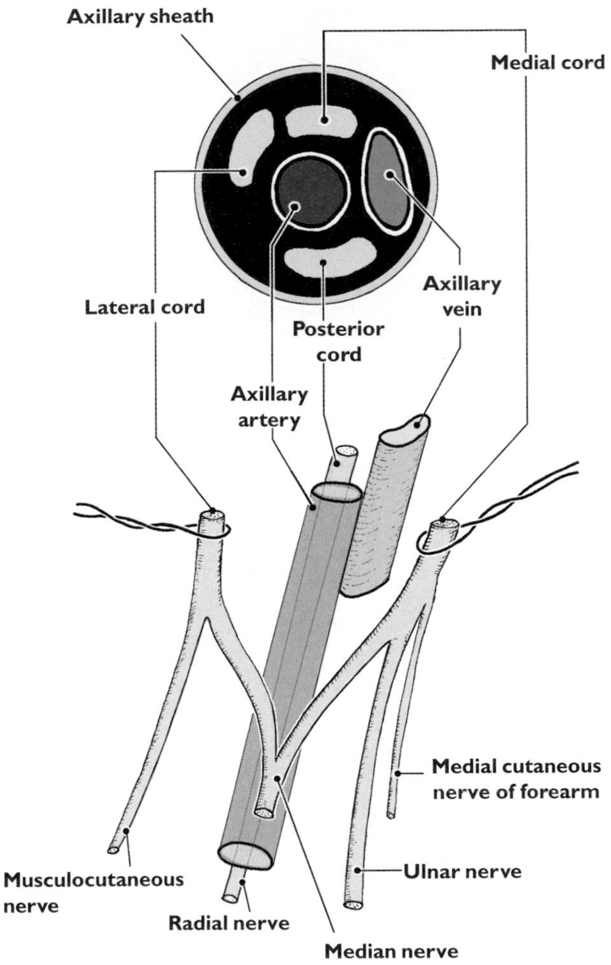

Figure 6.17. The brachial plexus and its relation to the axillary vessels.

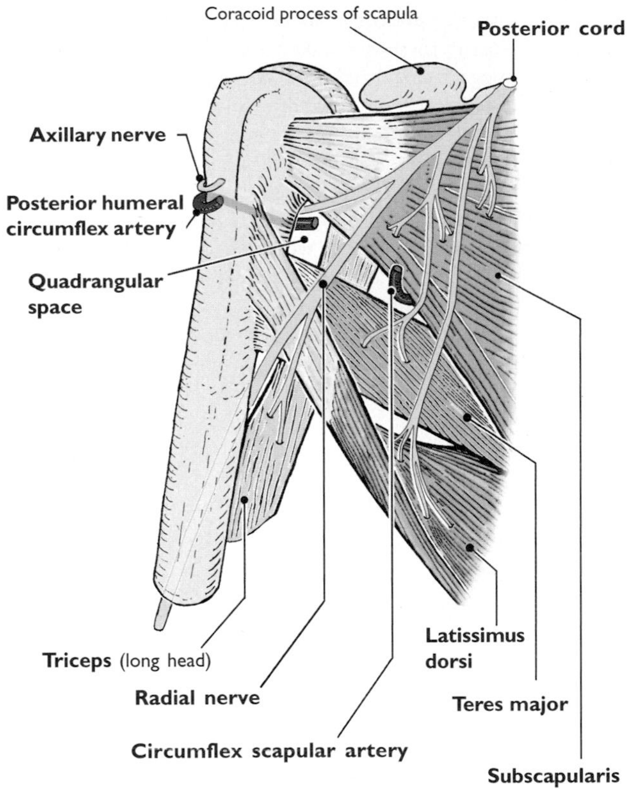

Figure 6.18. Posterior wall of axilla and posterior cord of brachial plexus.

- The axillary sheath passes about 2 cm inferior to it.
- All structures within the axillary sheath (artery; several nerves) may be easily severed here (stab wounds; piece of shrapnel).

GRANT'S 6.13
ROHEN 387
A.D.A.M. 6.29
NETTER 400
CLEMENTE 23, 24
A.V.A. 1: 1.09.52

Clinical Correlation: Injuries to the **brachial plexus** are of considerable clinical importance because the entire function of the upper limb depends on its integrity. Brachial plexus injuries are divided into groups: upper (superior to the clavicle or first rib) and lower (inferior to the clavicle or first rib) plexus injuries. Injuries may be caused by stab or bullet wounds to the neck or axilla, or they may be the result of excessive pressure or forceful stretching of the nervous tissue.

Upper brachial plexus injuries are more common. They occur when head, neck, and shoulder are forcefully stretched apart. Such trauma may occur in contact sports or when falling from a fast motorcycle or racing horse on the shoulder while the head and trunk continue to move in another direction. This excessive stretching and separation of head and upper limb often leads to tearing and laceration of the upper nerve plexus with severe neurologic deficits.

MOTOR NERVES TO BACK OF UPPER LIMB

(Spinal nerves C3 through C8)

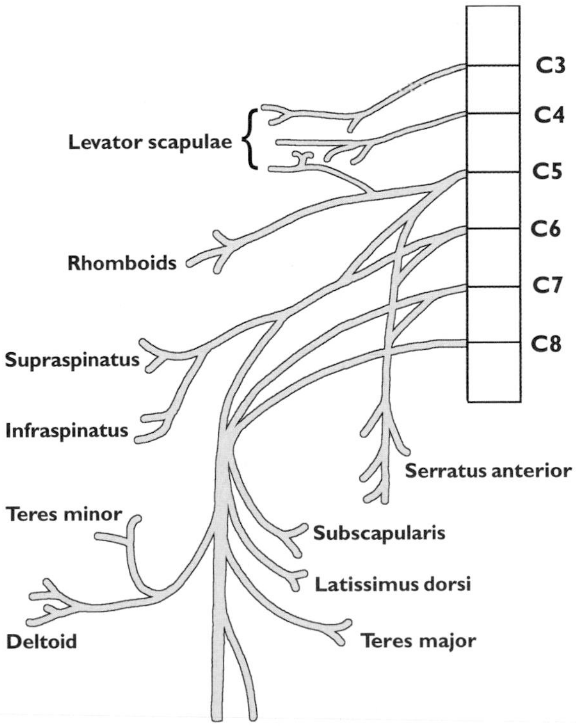

Figure 6.19. Distribution of motor nerves to the scapular and shoulder regions.

Lower brachial plexus injuries typically occur when the upper limb and torso are pulled apart. Such trauma may ensue during a fast fall, when the falling person is trying to break the descend and tumble by suddenly grasping onto a stationary object. Brachial plexus injuries can also be produced when the interval between first rib and clavicle is reduced, causing undue compression of the brachial plexus and its associated blood vessels. This **thoracic outlet syndrome** can be produced when the upper limb is pulled inferiorly, *i.e.*, when the clavicle is firmly pulled down on the first rib (*e.g.*, when carrying a heavy suitcase over extended periods of time). The syndrome my also result from the pressure of an improperly healed clavicular fracture or as the result from chronic pressure caused by an accessory cervical rib.

On the medial axillary wall (or lateral thoracic wall), free the **nerve to the serratus anterior**, also known as the **long thoracic nerve** (Fig. 6.20). Note the vertical course of this important nerve. Observe its branches to the various digitations of the serratus anterior muscle. Follow the nerve proximally and as far as possible to the apex of the axilla. This nerve originates separately from lower cervical segments (Fig. 6.19).

◁
GRANT'S 6.14, 6.22
ROHEN 389
A.D.A.M. 6.29
NETTER 400
CLEMENTE 24
A.V.A. 1:0.35.31

Study the attachments of the **serratus anterior** (Fig. 6.20). Proximally, the muscle is attached to the external surfaces of the lateral parts of ribs 1 to 8. Distally, the attachment site is the anterior surface of the medial border of the scapula. Verify this fact by placing your fingers into the interval between the subscapularis and serratus anterior muscles and by pushing posteriorly until stopped by the attachment of the serratus anterior to the medial border of the scapula. The serratus anterior is the essential protractor of the scapula (as when pushing). The muscle also abducts the arm above the horizontal plane.

◁
GRANT'S 6.22
A.D.A.M. TABLE 6.1
NETTER 177
CLEMENTE 252
A.V.A. 1: 0.14.04

Examine the **subscapularis muscle** (Fig. 6.21). Note that this thick, triangular muscle is attached to the costal surface (subscapular fossa) of the scapula. It contributes to the posterior wall of the axilla. Observe its distal attachment to the lesser tubercle of the humerus.

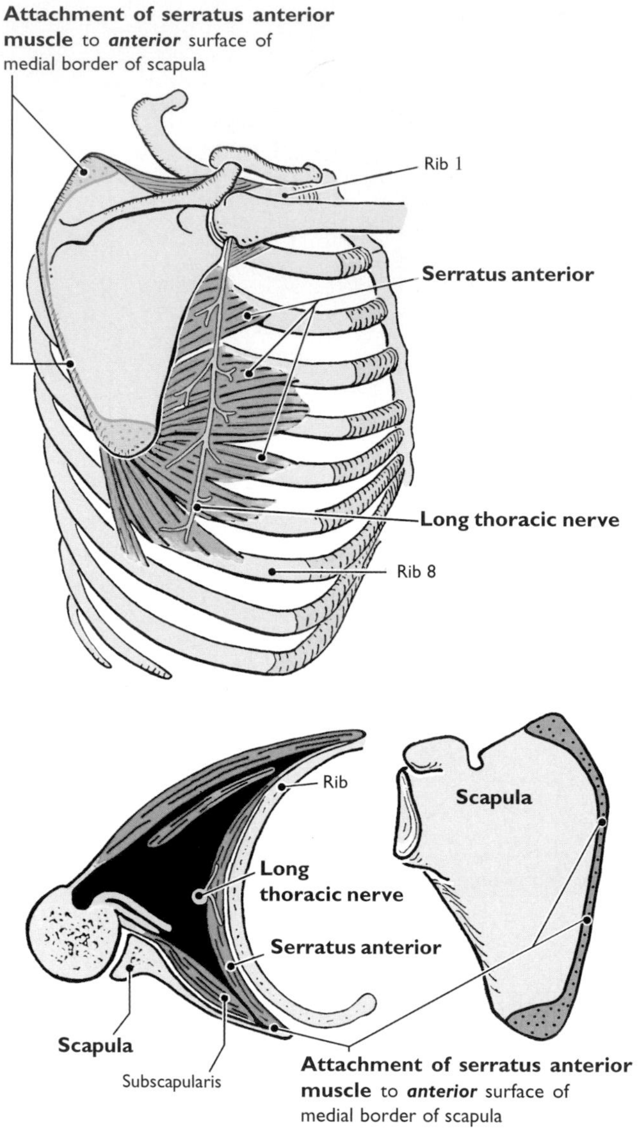

Figure 6.20. Serratus anterior and its attachment to ribs and scapula. Motor supply by the long thoracic nerve.

Clinical Correlation: Injuries to the **long thoracic nerve** will affect the important function of the serratus anterior muscle. The muscle can no longer protract the scapula or abduct the arm completely. When a patient with paralysis of the serratus anterior muscle is asked to push with both hands against a wall, the medial border of the scapula on the affected side becomes very prominent and protrudes, a condition known as "winged scapula." The long thoracic nerve can be injured in a number of ways. Its superficial and vertical course on the chest wall (Fig. 6.20) makes it fairly vulnerable to stab wounds or blunt, crushing injuries. Surgeons may damage the nerve inadvertently during thoracic surgery or during radical mastectomy, particularly when removing cancerous tissue from the axilla. Construction workers, who often carry long and heavy objects on their shoulders, may compress and damage the long thoracic nerve as it passes through the interval between first rib and clavicle.

Similarly, the **thoracodorsal nerve**, the nerve to the latissimus dorsi muscle (Fig. 6.18), is vulnerable to compression injuries and surgical trauma during mastectomy. When this nerve is injured, the latissimus dorsi can no

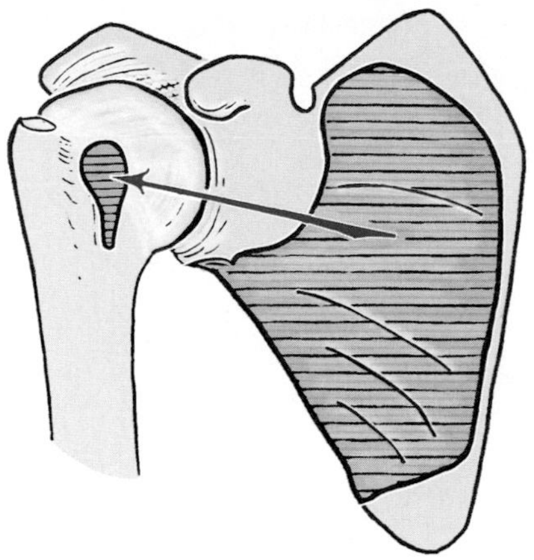

Figure 6.21. Attachments of the subcapularis muscle.

> longer extend, adduct, and medially rotate the humerus; this function essentially raises the body toward the arm during climbing.
>
> The **axillary nerve**, which winds around the neck of the humerus, may be injured during a fracture. The nerve may also be severely stretched and injured during a traumatic dislocation of the shoulder joint. Injury of the axillary nerve interferes with the important function of the deltoid muscle and also affects the teres minor muscle.

Review the essential anatomical features of the axilla. Examine additional cadavers to appreciate variations in the distribution of arteries and nerves. Study a transverse section through the axilla. Correlate your anatomical observations with a magnetic resonance image (MRI) of the shoulder. Review the scapular movements.

Arm and Cubital Fossa

General Remarks

The muscles of the arm or brachium are contained in two fascial compartments (Figs. 6.4 and 6.22). The posterior compartment contains one extensor muscle, the triceps brachii, and its nerves and vessels. The anterior compartment houses three muscles, their nerves, and vessels. The cubital fossa (L., *cubitus*, elbow) is related to the anterior aspect of the elbow.

Posterior Fascial Compartment

On the lateral aspect (side of thumb) of the forearm, identify the **brachioradialis muscle**. With your fingertips, explore the interval between brachioradialis, biceps, and brachialis. Deep in this interval, find the **radial nerve.**

GRANT'S 6.15B, 6.16B
NETTER 513-515
A.V.A. 1: 0.11.03

GRANT'S 6.33
A.D.A.M. 6.40
NETTER 406
CLEMENTE 132

GRANT'S 6.30, 6.31A
ROHEN 379
A.D.A.M. 6.34
NETTER 403
CLEMENTE 56, 57
A.V.A. 1: 1.10.12

GRANT'S 6.43
ROHEN 396
A.D.A.M. 6.41
NETTER 417
CLEMENTE 64
A.V.A. 1: 1.13.50

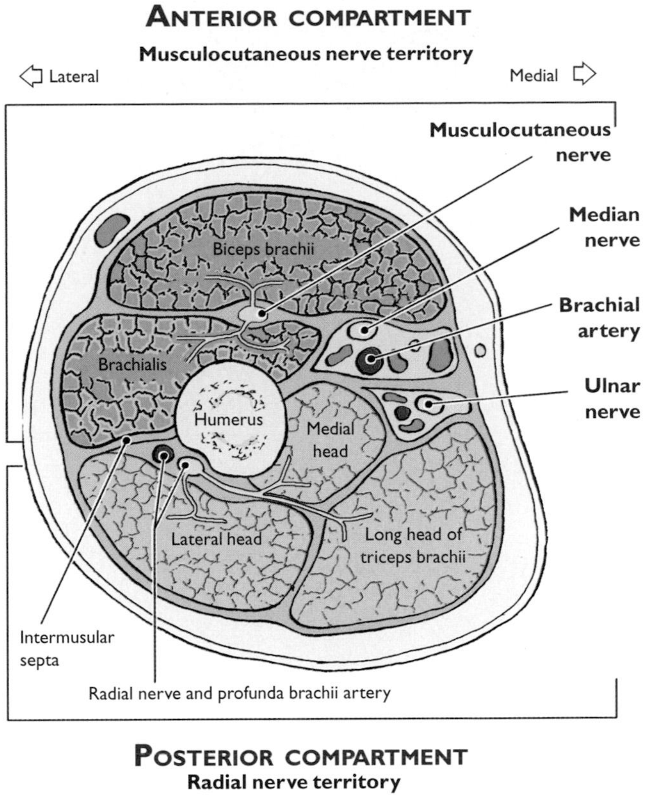

Figure 6.22. The two compartments of the arm with contents. The three heads of the triceps brachii occupy the posterior brachial compartment.

Follow the **radial nerve** proximally. The next objective is to expose the nerve where it is covered by the lateral head of the triceps brachii. Proceed as follows:

- To have better access to the triceps, rotate the arm medially.
- Push a probe proximally along the course of the radial nerve. The probe lies between the lateral head of the triceps and the humerus (Fig. 6.23A).
- Using the probe as a protective device to shield nerve and vessels, sever the lateral head of the triceps obliquely.
- Now, expose the **radial nerve** and the accompanying **profunda brachii artery** (Fig. 6.23B).

Establish the continuity of the radial nerve from the axilla to the elbow region. Observe that the radial nerve is in direct contact with the humerus. This area of contact is called the **sulcus for the radial nerve** or the **spiral groove**. In the area of this groove, the radial nerve can be easily injured during fracture of the humerus.

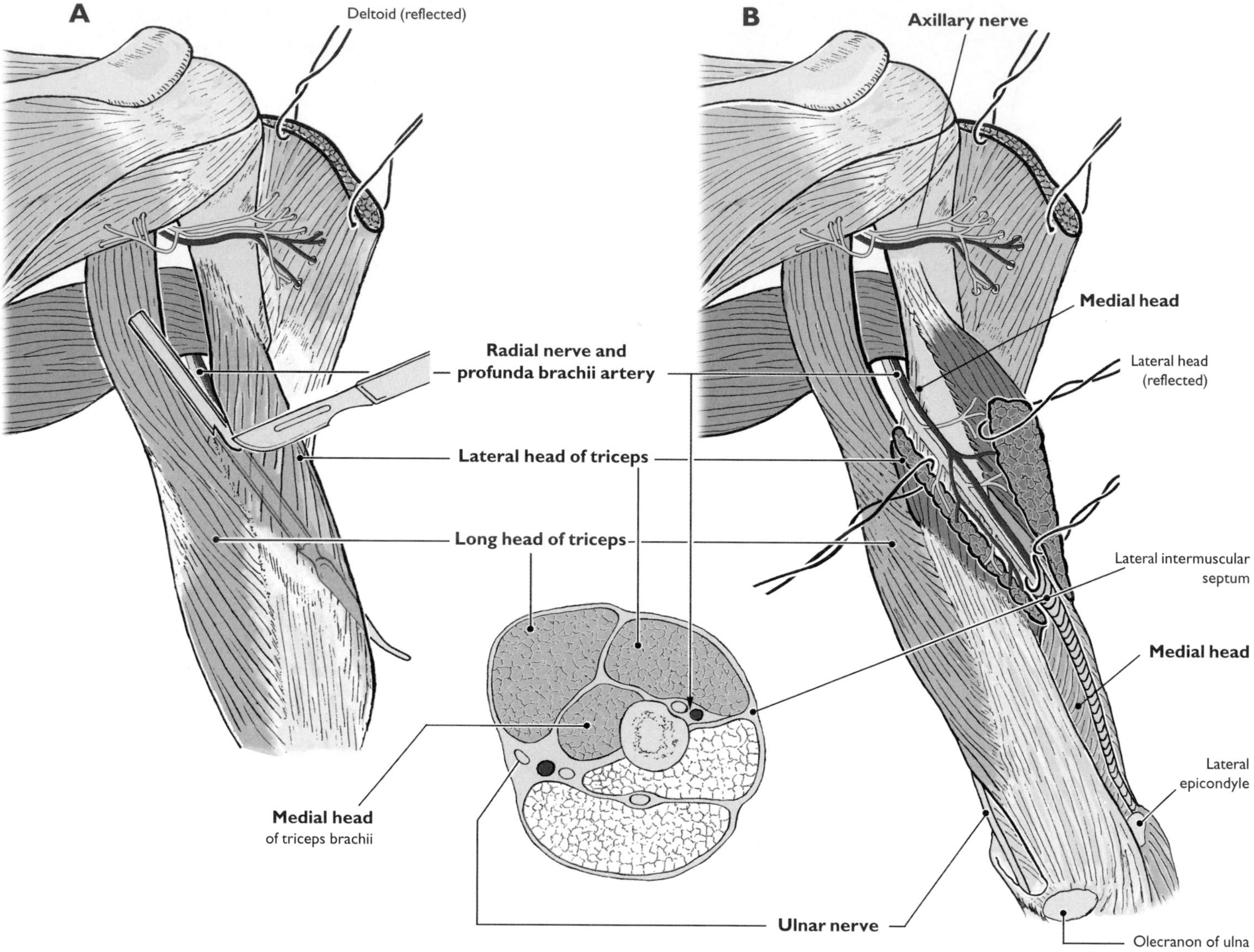

Figure 6.23. ***A,*** Division of the lateral head of the triceps brachii to expose the course of the radial nerve. ***B,*** Triceps brachii and its three related nerves.

Identify the **three heads of the triceps: long, lateral,** and **medial.** Observe that the triceps tendon inserts into the olecranon process of the ulna. Look for muscular branches of the radial nerve to the triceps. There is only one branch to the long head of the triceps. The other heads receive several branches. Correlate your observations with a transverse section of the arm (Figs. 6.22, 6.23).

GRANT'S 6.30, 6.31A, 6.44D
ROHEN 379
A.D.A.M. 6.34
NETTER 403
CLEMENTE 56, 57
A.V.A. 1: 1.57.54

Cubital Fossa

Cubital Fossa (Fig. 6.24A). Identify and define the **biceps brachii**. In the cubital fossa, note the **strong tendon of the biceps**. From its medial side, the tendon gives off a strong triangular aponeurosis, the **bicipital aponeurosis** (lacertus fibrosis). It passes obliquely into the deep fascia covering the flexor muscles of the forearm. Note that the bicipital aponeurosis bridges and protects the **median nerve** and the **brachial artery.** Cut across the aponeurosis, sever and reflect it (Fig. 6.24A).

GRANT'S 6.41, 6.42
ROHEN 364, 365
NETTER 402, 449
CLEMENTE 58, 60
A.V.A. 1: 1.10.35

Note the relative positions of bicipital tendon, brachial artery, and median nerve. Do not destroy the **lateral cutaneous nerve of the forearm** (the cutaneous branch of the musculocutaneous nerve). This nerve runs between biceps and brachialis, and reaches the cubital fossa lateral to the biceps tendon.

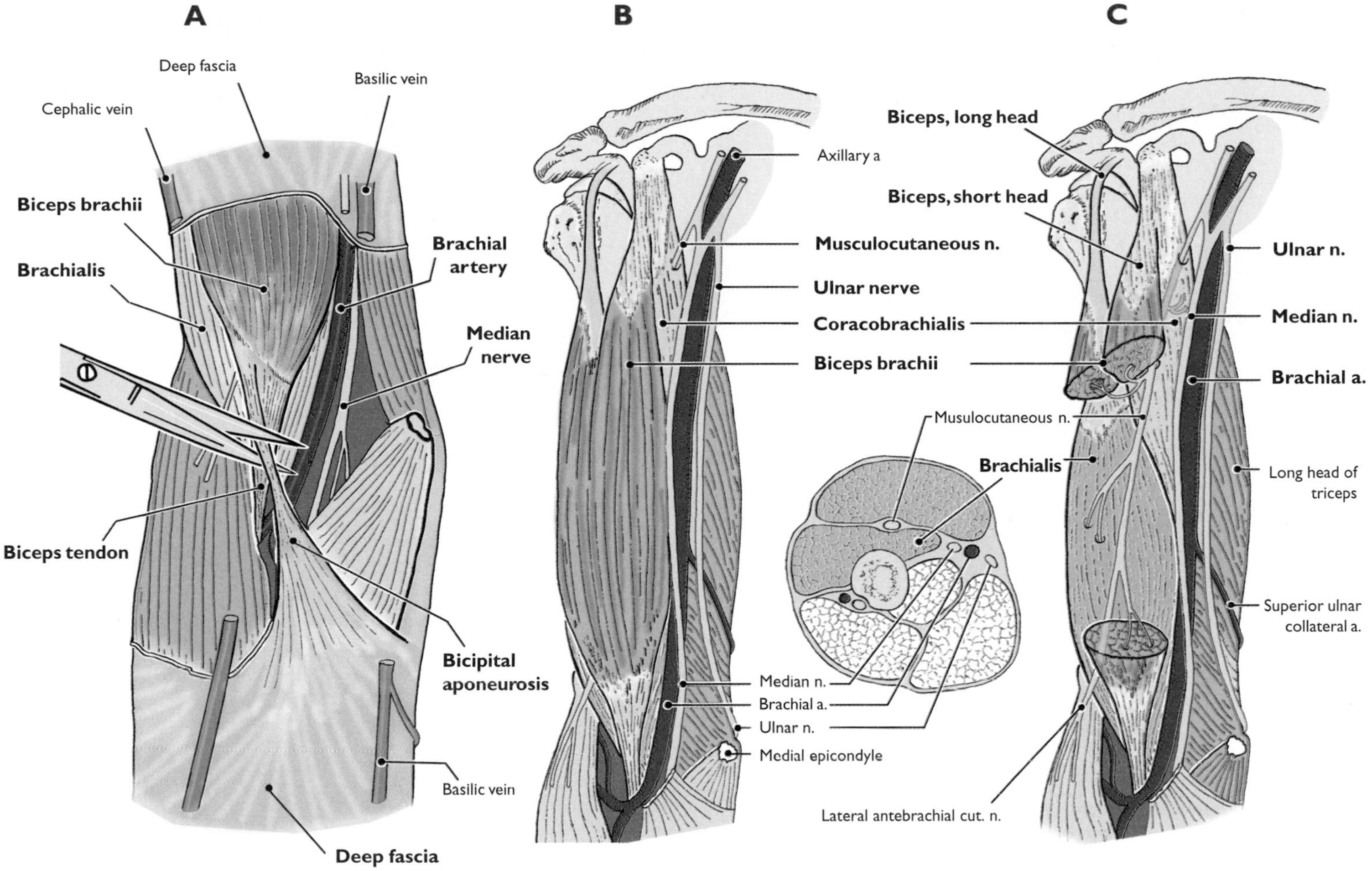

Figure 6.24. ***A,*** Cubital fossa. ***B,*** Muscles of the anterior compartment of the arm and related structures. ***C,*** Section of biceps brachii removed to demonstrate the course of the musculocutaneous nerve.

Anterior Fascial Compartment

Identify the **three muscles** in the **anterior compartment** of the **arm: coracobrachialis, brachialis,** and **biceps brachii** (Fig. 6.24B). Observe the tendon of the long head of biceps in the intertubercular sulcus (bicipital groove). Follow the tendon proximally, under the bridge of the transverse humeral ligament, and to the interior of the fibrous capsule of the shoulder joint. Note the attachment of the short head of the biceps to the coracoid precess of the scapula. Identify the musculocutaneous nerve and follow it distally into the substance of the coracobrachialis musle.

GRANT'S 6.42
NETTER 402
CLEMENTE 48
A.V.A. 1: 0.34.10, 0.55.19

GRANT'S 6.32
ROHEN 391
A.D.A.M. 6.37
NETTER 404
CLEMENTE 51
A.V.A. 1: 1.12.04

Sever the biceps about 5 cm proximal to the cubital region. Reflect the severed portions of the biceps. Now, the **musculocutaneous nerve** can be conveniently traced through the coracobrachialis and between biceps and brachialis muscles (Fig. 6.24C). Note nerve branches to the three muscles of the anterior brachial compartment (Figs. 6.24C, 6.25). Follow the nerve distally where it becomes the **lateral cutaneous nerve** of the **forearm**.

GRANT'S 6.43
ROHEN 365
NETTER 402
CLEMENTE 49
A.V.A. 1:1.11.36

Trace the **median nerve** from axilla to cubital fossa (Fig. 6.24). Next, follow the **ulnar nerve** from the medial cord to the medial epicondyle of the humerus. Note that the nerve is applied to the posterior aspect of the medial epicondyle. There, palpate the nerve. Verify that the median and ulnar nerves do not supply any muscles in the arm. Review the nerve territories of the brachial region (Fig. 6.22): The musculocutaneous nerve is responsible for the muscles in the anterior compartment. The radial nerve supplies the muscle of the posterior compartment, the triceps brachii.

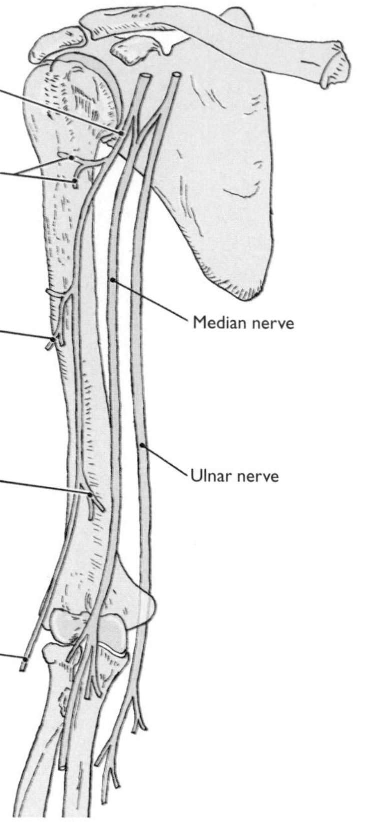

Figure 6.25. Scheme of motor distribution of the musculocutaneous nerve in the anterior compartment of the arm. Note that the median and ulnar nerves do not give off motor branches in the arm.

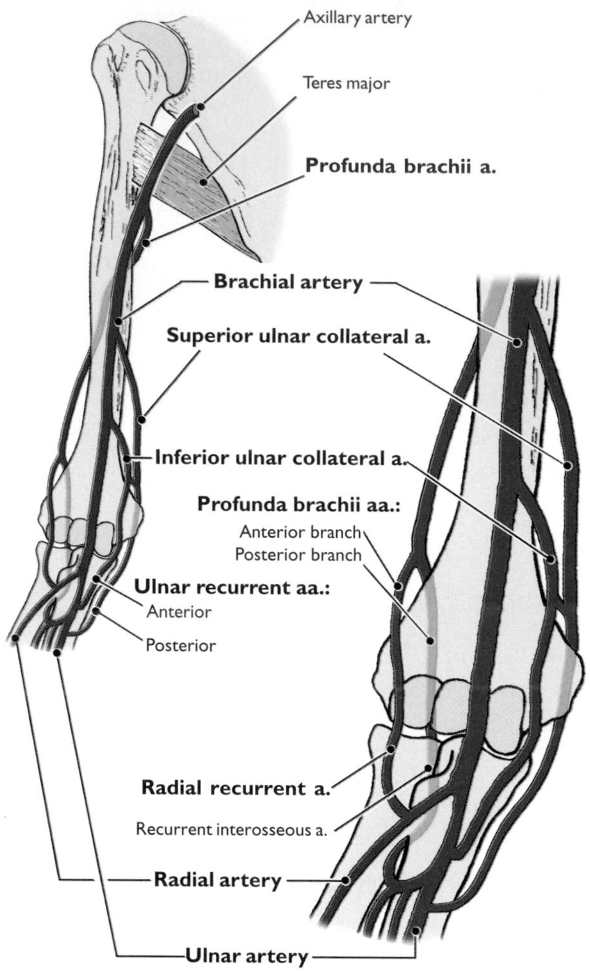

Figure 6.26. Brachial artery and branches. Anastomoses around the elbow.

The **brachial artery** is the continuation of the axillary artery. It begins at the inferior border of the teres major muscle. It ends at its bifurcation into the ulnar artery and radial artery (Fig. 6.26). Verify that the brachial artery is palpable throughout the arm. It runs with the median nerve, which is the only important structure to cross it. Identify:

- **Profunda brachii artery;** it is highest in origin; review its course;
- Several unnamed muscular branches;
- Superior and inferior ulnar collateral arteries.

GRANT'S 6.32
ROHEN 375, 395
A.D.A.M. 6.38
NETTER 404
CLEMENTE 51
A.V.A. 1: 1.10.06

Look for the superior ulnar collateral artery. This artery runs with the ulnar nerve posterior to the medial epicondyle where it anastomoses with the posterior ulnar recurrent artery. The important anastomotic connections around the elbow are often difficult to demonstrate. Collateral circulation occurs between small vessels, often within muscles. Limit the time spent in pursuit of these anastomotic connections.

Always keep in mind that the brachial artery lies medial to the biceps and its tendon. At this location, palpate the arterial pulse in yourself and in your partner. Where should you place the stethoscope when taking blood pressure and listening to the pulsations of the brachial artery?

Clinical Correlation: Understand the clinically and surgically important collateral circulation around the elbow joint (Fig. 6.26). The brachial artery may be tied off distal to the inferior ulnar collateral artery. Under these circumstances, sufficient blood reaches the ulnar and radial arteries via the existing anastomoses.

GRANT'S 6.6B
A.D.A.M. 6.13, 6.14
NETTER 405
CLEMENTE 66-68

Flexor Region of Forearm

General Remarks

The flexor muscles of the forearm can be divided into a superficial and a deep group. Study a transverse section through the middle of the forearm (Fig. 6.27). Note that the

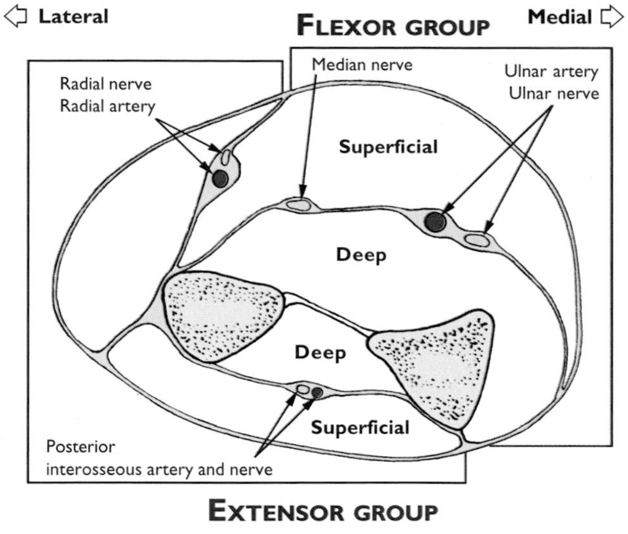

Figure 6.27. Schematic transverse section through the forearm.

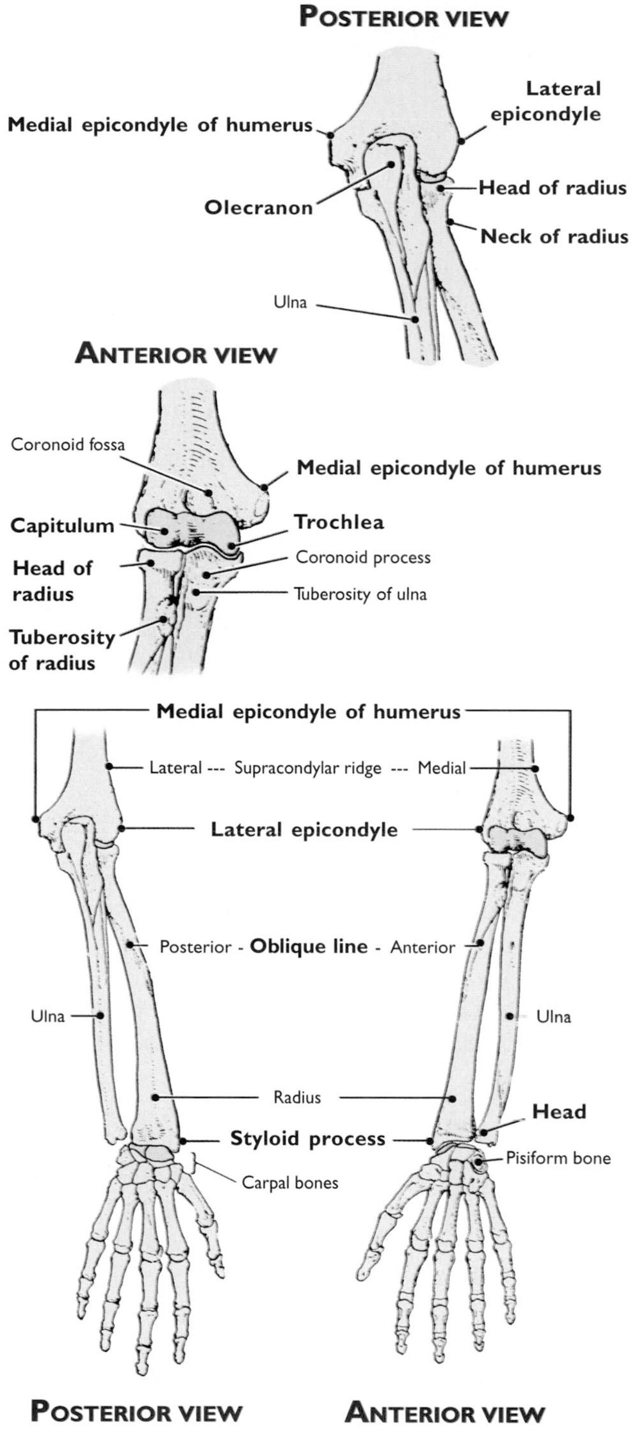

Figure 6.28. Bony landmarks of arm and forearm regions.

ulnar artery, ulnar nerve, and median nerve are located in an areolar septum. This septum separates the deep from the superficial flexors.

A.D.A.M. 6.44
ROHEN 403
NETTER 419
CLEMENTE 135

The superficial flexor muscles arise mainly on the medial side of the elbow from the medial epicondyle and its supracondylar ridge. The deep flexor muscles arise from radius and ulna. Their origin extends to the posterior border of the ulna. Thus, the posterior border of the ulna separates flexor region from extensor region (Fig. 6.27).

In the living subject, verify the following:

- Palpate the posterior border of the ulna throughout the forearm region. It lies subcutaneous and is not crossed by muscles or a motor nerve. Therefore, the posterior border of the ulna indicates a convenient "internervous line," where the surgeon may incise to reach deeper parts of the forearm.
- Flex your fingers (make a fist). Palpate the contraction of superficial and deep flexors. Note that the active muscle group originates from the medial region of the elbow and around the medial aspect of the forearm as far as the posterior border of the ulna.

Bony Landmarks

Refer to a skeleton and study pertinent bony landmarks of the humerus, radius, and ulna.(Fig. 6.28):

On the **humerus** identify:

GRANT'S 6.1
NETTER 392, 393
CLEMENTE 104, 105
A.V.A. 1: 0.06.39, 0.41.13

- **Medial epicondyle** and its medial supracondylar ridge for the attachment of the superficial flexor group;
- **Lateral epicondyle** and its lateral supracondylar ridge for the attachment of the extensor muscles;
- **Capitulum** for articulation with the radius;
- **Trochlea** for articulation with the ulna;
- **Olecranon fossa**.

On the **radius** identify:

- **Head** for articulation with humerus;
- **Neck**;
- **Tuberosity** for biceps tendon;
- **Anterior oblique line** for the origin of flexor digitorum superficialis;
- **Styloid process**;
- **Interosseous border** for attachment of the **interosseous membrane** between the radius and the ulna (Fig. 6.29).

GRANT'S 6.1
ROHEN 352
A.D.A.M. 6.5, 6.6
NETTER 407
CLEMENTE 110, 111
A.V.A. 1: 0.42.15

On the **ulna identify** (Fig. 6.28):

- **Olecranon**; observe that it fits into the olecranon fossa of the humerus and thus limits hyperextension of the forearm;
- Joint surface for articulation with trochlea of humerus;
- **Head**, the distal extremity of the ulna;
- **Interosseous border** for attachment of the interosseous membrane.

GRANT'S 6.1
ROHEN 352
A.D.A.M. 6.5, 6.6
NETTER 407
CLEMENTE 108, 109
A.V.A. 1: 0.42.17

It is essential to understand how the three bones (humerus; radius; ulna) articulate with each other. On the skeleton, examine the following (Fig. 6.28):

- Joint between the capitulum of the humerus and the head of the radius (humeroradial joint);
- Joint between the ulna and the trochlea of the humerus (humeroulnar joint);
- Proximal radioulnar joint, between the head of the radius and a corresponding notch on the proximal end of the ulna (Fig. 6.29);
- Distal radioulnar joint, between the head of the ulna and a corresponding notch on the distal end of the radius (Fig. 6.29);
- Observe the characteristic movements performed in the proximal and distal radioulnar joints. In the position of supination (anatomical position), the radius and the ulna are parallel; in the position of pronation, the two bones cross each other.
- On the palmar surface of the articulated hand, identify the pisiform bone (Fig. 6.28).

GRANT'S 6.52, 6.53
ROHEN 353
NETTER 409
CLEMENTE 118
A.V.A. 1: 0.42.00, 0.44.29

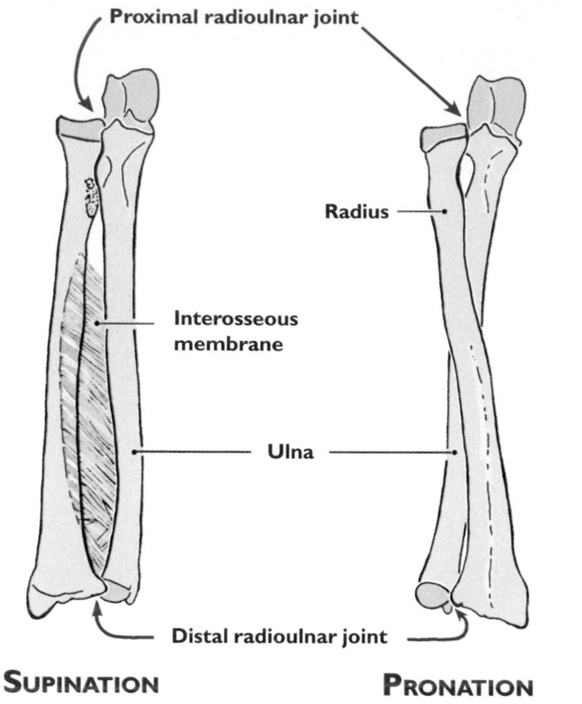

Figure 6.29. Anterior view of right ulna and radius in supination and in pronation. Note proximal and distal radioulnar joints.

Structures of Forearm

Before You Begin ...

At the level of the wrist, the relative positions of tendons, vessels, and nerves will be identified. After reflecting the superficial flexor group, the deep flexor group will be studied. The student should understand the relations of vessels, nerves, and muscles on transverse section (Fig. 6.27).

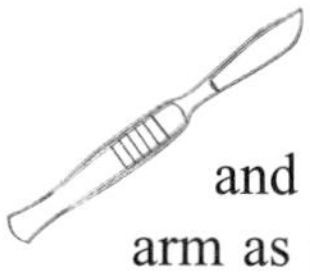

Dissection. Remove the superficial and deep fasciae from the anterior forearm as far around as the posterior border of the ulna. Expose the superficial flexor muscles. Follow them distally to the wrist. Be careful not to destroy arteries and nerves. From the lateral to medial side, identify the following structures at the level of the wrist (Fig. 6.30):

GRANT'S 6.55, 6.60
ROHEN 366
A.D.A.M. 6.41
NETTER 416
CLEMENTE 60, 63

- Tendons of **brachioradialis muscle** and **abductor pollicis longus**;
- **Radial artery**;
- Tendon of **flexor carpi radialis**;
- **Median nerve**;
- Tendon of **palmaris longus** (absent in 25%);

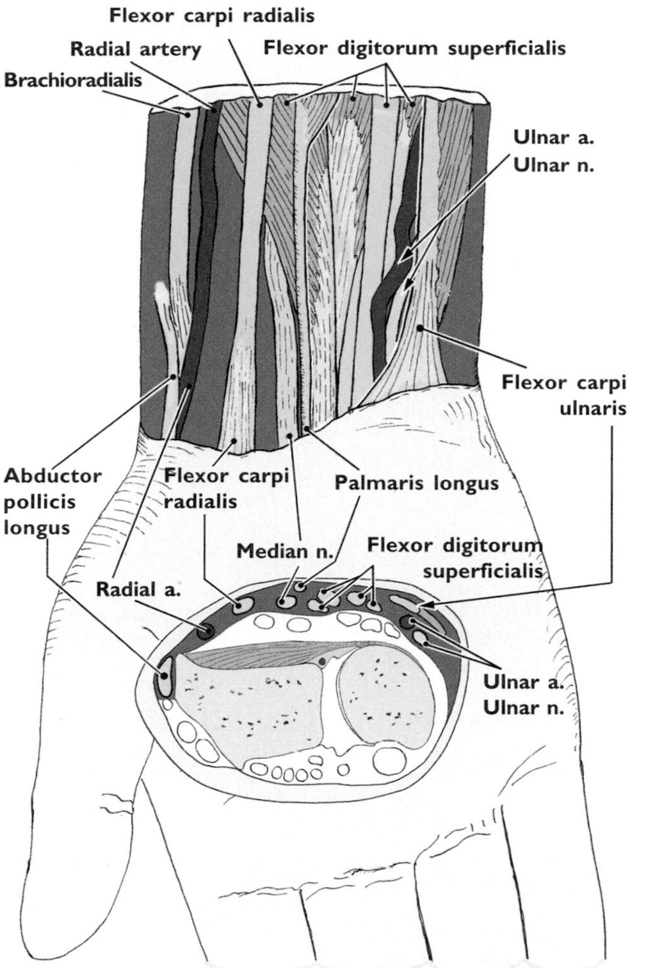

Figure 6.30. Structures at anterior aspect of wrist. Inset shows pertinent tendons, vessels, and nerves on transverse section.

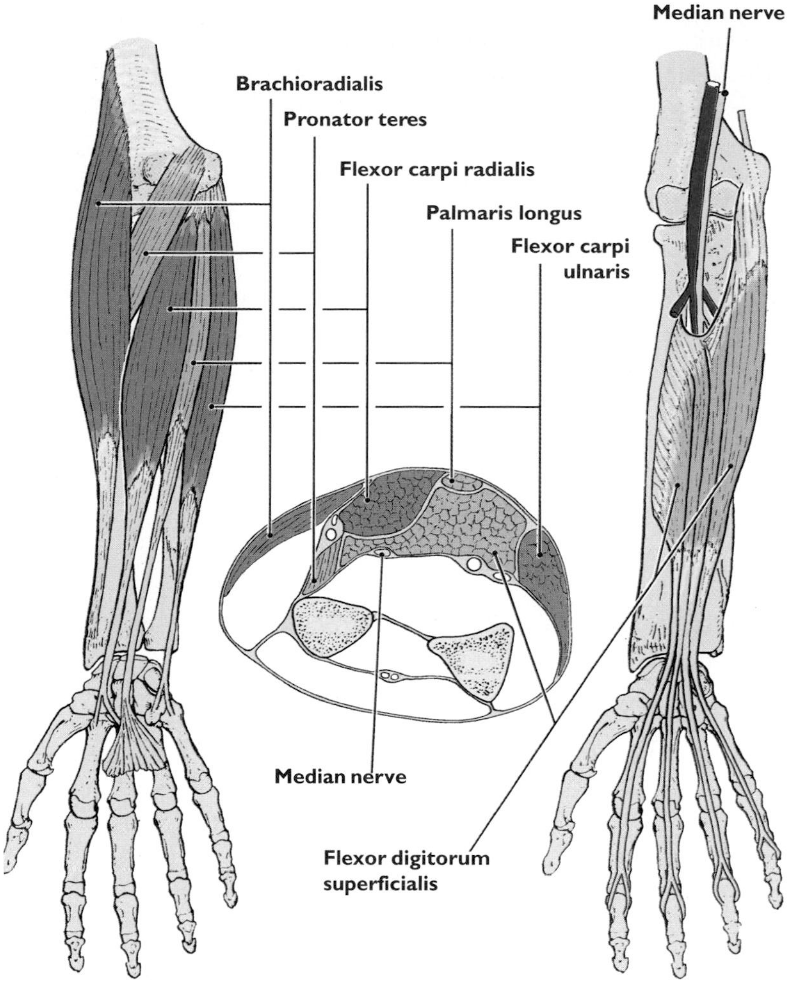

Figure 6.31. Superficial layers of anterior forearm muscles.

- The four tendons of the **flexor digitorum superficialis** (sublimis);
- **Ulnar artery** and **ulnar nerve**;
- Tendon of **flexor carpi ulnaris.**

> ***Clinical Correlation:*** Palpate these structures in your own wrist. Do you have a palmaris longus? Feel the pulse in the radial artery. Point to the site of the median nerve. Note that this important nerve can be easily injured in the wrist region. Palpate the insertion of the flexor carpi ulnaris tendon into the pisiform bone, and through it to the pisohamate and pisocarpal ligaments. In reference to the pisiform bone, where do you expect to find the ulnar nerve and artery?

Now, examine the **most superficial layer of the anterior forearm muscles** (Fig. 6.31):

- **Brachioradialis**;
- **Pronator teres**;

⇦
GRANT'S 6.55
ROHEN 366
A.D.A.M. 6.41
NETTER 416
CLEMENTE 63

- **Flexor carpi radialis**;
- **Palmaris longus**;
- **Flexor carpi ulnaris**.

⇨
GRANT'S 6.56
ROHEN 398
A.D.A.M. 6.41, 6.42
NETTER 417
CLEMENTE 64
A.V.A. 1: 0.57.26

Identify the **brachioradialis.** This muscle is a flexor of the elbow joint. Open the furrow medial to the brachioradialis. There, identify the **superficial branch of the radial nerve**. Follow the nerve proximally to the point where it arises from the radial nerve. Note that the **radial nerve** divides into its two end branches, **superficial branch** and **deep branch.** The deep branch and its relations will be examined later.

In the cubital region, pick up the **brachial artery.** Trace it distally to its subdivision into **ulnar and radial arteries**. Close to the origin of the radial artery, look for the radial recurrent artery. It is part of the anastomotic network around the elbow (Fig. 6.26). Follow the radial artery inferiorly to the wrist. Look for muscular branches. Note that no motor nerve crosses the radial artery; therefore, the course of the radial artery indicates a convenient "internervous line" where surgeons may incise to reach deeper parts of the forearm.

GRANT'S 6.56
ROHEN 396, 3.97
A.D.A.M. 6.43
NETTER 417
CLEMENTE 63, 64

In the cubital region, pick up the **median nerve**. It supplies most muscles of the flexor region of the forearm (Fig. 6.32). Observe that these branches arise from the medial side of the median nerve. Study a transverse section through the forearm (Figs. 6.27, 6.31, 6.33). Verify, on transverse section, that the median nerve runs in the plane between deep and superficial flexors. Correlate your anatomical observations with a transverse MRI of the forearm.

GRANT'S 6.56
ROHEN 397, 399
A.D.A.M. 6.43
NETTER 418
CLEMENTE 65
A.V.A. 1: 1.10.46, 1.56.35

To expose the median nerve, the most superficial layer of anterior forearm muscles must be reflected. Proceed as follows:

- Cut the tendon of **palmaris longus** about 3 cm proximal to the wrist; reflect it.
- Sever the **flexor carpi radialis** tendon about 5 cm proximal to the wrist; reflect it.

Now, the **flexor digitorum superficialis** (sublimis) is fully exposed (Fig. 6.31). This muscle constitutes the second layer of the superficial muscles of the anterior forearm. Pull on its four tendons and observe that the middle phalanges of fingers 2 to 5 are flexed. Note that the flexor digitorum superficialis is attached to the common flexor origin and to the anterior oblique line of the radius. Proceed as follows:

GRANT'S 6.56
ROHEN 398
NETTER 417
CLEMENTE 64
A.V.A. 1: 2.02.16

GRANT'S 6.56
ROHEN 399
A.D.A.M. 6.43
NETTER 445
CLEMENTE 65, 66
A.V.A. 1: 1.36.28

- Using scissors, detach the superficialis from the radius. Reflect the muscle medially.
- Identify the **pronator teres.** Understand its function of pronation. Divide this muscle close to its insertion into the radius.
- Observe the **median nerve** clinging to the deep surface of the flexor digitorum superficialis.
- Using a probe, free the median nerve and identify its muscular branches to palmaris longus, flexor carpi radialis, flexor digitorum superficialis, and pronator teres (Fig. 6.32).

GRANT'S 6.55
ROHEN 398
A.D.A.M. 6.41
NETTER 416
CLEMENTE 63
A.V.A. 1: 2.04.12

GRANT'S 6.5, 6.6C
ROHEN 375
NETTER 405, 418
CLEMENTE 43, 65, 68
A.V.A. 1: 0.59.10

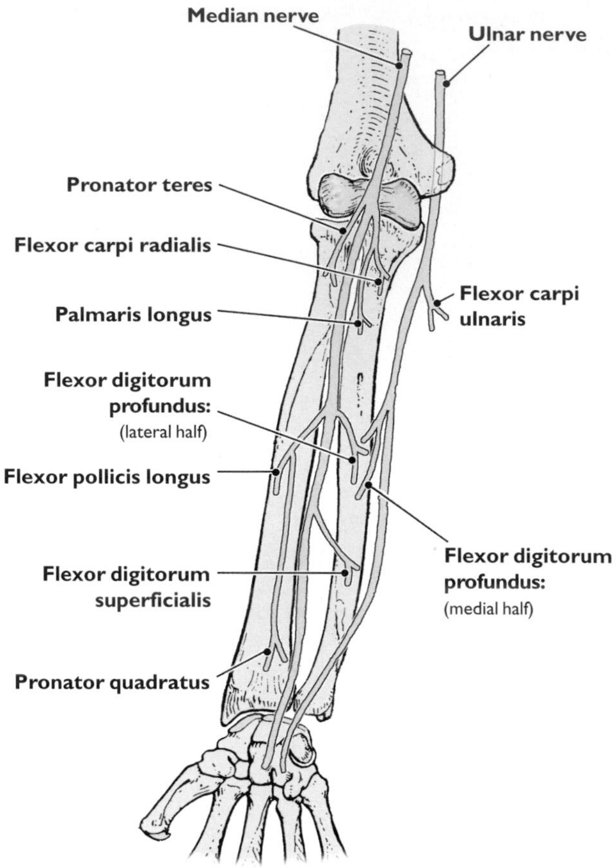

Figure 6.32. Scheme of motor innervation of anterior forearm muscles.

- Identify the **ulnar nerve** and follow it proximally to the elbow joint. Verify that the ulnar nerve sends a motor branch to the flexor carpi ulnaris (Fig. 6.32). The ulnar nerve branch to the medial half of the flexor digitorum profundus may be difficult to follow at this time.

With the flexor digitorum superficialis reflected, study the **ulnar artery** and its main branches. First, establish the continuity of the ulnar artery from cubital fossa to wrist. Note that the vessel passes deep to the flexor digitorum superficialis to reach the ulnar (medial) side of the forearm (Fig. 6.33). Refer to diagrams. Study the distribution of the **common interosseous artery.** Identify this vessel in the cadaver. The **anterior interosseous artery** descends on the anterior surface of the interosseous membrane. It gives off branches to the deep flexors and nutrient branches to the bones. Arterial twigs pierce the interosseous membrane to supply

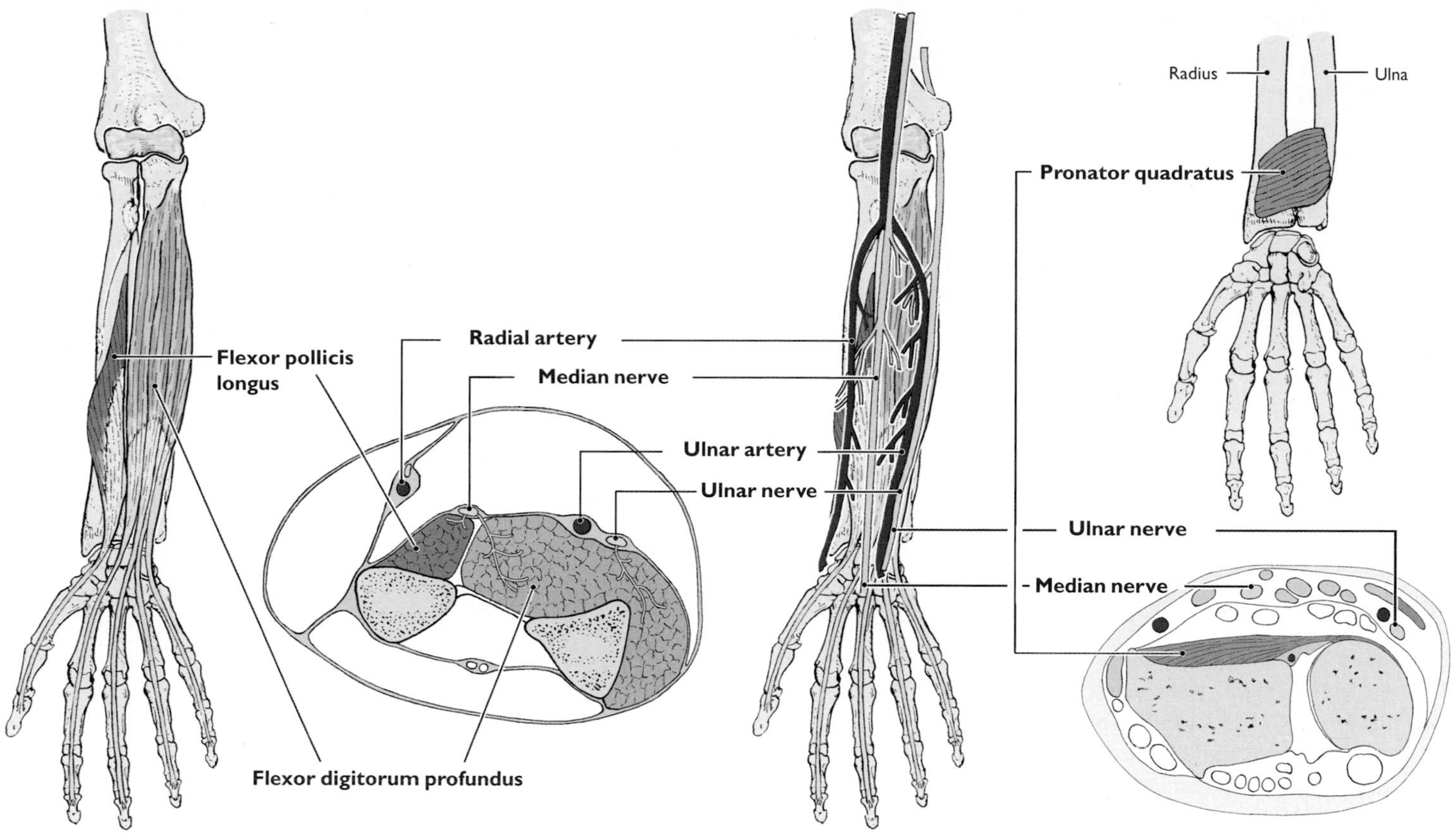

Figure 6.33. Deep layers of anterior forearm muscles.

the extensors. The **posterior interosseous artery** reaches the posterior aspect of the forearm and the extensor muscles. Identify the interosseous arteries.

GRANT'S 6.58
ROHEN 399
A.D.A.M. 6.10, 6.43
NETTER 418
CLEMENTE 62
A.V.A. 1: 1.35.55, 1.40.58

> ***Clinical Correlation:*** Occasionally (in about 3% of cases), the ulnar artery arises high from the brachial artery. When it does so, it runs almost invariably superficial to the flexor muscles. The artery may be mistaken for a vein. If certain drugs are injected into this vessel, the result may be disastrous: gangrene with subsequent partial or total loss of the hand.

The ulnar artery is joined by the **ulnar nerve**. Follow the nerve proximally and observe that it passes deep to the junction of the two heads of the flexor carpi ulnaris. Note the motor branch to this muscle. Verify that the ulnar nerve lies in a groove between the olecranon and the medial epicondyle. Here, the nerve is covered only by skin and fascia. In yourself, palpate the nerve. Understand the meaning of the popular term "funny bone."

GRANT'S 6.56
A.D.A.M. 375
NETTER 418
CLEMENTE 66, 67
A.V.A. 1: 2.04.12

GRANT'S 6.68
ROHEN 368, 371
A.D.A.M. 6.9, 6.43
NETTER 410, 418
CLEMENTE 65, 83
A.V.A. 1: 0.59.47

Study the **three deep flexor muscles** of the **forearm: flexor digitorum profundus, flexor pollicis longus,** and **pronator quadratus** (Fig. 6.33).

Pull on the tendon of the **flexor digitorum profundus** and observe the resulting flexion of the distal phalanges of digits 2 to 5. The profundus muscle receives a dual nerve supply from both the median and the ulnar nerve. Find the nerve branch of the median nerve that supplies the lateral half to the muscle. Similarly, identify the nerve branch from the ulnar nerve to the medial half of the flexor digitorum profundus. Pull on the tendon of the **flexor pollicis longus** and observe the resulting flexion of the distal phalanx of the 1st digit (thumb). The **pronator quadratus** runs transversely from ulna to radius in the inferior quarter of the forearm. Identify it.

Review the layers of the anterior forearm muscles and their nerve supply. The next objective is to follow tendons, nerves, and arteries from the forearm into the palm of the hand.

Palm of the Hand

General Remarks

There are two superficial muscle masses in the hand: the **thenar group** forming the ball of the thumb, and the **hypothenar musculature** forming the ball of the little (5th) finger. In the middle of the palm is a thick fibrous sheet, the palmar aponeurosis. Deep to the palmar aponeurosis are the tendons of the deep and superficial digital flexors. These tendons reach the palm through the carpal tunnel. Deep in the palm is a series of small muscles.

⇦ *GRANT'S 6.59A* A.D.A.M. 6.1 NETTER 428 CLEMENTE 40

The palm is supplied with blood by two arterial arches: the superficial arch is mainly derived from the ulnar artery and the deep arch from the radial artery. The nerve supply of the palmar (or volar) aspect of the hand is derived from the median and ulnar nerves.

Bony Landmarks

Refer to an articulated skeleton of the hand. As a group, identify the **eight carpal bones** (Fig. 6.34). Distal to the **carpus** (Gr. *karpos*, wrist) are the **five metacarpal bones.** Distal to the metacarpals are the **phalanges.** The thumb (digit 1) has only two phalanges: a proximal one and a distal one. Fingers 2 through 5 have three phalanges: proximal, middle, and distal.

⇦ *GRANT'S 6.81* ROHEN 354, 355 A.D.A.M. 6.5, 6.6 NETTER 426 CLEMENTE 112, 114 A.V.A. 1: 0.49.32, 1.17.25

Be able to **identify the eight carpal bones** in the articulated skeleton (Fig. 6.34). Identify the **pisiform bone** and the **hook of the hamate** on the medial side of the carpus. On the lateral side of the carpus, identify the **tubercle of the scaphoid** and the **tubercle of the trapezium.** These bony landmarks on both sides of the carpus are bridged by a thick fibrous band, the **flexor retinaculum (transverse carpal ligament).** Between carpal bones and flexor retinaculum is an important space, the **carpal tunnel** (Fig. 6.35). The carpal tunnel contains the median nerve and several tendons.

Note that the **scaphoid** and **lunate** are supported by the radius (Fig. 6.34). By necessity, any transmission of force from hand to forearm or vice versa must pass through these two carpal bones. This is a fact of clinical significance. Study a radiograph of the hand.

Structures of Palm of Hand

Before You Begin ...

The palmar aponeurosis and the flexor retinaculum will be examined. The ulnar nerve and artery will be traced into the palm. The carpal tunnel will be opened and its contents, the median nerve and the long flexor tendons, will be followed into the palm and on to the digits. Subsequently, the long flexor muscles will be severed and re-

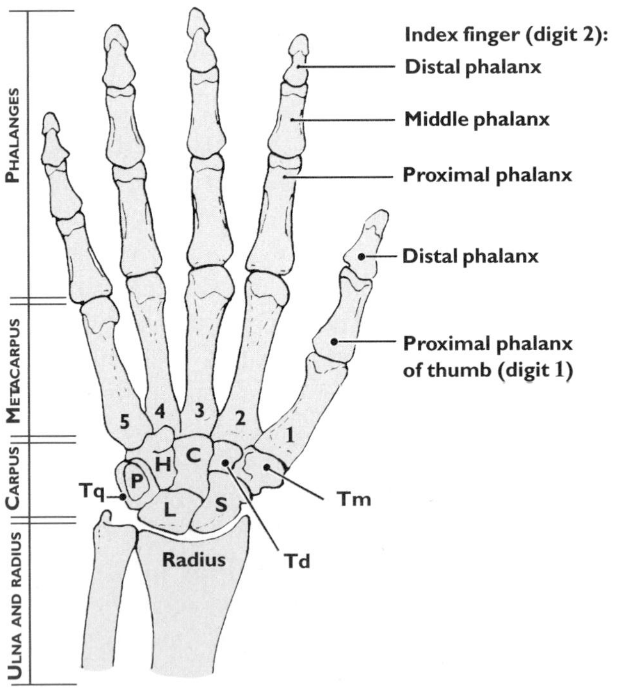

Figure 6.34. Important bony landmarks of the hand. The eight carpal bones include a distal row of four bones (*H*, hamate; *C*, capitate: *Td*, trapezoid; *Tm*, trapezium) and a proximal row of four bones (*Tq*, triquetrum; *P*, pisiform; *L*, lunate; *S*, scaphoid).

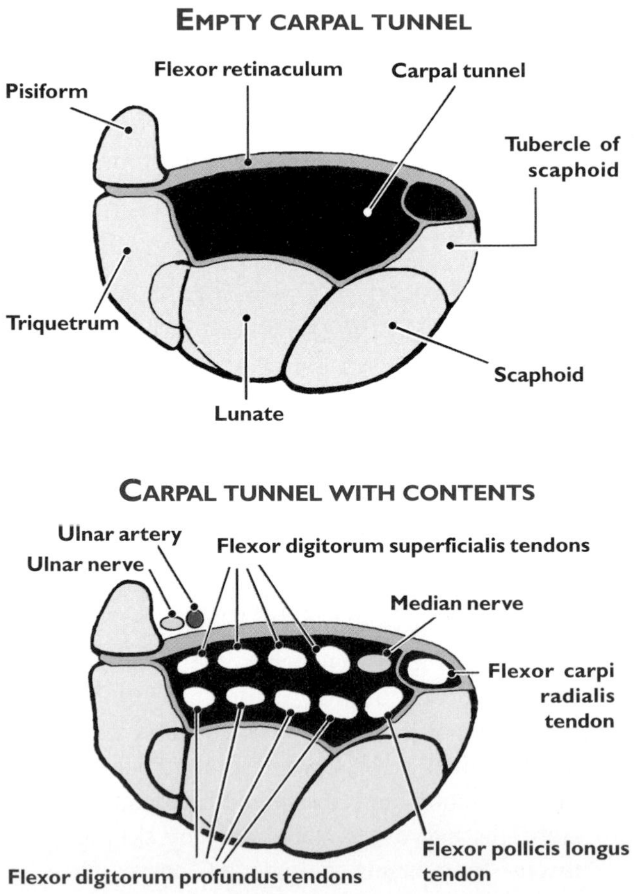

Figure 6.35. Transverse section through the right carpal tunnel.

flected distally. This procedure will allow convenient access to the deep structures of the palm (muscles, deep palmar arch, and deep branch of ulnar nerve).

Identify the **palmaris longus muscle**. It is absent in about 10-14% of cases. Follow the palmaris longus tendon distally into the palm and into the palmar aponeurosis. Clean the **palmar aponeurosis**. Observe four longitudinal bands of aponeurosis, one to each finger.

GRANT'S 6.55
ROHEN 366
A.D.A.M. 6.9
NETTER 416
CLEMENTE 60
A.V.A. 1: 1.03.14

Clinical Correlation: Nodular and fibrotic changes of the palmar aponeurosis may lead to a pulling down of one or more fingers via the longitudinal bands of the aponeurosis. This condition is known as Dupuytren's contracture.

Lateral to the palmar aponeurosis observe the fascia enveloping the **thenar muscles.** The palmaris brevis muscle arises from the medial aspect of the aponeurosis. Identify it.

GRANT'S 6.63
ROHEN 398
A.D.A.M. 6.55
NETTER 428
CLEMENTE 80
A.V.A. 1: 1.50.45

Carefully remove the palmar aponeurosis. Do not damage nerves and blood vessels deep to it. Detach the palmaris brevis from the palmar aponeurosis and reflect it medially. Now, the ulnar artery and nerve can be freely followed into the palm.

Study the arteries of the **superficial palmar arch** (Fig. 6.36). Identify the pisiform bone and verify that the ulnar artery and nerve lie lateral to it (anatomical position). Follow the **ulnar artery** into the palm. Dissect the superficial palmar arch and the digital arteries springing from it. Subsequently, dissect the **ulnar nerve.** Clean its **superficial branch,** which supplies the 5th and the medial part of the 4th finger. The **deep branch of the ulnar nerve** disappears under cover of two of the hypothenar muscles. Identify its initial portion. Note that it passes deep into the hand. Do not trace the deep branch of the ulnar nerve at this time.

GRANT'S 6.63
ROHEN 400
A.D.A.M. 6.55
NETTER 429
CLEMENTE 88
A.V.A. 1: 1.59.34

Review the flexor retinaculum and its role in the formation of the carpal tunnel (Fig. 6.35). Identify the **flexor retinaculum**. Starting at the forearm and wrist section, push a probe deep to the retinaculum through the **carpal tunnel** (Fig. 6.37). With a scalpel, cut through the retinaculum down onto the probe. This procedure will prevent injury to the contents of the carpal tunnel. Reflect the flexor retinaculum and open the carpal tunnel. Examine the **contents of the carpal tunnel** (Fig. 6.37). It consists of the median nerve and several digital flexor tendons.

GRANT'S 6.63, 6.65A
ROHEN 404, 405
A.D.A.M. 6.55
NETTER 435
CLEMENTE 88, 89
A.V.A. 1: 2.02.17

GRANT'S 6.66A, 6.67
ROHEN 405, 406
A.D.A.M. 6.58
NETTER 424, 430, 431
CLEMENTE 82, 83
A.V.A. 1: 1.28.20

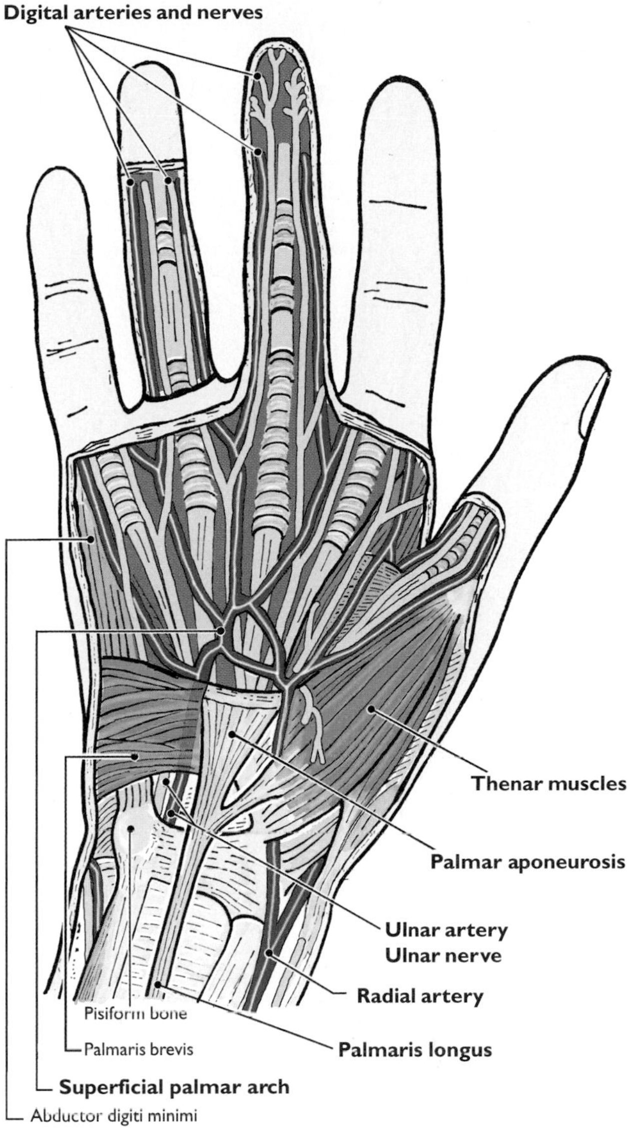

Figure 6.36. Superficial dissection of the palm.

Examine the extent of the synovial tendon sheaths deep to the retinaculum. The synovial sheaths can be more clearly demonstrated if phenol or water is injected; check with your instructor.

Dissect the **median nerve** and its branches (Fig. 6.38). Trace the small but important **recurrent branch of the median nerve** to the thenar muscles. The only two other muscles supplied by the median nerve in the hand are the 1st and 2nd lumbricals. Attempt to locate these two small muscular branches. Subsequently, follow the **digital branches** of the median nerve to the first 3½ digits. Study the cutaneous nerve supply of hand and fingers. Be aware of variations. Consult a useful diagram.

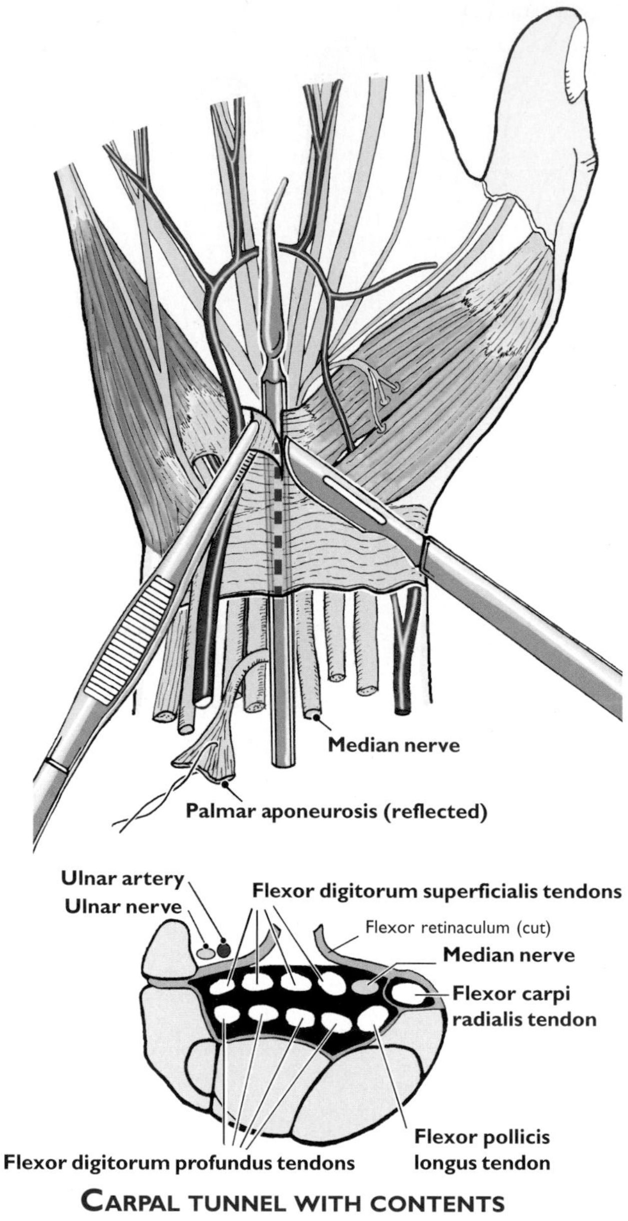

Figure 6.37. Opening of the carpal tunnel. The inserted probe protects the contents.

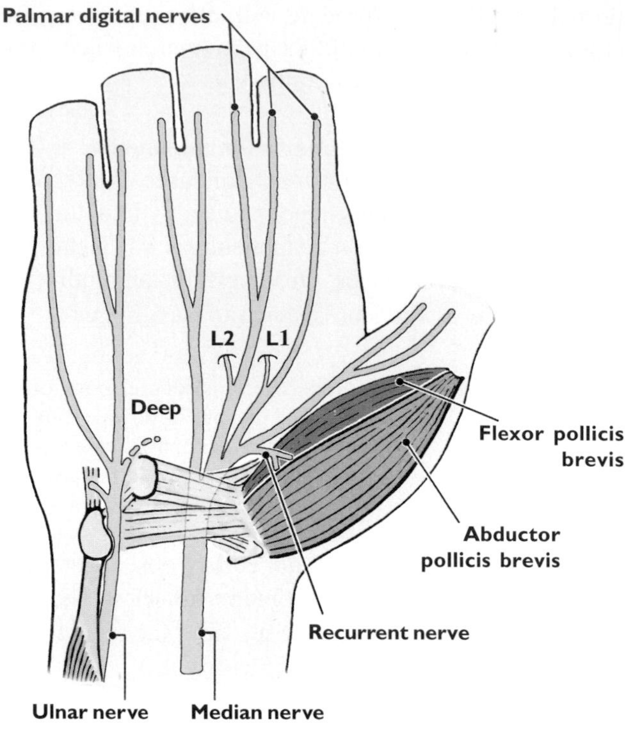

Figure 6.38. Essential nerves of the hand: median and ulnar nerves (*L1* and *L2*, lumbrical branches of median nerve).

> ***Clinical Correlation:*** The recurrent branch of the median nerve lies superficial. Therefore, it can be easily severed during "minor" cuts. If the nerve is injured, the thenar muscles are paralyzed and the thumb loses much of its usefulness. In the emergency room, never belittle superficial cuts over the thenar region. Always test the thenar muscles to make sure the important recurrent branch of the median nerve is intact.

Thenar Muscles (Gr., *thenar*, hand). Examine the three thenar muscles (Fig. 6.38):

- **Abductor pollicis brevis** (L. *pollex*, thumb; genitive, *pollicis*); raise the superficial muscle; sever it in the middle;
- **Opponens pollicis;** deep to the severed abductor;
- **Flexor pollicis brevis;** note the recurrent branch of the median nerve crossing over it.

GRANT'S 6.65A, 6.66A
ROHEN 405, 406
A.D.A.M. 6.56
NETTER 429, 434
CLEMENTE 89, 90
A.V.A. 1: 1.51.00

Hypothenar muscles. Identify:

GRANT'S 6.65A, 6.66A
ROHEN 405, 406
A.D.A.M. 6.56
NETTER 429, 430
CLEMENTE 89, 90
A.V.A. 1: 1.52.10

- **Abductor digiti quinti,** arising from the pisiform bone (Fig. 6.36);
- **Opponens digiti quinti;**
- **Flexor digiti quinti,** sometimes absent.

GRANT'S 6.66A
ROHEN 366, 367
A.D.A.M. 6.55, 6.56
NETTER 429
CLEMENTE 81
A.V.A. 1: 1.30.24

Clean the **fibrous digital sheaths** of the tendons (Fig. 6.39). Understand that the fibrous digital sheath and the phalangeal bones together form an **osseofibrous digital tunnel**. In this tunnel, the long flexor tendons are housed.

Turn your attention to the long flexor tendons that traverse the carpal tunnel. Note that these tendons are surrounded by synovial sheaths. These sheaths are lubricating devices. There are two sets of synovial sheaths:

- **Common synovial sheath** (sac) of the palm, within the carpal tunnel, and extending proximally and distally to it;

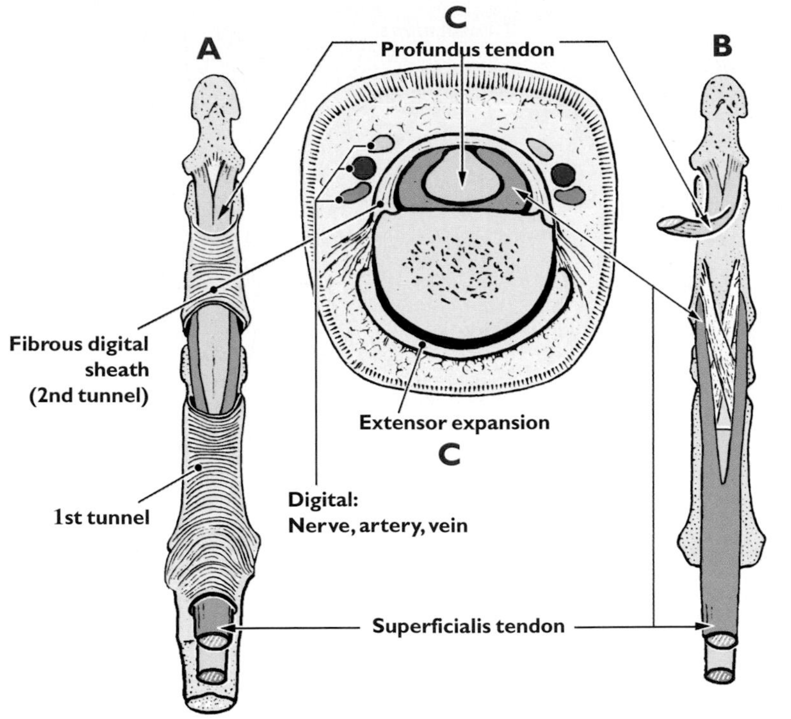

Figure 6.39. Long flexor tendons and their fibrous sheaths. ***A,*** fibrous digital flexor sheath showing the two osseofibrous tunnels; ***B,*** mode of insertion of the long digital flexors; ***C,*** transverse section of a finger showing the osseofibrous tunnel with tendons in it.

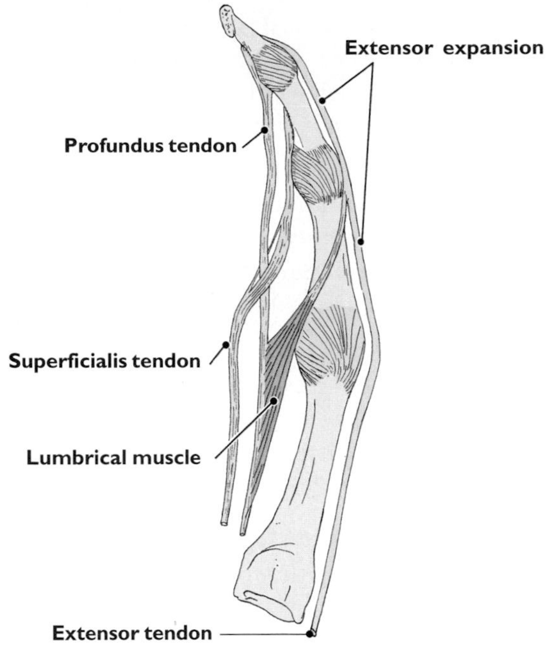

Figure 6.40. The profundus tendon pierces the superficialis tendon. The lumbrical muscles originate from the profundus tendon and insert into the extensor expansion.

- **Digital synovial sheaths,** within the osseofibrous digital tunnels; in most cases, the digital sheath of the little finger and thumb are connected to the common synovial sheath of the palm.

Clinical Correlation: Frequently, bacterial infection involves the synovial sheaths (bacterial tenosynovitis). The constant movements of the tendons within the synovial sheaths further enhance the spread of infection. Understand that a minor infection of the 5th finger may spread along the flexor tendon sheath, involve the common synovial sheath in the palm, and finally reach the thumb.

A swelling of the common synovial sheath (as in the nonbacterial tenosynovitis) may encroach on the available space in the carpal tunnel. As a result, movements of the flexor tendons are interfered with and the median nerve may be compressed (carpal tunnel syndrome; pain and paresthesia of thumb, index finger, and middle finger; weakness of thenar muscles). With these clinical comments in mind, study again the contents of the carpal tunnel (Figs. 6.35, 6.37).

With your fingers in the anterior forearm region, separate the **flexor digitorum superficialis** from the **profundus.** Cut across the fleshy part of the superficialis. Reflect the tendons distally. During this procedure, the common synovial sheath will be destroyed. To reflect the tendons even further, slit open the 1st osseofibrous tunnels of digits 2 through 5 (Fig. 6.39).

Now, the **flexor digitorum profundus** is exposed. Identify the four small **lumbrical muscles** originating from the profundus tendons (Fig. 6.40). Note that these muscles lie on the *radial* side of the corresponding digit. They insert into the dorsal or **extensor expansion** of the digits. Thus, they flex the metacarpophalangeal joints and extend the interphalangeal joints.

On the middle digit, open the fibrous digital sheath. Study the interactions of the tendons of flexor digitorum superficialis and profundus (Fig. 6.40). Note that the profundus tendon pierces the superficialis tendon. Verify that the superficialis tendon acts on the middle phalanx, whereas the profundus tendon acts on the distal phalanx of fingers 2 through 5.

⇦
GRANT'S 6.66
ROHEN 368, 369
A.D.A.M. 6.55, 6.56
NETTER 429-431
CLEMENTE 81, 88
A.V.A. 1: 1.37.20

⇨
GRANT'S 6.68, 6.69
ROHEN 370
A.D.A.M. 6.56
NETTER 432
CLEMENTE 82
A.V.A. 1: 1.49.22

⇨
GRANT'S 6.69
ROHEN 370, 371
A.D.A.M. 6.56
NETTER 433
CLEMENTE 83, 84
A.V.A. 1: 1.37.44

Now, identify the **flexor pollicis longus**. Leave it intact. Follow the tendon proximally through the carpal tunnel into the forearm. Observe that it is supplied by a branch of the median nerve.

Grant's 6.67A
Rohen 366, 368, 370
A.D.A.M. 6.55, 6.56
Netter 430, 431
Clemente 81, 83
A.V.A. 1: 1.40.58

Cut across the fleshy fibers of the **flexor digitorum profundus.** Reflect its tendons and the associated lumbricals as far distally as possible. Now, the **pronator quadratus** of the anterior forearm region is in full view, and the deep palmar space is exposed.

Grant's 6.68
Rohen 371
A.D.A.M. 6.57
Netter 410, 431
Clemente 83

Deep Structures in the Palm. The first objective is to follow the deep branches of the ulnar nerve and artery deep into the palm (Figs. 6.41, 6.42).

Grant's 6.68
Rohen 400
A.D.A.M. 6.57
Netter 434
Clemente 90
A.V.A. 1: 2.04.58

- Detach the flexor digiti quinti from the flexor retinaculum. Push a probe parallel to the ulnar nerve and accompanying ulnar artery as they pierce the opponens digiti quinti. Carefully remove the muscle tissue anterior to the nerve.
- Follow the **deep branch of the ulnar nerve** across the deep structures of the palm.
- Identify and clean the triangular **adductor pollicis**. This muscle draws the thumb toward the palm, a movement of considerable importance (see Fig. 6.43).
- Note the arteries of the **deep palmar arch**.

Identify the three **palmar interossei muscles** originating from the metacarpal bones of digits 2, 4, and 5.

Grant's 6.68, 6.69A
Rohen 370, 400
A.D.A.M. 6.12, 6.57
Netter 434, 435
Clemente 87, 90
A.V.A. 1: 1.42.20

- Note that the palmar interossei are inserted into the bases of the proximal phalanges and into the dorsal expansions.
- Understand the actions of these muscles (Fig. 6.43). They are adductors; they adduct the fingers toward an imaginary line drawn through the long axis of the middle finger.

Identify the four **dorsal interossei muscles**. Turn to the dosum of the hand and note that these muscles occupy the intervals between the metacarpal bones (Fig. 6.43).

Grant's 6.68, 6.69B
Rohen 370, 400
A.D.A.M. 6.12, 6.57
Netter 434
Clemente 86, 90
A.V.A. 1: 1.42.20

- Remove the fascia covering the muscles. The thin tendons of the dorsal interossei muscles insert into the extensor expansion.
- Understand the action of the muscles. They abduct the fingers from an imaginary line drawn through the axis of the middle finger.

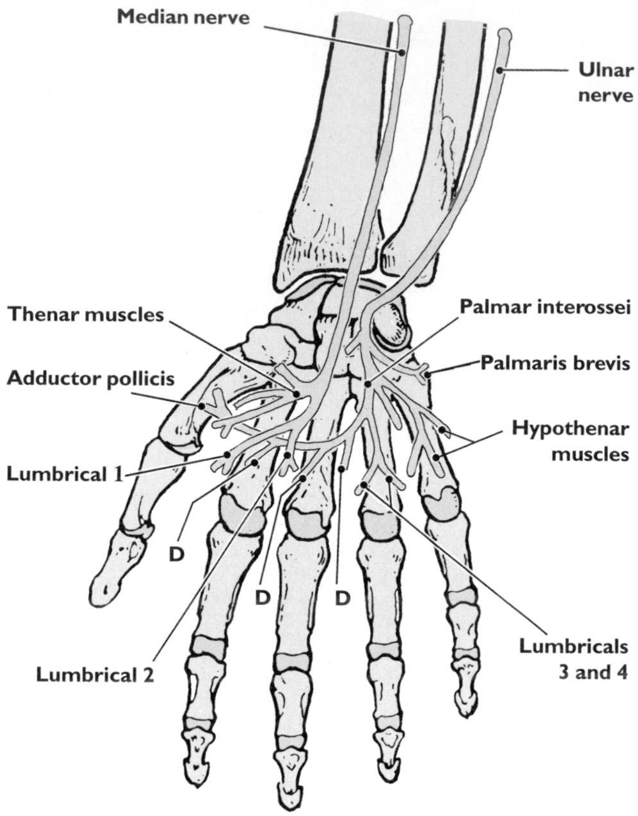

Figure 6.41. Ulnar and median nerve branches in palm of hand. Note that all seven interossei muscles are supplied by the ulnar nerve. D = Dorsal interossei.

The four dorsal interossei abduct. The three palmar interossei adduct. All seven interossei are supplied by the ulnar nerve (Fig. 6.41). That means: if the ulnar nerve is paralyzed, abduction, adduction, and full extension of the fingers is impossible.

Review the movements of fingers and thumb. Define flexion, extension, abduction, and adduction (Fig. 6.44). Which muscles are responsible for flexion? Which muscles are responsible for adduction of the fingers? Can you name the nerves that innervate these respective muscles? Review the motor branches of the median and ulnar nerves in the palm of the hand (Fig. 6.41).

Extensor Region of Forearm and Dorsum of Hand

General Remarks

The extensor muscles of the forearm can be divided into a superficial group and a deep group (see Fig. 6.45). The **superficial extensors** arise mainly on the lateral side of the elbow region; i.e., from the lateral epicondyle, supracondy-

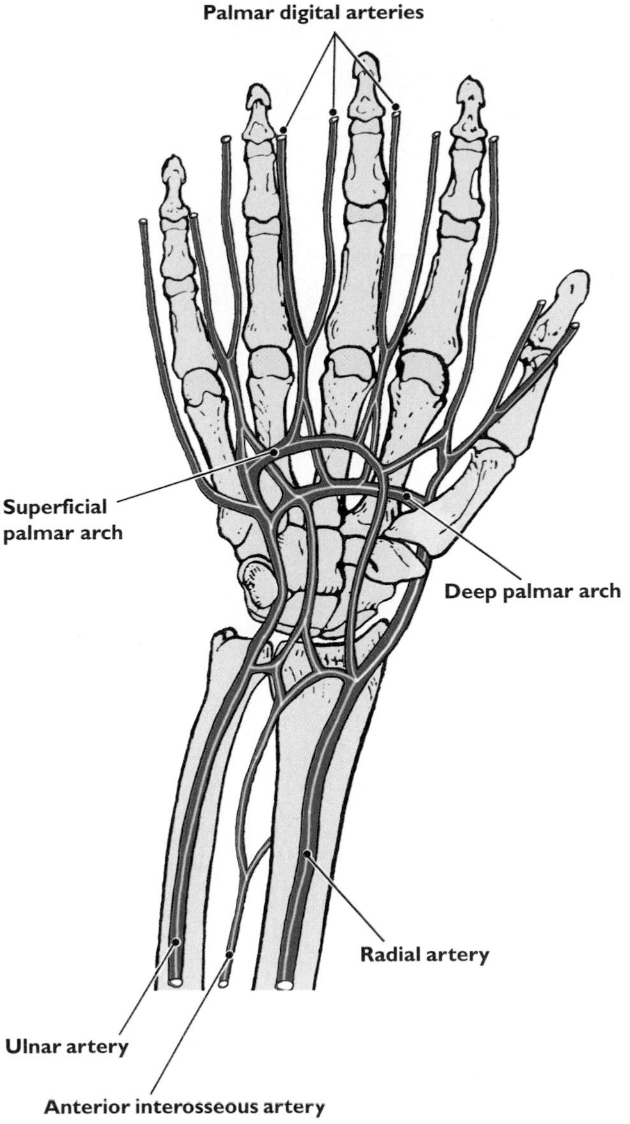

Figure 6.42. Palmar arterial arches.

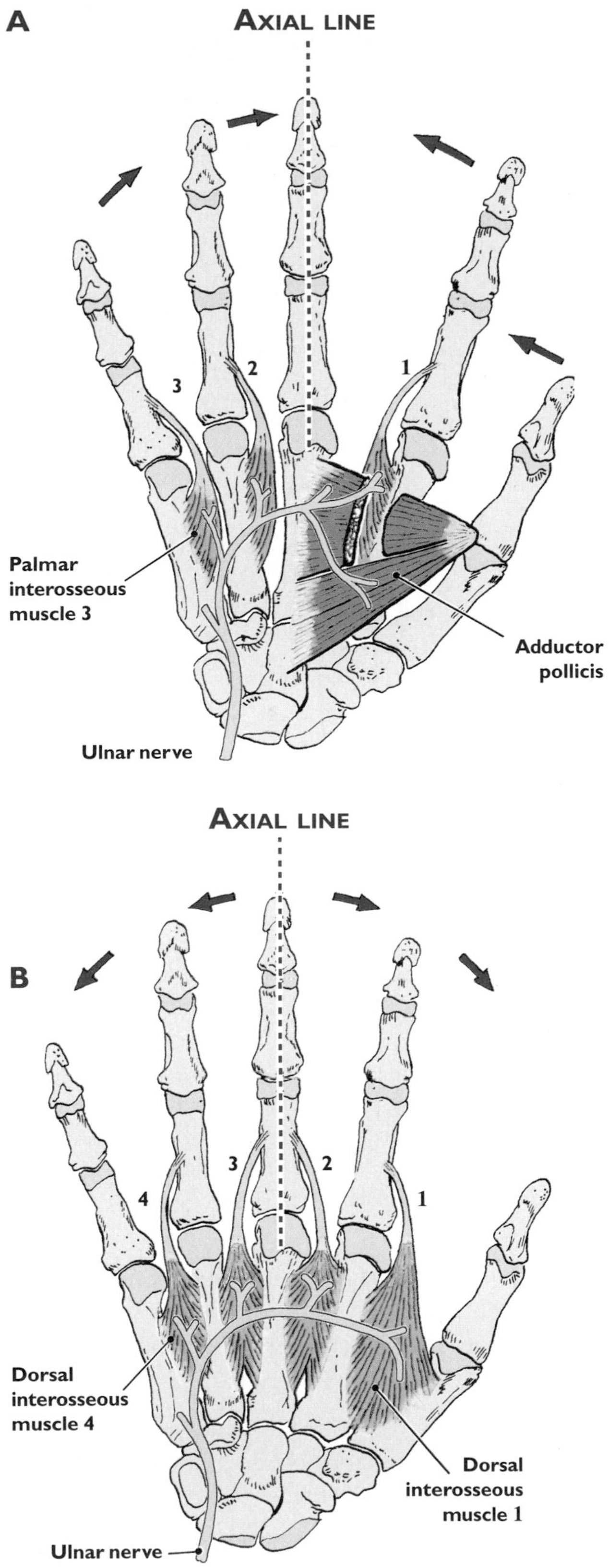

Figure 6.43. ***A,*** The three unipennate palmar interossei muscles and the adductor pollicis adduct the fingers in relation to the axial line. ***B,*** The four bipennate dorsal interossei muscles abduct the fingers. All muscles are supplied by the ulnar nerve.

lar ridge, and posterior border of the ulna. The tendons of these muscles reach across the posterior aspect of the wrist from side to side. They extend the carpus and the proximal phalanges.

The **deep extensors** arise mainly from the ulna and the posterior aspect of the interosseous membrane. This deep layer is chiefly concerned with supination of the radius and reposition of the thumb into the anatomical position.

The extensors are supplied by the deep branch of the radial nerve, the posterior interosseous nerve. Nerve and vessels of the extensor compartment run in the plane dividing the superficial from the deep group (Fig. 6.45).

On the back of the hand, the bones are almost superficial. There are no fleshy extensor fibers here; accordingly, no motor nerve supply is required. The cutaneous nerve supply to the back of the hand is shared by the radial, ulnar, and median nerves. Variations in the pattern of the cutaneous nerve supply are common.

⇦
GRANT'S 6.70, 6.73, 6.76
ROHEN 394
A.D.A.M. 6.51
NETTER 414, 439
CLEMENTE 71, 77

⇦
GRANT'S 6.72
ROHEN 392, 394
A.D.A.M. 6.19
NETTER 437, 441
CLEMENTE 39, 76

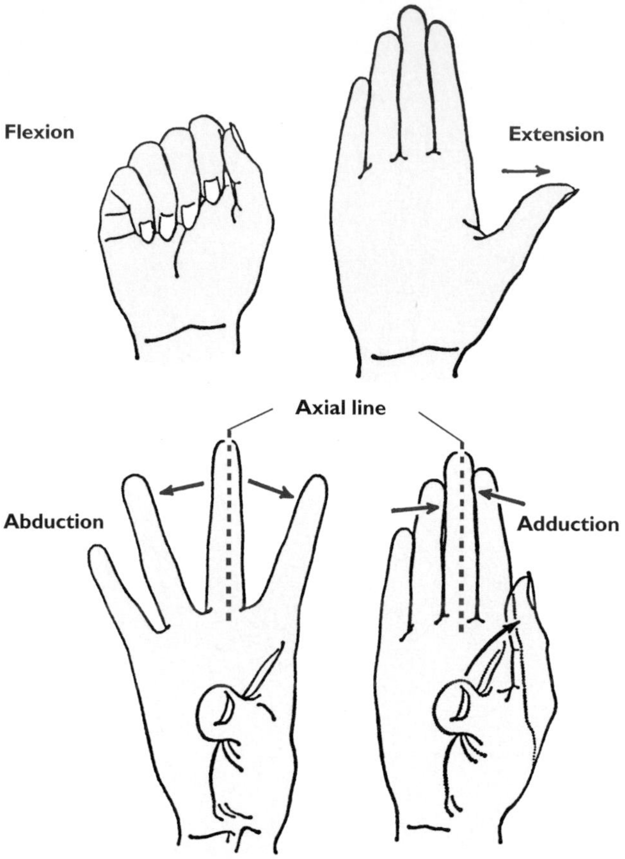

Figure 6.44. Movements of fingers and thumb.

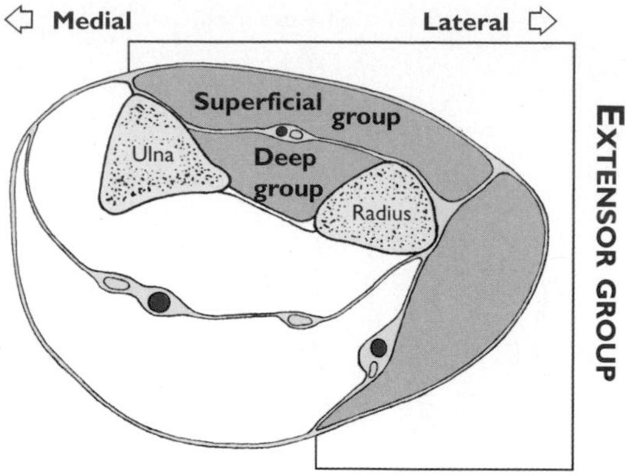

Figure 6.45. Extensor muscles of the forearm on transverse section.

Structures

Before You Begin ...

First, the anatomical "snuff box" will be defined and studied. Next, the superficial posterior forearm muscles will be identified and their tendons will be followed distally. Subsequently, the deep (outcropping) extensor muscles will be studied.

Anatomical "Snuff Box." Study its surface anatomy. Palpate it in a living person. Feel the pulsations of the radial artery within its boundaries.

In the cadaver, define the tendons that constitute the boundaries of the triangular "anatomical snuff box" (Fig. 6.46).

- The **abductor pollicis longus** and **extensor pollicis brevis** bound the snuff box anteriorly (*note the anatomical position*).
- The **extensor pollicis longus** bounds it posteriorly. These three tendons belong to muscles of the deep extensor group.

GRANT'S 6.79
ROHEN 370
A.D.A.M. 6.47
NETTER 436, 438, 439
CLEMENTE 75, 79
A.V.A. 1: 1.42.46, 1.57.10

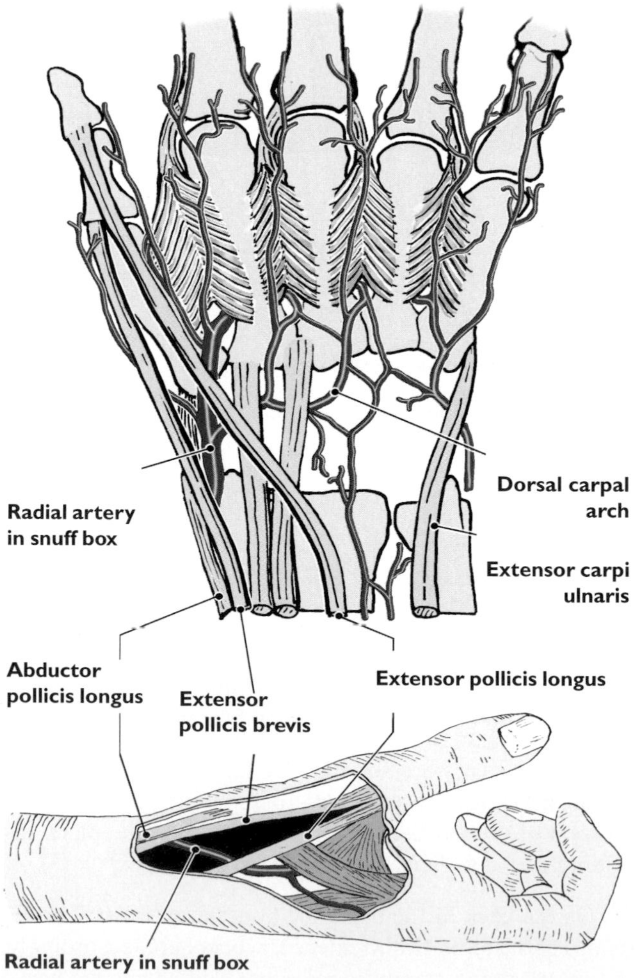

Figure 6.46. Radial artery in triangular "anatomical snuff box." Branches of radial artery on dorsum of hand (carpal bones removed.)

Clean the tendons. Deep within the snuffbox, find the **radial artery**. Trace it distally to where it disappears between the two heads of the **1st dorsal interosseous muscle.** Note that small arteries exist on the dorsum of the hand, but do not dissect them (Fig. 6.46).

⇨ *GRANT'S 6.71* ROHEN 373 A.D.A.M. TABLE 6.5 NETTER 410, 415, 447 CLEMENTE 71, 72 A.V.A. 1: 1.00.15

The deep fascia at the back of the wrist is thickened to form the **extensor retinaculum**. All tendons at the back of the wrist are enveloped in synovial sheaths; these extend distally and proximally to the extensor retinaculum.

⇦ *GRANT'S 6.70, 6.73* ROHEN 372, 373 NETTER 438, 439 CLEMENTE 77, 79 A.V.A. 1: 1.29.27

Trace the three tendons bounding the anatomical snuff box proximally into the forearm. The fleshy bellies of the corresponding muscles crop out along a furrow that divides the extensors into a lateral and a medial group. Open this furrow as far as the lateral epicondyle. In doing this, it is necessary to split the intermuscular septum between **extensor carpi radialis brevis** and **extensor digitorum.**

⇨ *GRANT'S 6.71* NETTER 415 CLEMENTE 74 A.V.A. 1: 2.01.34

⇦ *GRANT'S 6.71* ROHEN 373 A.D.A.M. 6.47 NETTER 414, 4.15 CLEMENTE 70 A.V.A. 1: 1.41.52

Identify the **supinator,** which is wrapped around the upper third of the radius. Proceed as follows:

- On the anterior aspect of the forearm, identify the deep branch of the radial nerve as it traverses the supinator.
- Push a probe along the nerve through the substance of the muscle. Turn the upper limb and look for the tip of the probe on the posterior aspect of the forearm.
- After traversing the supinator muscle, the deep branch of the radial nerve becomes the **posterior interosseous nerve.** This nerve sends motor branches to the extensor muscles. Once more, establish the continuity of the posterior interosseous nerve with the radial nerve in front of the elbow joint.

Muscles of the superficial extensor group. Identify, clean, and study the following muscles (Fig. 6.47):

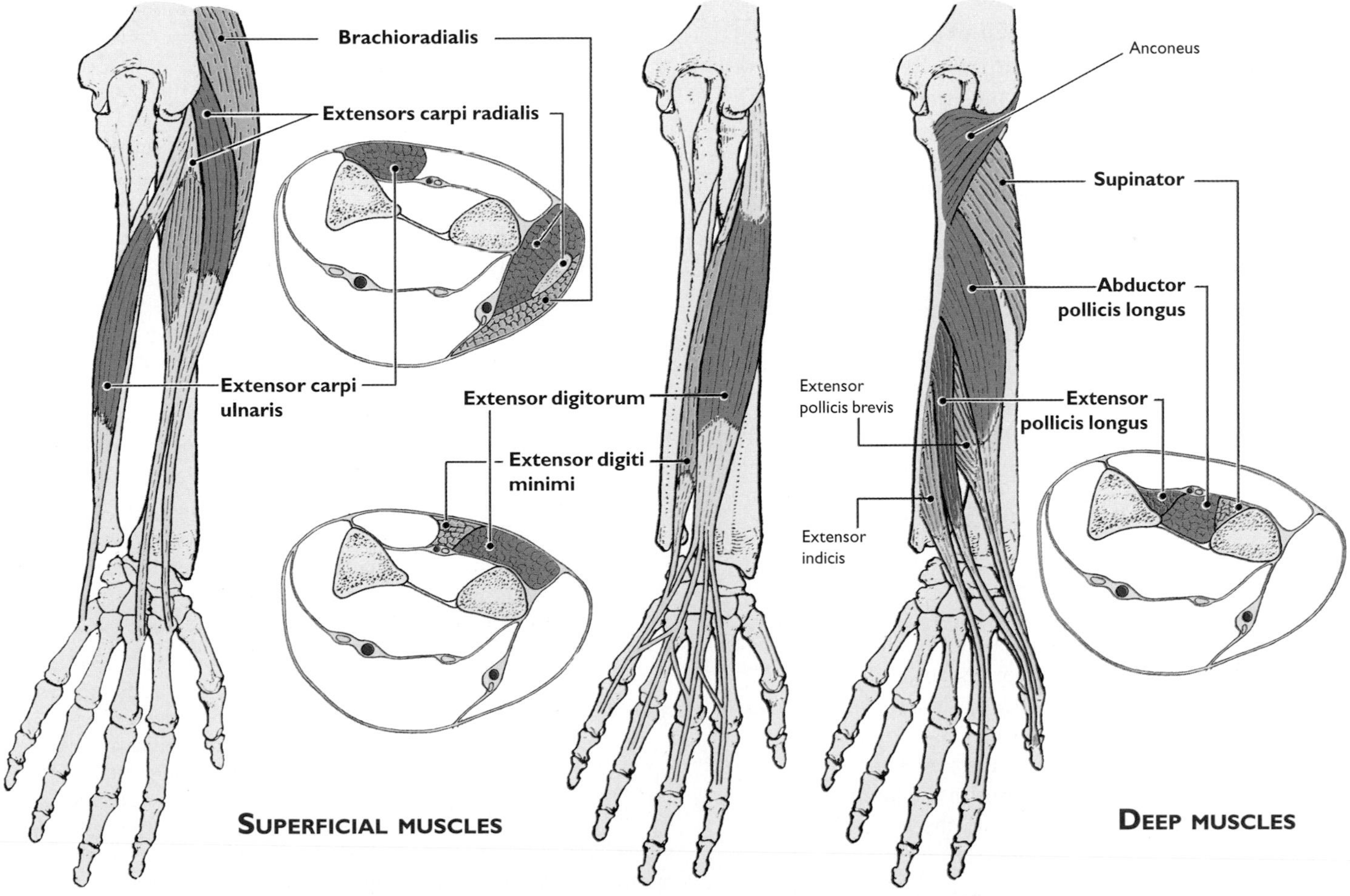

Figure 6.47. Superficial and deep muscles of the posterior forearm.

- Lateral to the outcropping of muscles of the anatomical snuff box find the **brachioradialis, extensor carpi radialis longus,** and **extensor carpi radialis brevis.**

- Medial to the outcropping muscles of the anatomical snuff box find the **extensor digitorum, extensor digiti minimi,** and **extensor carpi ulnaris.**

- Follow the flattened tendons of the **extensor digitorum** right to their insertions. Note their cross connections on the back of the hand.

- Cut through the extensor retinaculum, thus freeing the tendons of the extensor digitorum. Retract the tendons medially.

- Note that the tendons of these muscles are contained in special tunnels between the bones of the forearm and the extensor retinaculum.

- Look for **muscular branches of the radial nerve** (Fig. 6.48).

GRANT'S 6.70
ROHEN 393
A.D.A.M. 6.47
NETTER 414
CLEMENTE 69, 70
A.V.A. 1: 1.39.08

Muscles of the Deep Extensor Group. Now, the five muscles of the **deep extensor group** can be studied in their entirety. Identify, clean, and study the following muscles (Fig. 6.47):

- The three muscles bounding the snuff box (abductor pollicis longus; extensor pollicis brevis; extensor pollicis longus);

- The **supinator,** and the **extensor indicis** (i.e., the extensor for the 2nd or index finger).

- Note that the tendons of these muscles are contained in special tunnels between the bones of the forearm and the extensor retinaculum.

- Look for **muscular branches of the radial nerve** (Fig. 6.48).

GRANT'S 6.70
ROHEN 393
A.D.A.M. 6.47
NETTER 415
CLEMENTE 71, 72, 74
A.V.A. 1: 1.32.38

Extensor Expansion. The distal ends of the extensor tendons become flattened to the thickness of a tendinous sheath. This sheath is called the extensor expansion. It is wrapped around the dorsum and the sides of the proximal phalanx and the adjacent metacarpal bone. This hook-like expansion anchors the finger and retains the extensor tendon in the midline of the digit. The tendons of the lumbrical and interossei muscles are inserted into the extensor expansions.

GRANT'S 6.76-6.78
ROHEN 394
A.D.A.M. 6.47
NETTER 433
CLEMENTE 84
A.V.A. 1: 2.01.45

Review the insertions of flexor and extensor tendons into metacarpal bones and phalanges (Fig. 6.40). Note that

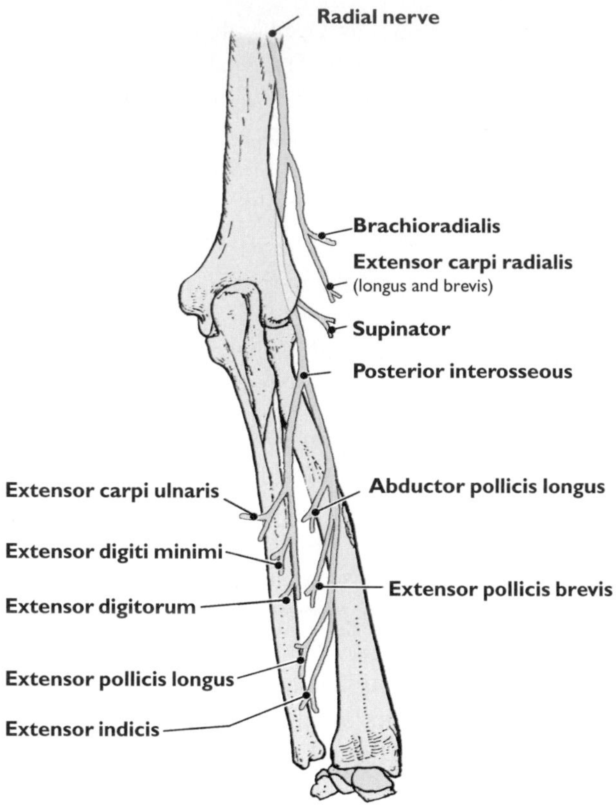

Figure 6.48. Motor distribution of the radial nerve to muscles in the posterior compartment of the forearm.

the strongest extensor tendons (extensor carpi radialis longus; extensor carpi radialis brevis; extensor carpi ulnaris) are inserted into the metacarpal bones. These three extensors of the wrist are the strongest because they work synergistically with the flexors of the digits. Understand and test on yourself: the firmly grasping hand requires an extended wrist. Review the extensor (dorsal) expansion of a finger.

GRANT'S 6.8
ROHEN 377
A.D.A.M. 6.23, 6.24
NETTER 444, 445, 447
CLEMENTE 65-67, 74

Review the **nerve territories** of the forearm (Fig. 6.49). The **median nerve** innervates the superficial and deep flexor muscles. The **ulnar nerve** supplies the flexor carpi ulnaris and the ulnar half (medial half) of the flexor digitorum profundus. The **radial nerve** supplies its territory with a superficial branch and a deep branch. Finally, review the motor nerve distribution to the entire upper limb.

Clinical Correlation: Read an account of the lymphatic drainage of the upper limb. Lymph vessels from the radial side of the hand and forearm drain directly into the axillary nodes. Some lymph channels from the ulnar side of the hand and forearm may drain into the cubital lymph nodes (located at the medial side of the cubital fossa) and from there into axillary nodes. Lymphangitis (i.e., inflammation of lymph vessels, as a result of an infection of the hand, for example) is characterized by red streaks in the skin leading proximally toward the axilla.

Joints of the Upper Limb

General Remarks

It is advantageous to dissect the joints in only one upper limb. Keep the soft structures of the other limb intact for review purposes.

Refer to the articulated bones of the upper limb. Identify the following joints.

- Sternoclavicular joint;
- **Shoulder joint**;
- **Elbow joint**
- Radioulnar joints (proximal, intermediate, distal);
- **Wrist joint** (radiocarpal joint);
- Joints of the digits.

If time is limited, dissect at least the following joints: **shoulder joint, elbow joint,** and **wrist joint.** If time permits, refer to the *Appendix* regarding the dissection of smaller joints.

GRANT'S 6.1
ROHEN 346
A.D.A.M. 6.3-6.6
NETTER 392, 408, 422
CLEMENTE 41

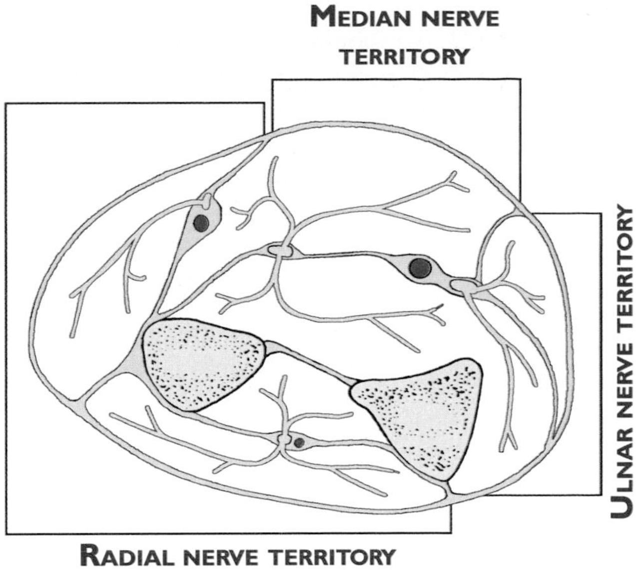

Figure 6.49. Nerve territories of the forearm.

Shoulder Joint

The **shoulder joint** (glenohumeral joint) is a multiaxial ball and socket type synovial joint with a wide range of motion. The shoulder joint has a greater degree of freedom of movement than any other joint in the body. By necessity, this freedom of movement requires laxity of the joint capsule; as a result, there is relative joint instability. Thus, functional stability of the shoulder joint depends largely on surrounding muscles and tendons, particularly the muscles of the rotator cuff (Fig. 6.50).

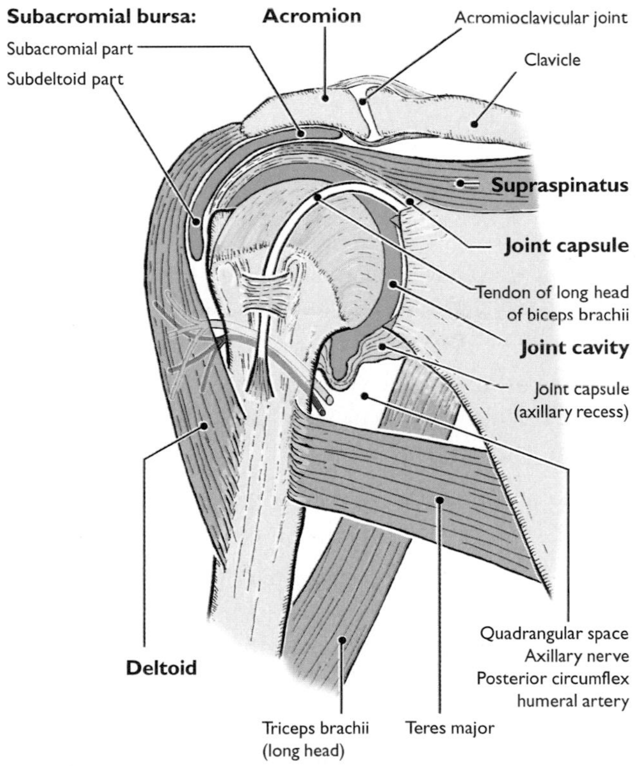

Figure 6.50. Anterior view of the right shoulder joint (coronal section)

Review the bony features pertinent to the **shoulder joint** (Fig. 6.51). Specifically, identify the **anatomical neck** and the **surgical neck** of the humerus.

GRANT'S 6.1
ROHEN 349-351
A.D.A.M. 6.3-6.6
NETTER 392, 393
CLEMENTE 92-96, 104, 105
A.V.A. 1: 0.06.43

- Remove the coracobrachialis, the short head of the biceps brachii, and the long head of the triceps.
- Clean the insertion of the subscapularis.
- Once again, observe that the tendons of the supraspinatus, infraspinatus, and teres minor muscles blend with the joint capsule. Cut these muscles.

GRANT'S 6.31A, 6.38A
ROHEN 363, 3.65
NETTER 394
CLEMENTE 98, 99
A.V.A. 1: 0.12.34

The **fibrous capsule** is now completely exposed, except in front where the subscapularis remains intact. Verify that the capsule is attached just proximal to the glenoid cavity. On the humerus, it is attached to the anatomical neck.

Approach the shoulder joint from its posterior aspect (Fig. 6.51). Remove the posterior portion of the joint capsule. With a saw or a hammer and chisel, remove the head of the humerus as close as possible to the anatomical neck. With a probe, explore the extent of the **synovial cavity** (Fig. 6.50). Identify the following structures (Fig. 6.51):

Grant's 6.30
A.D.A.M. 6.50
Netter 397
Clemente 99

- **Glenoid cavity;** around its margin, note a fibrocartilaginous rim, the **glenoid labrum**;
- Three bands reinforcing the front of the joint capsule (as seen from the posterior aspect), the **glenohumeral ligaments;** they converge on the supraglenoid tubercle;
- **Tendon of long head of biceps.**

Grant's 6.39
Rohen 356
Netter 394
Clemente 98

Define and clean the strong **coracoacromial ligament** from the coracoid process to the acromion. This ligament, together with acromion and coracoid process, forms a continuous ligamentous and bony protection, the **coracoacromial arch.** It prevents upward displacement of the head of the humerus. Finally, study radiographic images of the shoulder.

Grant's 6.37
Netter 394
Clemente 98
A.V.A. 1: 0.04.45

Grant's 6.40
A.D.A.M. 6.36
Clemente 103

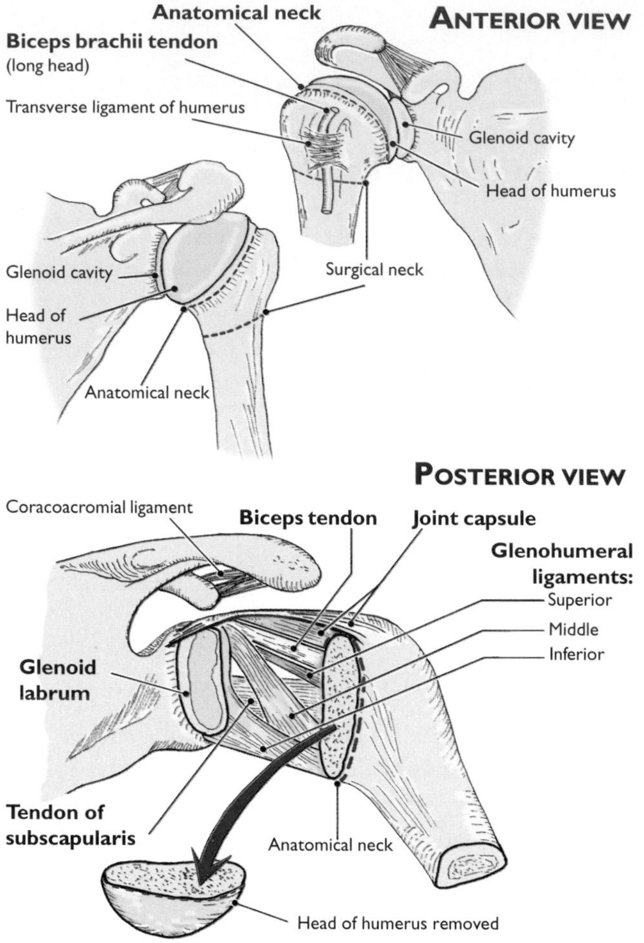

Figure 6.51. Interior of right shoulder joint exposed from posterior aspect.

Elbow Joint

Review the bony features of the elbow region (Fig. 6.52). In the articulated skeleton, verify that the joint consists of three different portions:

Grant's 6.48
Rohen 351-353
A.D.A.M. 6.5, 6.6
Netter 407
Clemente 104-111
A.V.A. 1: 0.41.58, 0.44.30

- The portion between the trochlea of the humerus and the trochlear notch of the ulna; it is a simple hinge joint (flexion and extension);
- The portion between the capitulum of the humerus and the head of the radius; it is a gliding joint;
- The portion between the circumference of the head of the radius and the radial notch of the ulna; rotation of the radius takes place here.

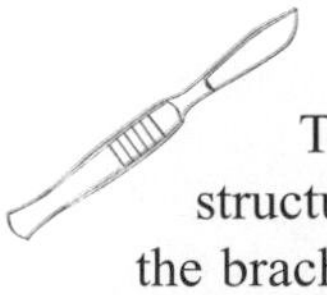

Turn to the cadaver. Remove the soft structures crossing the elbow joint. Dissect the brachialis off the capsule. Remove the triceps from the back of the thin capsule. Detach the tricipital aponeurosis from the olecranon. Remove the superficial flexor muscles of the forearm from the medial epicondyle.

On the medial side of the elbow joint, free the **ulnar collateral ligament** (Fig. 6.52). Observe that it consists of a strong anterior cord and a weaker posterior fan-like portion. Define the attachments of the ligament to humerus and ulna.

Grant's 6.51B
Netter 408
Clemente 116
A.V.A. 1: 0.45.00, 0.46.04

On the lateral side, detach the extensor muscles from their common tendon of origin. Remove the supinator. Expose the **radial collateral ligament**. It fans out from the lateral epicondyle to the anular ligament of the radius.

Grant's 6.49, 6.51
A.D.A.M. 6.45
Netter 408
Clemente 116-118
A.V.A. 1: 0.45.32

The **anular ligament** encircles the head of the radius. It is in circumferential continuity with the radial notch of the ulna (Fig. 6.52). Note that the radius can freely rotate in the anular ligament. Place the hand in the pronated position (radius and ulna crossed). Now, pull on the remains of the biceps tendon, which is attached to the radial tuberosity. Note the strong supinating action of the biceps brachii.

Grant's 6.51A
Rohen 357
Netter 408
Clemente 116
A.V.A. 1: 0.46.30

Open the joint capsule anteriorly by making a transverse cut through the capsule between the ulnar and radial collateral liga-

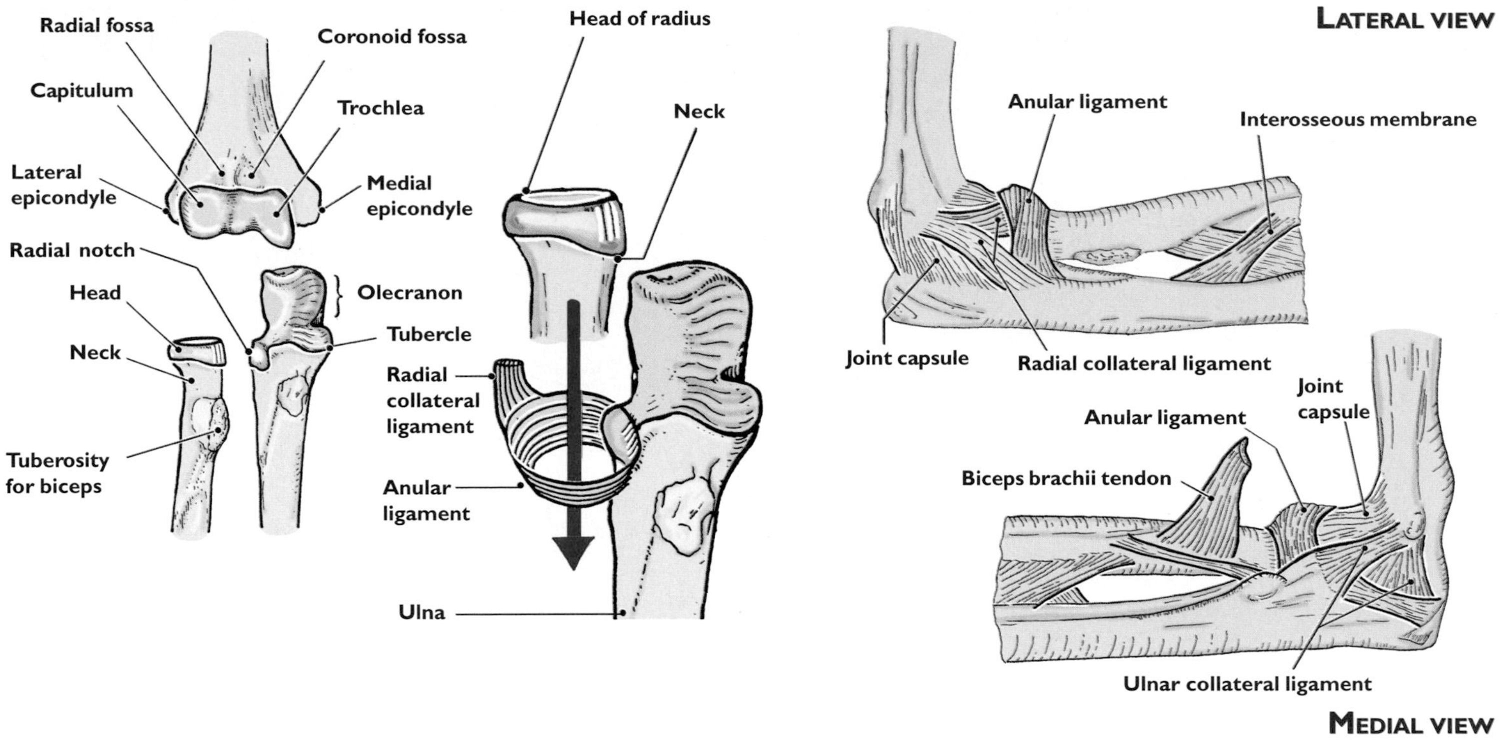

Figure 6.52. Bony landmarks of the elbow joint. The head of the radius is inserted into the anular ligament that holds the radius to the ulna. The joint capsule of the elbow joint is reinforced by ligaments.

ments. With a probe, explore the extent of the **synovial capsule**. Pass the probe (within the capsule) between the head of the radius and the anular ligament. Observe the smooth articular surfaces of the humerus, ulna, and radius. Notice the thin synovial fold and fatpads intervening between the head of the radius and the capitulum of the humerus. This fat pad may give radiologists a clue as to possible fractures in the elbow region. Review a transverse section through the elbow joint. Study radiographic images of the elbow region.

Wrist Joint

By definition, the **wrist joint or radiocarpal joint** is concerned with the movements between the **radius** and the **carpus.** Review the carpal bones. Note that the distal end of the radius has two joint surfaces for two carpal bones. In the articulated skeleton, observe that the radius articulates with the **scaphoid** and **lunate**.

Turn to the cadaver. Remove all soft structures crossing the wrist. On the anterior (palmar) aspect, observe a number of **radiocarpal ligaments** that hold radius and carpus together.

Force the hand backward (extend). Cut through the radiocarpal ligaments, and open the radiocarpal joint transversely. Leave the hand attached to the forearm by the dorsal part of the joint capsule.

Identify the smooth proximal surfaces of the **scaphoid, lunate, and triquetrum**. Study the corresponding articular surfaces of the radius and the **articular disc**. Verify that the articular disc holds the distal ends of the radius and the ulna firmly together. The articular disc forms part of the wrist joint. Note that it articulates with the triquetrum when adducted.

Perform the **principal movements** possible at the wrist joint: *flexion, adduction, extension,* and *abduction*. Carry out a *circumduction* by combining these movements in a consecutive fashion. Observe the articular surfaces during these movements.

Correlate your anatomical observations with radiographs and magnetic resonance images (MRIs) of the hand and wrist.

GRANT'S 6.50
A.D.A.M. 6.45
NETTER 408
CLEMENTE 119
A.V.A. 1: 0.46.44

GRANT'S 6.84-6.89
NETTER 425
CLEMENTE 128, 130

GRANT'S 6.48
A.D.A.M. 6.46
CLEMENTE 122-124

GRANT'S 6.1, 6.81
ROHEN 454, 355
NETTER 409, 422, 423
CLEMENTE 112, 114
A.V.A. 1: 0.49.12

GRANT'S 6.82A
CLEMENTE 125
A.V.A. 1: 0.51.06

GRANT'S 6.83
ROHEN 3.58, 3.59
A.D.A.M. 6.59, 6.60
NETTER 424, 425
CLEMENTE 126, 127

TEST 11

GAPP
GROSS ANATOMY PRACTICAL PRIMER

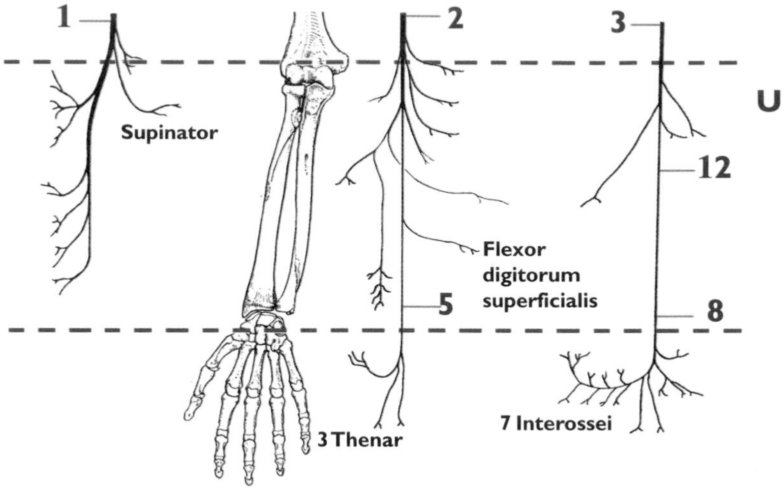

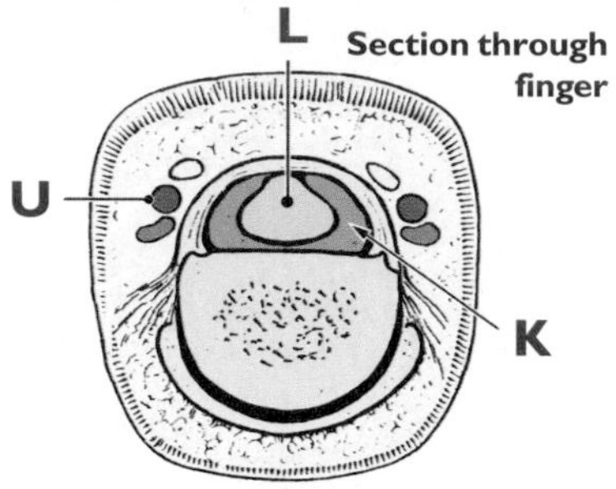

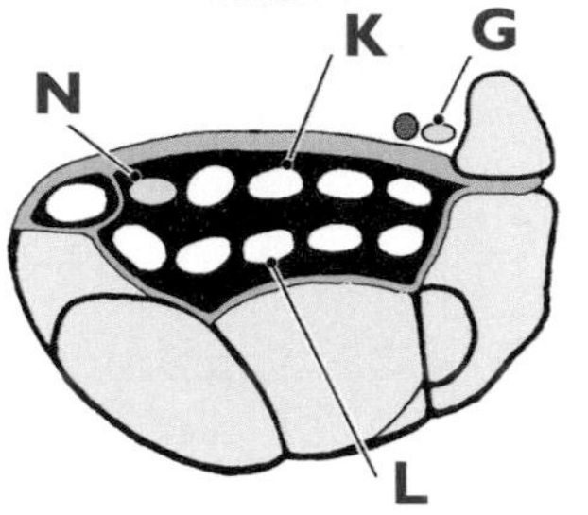

Carpal tunnel with contents

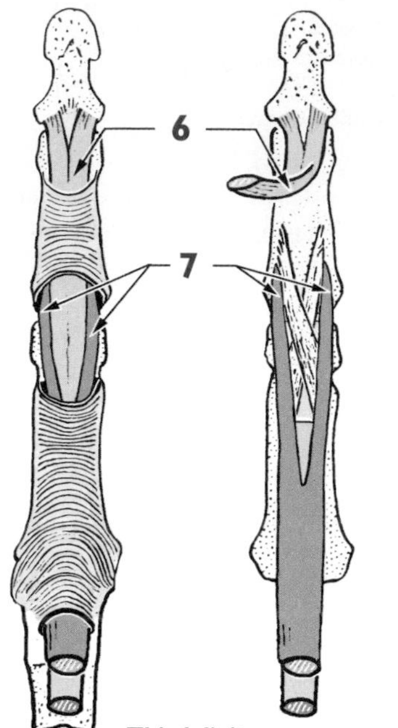

Third digit

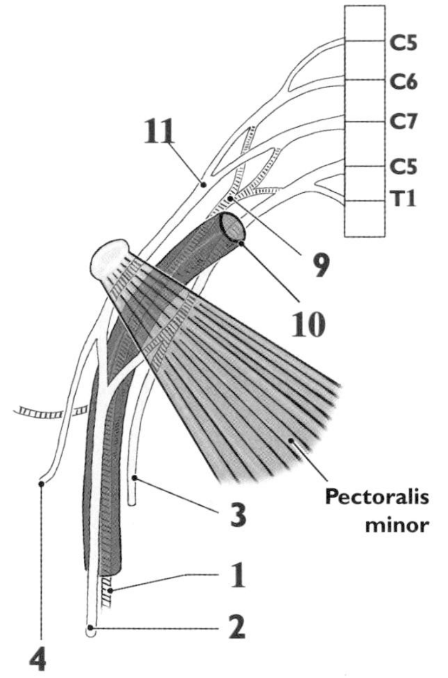

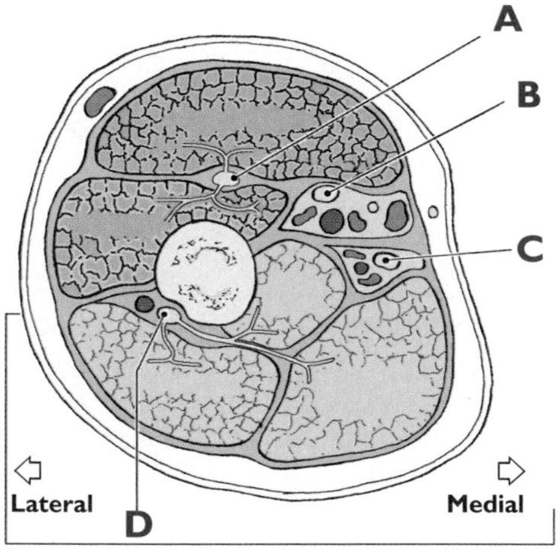

Posterior compartment

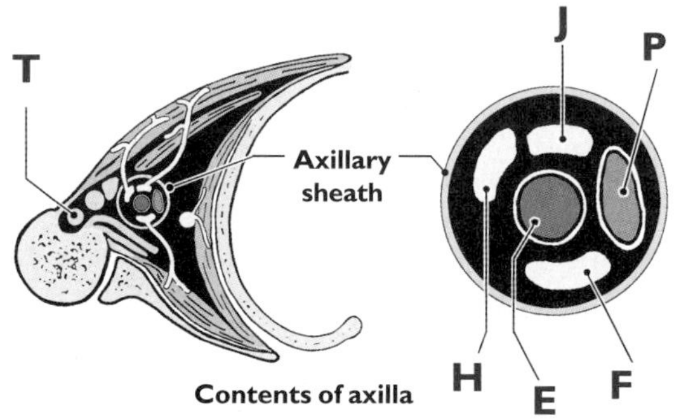

Contents of axilla

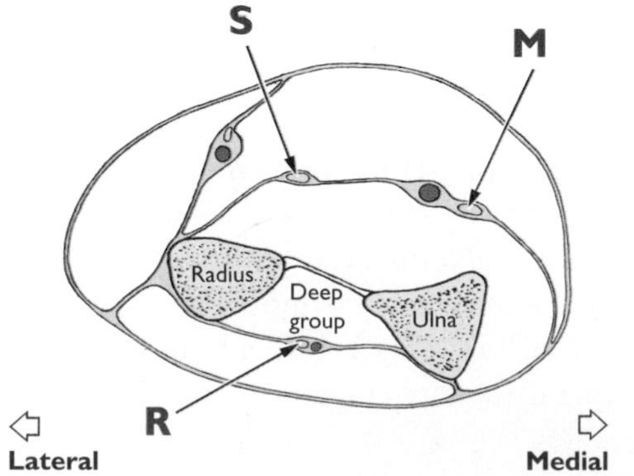

TEST YOUR 3-DIMENSIONAL CONCEPTUALIZATION.
MATCH THE NUMBERS WITH CORRESPONDING LETTERS:

1 ___	7 ___
2 ___	8 ___
3 ___	9 ___
4 ___	10 ___
5 ___	11 ___
6 ___	12 ___

GAPP TEST: IF YOU MADE AN ERROR, REVIEW AND GAIN A BETTER UNDERSTANDING OF THE CONCERNED 3-DIMENSIONAL ANATOMICAL CONCEPT. GAPP KEY: 1-D, 2-B, 3-C, 4-A, 5-N, 6-L, 7-K, 8-G, 9-F, 10-E, 11-H, 12-M.

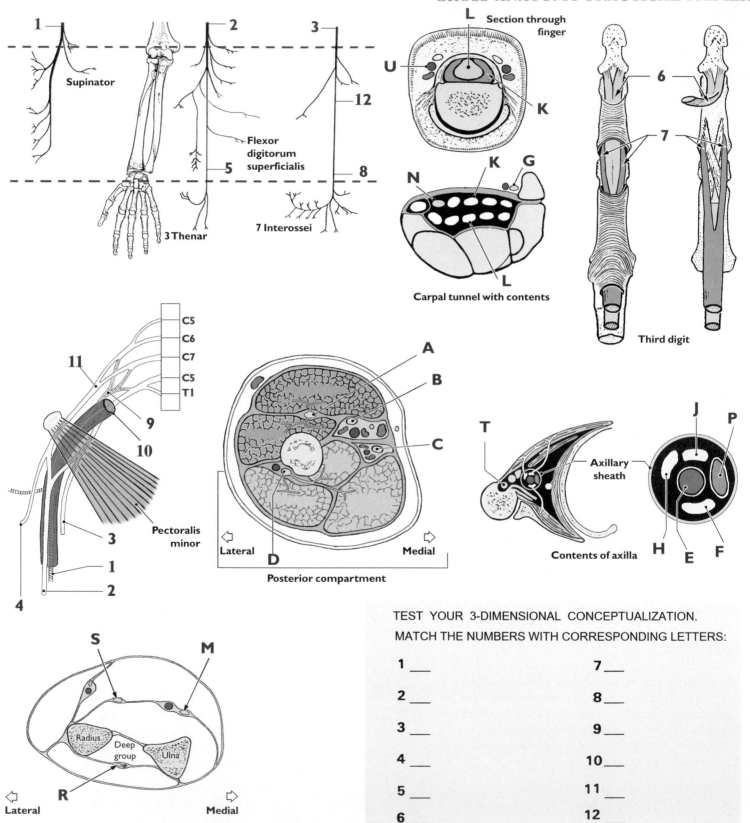

CHAPTER 7 THE HEAD AND NECK

GRANT'S ATLAS OF ANATOMY, 10TH ED.:	*GRANT'S FIG. #*
ROHEN, COLOR ATLAS OF ANATOMY, 4TH ED.:	ROHEN PAGE #
A.D.A.M. STUDENT ATLAS OF ANATOMY:	A.D.A.M. PLATE #
NETTER, ATLAS OF HUMAN ANATOMY, 2ND ED.:	NETTER PLATE #
CLEMENTE, ANATOMY, 4TH ED.:	CLEMENTE FIG. #
ACLAND'S VIDEO ATLAS OF HUMAN ANATOMY	**A.V.A. Vol: hr:min:sec**

Anterior Aspect of Skull and Face

General Remarks

Developmentally, the facial muscles of expression and the muscles of the scalp originate from the right and left *2nd* branchial arches. The nerve associated with the second arch is the **facial nerve or cranial nerve VII (CN VII).** This nerve innervates all muscles derived from the second arch including the facial muscles of expression, muscles of the scalp and external ear, and the platysma. The facial muscles are subcutaneous. Most of their fibers are inserted into the skin. They not only express a variety of emotions, but also act as sphincters and dilators for orifices (orbits; mouth; nostrils).

⇦
GRANT'S 7.13
ROHEN 60, 61
A.D.A.M. 8.11
NETTER 20, 21
CLEMENTE 728, 729
A.V.A. 5: 0.01.13

The nerve of the *1st* branchial arch is the **trigeminal nerve or cranial nerve V (CN V).** It supplies the muscles of mastication which are derived from the first arch. However, the main part of the trigeminal nerve is sensory. Each of the **three divisions** of cranial nerve V (V1, V2, V3) supplies an area of skin in the facial region (Fig. 7.1; *color coded*). In general, these areas of skin may be mapped out by drawing two lines:

⇦
GRANT'S 9.7
ROHEN 73
A.D.A.M. 8.7-8.9
NETTER 18, 116
CLEMENTE 734

- From the nose across the lateral angle of the eye;
- From the corner of the mouth to a point about midway between eye and ear.

The central V-shaped region (forehead, eyes, nose) is supplied by the **1st or ophthalmic division** of the trigeminal nerve (V1). The intermediate area (cheek) belongs to the **2nd or maxillary division** (V2). The lower part of the face (mandibular region) is supplied with sensory fibers from the **3rd or mandibular division** (V3). Sensory nerves from **cervical segments** supply the back of the head and parts of the mandibular area and of the ear (Fig. 7.1; *color coded*).

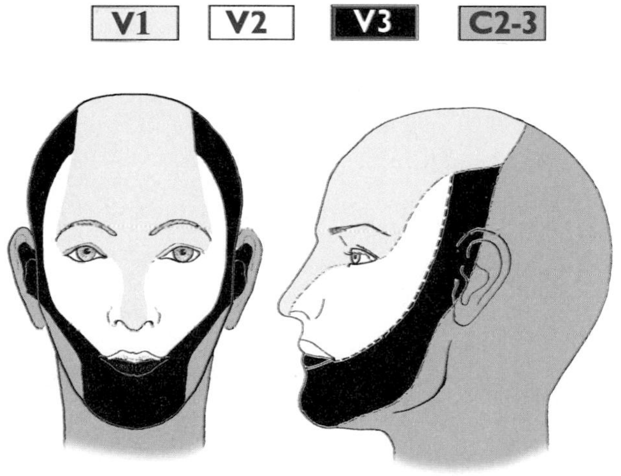

Figure 7.1. Cutaneous nerve distribution of the head and neck.

Bony Landmarks

> ***Note:*** Handle the skull with great care. Never hold a skull by placing your fingers into the orbital cavities. Their medial walls are paper thin. They are very easily broken.
>
> *Orientation:* Anatomists have agreed to examine skulls in the following position: The lower margins of the orbital apertures and the upper margins of the external acoustic (auditory) canals lie on a horizontal plane. This position approximates very closely the anatomical position.

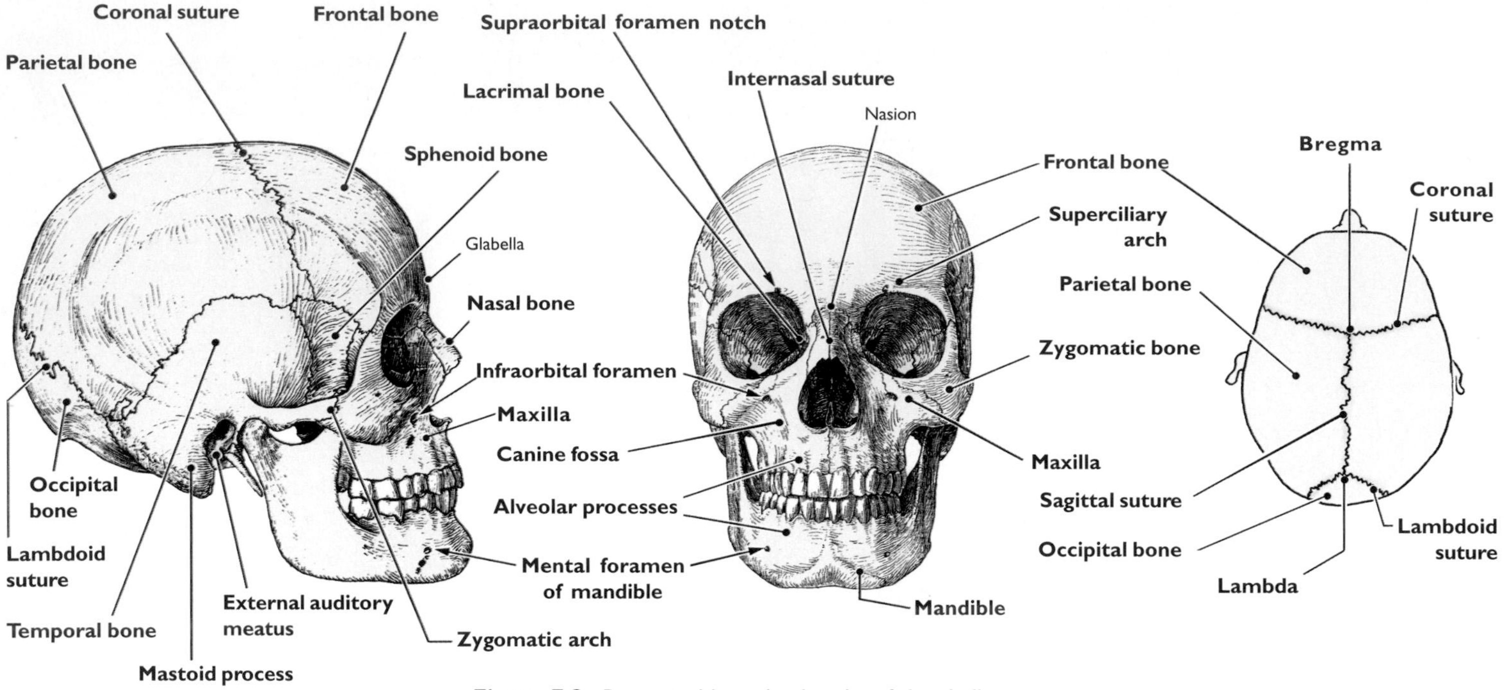

Figure 7.2. Bones and bony landmarks of the skull.

Skull on Anterior View (Norma Frontalis).

Examine the anterior aspect of a skull. Identify the following landmarks (Fig. 7.2):

- **Frontal bone;**
- **Maxilla;** it has a *frontal process* that joins the frontal bone;
- **Zygomatic bone;**
- **Mandible;**
- **Anterior nasal aperture** (piriform aperture); define its borders: two *nasal bones* superiorly; two *maxillae* laterally and inferiorly; *anterior nasal spine* of maxilla positioned inferiorly in the median plane;
- Nasion, the depression at the root of the nose;
- **Superciliary arch** (ridge);
- Glabella, the smooth eminence superior to the nasion and between the superciliary arches;
- **Orbital margin;** each of three bones (frontal; maxillary; zygomatic) forms approximately one-third of the orbital margin;
- **Lacrimal bone;** positioned at the anterior part of the medial orbital wall; together with the frontal process of the maxilla, it forms the **lacrimal fossa**; the lacrimal fossa is continuous inferiorly with the **nasolacrimal canal;** gently push a flexible wire through the canal into the nasal cavity;
- **Teeth**; if fully developed, the adult has 32 permanent teeth, 16 in the upper jaw (maxilla), and 16 in the lower jaw (mandible); the roots of the teeth are embedded in the **alveolar processes.**
- Briefly familiarize yourself with the primary or deciduous teeth (temporary; milk teeth). At the end of the 2nd year, there are normally 20 teeth, 10 in each jaw.

Grant's 7.1
Rohen 26, 27
A.D.A.M. 7.5
Netter 1
Clemente 752
A.V.A. 4: 0.35.30

Grant's 7.3
Rohen 33
Netter 4
Clemente 756, 757
A.V.A. 4: 0.03.15

Superior and Posterior Aspects of Skull

Identify the following bones and landmarks (Fig. 7.2):

- **Frontal bone**;
- Right and left **parietal bones**;
- **Coronal suture**, separating the frontal bone from the parietal bones;
- **Sagittal suture**, separating the two parietal bones;
- **Bregma**, the meeting point between coronal and sagittal suture;
- **Occipital bone**;
- **Lambdoid sutures**, separating the occipital bone from the parietal bones;
- **Lambda**, the meeting point of lambdoid and sagittal sutures.

Grant's 7.2
Rohen 25
A.D.A.M. 7.9
Netter 2, 11
Clemente 754
A.V.A. 4: 1.26.20

Lateral Aspect of Skull (Norma Lateralis)

Examine the lateral aspect of the skull. The following bony landmarks are of immediate interest:

- **Mandible;** identify its **body, ramus, angle,** and **posterior border;** the condylar process consists of the constricted **neck** and the **articular condyle or head;**

- **Temporomandibular joint (TMJ),** between head of mandible and a fossa on the temporal bone;
- **External auditory meatus** (canal), which is part of the temporal bone;
- **Zygomatic arch;** it is formed by two bony processes, the zygoma of the temporal bone and the temporal process of the zygomatic bone; note the suture line in the anterior third of the arch;

GRANT'S 7.2
ROHEN 25
A.D.A.M. 7.9
NETTER 2, 11
CLEMENTE 754
A.V.A. 4: 1.30.50

Identify the following foramina or openings (Fig. 7.2):

- On the frontal bone, the **supraorbital foramen** (or notch);
- On the maxilla, the **infraorbital foramen**;
- On the mandible, the **mental foramen**.

GRANT'S 7.5
ROHEN 23
A.D.A.M. 7.6, 7.8

> ***Clinical Correlation:*** Correlate the bony landmarks of the skull with appropriate radiographs. Realize that the radiographic images of several bony structures may be superimposed. For example, in a lateral view, right and left structures are more or less superimposed, depending on the accuracy of positioning and the direction of the x-ray beam. In the anteroposterior view, images of the posterior skull are superimposed with facial images. As you make progress and learn more about the bony details of the skull, refer back to these radiographs for correlation.

Before you begin ...

After reflection of the skin, the muscles of the face will be exposed. Branches of the facial nerve that are motor to these muscles will be identified as they emerge from the substance of the parotid gland. Two important sphincter muscles will receive particular attention: the orbicularis oris (mouth), and the orbicularis oculi (eye). The essential nerves responsible for the sensory supply of the facial skin will be exposed. Finally, the lacrimal apparatus will be explored.

Skin Incisions

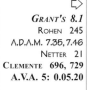

Make the following skin incisions (Fig. 7.3):

- In the midline, from vertex to chin (*A* to *B*); encircle the mouth at the margin of the lips.
- Start at the nasion (*C*), widely encircle the orbital margins, and return to the nasion.
- Make other incisions from the vertex, anterior to the ear, inferiorly to a point just posterior to the angle of the mandible (*A* to *D*).

First, reflect the skin between eyebrows and vertex. Notice that the skin is closely adherent to the thick and tough subcutaneous fascia. Leave this fascia intact; nerves and

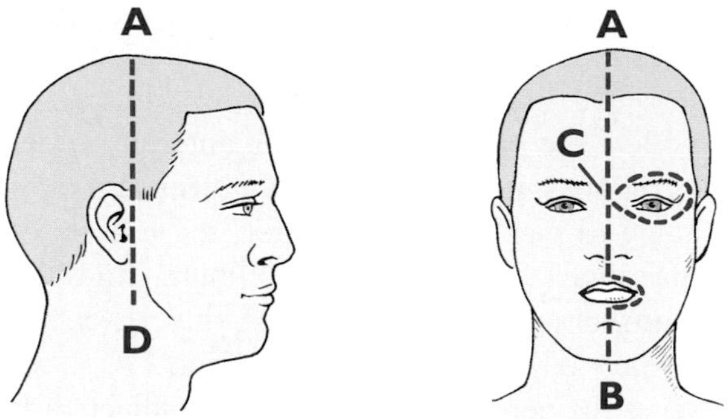

Figure 7.3. Skin incisions.

vessels run in it. Do *not* reflect the **frontalis muscle**. If the skin is raised without difficulty, you are probably in the areolar space deep to the frontalis and its aponeurosis.

The skin of the face is thin. There may be a considerable amount of subcutaneous fat. Reflect the skin carefully. Do not damage the underlying pale and inconspicuous facial muscles. Observe the thin and loose skin of the eyelids. Remove the skin at the margins of the eyelids. Reflect the skin of the face inferior and parallel to the inferior border of the mandible.

Facial Nerve, Vessels, and Related Structures

GRANT'S 8.1
ROHEN 245
A.D.A.M. 7.36, 7.46
NETTER 21
CLEMENTE 696, 729
A.V.A. 5: 0.05.20

The **platysma** reaches as far inferiorly as the 2nd rib. Demonstrate the superior attachment of the muscle sheet to the inferior border of the mandible. Subsequently, cut the posterior part of the platysma along the inferior border of the mandible, and reflect it toward the angle of the mouth.

GRANT'S 7.10
A.D.A.M. 7.44
NETTER 17, 19
CLEMENTE 731
A.V.A. 4: 1.36.54

Identify the rhomboid **masseter muscle** that extends from the zygomatic arch to the ramus of the mandible. About 2.0 to 2.5 cm inferior to the zygomatic arch, the **parotid duct** crosses the lateral aspect of the masseter muscle (Fig. 7.4). Identify the duct.

NETTER 45
A.V.A. 4: 2.03.47

> ***Clinical Correlation:*** The **parotid duct** opens into the oral cavity opposite the upper 2nd molar tooth. Usually, the opening is marked by a slight elevation of buccal mucosa, the **parotid papilla.** Palpate your own right or left parotid papilla with your tongue or your finger. Inspect the papilla in a fellow student. The parotid duct and the papilla transmit the saliva secreted by the parotid gland. Under certain conditions, the papilla may become inflamed. Also, a calculus (concretion) may develop in the parotid duct and then get impacted at the level of the parotid papilla.

The parotid duct is empty, collapsed, and flattened like a piece of narrow white tape. Follow the parotid duct to the anterior border of the masseter. Here, the duct turns at a right angle to pierce the buccinator, the muscle of the cheek. Superior to the duct, find the **transverse facial artery** and the *zygomatic branch* of the **facial nerve** (Fig. 7.4). Preserve the nerve. The artery, unless injected, is often difficult to trace.

Facial Nerve (Fig. 7.4)

After its emergence at the base of the skull, the facial nerve turns anteriorly and traverses the substances of the parotid gland. Within the gland, the nerve divides into various branches that radiate to the facial muscles of expression. To find these nerve branches, proceed by following the parotid duct posteriorly to the point where it emerges from the **parotid gland.** This point is about 5 to 7 mm anterior to the posterior border of the mandible.

- Raise the anterior border of the gland from the masseteric fascia.
- Find the white, flattened branches of the facial nerve issuing from the substance of the gland. Note that they run deep. They are separated from the masseter only by its fascia.
- Trace the **nerve branches of the facial nerve** to the muscles they supply.
- The highest of these radiating branches, the **temporal branch**, crosses the zygomatic bone.
- Identify the **zygomatic branch** and the **buccal branch**. Note that these branches may have interconnections.
- Identify the **mandibular branch** that runs just above the inferior margin of the jaw.
- The lowest branch, the **cervical branch**, runs below the angle of the mandible. This branch sends twigs to the platysma.

Define the free, anterior border of the **masseter** in its entire length. Anterior to the masseter is an extensive **buccal fatpad**. Remove this buccal fatpad to expose the underlying **buccinator muscle**. Once again, verify that the **parotid duct** pierces the buccinator. Notice that two different nerves enter the substance of the buccinator:

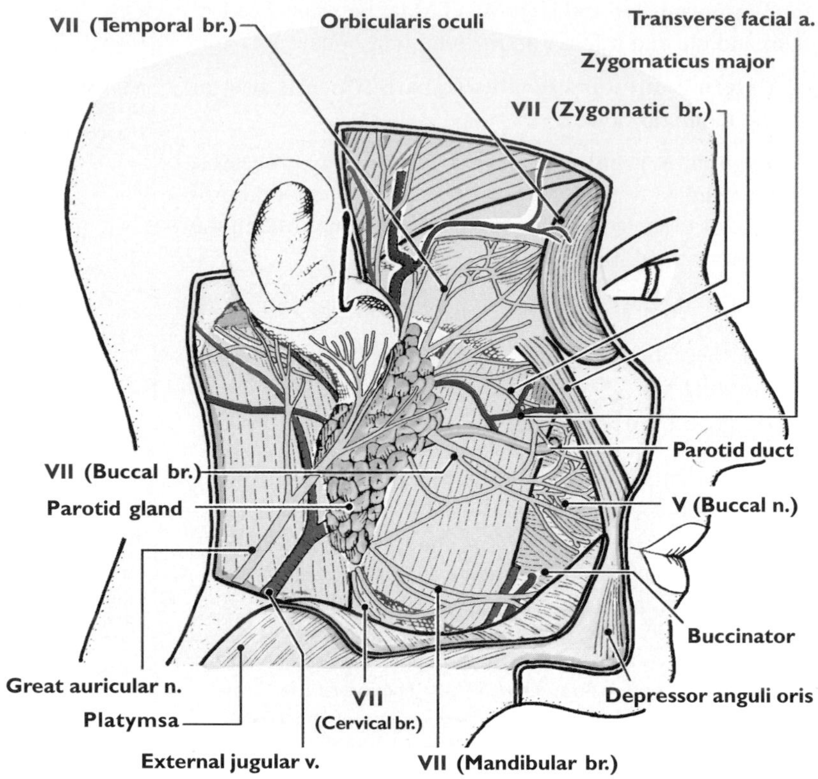

Figure 7.4. Dissection of the lateral aspect of the face. The branches of the facial nerve **(VII)** emerge from the parotid gland.

Grant's 7.10, 9.12
Rohen 76, 77
A.D.A.M. 8.11
Netter 19
Clemente 730, 736
A.V.A. 4: 2.02.50

Grant's 7.10
Rohen 72
Netter 18
Clemente 736
A.V.A. 5: 1.00.02

- The **buccal branch** of the **facial nerve;** it runs *lateral* to the masseter to supply the buccinator with motor fibers;
- The **buccal branch of the trigeminal nerve (V3);** it runs *medial* (deep) to the masseter. Observe its twigs. The nerve does *not* supply the buccinator muscle. It merely pierces the muscle to send sensory fibers to the buccal mucosa of the vestibule of the mouth. The buccal nerve also sends a small branch to the skin of the cheek. This cutaneous branch was destroyed during the skinning process.

Grant's 7.10
Rohen 76, 77
Netter 17, 19
Clemente 731, 736
A.V.A. 5: 0.03.26

Grant's 7.9
Rohen 76, 79
Netter 17
Clemente 735, 736
A.V.A. 5: 1.50.30

Facial Artery and Vein

On yourself, palpate the pulse of the **facial artery** (Fig. 7.5). This vessel crosses the mandible at the anterior border of the masseter. The accompanying **facial vein** lies posterior to the artery. Find these vessels in the cadaver. Trace the facial artery to the medial angle of the eye. In its course, the artery crosses successively the mandible, buccinator, and maxilla. Follow the corresponding facial vein to the medial angle of the eye.

Muscles of the Mouth

There are numerous muscles that alter the shape of the mouth and lips. Define the more important muscles (Fig. 7.5):

- **Depressor anguli oris**; it depresses the corners of the mouth; in this function, it is aided by the posterior fibers of the platysma;
- **Zygomaticus major,** descending from the zygomatic bone to the corner of the mouth; it draws the angle of the mouth superiorly and posteriorly;
- **Levator labii superioris,** descending from the infraorbital margin to the upper lip; it elevates the upper lip;
- **Orbicularis oris,** the important sphincter muscle of the mouth; demonstrate the circular arrangement of its muscle fibers. Note that the orbicularis oris intimately blends with the fibers of the other muscles of the mouth. If time permits, demonstrate additional muscles of facial expression (Fig. 7.5). Check with your instructor.

Clean the surface of the **buccinator**. Define its superior and inferior attachments to the lateral surfaces of the alveolar processes of maxilla and mandible. Note that the buccinator fibers blend with the orbicularis oris.

GRANT'S 7.9, 7.13A
ROHEN 60, 61
A.D.A.M. 7.21, 7.22
NETTER 20, 21
CLEMENTE 728, 729
A.V.A. 5: 0.02.42

SUPERFICIAL MUSCLES	DEEPER MUSCLES

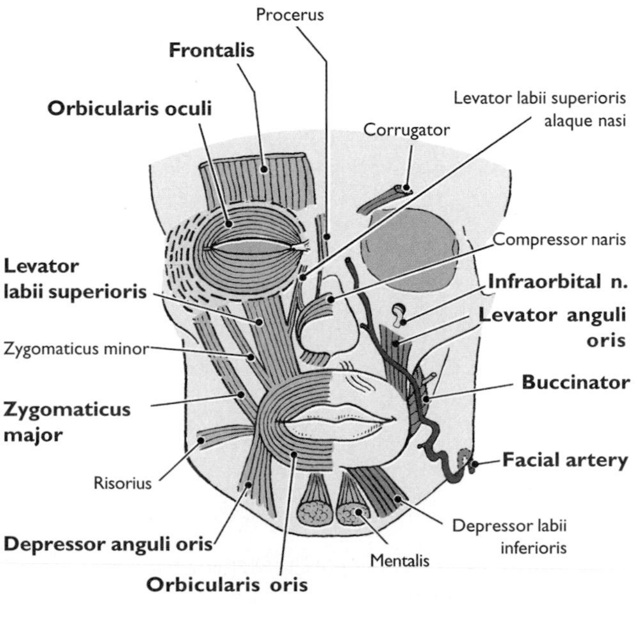

Figure 7.5. Muscles of the face.

With a probe, loosen the tissue deep to the levator labii superioris. Carefully cut horizontally through the muscle close to the infraorbital margin. Reflect the muscle inferiorly and thus expose the **infraorbital nerve**. Trace some of its branches to the inferior eyelid, side of the nose, and upper lip.

GRANT'S 7.13A, 9.9A
ROHEN 72, 73
A.D.A.M. 7.35, 8.8
NETTER 18
CLEMENTE 736
A.V.A. 5: 0.55.22

Clinical Correlation: Study the infraorbital foramen and canal in the skull. Pass a wire through the foramen into the canal. For purposes of local anesthesia, the infraorbital nerve is often infiltrated at the level of the foramen or in the canal. In the cadaver, palpate the foramen and push a probe through it.

Lower Lip, External Nose, and External Ear

Lower Lip

Make a midline incision through the entire thickness of the lower lip. Parallel to this incision, make a second vertical incision inferiorly from the angle of the mouth (do this on one side of the body only). Reflect the quadrangular piece of lip inferiorly. Cut through the mucous membrane along the line of its reflection from lips to gums. Dissect the mucous membrane from the underlying muscle fibers up to the red line of the lip.

A.D.A.M. 7.30
NETTER 63, 64
CLEMENTE 843

Observe the small **labial glands** immediately deep to the mucous membrane. At the red line of the lip, see the **inferior labial artery** (the cut end of the artery may, of course, be seen in the cut edge of the flap). This artery is a branch of the facial artery. The nerve fibers that ascend in the flap are branches of the **mental nerve.** Now, strip the flap from the bone and locate the **mental foramen.** It is located approximately 3 cm from the median plane. Observe that the mental nerve traverses the foramen.

GRANT'S 7.13A, 9.10A
ROHEN 72, 73
A.D.A.M. 7.35, 8.9
NETTER 18
CLEMENTE 736
A.V.A. 5: 1.01.52

Clinical Correlation: The mental nerve (mental; L. *mentum*, chin) is a branch of the inferior alveolar nerve. The inferior alveolar nerve runs within the substance of the mandible. Dentists frequently anesthetize the inferior alveolar nerve and, therefore, also the mental nerve. The resulting local anesthesia of the mental nerve involves the region of the chin and the lower lip on the concerned side.

External Nose

The nose is held in shape by the **nasal cartilages** that consist of hyaline cartilage (Fig. 7.6). Palpate the inferior borders of the two nasal bones. Adjacent to these bony borders, identify the paired **lateral nasal cartilages.** They are not independent structures, but merely triangular expansions of the large **septal cartilage.** This median, unpaired septal cartilage extends between the right and left nasal cavities. It forms the anterior part of the nasal septum.

On each side of the septal cartilage is an **alar cartilage** (Fig. 7.6). These U-shaped cartilages are responsible for the formation of the nares (nostrils). Make a small midline incision at the tip of the nose. Separate the two alar cartilages from the septal cartilage. Follow the free inferior edge of the septal cartilage to the anterior nasal spine.

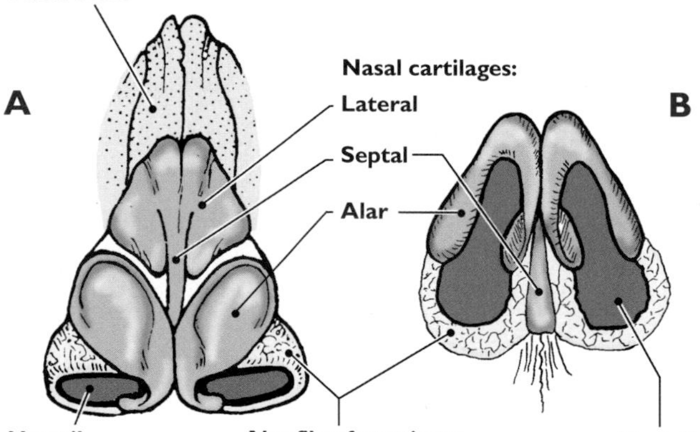

Figure 7.6. Framework of the external nose in anterior view *(A)* and in inferior view *(B)*.

External Ear

The external ear consists of the **auricle** and the **external acoustic meatus** (external ear canal). The characteristic shape of the auricle is maintained by a single piece of elastic cartilage. There is no cartilage in the lobule. Examine the **auricle** and identify the following parts:

- **Helix**, the prominent rim;
- **Antihelix**, the curved prominence anterior to the helix;

GRANT'S 7.80
ROHEN 49, 58
NETTER 31
CLEMENTE 825
A.V.A. 4: 1.15.57

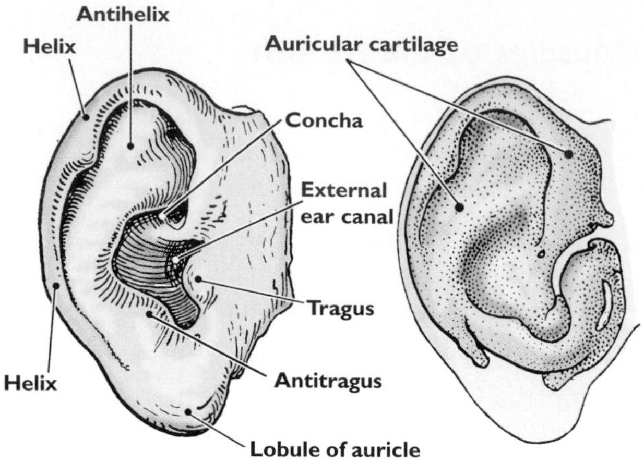

Figure 7.7. External ear and auricular cartilage.

GRANT'S 7.94A
ROHEN 118, 120
A.D.A.M. 7.3
NETTER 88
CLEMENTE 915-918
A.V.A. 5: 2.21.14

- **Concha**;
- **Tragus**, usually showing hairs on its medial surface;
- **Antitragus**;
- **Lobule** of auricle.

You may not have enough time for a detailed dissection of the auricle, its cartilage, and its six tiny intrinsic muscles. Palpate the auricular cartilage on yourself. By palpation, verify that the cartilage is continuous with the cartilage of the external acoustic meatus.

Inspection of Eye and Eyelids

GRANT'S 7.13
ROHEN 131
A.D.A.M. 7.3
NETTER 76
CLEMENTE 783, 784
A.V.A. 5: 2.13.20

Inspect or palpate the living eye. Your own eye can be examined with the aid of a mirror. Identify the following structures:

- **Palpebral commissures,** uniting the eyelids medially and laterally;
- **Palpebral rima or fissure,** the opening between the lids;
- **Medial and lateral angles (canthi)** of the fissure;
- **Cornea,** the transparent anterior 1/6 of the outer coat of the eyeball;
- **Sclera,** the whitish, opaque, posterior 5/6 of the outer coat of the eyeball;
- **Iris,** the varied colored diaphragm seen through the cornea;
- **Pupil,** the aperture in the center of the iris;
- **Conjunctival sac,** the potential space between the eyeball and the eyelids;
- **Conjunctiva,** the membrane lining the sac;

GRANT'S 7.94A
ROHEN 118, 120
NETTER 88
CLEMENTE 915-918
A.V.A. 5: 2.21.08

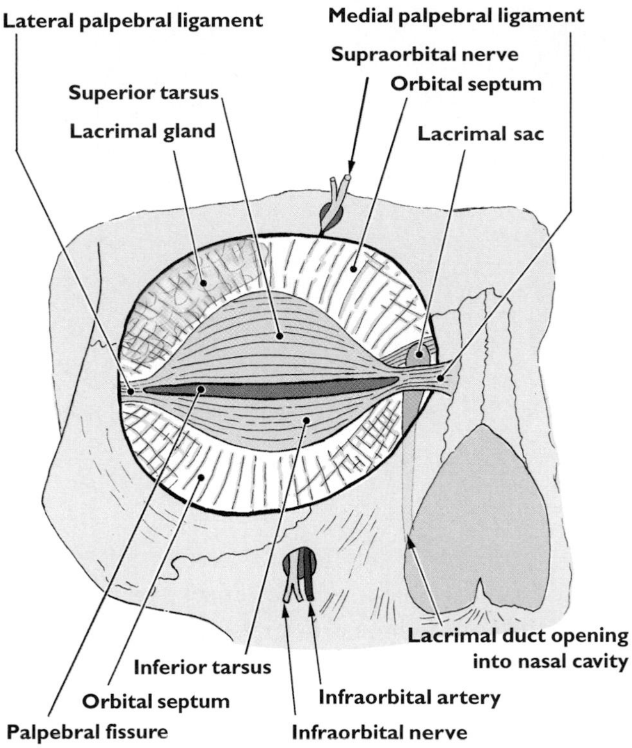

Figure 7.8. Structures related to the orbital region.

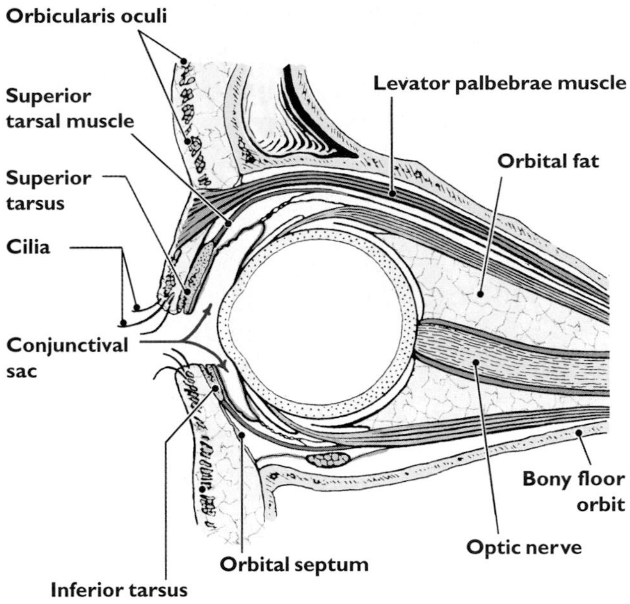

Figure 7.9. Parasagittal section through the orbit showing the eyelids and the conjunctival sacs.

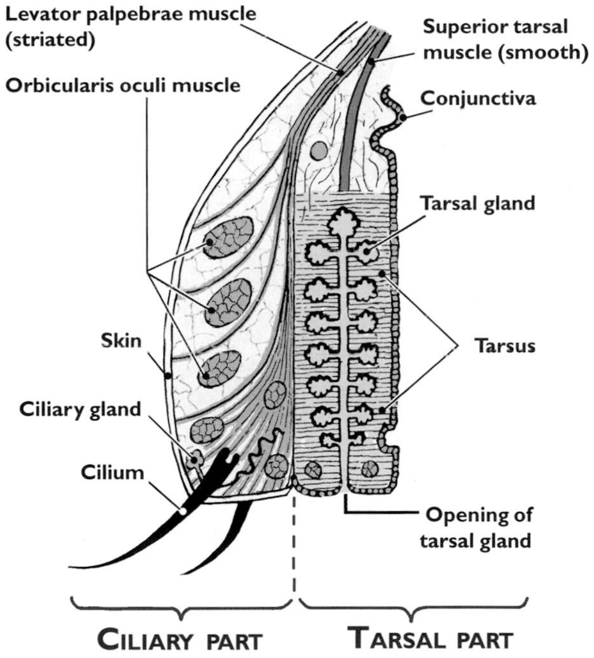

Figure 7.10. Schematic, parasagittal section through the upper eyelid.

- **Fornices** (L., *fornix*, arch; one fornix; two fornices), the regions of conjunctival reflection from the eyelid to the eyeball.

GRANT'S 7.43, 7.44
A.V.A. 5: 2.14.15

In the cadaver, identify the following (Figs. 7.8, 7.9):

- **Tarsus,** superior and inferior.
- **Medial palpebral ligament,** a fibrous band deep to the medial commissure. It becomes conspicuous and palpable when the skin at the lateral commissure is pulled laterally (Fig. 7.7).

GRANT'S 7.13
ROHEN 138
A.D.A.M. 7.69
NETTER 76
CLEMENTE 795, 796
A.V.A. 5: 2.14.50

Inspect the **margins of the eyelids** (Fig. 7.10). The margins are flat and thick. They carry double or triple irregular rows of **eyelashes or cilia.** Observe the lack of cilia close to the medial angle of the eye. Posterior to the cilia are the pinpoint orifices of the **tarsal glands.** Examine the inner surfaces of the eyelids. Note yellowish streaks shining through the conjunctiva. These are the tarsal glands.

GRANT'S 7.48C
NETTER 76
CLEMENTE 798
A.V.A. 5: 2.16.33

Inspect the **medial palpebral commissure** or medial canthus (Fig. 7.11). Here, the upper and lower lids are separated by a triangular space, the **lacus lacrimalis** or **lacrimal lake** (L., *lacus*, lake; *lacrima*, tear; "lake of tears"). The lacus contains a small reddish prominence, the **caruncula.** Focus your attention on the area where the base of the triangular lacus lacrimalis meets the eyelids. On both eyelids, find a small elevation, the **lacrimal papilla.** Each papilla has a minute orifice, the **lacrimal punctum.** It is the opening of the **lacrimal**

GRANT'S 7.44
ROHEN 138
NETTER 77
CLEMENTE 784, 798
A.V.A. 5: 2.17.37

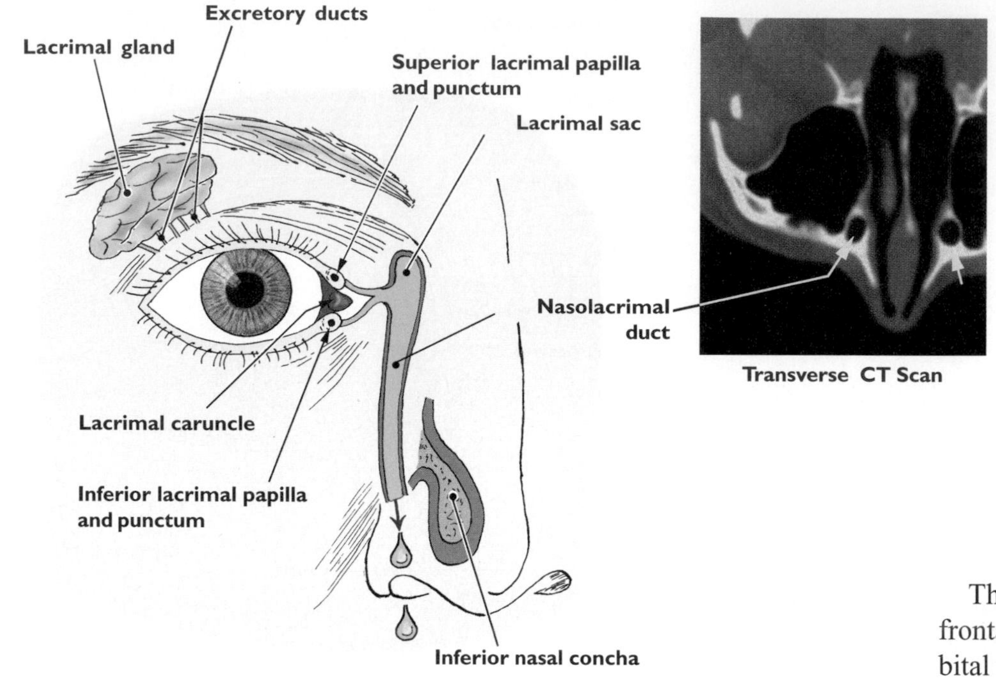

Figure 7.11. Lacrimal apparatus.

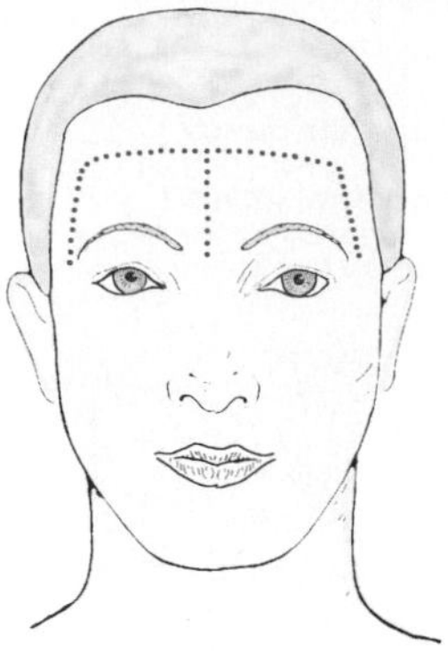

Figure 7.12. Muscle flaps to be reflected.

canaliculus that drains lacrimal fluid into the **lacrimal sac** (Fig. 7.11).

GRANT'S 7.44
ROHEN 138
NETTER 77
CLEMENTE 784, 798
A.V.A. 5: 2.18.06

Orbital Region

Dissect the circularly disposed fibers of the **orbicularis oculi** (Fig. 7.5). Note that this sphincteric muscle consists of two parts:

GRANT'S 7.9
A.D.A.M. 7.21, 7.22
NETTER 20, 21
CLEMENTE 786
A.V.A. 5: 0.01.34

- A thick *orbital portion*, which surrounds the orbital margin and is responsible for the tight closure of the eye;
- A thin, pale *palpebral portion*, which is contained in the eyelids and is involved in the usual blinking of the eye (Fig. 7.10).

The orbicularis oculi originates from the medial part of the bony orbital margin and from the medial palpebral ligament.

- Raise the lateral part of the muscle and reflect it medially.
- Raise the thin palpebral portion off the underlying tarsus, and also turn it medially.
- Examine the **medial palpebral ligament** (Fig. 7.8). Its lower border is free. Fibers of the orbicularis oculi arise from its upper border.

GRANT'S 7.9
ROHEN 138
NETTER 20, 21
CLEMENTE 785, 795
A.V.A. 5: 2.14.50

The next objective is to reflect part of the frontalis muscle and to expose the supraorbital nerve. Proceed as follows (Fig. 7.12):

From the nasion to a point 3 cm above the glabella, make a midline incision through *all* layers of the scalp right down to the bone. Subsequently, make three incisions, two parallel and one horizontal. Reflect the quadrangular flap inferiorly.

In the flap, identify the following structures:

- **Frontalis muscle,** interlacing with the orbicularis oculi;
- **Supraorbital nerve (V1) and vessels.** These emerge from the **supraorbital foramen** (or notch).

GRANT'S 7.13, 7.14, 9.8
ROHEN 138
A.D.A.M. 8.7
NETTER 18
CLEMENTE 735, 785
A.V.A. 5: 0.51.45

Turn the flap inferiorly as far as the supraorbital margin and the medial palpebral ligament. Then, remove the flap entirely.

Now, examine the **orbital septum** (palpebral fascia). It is an oval membranous sheet that is attached to the margin of the orbit (Fig. 7.8). It is continuous with the periorbita (the periosteum of the orbital cavity).

Examine the tarsi. Each **tarsus** is a condensed thickening of the orbital septum, designed to stiffen the eyelid. Evert the larger superior lid and study its free margin. Note the cilia. With the handle of the scalpel, stroke the posterior surface of the upper lid firmly toward its margin. This action will extrude secretions from the **tarsal glands** (Fig. 7.10).

> ***Clinical Correlation:*** There are about 20 to 30 **tarsal or Meibomian glands** in each tarsus (Fig. 7.10). These are sebaceous glands that secrete an oily substance onto the free margin of the eyelids. This lipid prevents an overflow of lacrimal fluid under normal conditions.
>
> If the duct of a tarsal gland becomes obstructed, a cyst will develop. This is a **chalazion.** Understand that a chalazion will be located between tarsal plate and conjunctiva. The chalazion must be distinguished from a **hordeolum** (sty), which involves an inflammation of a small sebaceous gland around the follicle of a cilium.

Cut through the orbital septum in its superior lateral quadrant close to the orbital margin. Pass a probe through the incision. Keep the probe close to the bony orbital roof and free the **lacrimal gland**. Attempt to find some of the 6 to 10 ducts that connect the gland to the fornix of the upper part of the conjunctival sac (Fig. 7.11).

The next objective is to study the structures that collect and drain the lacrimal fluid. Refer to the bony skull and identify the **lacrimal fossa** for the **lacrimal sac**. Observe the *anterior crest* of the fossa. The **medial palpebral ligament** is attached to this crest. The lacrimal sac lies just posterior to the ligament (Fig. 7.8).

Turn to the cadaver. With a probe, puncture the lacrimal sac just below and posterior to the medial palpebral ligament. Explore the extent of the sac. Use a stiff wire or a thin probe and push the instrument downward within the sac. The instrument will traverse the **nasolacrimal duct** and enter the inferior meatus of the nose (Fig. 7.11). Looking through the nostril on the corresponding side, you may or may not be able to see the tip of the probe (depending on the configuration of the nasal structures in each particular specimen).

> ***Clinical Correlation:*** The normal flow of lacrimal fluid is conducted obliquely across the eye, from the ductules of the lacrimal gland (i.e., the lateral portion of the superior fornix) to the medial angle of the eye (i.e., to the point of drainage; Fig. 7.11). Increased tear production and drainage via the two lacrimal canaliculi (canals) and the nasolacrimal duct into the nose will induce the characteristic sniffing during crying. Also, during crying, the excessive amount of lacrimal fluid cannot be sufficiently emptied through the lacrimal drainage system, and tears flow over the lower eyelids and the cheeks.

GRANT'S 7.48
NETTER 76
A.V.A. 5: 2.16.33

GRANT'S 7.13A, 9.8-9.10
ROHEN 72
A.D.A.M. 7.34, 7.35
NETTER 18
CLEMENTE 735, 736

GRANT'S 7.43
ROHEN 138
NETTER 77
CLEMENTE 795-797
A.V.A. 5: 2.17.18

GRANT'S 7.14A, 9.8
ROHEN 72
A.D.A.M. 7.34, 7.35
NETTER 18
CLEMENTE 735, 736
A.V.A. 5: 0.58.49

GRANT'S 7.43, 7.44
ROHEN 138
A.D.A.M. 7.68, 7.69
NETTER 77
CLEMENTE 796
A.V.A. 5: 2.18.24

GRANT'S 7.44
ROHEN 138
A.D.A.M. 7.69
NETTER 77
CLEMENTE 798-800
A.V.A. 4: 1.09.00

> The upper and lower lacrimal punctum and the corresponding lacrimal canaliculi may be obstructed or not sufficiently open. This condition is not uncommon in the newborn child.

Sensory Nerves of the Face

Review the sensory nerves of the face that are derived from the three divisions of the trigeminal nerve (Fig. 7.13). Positively identify the following structures in the cadaver:

- **Supraorbital nerve,** a branch of the ophthalmic division (V1);
- **Infraorbital nerve,** a branch of the maxillary division, (V2);
- **Mental nerve,** a branch of the mandibular division, (V3).
- Note that the skin of the nose is supplied by the **external nasal nerve,** a branch of V1.
- There are several smaller branches of the trigeminal nerve (lacrimal; infratrochlear; zygomaticofacial; zygomaticotemporal). Do not dissect these twigs. The auriculotemporal nerve (V3) will be dissected later.

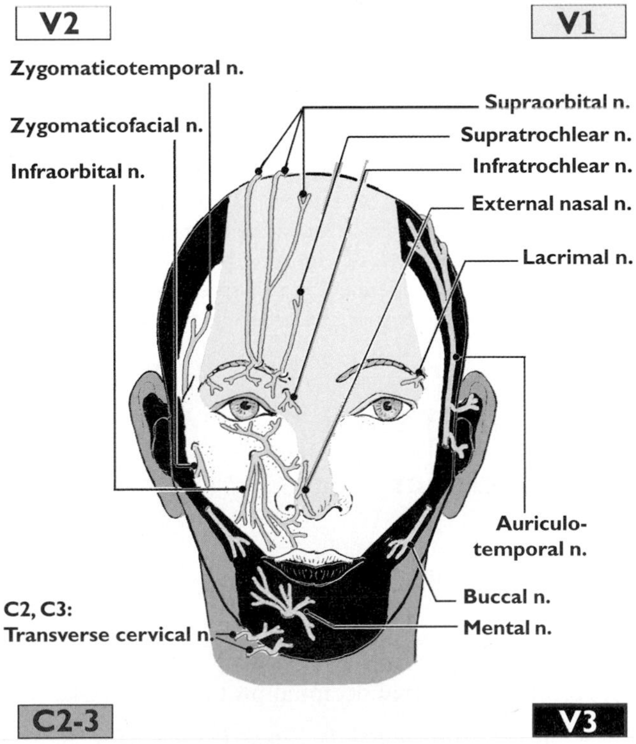

Figure 7.13. Sensory nerves of the face.

Scalp

General Remarks

The scalp is the covering of the cranial vault. It consists of three layers that are firmly bound together (Fig. 7.14):

- **Skin,** usually covered with hair;
- **Superficial fascia** (subcutaneous tissue), which is exceedingly tough and dense; vessels and nerves run in it;
- **Muscular layer,** consisting of the **frontalis muscle** anteriorly and the **occipitalis muscle** posteriorly; the two muscles are united by a broad aponeurosis, the **epicranial aponeurosis** or **galea aponeurotica**.

The bones of the cranial vault are intimately covered with **pericranium** or periosteum. The pericranium is separated from the three layers of the scalp by very **loose areolar tissue.** This loose areolar layer permits the frontalis and occipitalis muscles to produce a limited amount of movement.

GRANT'S 7.18
ROHEN 85
A.D.A.M. 7.44, 7.66
NETTER 17, 21
CLEMENTE 731, 733
A.V.A. 5: 0.06.02

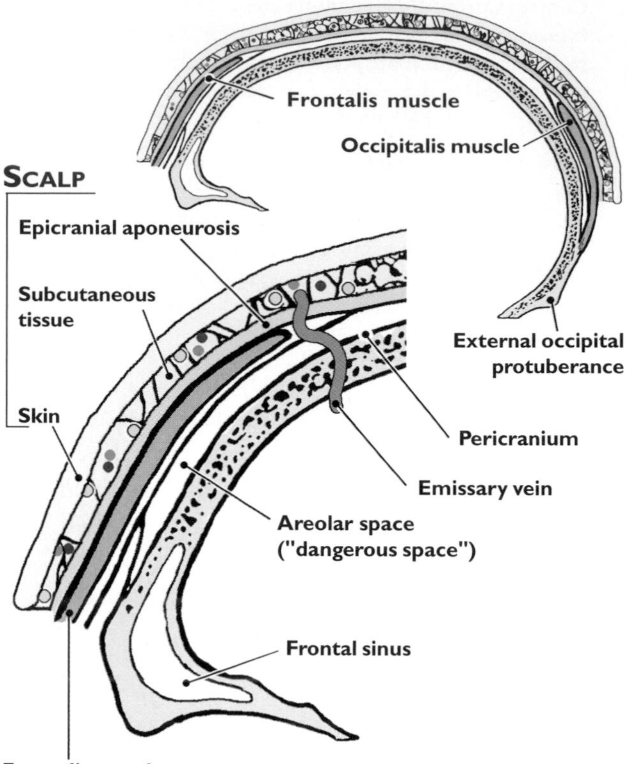

Figure 7.14. Sagittal section of the skull cap and overlying tissues.

Blood vessels and sensory nerves reach the scalp from all around its periphery. These structures are contained in the exceedingly tough superficial fascia. You may not have time for the dissection of nerves and vessels in the scalp region. However, be aware of the fact that a rich nerve and blood supply exists (Fig. 7.15).

GRANT'S 7.14B
ROHEN 85
A.D.A.M. 7.30, 7.32, 7.44
NETTER 17
CLEMENTE 735, 736
A.V.A. 5: 0.08.33

> ***Clinical Correlation:*** The loose areolar layer between the scalp and the pericranium is of clinical importance. Once an infection has reached the loose layer, it can spread readily in it. Therefore, this layer has been called the "dangerous area" (Fig. 7.14). From the "dangerous area," the infection is easily carried along veins that traverse the bony vault. As a result, the infection may spread to the substance of the bones, to venous channels within the cranial cavity, or to the brain. At the level of the zygomatic arch and at the superior nuchal line in the occipital region, the loose areolar layer is closely adherent to bone; that means, infections of the scalp cannot readily spread beyond these areas. The physician must be aware of this fact and its anatomical basis.

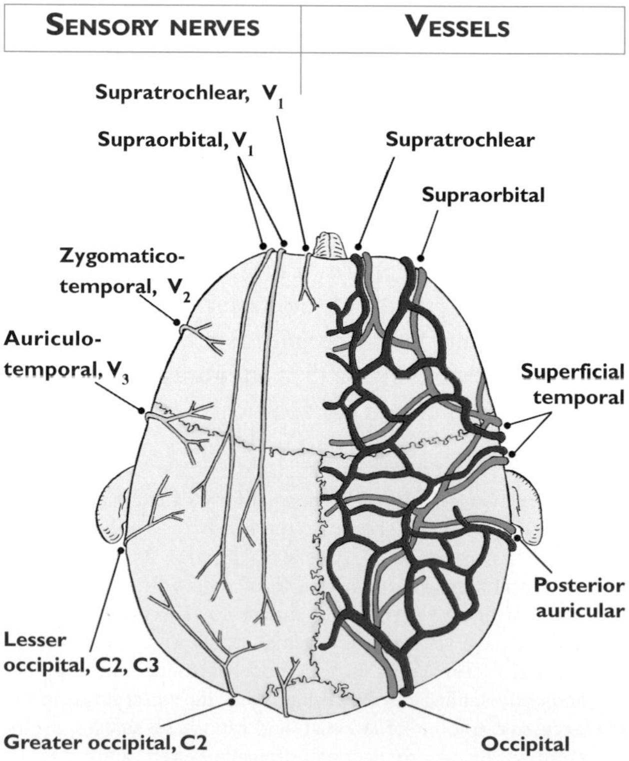

Figure 7.15. Sensory nerves and vessels of the scalp.

Structures of Scalp

Skin Incisions

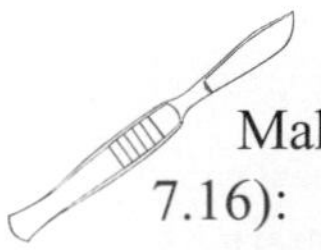

Make the following skin incisions (Fig. 7.16):

- In the midline, from nasion (*A*) to vertex (*B*), and on to the external occipital protuberance (*C*);
- On the right and left sides, from vertex to a point just above and in front of the ear (*B* to *D*);

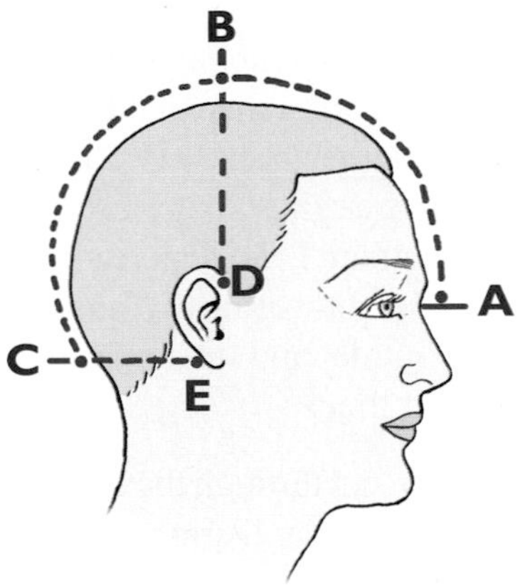

Figure 7.16. Skins incisions.

• On the right and left sides, from external occipital protuberance transversely to the mastoid process (*C* to *E*).

Reflect the four flaps of scalp inferiorly. Do this by working in the loose areolar space ("dangerous area") with your fingers or the handle of the scalpel. On the side of the skull, reflect the scalp from the underlying **temporalis fascia,** which covers the temporalis muscle.

GRANT'S 7.9, 7.18
ROHEN 85
A.D.A.M. 7.44
NETTER 17
CLEMENTE 731, 733
A.V.A. 5: 0.07.29

The nerves and vessels are contained within the flaps of scalp. The **occipitalis muscle** is contained in the posterior flap. The anterior flap contains the **frontalis muscle**. Examine the **epicranial aponeurosis** (galea aponeurotica), which unites these two muscles (Fig. 7.14). Verify the existence of a rich blood supply to the scalp (Fig. 7.15).

GRANT'S 7.2
ROHEN 33
A.D.A.M. 7.2
NETTER 4, 8
CLEMENTE 756
A.V.A. 4: 0.03.00

Next, observe the **pericranium** that intimately covers the skull cap. With a sharp instrument, scrape off the pericranium superior to the attachment of the temporalis fascia. Do not remove the temporalis fascia. Now, the **suture lines** separating the individual bones can be seen. In the cadaver and the bony skull, identify the following (Figs. 7.17, 7.18):

• **Coronal suture,** separating the large unpaired frontal bone from the two parietal bones;

• **Sagittal suture,** separating the two parietal bones;

• **Bregma,** the point where sagittal and coronal sutures meet;

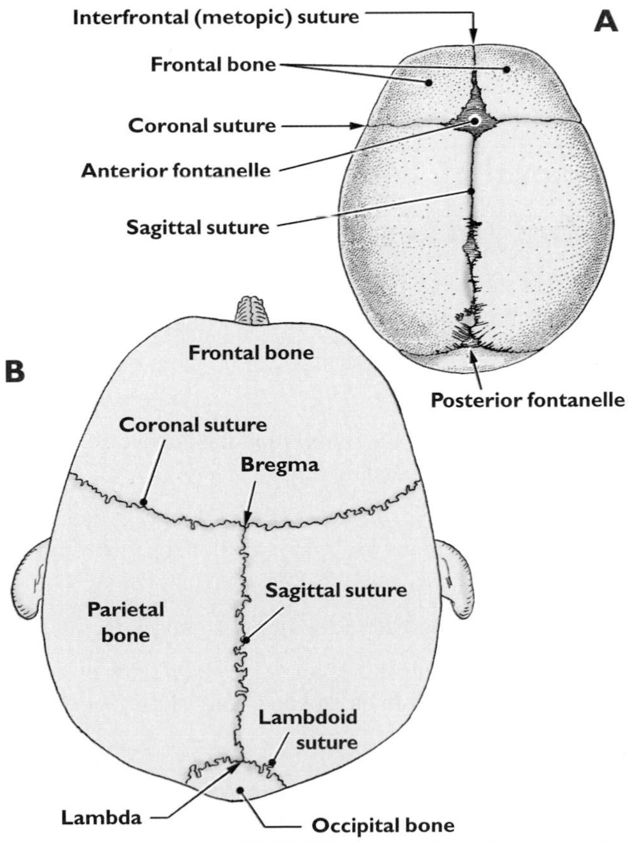

Figure 7.17. Suture lines (superior view) of the infant skull ***(A)***, and the adult skull ***(B)***.

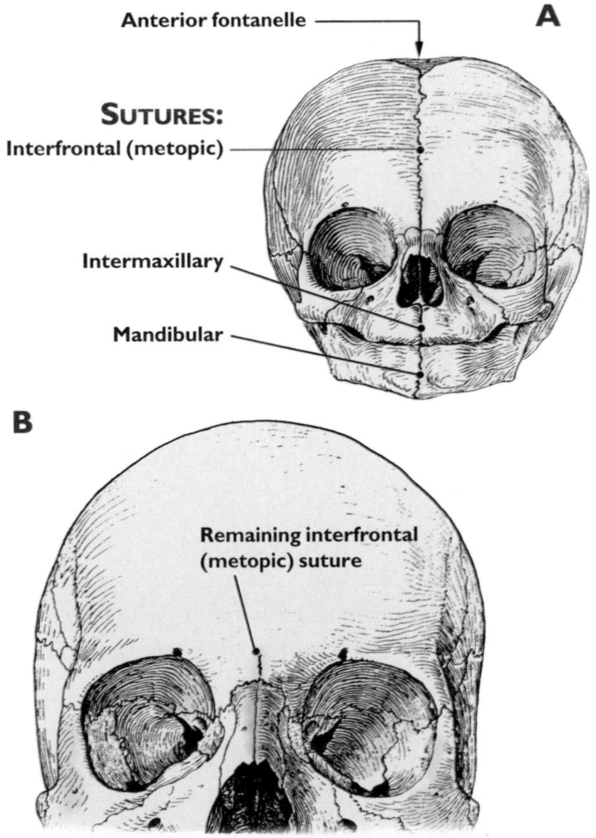

Figure 7.18. Suture lines (anterior view) of the infant skull ***(A)***, and the adult skull ***(B)***.

- **Lambdoid suture,** separating the unpaired occipital bone from the two parietal bones;
- **Lambda,** the point where sagittal and lambdoid sutures meet;
- Remains of the **metopic suture**, extending a short distance superiorly from the nasion (Fig. 7.18).

> ***Clinical Correlation:*** In the skull, identify the large unpaired frontal bone. Note the remains of the **metopic** or **interfrontal suture** extending a short distance superiorly from the nasion (Fig. 7.18). In about 2% of the population, the frontal bone of the adult is paired, as is normally the case in infants up to 2 years of age. In the mentioned adult cases, the persisting frontal or metopic suture is of radiological importance. It must not be mistaken for a fracture line.

Interior of Skull

Removal of Skull Cap (Calvaria)

Refer to the bony skull of a skeleton. Lift up the calvaria. Note that the bones of the roof of the skull consist of three parts:

- A compact *outer lamina*;
- A compact and very hard *inner lamina*;
- The *diploe*, a layer of spongy bone that is sandwiched in between the outer and inner laminae. The diploe contains diploic veins. Observe that there is no diploe in the temporal region (here the bones are covered with the thick and fleshy temporalis muscle).

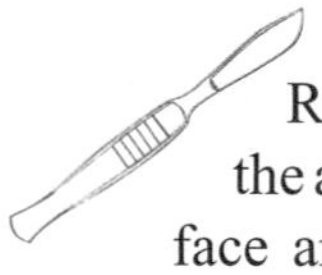

Return to the cadaver specimen. Pull the anterior half of the scalp well over the face and the posterior half well over the nuchal region of the occipital bone. Reflect the temporalis muscles in the following manner:

- With a sharp scalpel, incise the temporalis fascia along the temporal lines, i.e., incise it in a semicircular fashion along the superior and posterior margins of the temporalis muscle.
- Insert the handle of the scalpel between muscle and bones. Lift off the temporalis muscle. Reflect it inferiorly to the level of the zygomatic arch.
- Scrape the bones clean.

Grant's 7.2
Rohen 33
A.D.A.M. 7.2
Netter 4, 8
Clemente 756, 760

Place an elastic rubber band or a string around the circumference of the skull. Anteriorly, the band must be at least 2 cm above the supraorbital margin. Posteriorly, place the rubber band about 2 cm superior to the external occipital protuberance (inion). Use the band as a guide and encircle the calvaria with a pencil line.

Grant's 7.6
Rohen 44, 54

With a saw, cut through the external lamina along the pencil line. During the sawing, turn the body alternately on the back or the face. Moist red bone indicates that the saw is well within the diploe. Be particularly careful on the sides where the bones are thin. If you saw through the inner table, you are liable to damage the underlying dura mater or even the brain. Therefore, break the inner table by repeatedly inserting a chisel into the saw cut and by striking the chisel gently with a mallet. Continue with this procedure until the calvaria can be pried loose. Remove the calvaria by gently detaching it from the dura mater. Use your fingers, the handle of a scalpel, or a pair of forceps. Do not use more force than necessary. Violent pulling will frequently result in tearing of the dura and in damage to the brain.

Grant's 7.18
Rohen 34
A.D.A.M. 7.38, 7.66
Netter 4
Clemente 758
A.V.A. 5: 0.06.12

Removal of Wedge of Occipital Bone

Before you begin . . .

At this stage, the removal of a large wedge-shaped area of the occipital bone offers many advantages:

- The brain and its coverings can be more easily examined *in situ*.
- The confluens of the sinuses and the transverse sinuses can be demonstrated *in situ*.
- After removal of the cerebellum, the brain stem and the cranial nerves emerging from it can be studied *in situ*.
- Finally, the removal of the brain is greatly facilitated.

Grant's 7.2
Rohen 34
A.D.A.M. 7.12
Netter 6, 7
Clemente 779, 780
A.V.A. 4: 0.06.56

Also, prior to removal of part of the occipital bone, study pertinent landmarks in an isolated bony skull:

- **Mastoid process**;
- **External occipital protuberance or inion;**
- Foramen magnum;
- Examine the internal surface of the **occipital bone** (Fig. 7.19): **groove for superior sagittal sinus; grooves for**

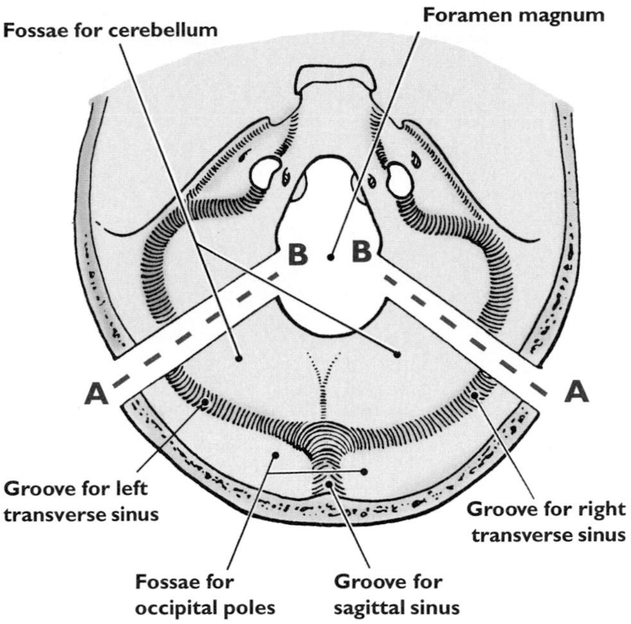

Figure 7.19. Internal surface of the occipital bone. Demarcation of the wedge-shaped area that is to be removed from the occipital bone.

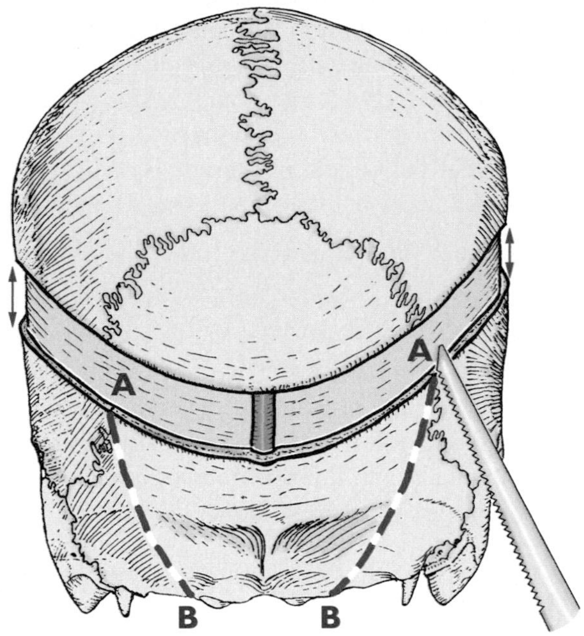

Figure 7.20. After removal of the calvaria, make two saw cuts from ***A*** to ***B*** to remove a large wedge from the occipital bone.

right and left transverse sinuses; two fossae for cerebellum, inferior to the grooves for the transverse sinuses; **two fossae for the occipital poles** of the cerebral hemispheres, superior to the grooves for the transverse sinuses.

GRANT'S *7.4*
ROHEN 34
A.D.A.M. 7.12
NETTER 6, 7
CLEMENTE 779, 780
A.V.A. 5: 1.43.15

In the isolated skull, mark with a pencil the point where the cut edge of the skull intersects with the lambdoid suture (suture between occipital and parietal bone; *A*). Next, identify the lateral margin of the foramen magnum (*B*). On the right and left sides, connect points (*A*) and (*B*) with pencil lines. You have now demarcated on the *isolated* skull the wedge that is to be removed in the cadaver (Fig. 7.19; *see also* Fig. 7.21).

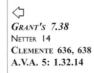

Turn to the cadaver, which must be in the prone position (face down). Proceed:

- Detach all muscles from the occipital bone.
- Clearly identify the interval between **occipital bone** and **atlas** (C1).
- Preserve the **vertebral arteries**.
- Using fine scissors, carefully incise the **posterior atlanto-occipital membrane** transversely from vertebral artery to vertebral artery.
- Scrape the occipital bone clean of muscle remains and pericranium.
- With pencil lines, mark the bony wedge between points *A* and *B* as shown in Figure 7.20.

GRANT'S *7.38*
NETTER 14
CLEMENTE 636, 638
A.V.A. 5: 1.32.14

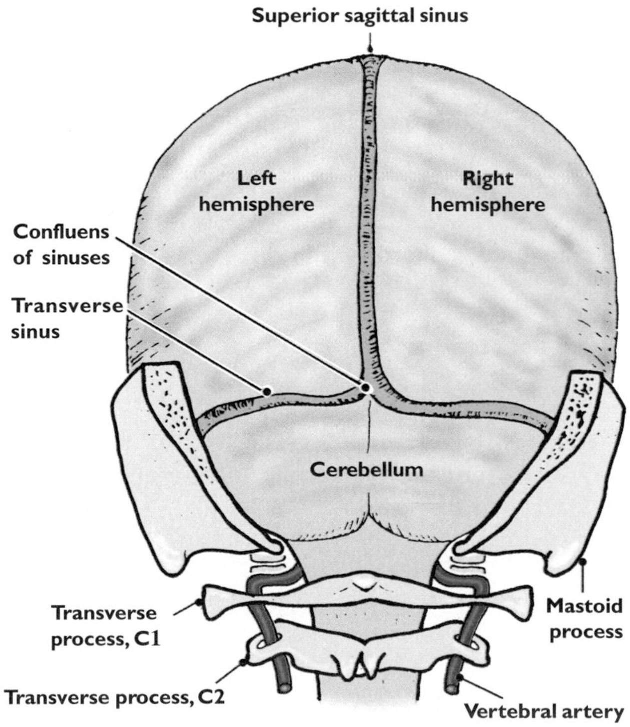

Figure 7.21. Calvaria and large wedge of occipital bone removed to expose the posterior aspect of the brain and venous sinuses.

- Cut along these lines with a small saw. As in the removal of the calvaria, do not cut through the inner compact layer of bone. Loosen the bony wedge with chisel and mallet. Carefully pry it loose from the moistened dura mater. Protect the vertebral arteries. Be sure to extend the saw cut into the foramen magnum.
- Remove the wedge (Fig. 7.21).

Examine the inner surface of the removed bony wedge. Verify that the two **cerebellar fossae** were in contact with the dura mater overlying the **cerebellum.** Demonstrate that the **grooves for the transverse sinuses** were in contact with these venous channels. Save the wedge of occipital bone.

⇦
GRANT'S 7.4
ROHEN 34, 35
A.D.A.M. 7.12
NETTER 6, 7
CLEMENTE 779, 780
A.V.A. 5: 1.43.15

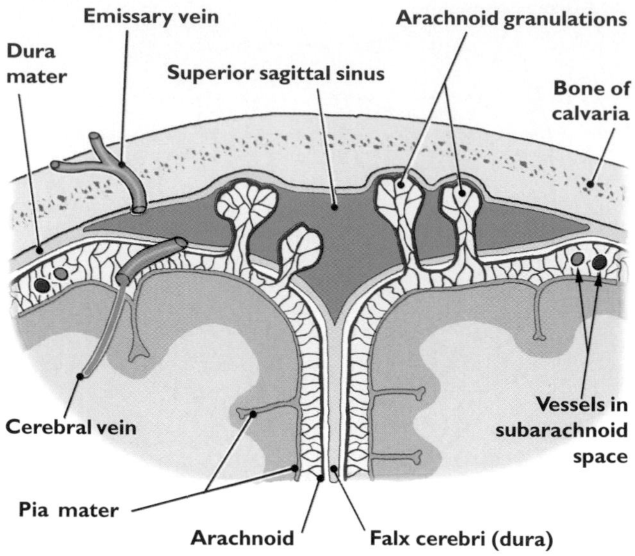

Figure 7.22. Meninges of the brain. Coronal section through the superior sagittal sinus and related structures.

Meninges of Brain

The brain is covered with three membranes, the meninges (Gr., *meninx*, membrane). These are (Fig. 7.22):

- **Dura mater,** the outer tough membrane;
- **Arachnoid,** the intermediate membrane with spiderweb-like processes toward the pia mater;
- **Pia mater,** a soft delicate membrane that is closely applied to the brain tissue.

⇦
GRANT'S 7.18
ROHEN 85
NETTER 94
CLEMENTE 765
A.V.A. 5: 1.15.17

⇨
GRANT'S 7.4A
ROHEN 36, 88
NETTER 95
CLEMENTE 758
A.V.A. 5: 1.53.43

Explanation of Terms

The **dura mater** (Lat., *dura*, hard) is also known as pachymeninx (Gr., *pachys*, thick). The two soft membranes, **arachnoid** and **pia mater**, are also collectively called **leptomeninx** (Gr., *leptos*, thin; delicate). The meninges of the brain are continuous with those covering the spinal cord (Chapter 4).

Dura Mater

The **dura mater** consists of two layers:

- A rough, outer layer; it is adherent to the cranial bones where it forms an endocranium (periosteal covering for the bone);
- A smooth inner layer.

The two dural layers are indistinguishable except where they separate to enclose the venous sinuses (Fig. 7.22).

⇦
GRANT'S 7.19
ROHEN 85, 88
A.D.A.M. 7.66
NETTER 94, 95
A.V.A. 5: 0.14.20

In the cadaver, examine the rough, outer layer of the dura mater that covers the cerebral and cerebellar hemispheres. In the outer dural layer, observe the branches of the important **middle meningeal artery**. This vessel supplies the dura mater. The bulk of blood, however, reaches the adjacent cranial bones. Examine the internal surface of the removed calvaria. Note the distinct grooves for the branches of the middle meningeal artery. In the immediate vicinity of these grooves, observe numerous, tiny nutrient foramina leading to the substance of the bones. The use of a magnifying glass is helpful!

> ***Clinical Correlation:*** The **middle meningeal artery** is of great clinical importance. If it is torn in a head injury, blood will quickly accumulate between the bony skull and dura mater (epidural hematoma). The expanding hematoma may exert fatal pressure on the brain unless it is promptly recognized and surgically treated. Surgeons must be aware of the course of the middle meningeal artery and its projection on the surface of the cranium. In the interior of a skull, examine the **groove for the middle meningeal artery.** Note that its **anterior branch** crosses the area of the **pterion**. Identify the pterion on the outside of a skull. Fractures through this area are likely to result in tearing of the middle meningeal artery with the consequence of an epidural hematoma.

⇦
GRANT'S 7.19
ROHEN 88
NETTER 95
CLEMENTE 766
A.V.A. 5: 1.53.51

In certain areas, the two layers of dura split to enclose the venous sinuses. Identify the **superior sagittal sinus** and the right and left **transverse sinuses** (Fig. 7.21). With scissors, slit these sinuses open. Examine closely the superior sagittal sinus and verify that:

- It increases in caliber as it passes posteriorly (direction of venous blood flow);
- It is triangular on transverse section (Fig. 7.22);
- It has lateral expansions, the **lacunae laterales**.

In relation to the superior sagittal sinus and its lacunae, observe numerous cauliflower-like masses, the **arachnoid granulations**.

GRANT'S 7.19-7.21
ROHEN 86, 87
A.D.A.M. 7.66
NETTER 96, 97
CLEMENTE 766, 767
A.V.A. 5: 1.41.36

Clinical Correlation: As a complication of head injury, bleeding into the potential space between the dura mater and the arachnoid may occur. This hemorrhage is called a **subdural hematoma**.

Because the potential space is only limited by the falx cerebri and the tentorium cerebelli, a subdural hemorrhage may spread thinly and widely over a hemisphere. The subdural hematoma, which is venous in origin, is a serious and insidious complication of head injuries. It must be distinguished from the epidural hematoma.

Clinical Correlation: The **arachnoid granulations** (Fig. 7.22) are projections of the subarachnoid space filled with **cerebrospinal fluid (CSF)**. The CSF is constantly produced by the choroid plexuses in the ventricular system of the brain. To avoid undue and harmful pressure, any excess of CSF must be removed. This is accomplished by the arachnoid granulations. They empty the CSF into the venous sinuses by diffusion.

The arachnoid granulations are responsible for small shallow depressions on the inner aspect of the calvaria. Examine the removed calvaria. Note these depressions, the *foveolae granulares*, in the vicinity of the sulcus for the superior sagittal sinus.

GRANT'S 7.18
ROHEN 89
NETTER 96
CLEMENTE 765
A.V.A. 5: 0.15.54

Arachnoid (Gr., *arachne*, spider; referring to the fine spiderweb-like processes between arachnoid membrane and pia). The arachnoid is a thin, nonvascular membrane that surrounds the brain loosely (Fig. 7.22).

NETTER 4, 96
CLEMENTE 758
A.V.A. 5: 1.45.10

The **subarachnoid space** is a real space that contains cerebrospinal fluid. In the living, this fluid-filled space acts as an effective shock absorber. In the embalmed cadaver, the CSF is absent. Restore it artificially over a limited area of the cerebral hemisphere as follows:

ROHEN 85
NETTER 96
CLEMENTE 765
A.V.A. 5: 0.16.18

On both sides, **reflect the dura mater** from the cerebral and cerebellar hemispheres in the following manner:

NETTER 96

- Use a syringe with a fine needle. Puncture the arachnoid membrane obliquely.
- Inject 5 to 10 ml of fluid (colored or plain water) into the subarachnoid space. An effective fluid cushion is being formed that covers several gyri and sulci.
- Note that the arachnoid smoothly covers all gaps and fissures of the brain surface.

- Make an incision through the dura corresponding to the coronal suture. Be very careful not to injure the underlying arachnoid. With a forceps, produce a small fold of dura, nick it, and insert the scissors.
- Cut the dura parallel to the superior sagittal and transverse sinuses. Stay about 2 cm clear of the venous channels. Now, expose the cerebral hemispheres by reflecting the dural flaps inferiorly. Note the smooth inner surface of the dura.
- Cut the dura just inferiorly to the transverse sinuses. Then, cut it along the margins of the removed bony wedge.
- You may enlarge the exposed area by carefully resecting the posterior arch of the atlas.
- Remove the dura, but leave a small, sickle-shaped dural fold between the two cerebellar hemispheres. This is the **falx cerebelli**.

Now, with the dura mater reflected, the arachnoid is widely exposed. Note that there is an extensive potential space between the dura mater and the delicate membrane of the arachnoid.

ROHEN 86, 110, 141
NETTER 103
A.V.A. 5: 0.16.34

Substantial intervals between pia and arachnoid are known as cisternae. Find the largest of these, the **cisterna cerebellomedullaris (cisterna magna).** It is the enlarged subarachnoid space between the caudal part of the cerebellar hemispheres and the medulla oblongata.

GRANT'S 7.18
ROHEN 85, 89
NETTER 96
CLEMENTE 765
A.V.A. 5: 0.15.17

Pia Mater (Lat., *pius*, tender; faithful). On part of one cerebral hemisphere, remove the arachnoid. Identify the pia. It is a delicate membrane that follows (faithfully) the brain tissue in between all sulci and fissures. The pia carries the blood vessels that supply the brain (Fig. 7.22). Observe the **cerebral veins** that empty into the superior sagittal sinus.

Exposure of Brain Stem and 4th Ventricle

It is desirable to maintain the structural integrity of the brain so that it can be used for future detailed studies (courses in neuroanatomy or the neurosciences). If it is not necessary to preserve the brain, follow special directions from your instructors. Only half of the cerebellum will be sacrificed to expose the brain stem and the 4th ventricle.

The objective is to expose the brain stem and the cranial nerves emerging from it. The cerebellum covers the brain stem posteriorly (Fig. 7.23). Remove the *right half* of the cerebellum *only* in the following manner:

GRANT'S 7.38
ROHEN 69
A.V.A. 5: 0.28.10

- With a scalpel, carefully split the narrow median portion (vermis) of the cerebellum in the midsagittal plane. Start just inferior to the confluens of the sinuses (Fig. 7.21) and just to the right of the falx cerebelli. Avoid cutting into the medulla.
- Next, make a parasagittal cut about 5 mm lateral to the midsagittal incision. Remove the narrow slice of cerebellar tissue.
- Gently force the two cerebellar hemispheres apart to obtain a partial view of the 4th ventricle.
- Remove several more thin slices of cerebellum. Finally, cut through the attachments of the right cerebellar hemisphere to the brain stem and remove the remains of the right half of the cerebellum.
- The *right half* of the brain stem and of the 4th ventricle is now exposed.

On the *right side only*, identify the following important structures:

GRANT'S 7.38
ROHEN 69
A.V.A. 5: 0.45.23

- **Vertebral artery,** entering the cranial cavity through the foramen magnum;
- **Trochlear nerve (IV);** it is the most delicate of the cranial nerves; see it just caudal to the colliculi of the midbrain;
- **Trigeminal nerve (V);** it is the largest of the cranial nerves emerging from the brain stem;
- **Facial nerve (VII)** and **vestibulocochlear nerve (acoustic nerve; VIII),** taking a common course toward the internal acoustic meatus;

GRANT'S 7.40
ROHEN 69, 87
A.D.A.M. 7.67
CLEMENTE 777
A.V.A. 5: 0.13.12

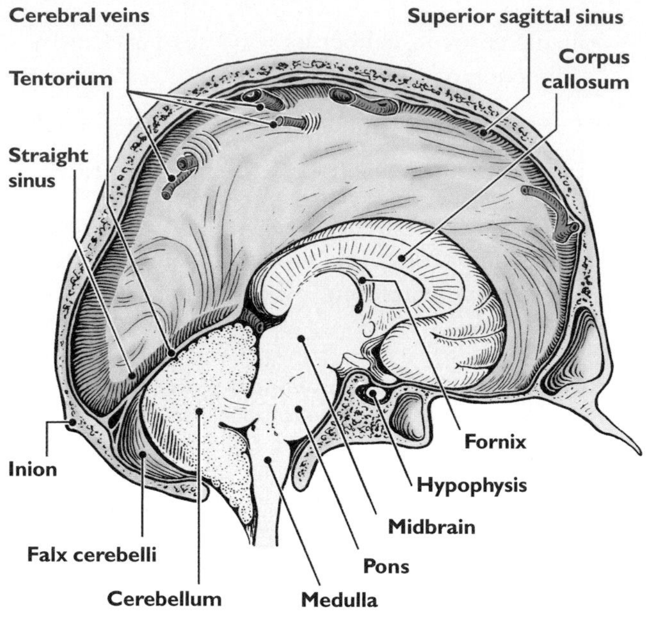

Figure 7.23. Folds of dura matter and related structures.

GRANT'S 7.38
ROHEN 69
NETTER 98
A.V.A. 5: 1.10.23

- Three cranial nerves that converge on the **jugular foramen: glossopharyngeal nerve (IX), vagus nerve (X),** and **accessory nerve (XI).**

Folds of Dura Mater

GRANT'S 7.20
ROHEN 69, 87
NETTER 97
CLEMENTE 765, 767
A.V.A. 5: 0.12.52

The *inner layer* of dura mater forms inwardly projecting folds that serve as incomplete partitions of the cranial cavity. Three of these folds will be examined now (Fig. 7.23):

- **Tentorium cerebelli**;
- **Falx cerebelli**;
- **Falx cerebri**.

Tentorium Cerebelli (L., *tentorium*, tent).

In the cadaver, examine the inferior surface of the tentorium where the right cerebellar hemisphere was removed. Verify that it separates the cerebellar lobe from the corresponding occipital pole of the cerebral hemisphere. In fact, in the anatomical position, the tentorium supports the weight of the occipital poles. Observe the *posterior convex border* of the tentorium. It encloses the transverse sinuses. Review its attachments to the inner surface of the occipital bone along the grooves for the transverse sinuses. The *anterior and medial borders* of the tentorium are free and concave and form the tentorial notch that surrounds the midbrain.

Falx Cerebelli (L. *falx*, sickle).

It is small. Observe its anterior free border that projects between the cerebellar hemispheres in the median plane (Fig. 7.23).

GRANT'S 7.20
ROHEN 88
A.D.A.M. 7.67
NETTER 97
CLEMENTE 767

Falx Cerebri

This large, sickle-shaped membrane lies in the midsagittal plane between the two cerebral hemispheres (Figs. 7.23, 7.24). Anteriorly, it is attached to the *crista galli* of the ethmoid bone. Posteriorly, it is fused with the tentorium cerebelli. The superior convex border encloses the **superior sagittal sinus**. Review its attachments to the inner surface of the calvaria, along the groove for the superior sagittal sinus. On the right and left sides, cut the **cerebral veins** that empty into the superior sagittal sinus. Free the falx cerebri. Gently pull the cerebral hemispheres apart and observe the free inferior border of the falx cerebri. It lies superior to the *corpus callosum* of the brain (Fig. 7.23).

GRANT'S 7.20
ROHEN 69, 87
A.D.A.M. 7.67
NETTER 97
CLEMENTE 767
A.V.A. 5: 0.13.48

The inferior concave border of the falx cerebri encloses the **inferior sagittal sinus** (Fig. 7.24). This sinus joins the great cerebral vein (of Galen) to form the **straight sinus.** The straight sinus runs obliquely between the falx cerebri and the tentorium cerebelli. Find the straight sinus as it empties into the **confluens of the sinuses**. Push a thin probe from the confluens of the sinuses (confluens sinuum) into the straight sinus.

Review the folds of dura mater and obtain a clear concept of their arrangements. These dural folds will be detached during removal of the brain from the cranial cavity.

Removal of Brain

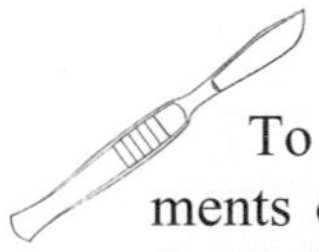

To remove the brain skillfully, all attachments of the brain to the cranium must be freed. With the cadaver in the prone position (face down), begin with the transection of the following three structures:

GRANT'S 7.4
ROHEN 34, 35
A.D.A.M. 7.12
NETTER 6, 7
CLEMENTE 779, 780
A.V.A. 4: 0.39.27

The **spinal cord** at the level of the atlas (C1);

- Both **vertebral arteries,** anywhere between the foramen magnum and the transverse processes of the atlas;

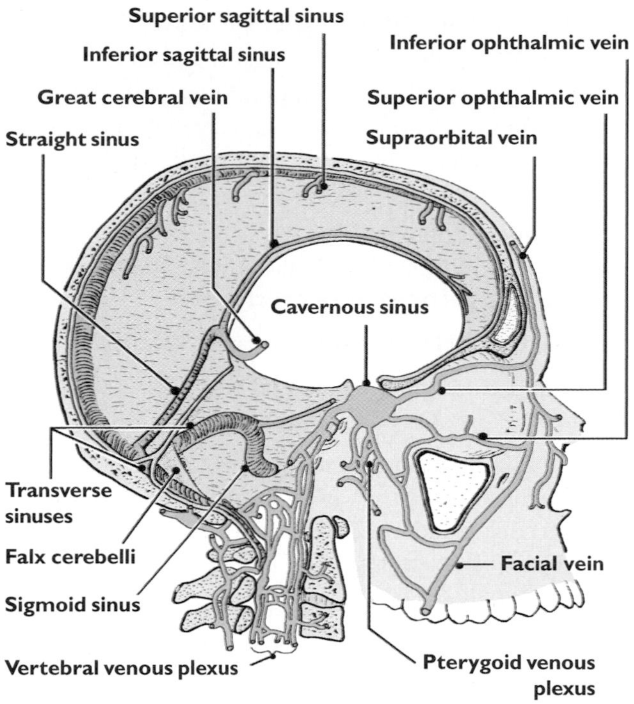

Figure 7.24. Folds of dura mater and venous sinuses.

GRANT'S 7.38
ROHEN 69
NETTER 98
CLEMENTE 777, 778
A.V.A. 5: 0.24.20

- On the right side, where the cerebellum has been removed, cut with fine scissors the following **cranial nerves** close to the brain stem: **IV, V,** and **VII** through **XI**. Reflect cranial nerves **X** and **XI** posteriorly, and expose the fiber bundles of the **hypoglossal nerve (XII)**. Sever this nerve.

Which structures must still be severed to completely mobilize the brain?

- Cranial nerves I, II, III, and VI on the right side;
- All cranial nerves on the left side;
- Blood vessels;
- Attachments of dural folds.

At this stage, and in preparation for the removal of the brain, familiarize yourself with **relevant bony landmarks** and certain soft structures. In the interior of the isolated **bony skull**, identify the following:

- **Crista galli;** a triangular plate of the ethmoid bone projecting into the interior of the skull in the median plane;
- **Cribriform plate** (L., *cribrum*, sieve); a plate on either side of the crista galli; its numerous foramina transmit the filaments of the olfactory nerve; the olfactory bulb rests on the cribriform plate;
- **Optic foramen** (canal); a round opening traversed by the optic nerve and the ophthalmic artery; view this foramen from the orbital cavity;

- **Groove for the internal carotid artery;** just inferior to the optic canal;
- **Petrous portion of the temporal bone**; note its sharp **superior margin;** the tentorium cerebelli is attached here; the margin also contains a small groove for the superior petrosal sinus.

In addition, examine the base of a brain (demonstration specimen) or at least a good atlas illustation and identify the following **pertinent soft structures**:

GRANT'S 7.34
ROHEN 68
A.D.A.M. 7.36
NETTER 112
CLEMENTE 778
A.V.A. 5: 0.33.36

- **Olfactory bulbs and tracts** (cranial "nerve" **I**);
- Right and left **optic nerves** (cranial "nerve" **II**); they unite to form the optic chiasma;
- **Infundibulum,** just posterior to the optic chiasma; essentially, it is the stalk of the hypophysis cerebri (pituitary); the gland must be severed from its stalk during removal of the brain;
- Right and left **internal carotid arteries,** lying in their grooves just inferior to the optic nerves;
- **Oculomotor nerve (III),** just cranial to the pons;
- **Abducent nerve (VI),** just caudal to the pons.

Dissection Procedure

Turn the cadaver into the supine position (face up). Ask your partner to support the brain posteriorly with one or two hands. Preceed as follows:

- Gently separate the frontal poles of the cerebral hemispheres. Cut the **falx cerebri** close to the **crista galli**. Pull the falx superiorly and posteriorly.
- Gently lift up the frontal poles. To both sides of the crista galli, note the **olfactory bulbs and tracts.** Dislodge the bulbs from the cribriform plates. Accomplish this with the aid of forceps and probe.
- Elevate the brain further until you see the **infundibulum** just posterior to the **optic chiasma.** Cut across the infundibulum.
- Next sever the **optic nerves** and the two **internal carotid arteries** close to the optic foramina. Lift up the brain further.
- Identify the two **oculomotor nerves** and cut them.
- With a scalpel, **detach the tentorium cerebelli** on both sides. Start the cut at the free border of the tentorial notch. Carry the cut posteriorly, close to the **superior margin of the petrous bone.** Complete the detachment by cutting all the way to the free margin of the excised occipital wedge. Ask your partner to support the weight of the brain.
- Next, identify and cut the two **abducent nerves.**
- Subsequently, sever the remaining cranial nerves on the *left side* (IV, V, VII through XII).
- Pull the brain gently posteriorly, and remove it from the cranial cavity.

Gross Examination of the Brain

GRANT'S 7.24
ROHEN 68, 89
A.D.A.M. 7.37
NETTER 99
CLEMENTE 778
A.V.A. 5: 0.30.30

Examine the **cerebral hemispheres** and identify the following (Fig. 7.25):

- **Frontal pole;**
- **Temporal pole;**
- **Occipital pole;**
- **Lateral sulcus** (lateral cerebral fissure; fissure of Sylvius);
- **Central sulcus** (fissure of Rolando);
- **Frontal lobe,** the largest of the lobes; it is bounded posteriorly by the central sulcus, inferiorly by the lateral sulcus.

GRANT'S 7.4B
ROHEN 34, 35
A.D.A.M. 7.12
NETTER 6
CLEMENTE 779, 780
A.V.A. 5: 0.38.50

Refer to a skull and identify the **three cranial fossae:** *anterior, middle, and posterior.* By placing the brain back into the cranial cavity of the cadaver, verify the following (Fig. 7.25):

- The frontal pole and part of the **frontal lobe** are located in the **anterior cranial fossa**.
- The temporal pole and part of the **temporal lobe** fit into the **middle cranial fossa**.
- The occipital pole and part of the **occipital lobe** are located in the **posterior cranial fossa** (superior to the grooves for the transverse sinuses).
- The **cerebellum** is also located in the **posterior cranial fossa** (inferior to the grooves for the transverse sinuses).

ROHEN 94
A.D.A.M. 7.36, 7.37
NETTER 132
CLEMENTE 775
A.V.A. 5: 1.36.54

Examine the base of the brain. Note that it is covered with arachnoid. Remove the arachnoid. Note the arteries at the base of the brain (Fig. 7.26). The two vertebral and the two internal carotid arteries supply the brain. These arteries join to form the **cerebral arterial circle** (of Willis). Verify the following:

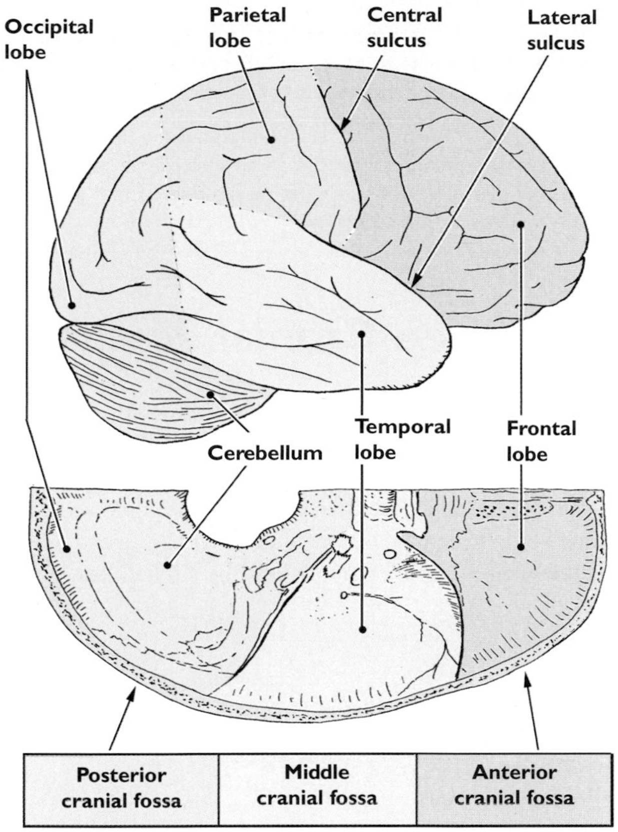

Figure 7.25. The brain and its relation to the three cranial fossae.

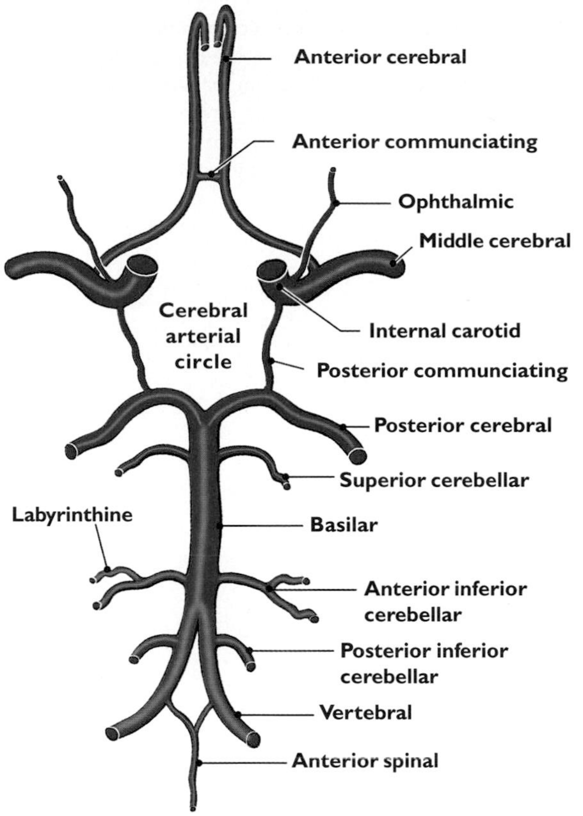

Figure 7.26. Cerebral arterial circle (of Willis) at the base of the brain.

- The right and left **posterior inferior cerebellar arteries** arise from the respective **vertebral arteries**.
- The right and left **vertebral arteries** join to form the **basilar artery**.
- The **basilar artery** gives off several branches: anterior inferior cerebellar, superior cerebellar, and posterior cerebral.
- Note the **oculomotor nerve** (III) emerging between **posterior cerebral artery** and **superior cerebellar artery**.
- After giving off the ophthalmic artery, each **internal carotid artery** terminates by dividing into a **middle cerebral artery** and an **anterior cerebral artery**.
- The **arterial circle** (Fig. 7.26) is completed by communicating arteries. Anteriorly, the two anterior cerebral arteries are united by the unpaired and very short **anterior communicating artery**. Posteriorly, the **posterior communicating arteries** connect the internal carotid arteries with the posterior cerebral arteries.

⇦
GRANT'S 7.34
ROHEN 94
NETTER 132,133
CLEMENTE 775
A.V.A 5: 1.35.08

Observe that the flat *medial surfaces* of the cerebral hemispheres are supplied by the anterior and posterior cerebral arteries. Specifically, the **anterior cerebral artery** supplies the anterior and superior aspects of the medial surface. The **posterior cerebral artery** supplies the posterior aspect of the medial surface and the inferior surface of the hemisphere.

⇨
GRANT'S 7.34
ROHEN 94
NETTER 132, 134
CLEMENTE 775
A.V.A 5: 1.39.03

Follow the large **middle cerebral artery** through the lateral sulcus. Gently widen the sulcus by retracting the gyri, which bound it superiorly and inferiorly. This procedure will expose the **insula**. Note that the insula is supplied by branches of the middle cerebral artery. Follow the artery on to the convex aspect of the hemisphere. Note that the superolateral surface of the cerebral hemisphere is predominantly supplied by branches of the middle cerebral artery. Correlate the course of these dissected vessels with a carotid arteriogram. Also study a vertebral arteriogram.

⇦
GRANT'S 7.34
ROHEN 94, 95
A.D.A.M. 1.29, 7.31
NETTER 133
CLEMENTE 776
A.V.A 5: 1.36.17

> ***Clinical Correlation:*** If time permits, examine more closely the middle cerebral artery within the lateral cerebral fissure. Observe several small but important branches that supply the corpus striatum and the internal capsule. These branches are also known as "arteries of cerebral apoplexy" since they are frequently involved in apoplexy (stroke).

GRANT'S 7.34
NETTER 134

At the base of the brain, identify all **12 cranial nerves** by names and numbers (Fig. 7.27):

GRANT'S:

- **CN I**, olfactory; — 9.3
- **CN II**, optic; — 9.4
- **CN III**, oculomotor; — 9.5
- **CN IV**, trochlear; — 9.5
- **CN V**, trigeminal; — 9.7-9.10
- **CN VI**, abducent; — 9.5
- **CN VII**, facial; — 9.11
- **CN VIII**, vestibulocochlear; — 9.12
- **CN IX**, glossopharyngeal; — 9.13
- **CN X**, vagus; — 9.14
- **CN XI**, accessory; — 9.15
- **CN XII**, hypoglossal. — 9.16

GRANT'S 7.22
ROHEN 68
A.D.A.M. 7.36
NETTER 112
CLEMENTE 778

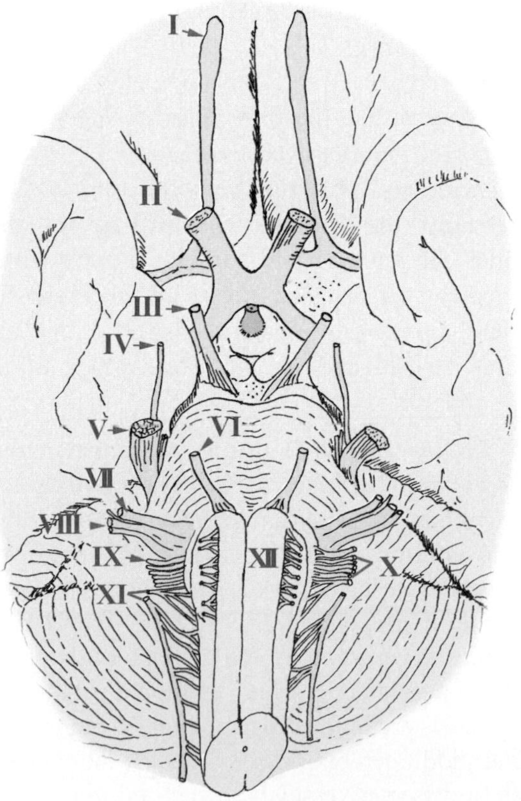

Figure 7.27. Cranial nerves **(CN)** at the base of the brain. The ***red*** numerals denote the various cranial nerves.

> ***Note:*** Later, the peripheral path of each cranial nerve will be followed from its point of entry through a specific opening in the skull to its peripheral destination.
>
> After completion of your studies, moisten the brain with embalming fluid and store it in an airtight plastic bag. Detailed studies of the brain must be conducted in a separate neuroanatomy course.

The Three Cranial Fossae

The interior of the base of the skull can be divided into three parts, each forming a **fossa** (Fig. 7.28): **anterior**, **middle**, and **posterior**. The anterior and posterior cranial fossae will be discussed first. The middle cranial fossa, which lies between the between the other fossae and which is anatomically more complex, will be studied last.

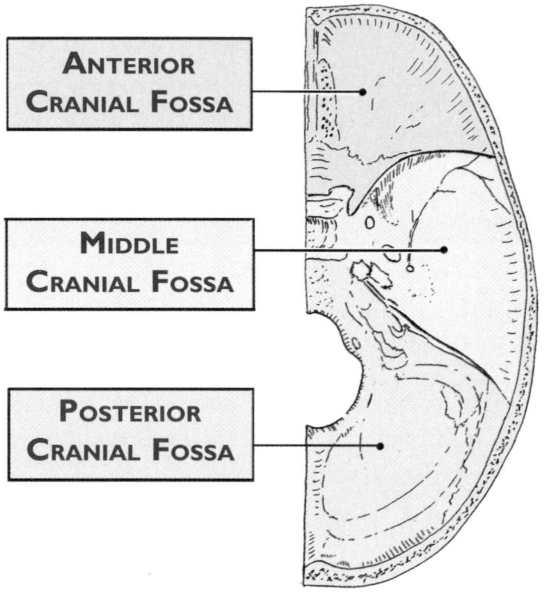

Figure 7.28. The three cranial fossae.

Anterior Cranial Fossa

GRANT'S 7.4
ROHEN 34, 35
A.D.A.M. 7.12
NETTER 6
CLEMENTE 779, 780
A.V.A. 4: 0.38.50

Refer to the bony skull and observe the following (Fig. 7.29): The **anterior cranial fossa** is sharply marked off from the middle cranial fossa by three concave crests: the sharp posterior borders of the right and left lesser wings of the sphenoid bone, and the anterior margin of the optic (chiasmatic) groove.

Identify the three bones that participate in the formation of the anterior cranial fossa: sphenoid bone; crista galli and cribriform plate of ethmoid bone; orbital plates of frontal bone, forming the roofs of the orbital cavities.

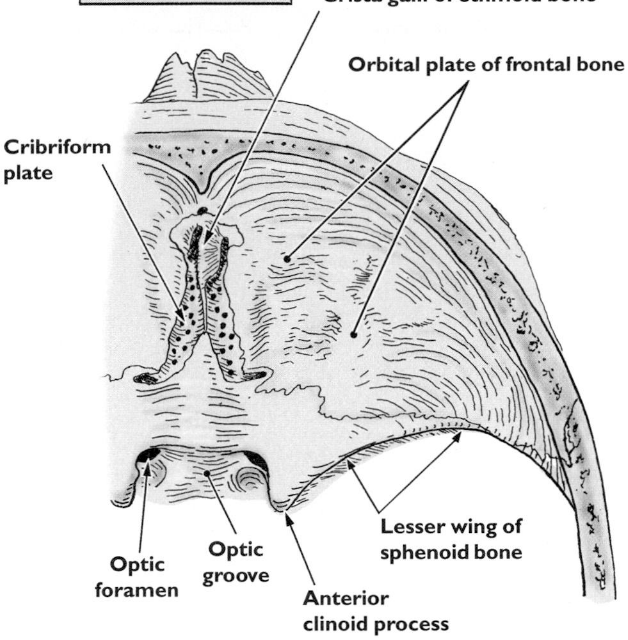

Figure 7.29. Bony landmarks of the anterior cranial fossa.

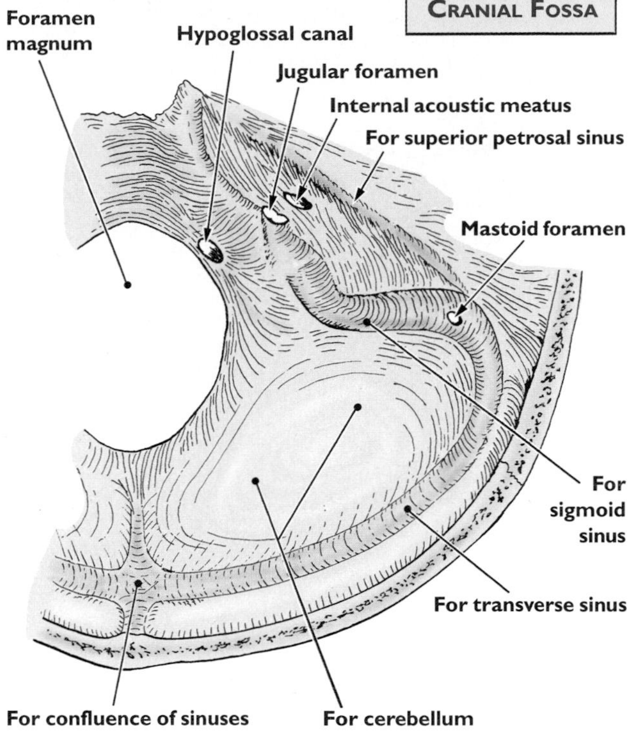

Figure 7.30. Bony landmarks of the posterior cranial fossa.

Recall the topographic relations of soft structures and bony landmarks. The olfactory bulbs rest on the cribriform plates. The falx cerebri is attached to the triangular crista galli. The frontal poles of the cerebral hemispheres rest on the orbital plates of the frontal bone.

Posterior Cranial Fossa

Refer to the bony skull and observe the following (Fig. 7.30): The **posterior cranial fossa** is the largest and the deepest of the three fossae. It is separated from the middle fossa by the dorsum sellae and the superior borders (margins) of the right and left petrous bones.

GRANT'S 7.4
ROHEN 34, 35
A.D.A.M. 7.12
NETTER 6
CLEMENTE 779, 780
A.V.A. 4: 0.38.56

The posterior cranial fossa is dominated by the enormous unpaired **foramen magnum**, which is oval in shape. At the level of this foramen, the medulla oblongata becomes continuous with the spinal cord. The inclining bony surface anterior to the foramen magnum is the clivus. It is topographically related to the pons and to the medulla oblongata. The fossae for the cerebellum and the occipital poles of the cerebral hemispheres were examined earlier.

GRANT'S 7.23
ROHEN 87
A.D.A.M. 7.33
NETTER 98
CLEMENTE 767, 768, 773
A.V.A. 5: 1.43.40

In the bony skull, identify the following openings (Fig. 7.30):

- **Hypoglossal canal** for cranial nerve XII;
- **Jugular foramen**, which transmits cranial nerves IX, X, XI, and the sigmoid sinus;
- **Internal acoustic meatus** for cranial nerves VII and VIII.

GRANT'S 7.34
ROHEN 34, 35
A.D.A.M. 7.12
NETTER 7
CLEMENTE 779, 780
A.V.A. 4: 0.09.25

Turn to the cadaver. In the posterior cranial fossae, identify the stumps of **cranial nerves** VII through XII and follow them to their respective foramina (Figs. 7.31). Note the large trigeminal nerve (V) as it curves superior to the most medial part of the superior margin of the petrous bone. The nerve passes inferior to the attached margin of the tentorium into the middle cranial fossa to enter the trigeminal cave.

- Slit open the transverse sinus.
- After leaving the tentorium, the transverse sinus becomes the sigmoid sinus.
- Open the sigmoid sinus.
- Verify that it leads to the jugular foramen.
- Slit open the superior petrosal sinus. Note that it runs in the attachment of the tentorium cerebelli to the superior margin of the petrous bone. This small sinus connects the large cavernous sinus with the transverse sinus.
- Finally, identify the stump of the abducent nerve (VI). It pierces the dura within the posterior cranial fossa.

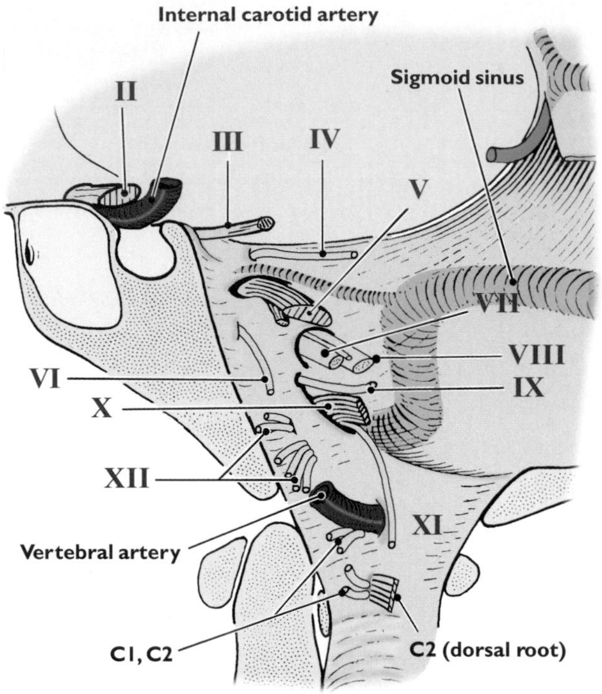

Figure 7.31. Stumps of nerves and vessels in the posterior and middle cranial fossae. Cranial nerves VII through XII are located in the posterior cranial fossa.

Refer to Figure 7.31 above and identify the following cranial nerves by names and numbers:

- **CN II**, optic; 9.4
- **CN III**, oculomotor; 9.5
- **CN IV**, trochlear; 9.5
- **CN V**, trigeminal; 9.7-9.10
- **CN VI**, abducent; 9.5
- **CN VII**, facial; 9.11
- **CN VIII**, vestibulocochlear; 9.12
- **CN IX**, glossopharyngeal; 9.13
- **CN X**, vagus; 9.14
- **CN XI**, accessory; 9.15
- **CN XII**, hypoglossal. 9.16

GRANT'S:

Middle Cranial Fossa

Refer to the bony skull and observe the following (Fig. 7.32): The main part of the **middle cranial fossa** is composed of two bones, the sphenoid bone and the temporal bone. On each side, the greater wing of the sphenoid contains a crescent of foramina. The right and left middle cranial fossae are occupied by the temporal poles and lobes of the cerebral hemispheres. Identify the following important openings or landmarks:

GRANT'S 7.34
ROHEN 34, 35
NETTER 6, 7
CLEMENTE 779, 780
A.V.A. 4: 0.49.45

- **Superior orbital fissure**, which transmits cranial nerves III, IV, V_1, VI, sympathetic nerve fibers, and the superior ophthalmic vein;

GRANT'S 7.22, 7.23, 7.41
ROHEN 86, 87
NETTER 98
CLEMENTE 773, 774
A.V.A. 5: 0.37.00

MIDDLE CRANIAL FOSSA

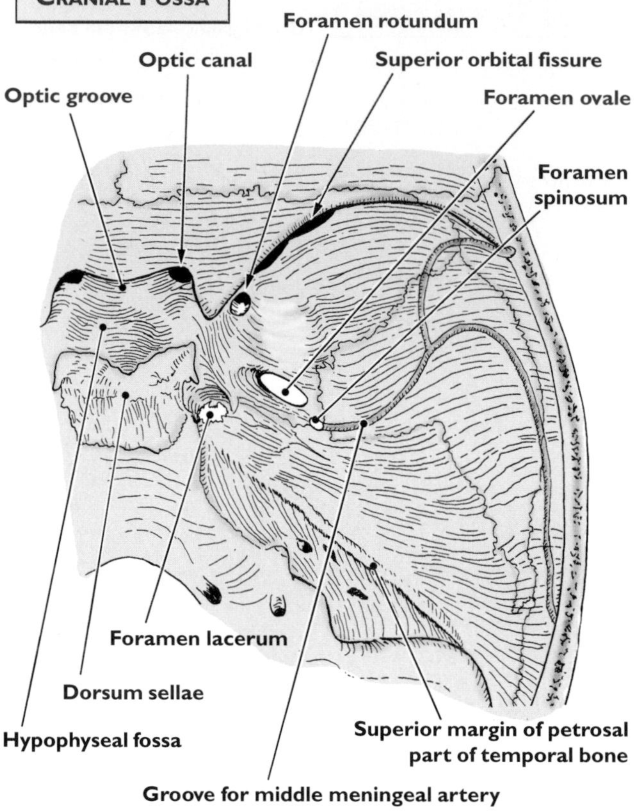

Figure 7.32. Bony landmarks of the middle cranial fossa.

- **Foramen rotundum** for cranial nerve V2;
- **Foramen ovale** for nerve V3;
- **Foramen spinosum** for the middle meningeal vessels; the groove for the middle meningeal artery leads from it.
- **Hypophyseal fossa** for the hypophysis cerebri (pituitary gland);
- **Optic groove** (chiasmatic sulcus), leading on each side to the optic canal;
- **Optic canal**, for the optic nerve and ophthalmic artery;
- **Dorsum sellae**;
- **Foramen lacerum**, situated between hypophyseal fossa and apex of petrous bone;
- **Carotid groove** for the internal carotid artery.

Turn to the cadaver. Identify the **optic nerve**, which traverses the optic canal. During removal of the brain, the **hypophysis cerebri** (pituitary gland) was severed from its stalk. This small but important master gland lies inferior to a circular dural fold, which covers the hypophyseal fossa. This fold is the **diaphragma sellae**. With a probe, define the circular aperture of the diaphragma sellae. Enlarge the opening and scoop out the pituitary gland.

Certain soft structures of the middle cranial fossa lie between two layers of dura. With a probe and forceps:

- Slit the dura and expose vessels and nerves.
- Incise the **superior petrosal sinus**.
- Carry the cut anteromedially into the **cavernous sinus**.

The cavernous sinus is large and important. Study a coronal section through the cavernous sinus. Observe that this venous sinus is actually traversed by the **internal carotid artery** and by cranial nerves (Fig. 7.33).

Clinical Correlation: The relation of the cavernous sinus and the internal carotid artery is of considerable clinical significance. In fractures of the base of the skull, the internal carotid artery may rupture within the cavernous sinus. As a result, an arteriovenous fistula (shunt) occurs. This creates an abnormal reflux of blood from the cavernous sinus into the ophthalmic veins, which normally drain the contents of the orbital cavity. As a result, the eye is protruded, engorged, and is pulsating in synchrony with the radial pulse (pulsating exophthalmos). During injuries or infections of the cavernous sinus, the cranial nerves traversing it may also be affected.

ROHEN 86
A.D.A.M. 7.66
NETTER 98
CLEMENTE 773
A.V.A. 5: 0.18.41

GRANT'S 7.41
ROHEN 86
NETTER 98, 133
CLEMENTE 770, 771, 773
A.V.A. 5: 1.45.41

GRANT'S 7.39, 9.7A
ROHEN 87, 95
A.D.A.M. 8.7-8.9
NETTER 98, 116
CLEMENTE 777
A.V.A. 5: 0.49.58

GRANT'S 7.39-7.41
NETTER 98, 115, 125
CLEMENTE 771
A.V.A. 5: 1.29.39

Pick up the **abducent nerve** (VI) in the posterior cranial fossa. Slit open the dura. Follow the nerve into the cavernous sinus. Trace the **oculomotor nerve** (III) anteriorly by slitting the dura. Identify a portion of internal carotid artery within the cavernous sinus.

Pick up the **trigeminal nerve** (V) where it crosses the superior border of the petrous bone. Here, the nerve lies in a 1-cm long cave that is lined with arachnoid. Slit open the roof of the cave. In doing so you will necessarily cut across the superior petrosal sinus. Remove the dura from the greater wing of the sphenoid to expose the **trigeminal ganglion** and the **three trigeminal divisions**. Trace the **mandibular division** (V_3) to the **foramen ovale**. Follow the **maxillary division** (V_2) to the **foramen rotundum**. Trace the small **ophthalmic division** (V_1) toward the **superior orbital fissure**.

Clean the **internal carotid artery** and demonstrate its sinuous course. In Figure 7.34 observe its close relations to cranial nerves **III**, **IV**, and **VI**.

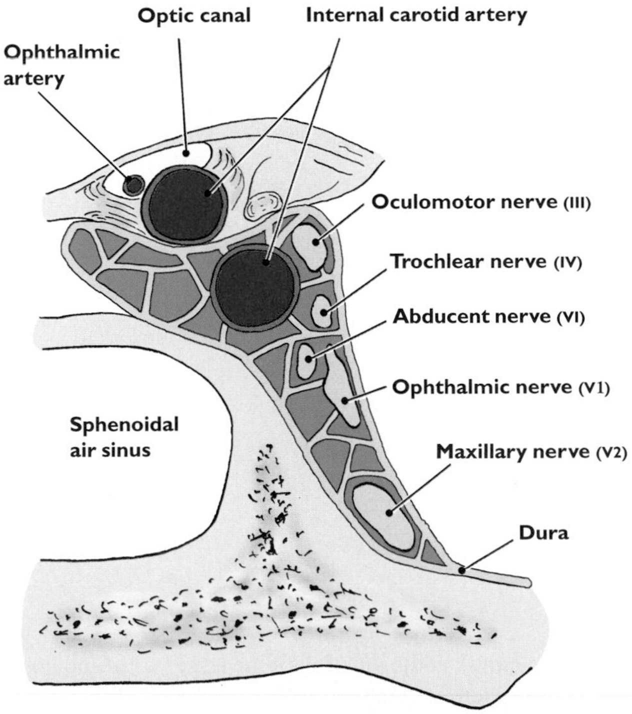

Figure 7.33. Cavernous sinus and related structures (coronal section).

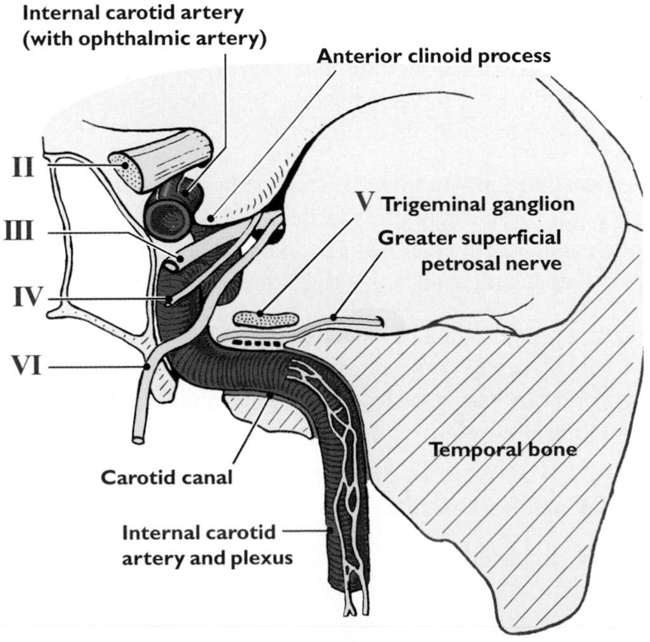

Figure 7.34. Internal carotid artery and its close relations to cranial nerves. The ***red*** numerals denote the various cranial nerves.

The **middle meningeal vessels** are embedded in the outer layer of the dura mater. Follow these vessels to the foramen spinosum.

If you have time, look for a small branch of the facial nerve, the **greater petrosal nerve**. It carries important parasympathetic fibers to the pterygopalatine ganglion. The nerve lies extradurally. Therefore, remove the moistened dura in the vicinity of the foramen lacerum. Be sure the dura is moist. If it is dry, it will break. The fine nerve may be seen running from the hiatus for the greater petrosal nerve in the petrous bone to the foramen lacerum. After traversing this foramen, the nerve enters the pterygoid canal.

The tiny lesser petrosal nerve carries parasympathetic fibers to the otic ganglion. The nerve runs lateral to the greater petrosal nerve to the foramen ovale or to a tiny foramen just posterior to the foramen ovale.

⇦
Grant's 7.4A, 7.19
Netter 95
Clemente 766-768
A.V.A. 5: 1.53.42

⇦
Grant's 7.39A, 9.11B
Rohen 143
A.D.A.M. 8.12
Netter 81, 125
Clemente 771
A.V.A. 5: 1.37.34

⇦
Grant's 7.39A, 9.13
Rohen 143
A.D.A.M. 8.15
Netter 81, 125
Clemente 769

Read an account of the dural sinuses and review them in the cadaver. Correlate your anatomical observations with a venogram of the sinuses. Study an outline of the cranial nerves. In the bony skull, review the openings (foramina; fissures) through which the cranial nerves pass.

⇦
Grant's 9.1-9.16
A.D.A.M. 8.1-8.23
Netter 112-122
Clemente 778

Orbit and Contents

General Remarks

The two orbits are deep bony sockets for the eyeballs and their related structures (muscles; nerves; vessels). Certain vessels and nerves traverse the orbit in close contact with its roof or floor to reach the scalp or face.

Each orbit is pyramidal in shape (Fig. 7.35). It has four walls. The orbital margin is at the base. The apex is at the optic canal. The medial walls are parallel and about 25 mm apart. The lateral walls are at right angles to each other.

⇦
Grant's 7.45
Rohen 117
Netter 78
Clemente 801, 802
A.V.A. 5: 2.00.48

The eyeball is about 25 mm long; i.e., it is half as long as the orbit. It occupies the anterior half of the orbit (Fig. 7.35). The posterior half of the orbit is largely filled with muscles and loose fatty tissue.

Bony Landmarks

Refer to a skull. Verify that a number of different bones participate in the formation of the orbital cavity (Fig. 7.36):

⇦
Grant's 7.42
Rohen 47, 128
Netter 1
Clemente 787, 788
A.V.A. 5: 2.02.21

- **Maxilla**;
- **Zygomatic bone**;

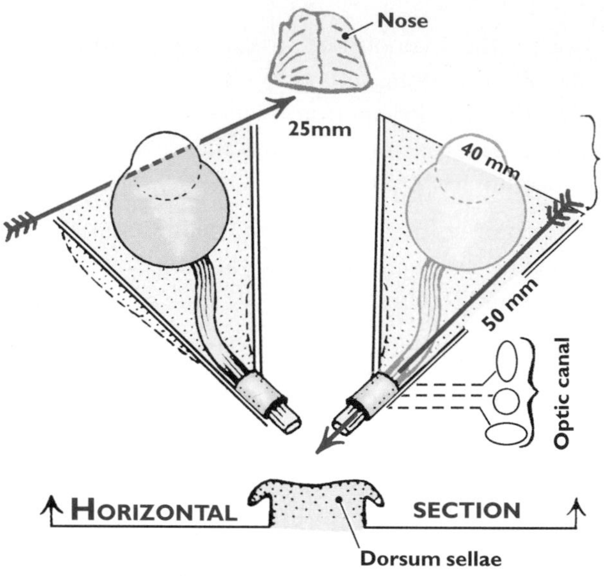

Figure 7.35. The orbital cavities and their dimensions (transverse section).

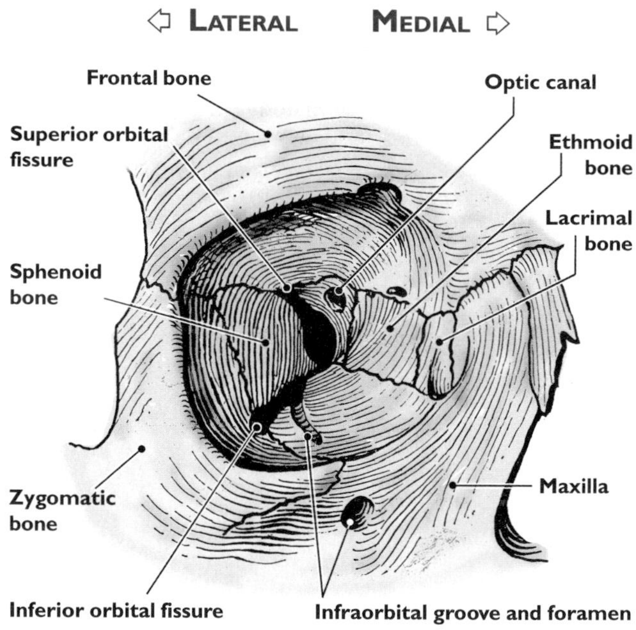

Figure 7.36. The bony walls of the orbital cavity.

- **Frontal bone**;
- **Lacrimal bone**;
- **Ethmoid bone**;
- **Sphenoid bone**.

In addition, observe the following details:

- **Optic canal**, at the junction of the lesser wing and body of the sphenoid bone;
- **Superior orbital fissure**, positioned between the greater and the lesser wings of the sphenoid;

- **Inferior orbital fissure**, a gap between the maxilla and the greater wing of the sphenoid;
- **Infraorbital groove**, continuous with the infraorbital canal and continuing anteriorly to the **infraorbital foramen**;
- Anterior and posterior ethmoidal foramina, on the medial wall of the cavity (a passageway for small nerves between the orbit and the anterior cranial fossa);
- The lateral wall of the orbit is stout and strong.

Examine the topographic relations of the orbit. Understand the following (Fig. 7.37):

- An object pushed through the roof of the orbit will enter the anterior cranial fossa.
- An object pushed through the floor or the orbit will enter the large maxillary sinus.
- An object pushed through the paper-thin medial wall of the orbital cavity, the lamina papyracea of the ethmoid bone, will enter the ethmoidal sinuses of the nasal cavity.

> ***Clinical Correlation:*** Keeping in mind the topographic relations of the orbit, explore this realistic possibility: a sharp object (pencil, nail, or a bullet) entering the orbit in an anteroposterior direction will traverse the superior orbital fissure and enter the middle cranial fossa. The physician will be confronted with such penetrating injuries; he or she must understand which anatomical substrates may have been injured.

⇦
GRANT'S 7.42
ROHEN 47, 128
A.D.A.M. 7.5
NETTER 1
CLEMENTE 787, 788
A.V.A. 5: 2.03.05

⇨
NETTER 78
CLEMENTE 801, 815

⇦
GRANT'S 7.92
ROHEN 144, 145
A.D.A.M. 8.2, 8.3
NETTER 42
CLEMENTE 788, 790
A.V.A. 4: 0.58.50

The bones of the orbital cavity are lined with periosteum called periorbita. At the optic canal and the superior orbital fissure, the periorbita is continuous with the dura mater of the cranial cavity.

Before you begin ...

Do not dissect at this time. It is recommended that the right orbital cavity be approached superiorly (from above) through its roof. The orbital plate of the frontal bone must be removed (Fig. 7.38). This procedure will reveal nerves, vessels, and muscles that are in contact with the roof of the orbit. The extraocular muscles will be studied. Two muscles will be divided and reflected to expose various important nerves and vessels located in the posterior half of the cavity. It will be demonstrated that the optic canal transmits the optic nerve and the ophthalmic artery. The ophthalmic vein and nerves III, IV, V_1, and VI will be followed through the superior orbital fissure.

The left orbital cavity should be dissected by using the anterior (or surgical) approach. General knowledge of the topographic anatomy in the orbit is a prerequisite for this most useful exercise. Eventually, the dissection is concluded with the enucleation of the eyeball. Subsequently, the interior of the removed eye may be dissected.

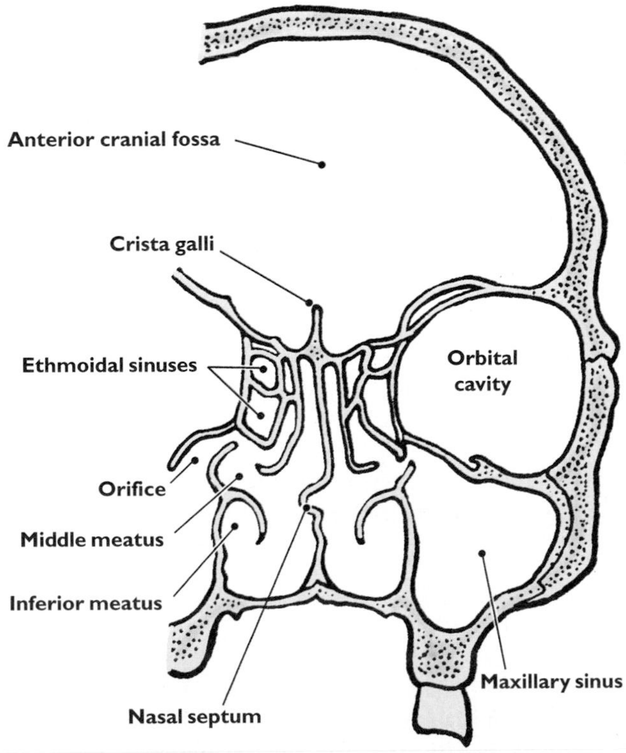

Figure 7.37. Coronal section of the skull at the level of the orbits.

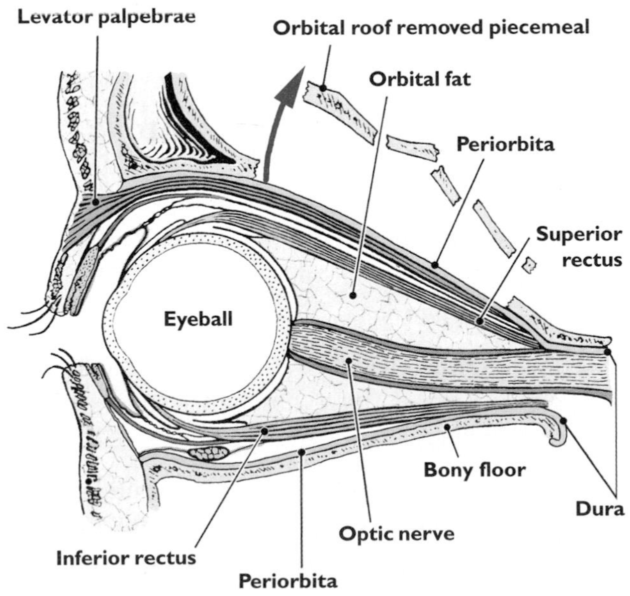

Figure 7.38. Orbital contents on sagittal section. The orbital plate of the frontal bone must be removed to allow the superior approach to the orbital contents.

Right Orbit, Superior Approach

> ***Dissection Note:* Special Dissection Technique**. In most cases, the eyeball is partially collapsed. Distend it by injecting preservative fluid or glycerine into it with a fine needle attached to a syringe. Insert the needle very obliquely through the transparent cornea in front of the pupil. This procedure will make the dissection of the orbital contents easier.

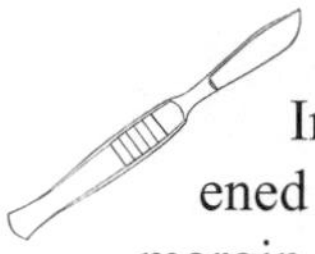

In the cranial cavity, incise the moistened dura mater along the posterior sharp margin of the lesser wing of the sphenoid and along the lateral margin of the cribriform plate. Now, strip the dura from the anterior cranial fossa (roof of the orbital cavity).

Remove the **roof of the orbit** (Fig. 7.38). With a chisel or another suitable metal instrument, break the center of the roof of the orbit. With bone forceps, nibble away the whole roof piece by piece.

Anteriorly, the bone is hollow. The exposed spaces belong to the frontal sinus. Observe its mucosal lining. Remove the roof of the orbit as far anteriorly as possible, but leave the superior orbital margin intact.

Medially, the roof may also be hollow. Here, the anterior and posterior ethmoidal air cells will be exposed. Understand that the ethmoidal cells have a tendency to invade the adjacent frontal bone. Observe the mucosal lining of these cells. At this stage, identify the tough membrane just inferior to the removed roof of the orbit. This is the **periorbita** that envelops the contents of the orbital cavity.

GRANT'S 7.45
ROHEN 131
NETTER 78, 81
CLEMENTE 802, 809
A.V.A. 5: 0.43.08

Posteriorly and laterally, the lesser wing of the sphenoid must be removed. This procedure will expose the superior orbital fissure and the optic canal.

- Push a probe between the bony roof and the periorbita posteriorly through the superior orbital fissure.
- With the probe still in a guiding position, remove the lesser wing of the sphenoid, which forms the upper margin of the superior orbital fissure.
- Next, with the aid of a probe, carefully break away the roof and the lateral wall of the optic canal. Finally, remove the anterior clinoid process. Shell it out of the investing dura with a pair of forceps.
- Incise the periorbita transversely near the anterior margin of the orbit.
- Make a second incision in an anteroposterior direction, but only as far posterior as the periorbita is free.
- Reflect or remove the flaps. Now, the most superior parts of the orbital contents are exposed (Fig. 7.39).

GRANT'S 7.39
ROHEN 136, 137
A.D.A.M. 7.74
NETTER 81, 115
CLEMENTE 803, 804
A.V.A. 5: 0.46.09

- Locate the intracranial stump of the delicate **trochlear nerve**. Carefully follow it anteriorly.
- Observe the nerve along the lateral wall of the cavernous sinus and lateral to the internal carotid artery. In the superior orbital fissure, the nerve is in intimate contact with the frontal nerve.

GRANT'S 7.45
ROHEN 136, 137
A.D.A.M. 7.74
NETTER 81
CLEMENTE 803-806
A.V.A. 5: 0.48.28

- Separate the nerves with a delicate instrument, such as fine sharp-sharp scissors. Follow the trochlear nerve to the superior border of the **superior oblique muscle** in the orbit (Fig. 7.39).
- Trace the **frontal nerve** from the 1st trigeminal division through the superior orbital fissure. In the orbit, trace the nerve anteriorly to its division into the small supratrochlear nerve and the larger **supraorbital nerve**.

GRANT'S 7.39, 7.45A
ROHEN 136, 137
A.D.A.M. 7.74
NETTER 81
CLEMENTE 803
A.V.A. 5: 0.50.52

- Push a probe through the supraorbital notch or foramen, and establish the continuity of the nerves onto the forehead and scalp region. At this stage, you may extend the dissection field. If you wish to do so, carefully remove the part of the frontal bone that forms the superior orbital margin. This procedure completely exposes the upper eyelid and the levator palpebrae superioris.

GRANT'S 7.45
ROHEN 136, 137
A.D.A.M. 7.74
NETTER 81
CLEMENTE 803, 804
A.V.A. 5: 0.51.06

The delicate **lacrimal nerve** enters the superior orbital fissure lateral to the frontal nerve.

- In the orbit, trace the nerve anteriorly to the lacrimal gland. Arteries accompany the frontal and lacrimal nerves.

GRANT'S 7.45A
ROHEN 136, 137
NETTER 81
CLEMENTE 803, 804
A.V.A. 5: 2.11.13

- With forceps, pick out fine lobules of loose fatty tissue and expose the surface of the most superiorly positioned muscle, the **levator palpebrae superioris**.

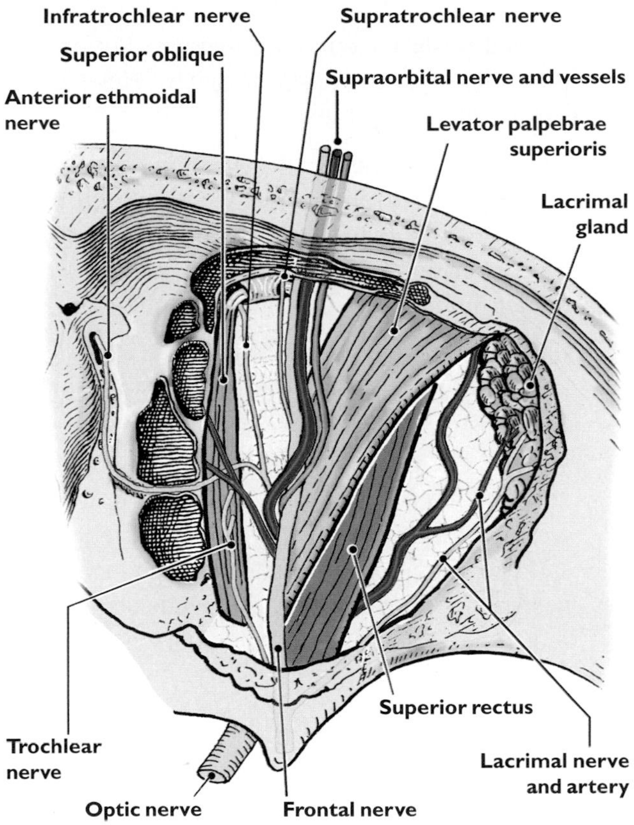

Figure 7.39. Superior structures of the orbital cavity.

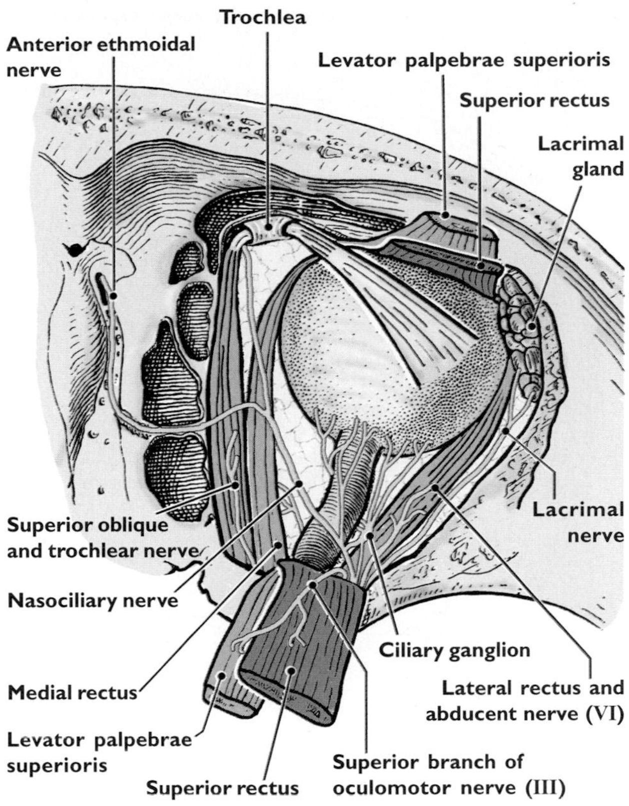

Figure 7.40. Dissection of the orbital cavity (superior approach).

Examine this muscle. Gently pull on it. Verify that it raises the upper eyelid. Understand that various layers of the muscle are inserted into different parts of the lid.

- Cut the muscle as far anteriorly as possible and reflect it posteriorly. Now, the underlying **superior rectus** lies exposed.
- Clean it. Observe that the muscle is attached to the eyeball by a tendinous expansion.
- Cut the superior rectus close to the eyeball and reflect it posteriorly (Fig. 7.40). Note that a branch of the oculomotor nerve (III) reaches its deep surface.
- Examine the **superior oblique muscle** and trace it forward to its pulley, the **trochlea**. Observe that the tendon of the superior oblique muscle bends at an acute angle and passes to its insertion into the lateral and posterior portion of the eyeball.

At this stage, the origin of the **four recti muscles** must be considered. They arise from a tough tendinous ring or cuff, the **anulus tendineus** (Fig. 7.41). This fibrous ring surrounds the optic canal and its contents. In addition, the ring partially includes the superior orbital fissure. The two heads of the lateral rectus are attached to the ring. The narrow interval overlying the superior orbital fissure, encircled by the fibrous ring and bounded by the heads of the lateral rectus, is of strategic importance. Several structures pass through this gap: nasociliary nerve, abducent nerve, oculomotor nerve, and ophthalmic vein (Fig. 7.41).

⇨
GRANT'S 7.46, 7.47
ROHEN 131, 137
NETTER 79
CLEMENTE 808, 809, 815
A.V.A. 5: 2.07.08

⇦
GRANT'S 7.45
ROHEN 136, 137
A.D.A.M. 7.73
NETTER 79, 81
CLEMENTE 804
A.V.A. 5: 2.06.39

⇦
GRANT'S 7.45
ROHEN 136, 137
A.D.A.M. 7.74
NETTER 81
CLEMENTE 806
A.V.A. 5: 2.09.05

⇨
GRANT'S 7.45A, 7.46
ROHEN 137
A.D.A.M. 7.75, 8.7
NETTER 81
CLEMENTE 805
A.V.A. 5: 0.51.26

In the dissection field, identify the **lateral rectus** and its superior head (Fig. 7.41).

- Gently push a probe through the interval between the two heads of the muscle.
- Carefully sever the superior head and the anulus tendineus. Now, all structures passing through the narrow interval can be studied.

Nasociliary Nerve (Fig. 7.40)

It is a branch of the 1st trigeminal division (V_1). Follow it into the orbit. As the nerve crosses the optic nerve, it gives off two or three delicate **long ciliary nerves** to the posterior part of the eyeball. Subsequently, the nasociliary nerve runs obliquely toward the medial wall of the orbit, at the level between the superior oblique and the medial rectus. To clarify the dissection field, pick out the numerous tiny lobules of

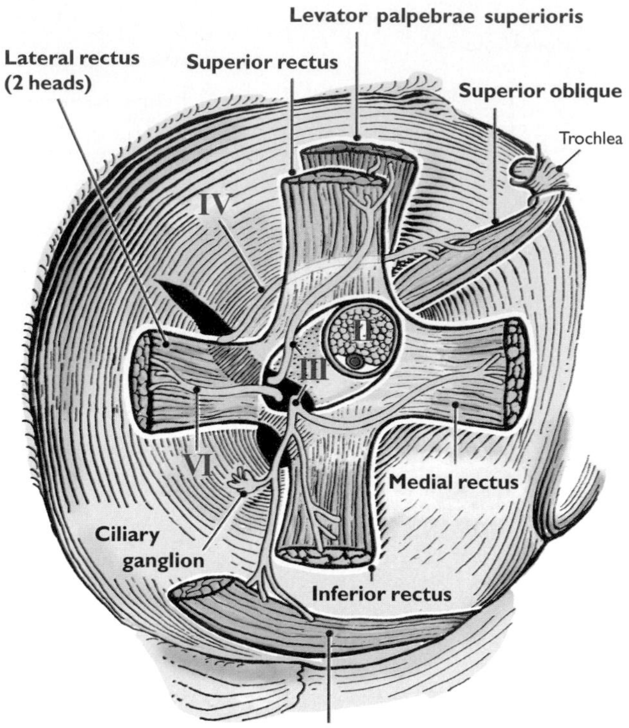

Figure 7.41. Right orbit (anterior view). The fibrous cuff (anulus tendineus) and its relation to the four recti muscles and cranial nerves **II, III, IV,** and **VI**.

loose fatty tissue that fill the interval between muscles, nerves, and vessels.

A small branch of the nasociliary nerve, the **anterior ethmoidal nerve**, passes through the anterior ethmoidal foramen. The nerve enters the cranial cavity, runs lateral to the cribriform plate, and enters the ethmoid bone to reach the nasal cavity. It supplies part of the mucous membrane in the nasal cavity. Finally, it sends a terminal twig to the tip of the nose as the external nasal nerve.

Abducent Nerve (VI)

Identify its intracranial stump and follow it through the cavernous sinus. Subsequently, trace it lateral to the internal carotid artery to the superior orbital fissure. In the orbital cavity (Fig. 7.40), find the nerve applied to the medial surface of the lateral rectus.

Oculomotor Nerve (III)

In the cranial cavity, identify the nerve where it pierces the dura between the anterior and posterior clinoid processes. Follow it to the superior orbital fissure. Here it divides into two divisions.

⇨
Grant's 7.39A, 7.45, 9.5
Rohen 136, 137
A.D.A.M. 7.75, 8.4
Netter 81, 115
Clemente 805, 806
A.V.A. 5: 0.46.06

- Identify the superior division, which supplies the reflected levator palpebrae superioris and the superior rectus (Fig. 7.40). The inferior division supplies the medial rectus, inferior rectus, and inferior oblique.

⇨
Grant's 7.45, 7.46, 9.5
Rohen 132
A.D.A.M. 7.73, 8.4
Netter 81, 115
Clemente 805, 807

- Identify the **ciliary ganglion**, which receives parasympathetic fibers from the inferior division of the oculomotor nerve (III). This parasympathetic ganglion is only 1 to 2 mm in diameter. Find it lateral to the optic nerve, about 1 cm anterior to the apex of the orbit. Delicate short ciliary nerves connect the ganglion to the posterior portion of the eyeball. Understand the functional importance of the ciliary ganglion and the ciliary nerve.

⇨
Grant's 7.53B
A.D.A.M. 7.33, 7.74
Netter 80
Clemente 747

- Look for the **superior ophthalmic vein**. At the medial angle of the eye, this vein anastomoses with tributaries of the facial vein.

In the orbit, the superior ophthalmic vein and its tributaries accompany the ophthalmic artery. Identify the vein on the basis of two facts:

- It passes through the superior orbital fissure;
- It drains into the cavernous sinus.

⇦
Grant's 7.45, 9.8
Rohen 137
A.D.A.M. 7.74, 8.7
Netter 81
Clemente 805, 806
A.V.A. 5: 0.51.17

Clinical Correlation: The anastomoses between facial vein and ophthalmic veins are of clinical importance. Infections (boils) of the nasal cavity, upper lip, cheeks, and forehead region may spread along venous channels into the ophthalmic veins and on into the cavernous sinus. The resulting cavernous sinus thrombosis is a most dangerous complication.

Optic Nerve

⇨
Grant's 7.39A, 7.45-7.47, 9.4
Rohen 134
A.D.A.M. 7.74, 7.75, 8.3
Netter 78-81, 114
Clemente 805, 806
A.V.A. 5: 0.43.47

Open the roof of the optic canal. The optic "nerve" is actually a brain tract. Therefore, it is surrounded with the three meningeal layers: dura, arachnoid, and pia.

⇦
Grant's 7.39A, 7.45, 9.5
Rohen 136, 137
A.D.A.M. 7.74, 8.10
Netter 81, 115
Clemente 804
A.V.A. 5: 0.48.36

- Pass a thin probe underneath the external (dural) sheath and slit it open. Cut across the optic nerve inside the sheath. Lift up the nerve.
- Examine the cut surface of the nerve, and identify a dark spot at the center. This is the sectioned central artery of the retina.

Ophthalmic Artery (Fig. 7.42)

Identify the artery where it arises from the internal carotid artery. In the optic canal, the vessel lies inferior and lateral to the optic nerve.

- With the tip of a probe, elevate the optic nerve slightly and observe the ophthalmic artery.
- Follow the artery into the orbital cavity.
- Note that it curves superior to the optic nerve and, subsequently, reaches the medial wall of the orbit.
- Observe the fine ciliary arteries to the eyeball. If time permits, examine other branches of the ophthalmic artery.

GRANT'S 7.53A
ROHEN 130
A.D.A.M. 7.31
NETTER 80
CLEMENTE 806, 807
A.V.A. 5: 1.30.40

The **central artery of the retina** was already seen on the sectioned surface of the optic nerve. The artery enters the nerve about 13 mm posterior to the eyeball, runs in the center of the nerve, pierces the sclera, and reaches the retina. Its occlusion leads to instant and total blindness of the concerned eye.

GRANT'S 7.47, 7.53A
ROHEN 129, 130
NETTER 86
CLEMENTE 806, 817

- Remove the optic nerve and its sheath. Now, the muscles at the floor of the orbital cavity can be observed.

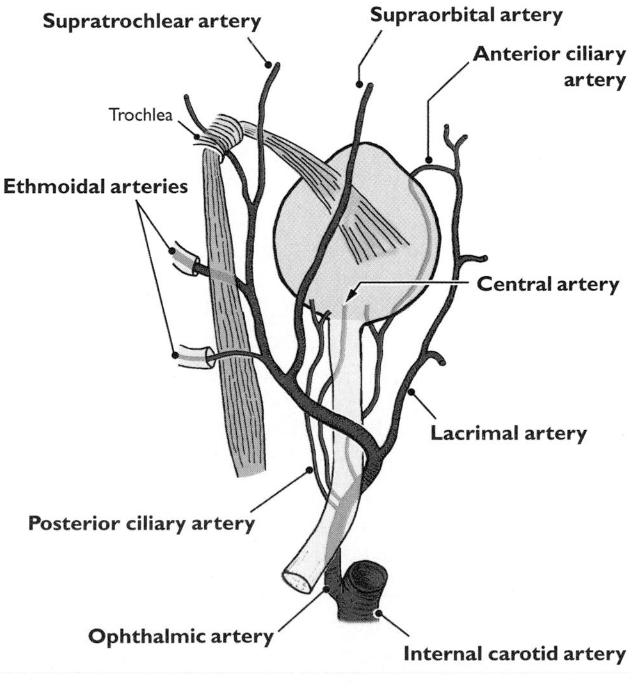

Figure 7.42. Ophthalmic artery and branches in the orbital cavity.

GRANT'S 7.49, 7.50
ROHEN 131
A.D.A.M. 8.3
NETTER 79
CLEMENTE 808-816
A.V.A. 5: 2.07.03

- Identify the **inferior rectus**. Raise the posterior pole of the eyeball, and observe the insertion of the inferior oblique into the sclera.
- Identify and study the **medial rectus**. Review the distribution of the superior and inferior divisions of the oculomotor nerve.

Review the insertion of the extraocular muscles (Fig. 7.43): the four recti muscles are inserted by thin, wide tendons into the scleral coat near the cornea. The two oblique muscles are also inserted by thin wide tendons; but they are attached to the sclera of the posterior half of the eyeball.

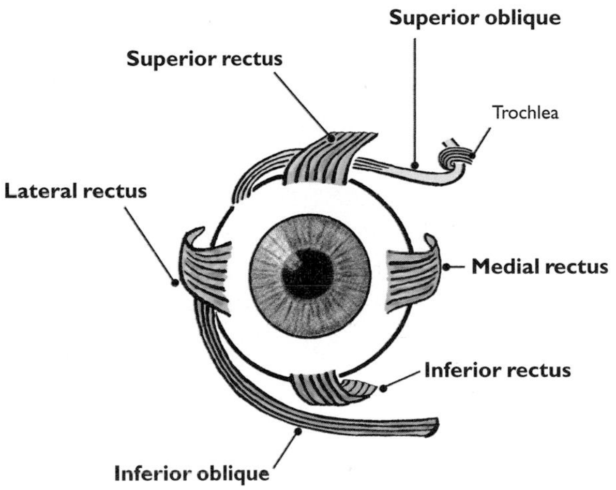

Figure 7.43. The six extraocular muscles; frontal view of the right eye.

Left Orbit from Facial Aspect (Surgical Approach)

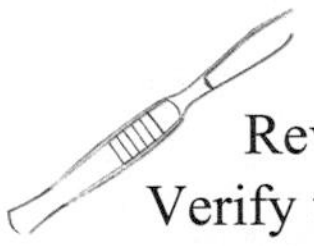

Review the extent of the conjunctival sac. Verify that the conjunctiva is firmly adherent to the cornea, but loosely attached to the sclera.

- With a sharp scalpel, make a complete circular incision through the conjunctiva, about 6 to 8 mm from the sclerocorneal junction.
- Push a probe through the incision, and find at least one of the recti muscles.

GRANT'S 7.13
ROHEN 138
A.D.A.M. 7.68-7.70
NETTER 76
CLEMENTE 795
A.V.A. 5: 2.16.53

To facilitate the dissection, remove both eyelids and the orbital septum. Compare your field of dissection with appropriate atlas illustrations (illustrations may depict the right orbit; you are dissecting the left one). Examine three corners of the orbit (*see* Fig. 7.11). Observe:

- Superior and lateral lies the lacrimal gland;
- Superior and medial is the trochlea for the superior oblique;
- Inferior and medial are the origin of inferior oblique and the lacrimal sac.

Observe the insertion of the four recti muscles. Study the insertions of the superior and inferior obliques. Notice that the obliques pass inferior to the corresponding recti.

GRANT'S 7.44
ROHEN 138
A.D.A.M. 7.68, 7.69
NETTER 77
CLEMENTE 795-798

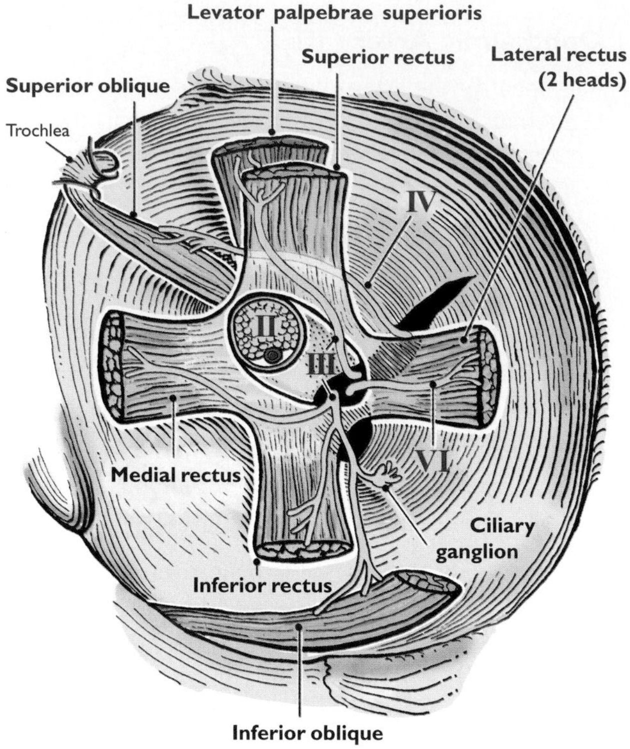

Figure 7.45. Left orbit (anterior view). The fibrous cuff (anulus tendineus) and its relation to the four recti muscles and cranial nerves **II, III, IV,** and **VI.**

Enucleation of Eyeball

With a probe, hook up each rectus tendon and cut across it (Fig. 7.44). Cut all four recti. Adduct the eyeball (turn medially) and pull it anteriorly. Insert a cutting instrument (preferably long, curved scissors) into the orbit from the lateral side. Cut the optic nerve. Now, pull the eyeball anteriorly and sever the two oblique muscles. Remove the eyeball. Keep it moist, and store it in a small plastic bag.

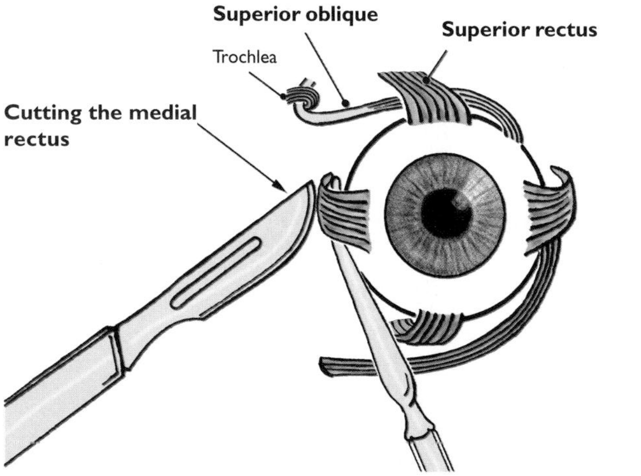

Figure 7.44. Frontal view of the left eye cutting the recti muscles.

Study the socket (Fig. 7.45). Remove the loose fatty tissue from the posterior portion of the orbital cavity. Pick up the nerve to the inferior oblique and follow it posteriorly as far as possible. Trace the four recti to their origin from the anulus tendineus. Identify the structures that pass between the two heads of the lateral rectus: nerve VI, inferior and superior divisions of nerve III, and nasociliary nerve.

GRANT'S 7.47
ROHEN 131, 132
A.D.A.M. 7.70, 8.3
NETTER 78
CLEMENTE 808, 815, 816

Dissection of the Human Eyeball

GRANT'S 7.51
ROHEN 129
A.D.A.M. 7.71
NETTER 82-86
CLEMENTE 817-824

In most cases, the removed human eyeball is not well preserved enough to warrant its dissection. If the eye is in acceptable condition, cut it into two halves along a sagittal plane. Use a sharp scalpel (new blade!). Carefully remove the remains of the vitreous body. Gently wash it out, if necessary. Note the following essential features:

- External or fibrous coat, consisting of sclera (posterior 5/6) and cornea (anterior 1/6); the cornea is more convex than the sclera.
- Middle or vascular coat, consisting of choroid, ciliary body, and iris; blood vessels and the ciliary nerves are contained in this coat.
- Internal or retinal coat; in the cadaver, the retina is gray and partially detached. In well preserved specimens, you may find the macula. Identify the region where the optic nerve and retinal vessels enter or leave. This is the optic papilla or disc.

- Two of the four refractive media are still present: cornea and lens. The now empty space between the cornea and the lens is normally filled with aqueous humor. The jelly-like vitreous body has been removed earlier.

The principal gross anatomical structures of the eye can be conveniently examined in the large and fresh eye of the bull. If a detailed dissection of the eye is on your agenda, refer to the APPENDIX.

Posterior Triangle of Neck

General Remarks

The boundaries of the posterior triangle of the neck are (Fig. 7.46A):

- Anteriorly, the posterior border of the sternocleidomastoid muscle;
- Posteriorly, the anterior border of the trapezius muscle;
- Inferiorly, the middle third of the clavicle.

GRANT'S 8.3
ROHEN 153
A.D.A.M. 7.21
NETTER 18
CLEMENTE 693

The **posterior triangle** has a **fascial roof** of deep fascia that stretches between the two muscles forming its boundaries (Fig. 7.46B). This fascia splits to envelop the trapezius and the sternocleidomastoid. Superficial veins lie superficial to the fascial roof; however, at the inferior border of the triangle, the external jugular vein pierces the roof and then lies deep to it. The fascial roof is also pierced by cutaneous nerves.

GRANT'S 8.2A
ROHEN 150
A.D.A.M. 7.29
NETTER 21
CLEMENTE 704

The **floor of the triangle** is covered with the anterior continuation of the prevertebral fascia (Fig. 7.46B). Following removal of this fascial floor, the deep muscles of the posterior triangle are exposed. The contents of the posterior triangle consist largely of nerves and vessels connecting the neck region with the upper limb.

GRANT'S 8.5
ROHEN 172
A.D.A.M. 7.35
NETTER 30
CLEMENTE 705

Superficial Structures and Contents of Posterior Triangle

Before you begin ...

Following reflection of the skin and a portion of the platysma, the posterior triangle will be fully exposed. First, the accessory nerve, an important guiding structure for dissection, must be identified (Fig. 7.46). Subsequently, a number of sensory nerves radiating from the posterior border of the sternocleidomastoid muscle will be dissected. At the base of the triangle, tributaries of the external jugular vein and branches of the thyrocervical trunk will be observed. Dissection in this area will be greatly facilitated by partial resection of the clavicle. Finally, the fascia forming the floor of the triangle will be removed and the underlying muscles will be exposed. The important brachial plexus will be followed from the neck into the axilla.

GRANT'S 8.5
ROHEN 172, 173
A.D.A.M. 7.44
NETTER 18
CLEMENTE 698
A.V.A. 5: 1.22.45

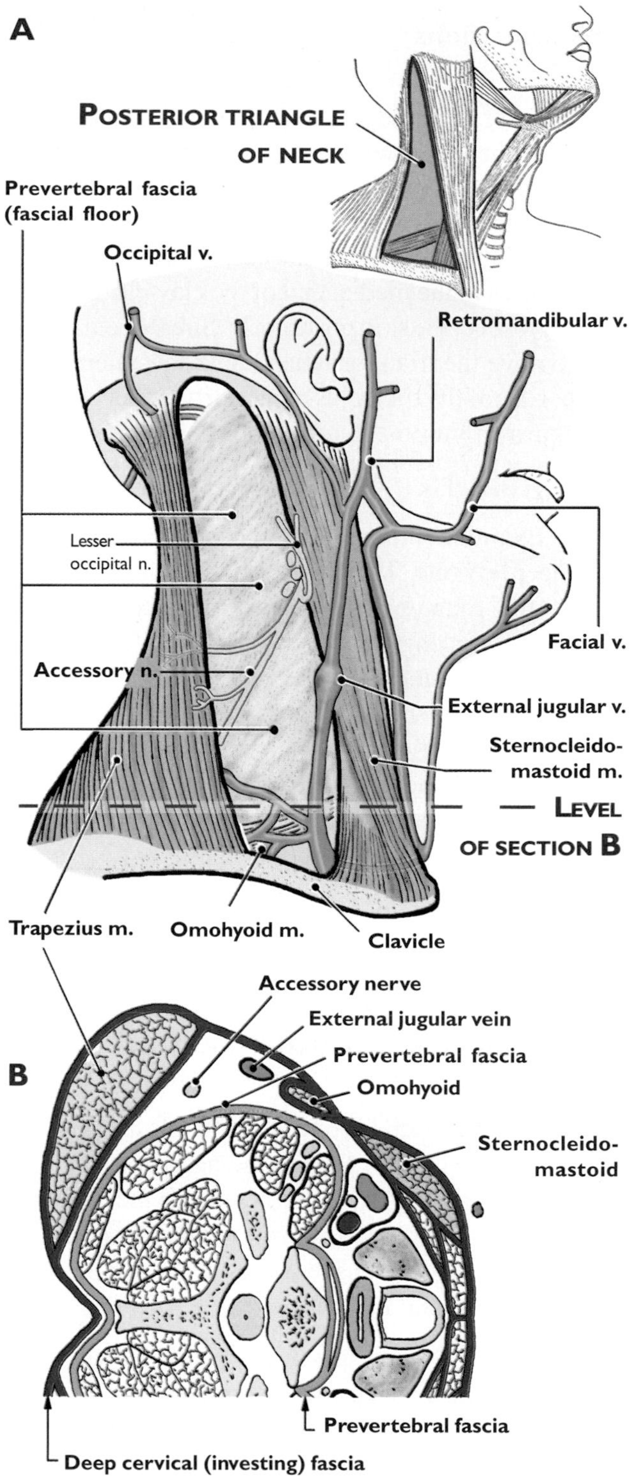

Figure 7.46. Posterior triangle of neck. ***A***, The accessory nerve and external jugular vein lie superficial to the fascial floor. ***B***, Transverse section through neck shows the fascial floor (prevertebral fascia) and the fascial roof (investing fascia) of the triangle.

Skin Incisions

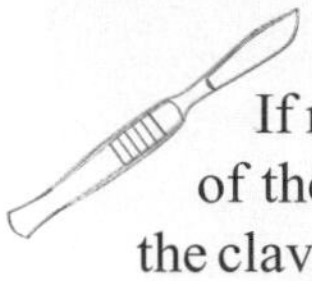

If not already done during the dissection of the upper limb, make an incision along the clavicle from its medial end to a point 3 cm beyond the acromion. Refer to Figure 7.47. Make an incision from the base of the mastoid process to the medial end of the clavicle (E to F). Reflect the skin posteriorly. Subsequently, remove the triangular flap along the anterior border of the trapezius. Anteriorly, reflect the skin overlying the sternocleidomastoid muscle.

Platysma (Fig. 7.48)

Examine the posteroinferior portion of the **platysma**, which covers the basal part of the triangle. The platysma passes over the whole length of the clavicle. The **supraclavicular nerves**, which cling to the deep surface of the platysma, also cross the clavicle. Reflect the platysma upward. Do not injure the supraclavicular nerves.

⇦
GRANT'S 8.1, 8.5
ROHEN 172
A.D.A.M. 7.34, 7.35
NETTER 18, 21, 26
CLEMENTE 696, 698, 699
A.V.A. 5: 1.22.52

Find the **accessory nerve** (Fig. 7.46). Its approximate course is marked by a line connecting two points:

⇦
GRANT'S 8.5
ROHEN 173
A.D.A.M. 7.35, 7.44, 8.22
NETTER 27
CLEMENTE 698
A.V.A. 5: 1.18.10

- A point slightly superior to the middle of the posterior border of the sternocleidomastoid;
- A point about 5 cm superior to the clavicle at the anterior border of the trapezius.
- Incise the fascial roof of the triangle along the course indicated. Spread the tissue with scissors along the expected course of the accessory nerve (XI). Find the nerve and free it from its surrounding tissue. Be aware of the function of cranial nerve XI.

Search for the **lesser occipital nerve**. It emerges from the posterior border of the sternocleidomastoid in close proximity to cranial nerve XI (Fig. 7.46A). Trace the lesser occipital nerve superiorly along or near the posterior border of the sternocleidomastoid. The nerve supplies the scalp. At the apex of the posterior triangle, identify the occipital artery.

⇦
GRANT'S 8.5
ROHEN 172, 173
NETTER 18, 27
CLEMENTE 699
A.V.A. 5: 1.23.12

In addition to the accessory nerve and the lesser occipital nerve (C2, C3), three other nerves radiate from the posterior border of the sternomastoid:

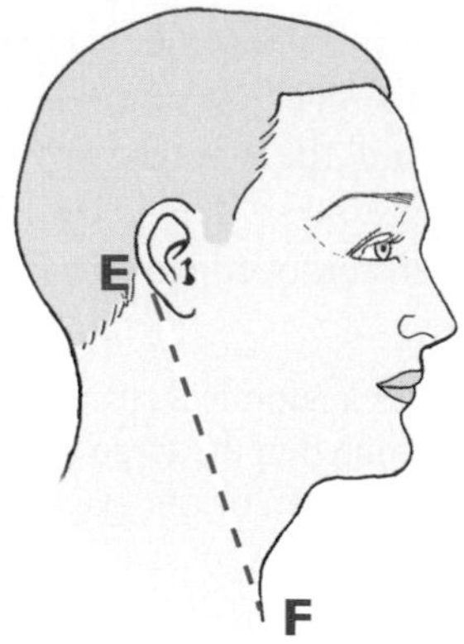

Figure 7.47. Skin incisions.

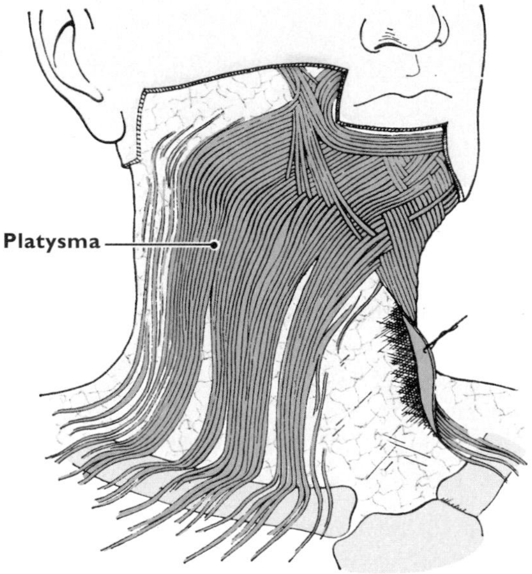

Figure 7.48. The platysma and its interdigitations with other muscles of facial expression.

- **Great auricular nerve** (C2, C3). Together with the external jugular vein, it ascends vertically on the surface of the sternocleidomastoid. The nerve supplies the back of the auricle and a cutaneous area extending from the angle of the mandible to the mastoid process.

⇨
GRANT'S 8.5
ROHEN 172, 173
A.D.A.M. 7.25, 7.44
NETTER 18
CLEMENTE 699
A.V.A. 5: 1.22.58

- **Transverse cervical nerve** (C2, C3). Follow it transversely across the middle of the sternocleidomastoid. It supplies the skin of the anterior triangle of the neck.
- **Supraclavicular nerves** (C3, C4). Observe medial, intermediate, and lateral branches.

External Jugular Vein

This vein runs superficially from an area posterior to the angle of the mandible to a point about 3 cm superior to the clavicle. At this point, the vein pierces the fascial roof of the posterior triangle. Clean the vein and follow it through the fascia. Then, remove the remains of the fascial roof.

Resection of Middle Portion of Clavicle

With a small saw, cut through the clavicle at two points:

- Laterally, close to the anterior attachments of the trapezius and deltoid muscles;
- Close to the medial end of the clavicle.

Next, detach the clavicular head of the sternocleidomastoid as far as necessary. Remove the middle portion of the clavicle. Observe the slender **subclavius muscle** inferior to the clavicle. Now, the structures at the base of the posterior triangle can be displayed.

Examine the slender **omohyoid muscle**. Its inferior (posterior) and superior bellies are separated by an **intertendon** (Fig. 7.49). This intertendon is held down to the clavicle by a fibrous expansion. Observe this fibrous band (omohyoid fascia) deep to the clavicular attachment of the sternocleidomastoid. Remove the omohyoid fascia, thereby exposing the blood vessels at the base of the posterior triangle.

Blood Vessels

Follow the **external jugular vein** through the omohyoid fascia to the subclavian vein (Fig. 7.49). Note the suprascapular vein that runs posterior to the clavicle. Observe the **transverse cervical artery** running about 2 to 3 cm superior to the clavicle and deep to the omohyoid (Fig. 7.49). This artery heads toward the levator scapulae. The **suprascapular artery** takes a posterior course to reach the suprascapular notch. Review the origin and destination of the two arteries. Observe that both arteries pass anterior to the scalenus anterior. Variations in the origin of the transverse cervical and suprascapular arteries are common (*see* Chapter 6, p. 191). In over 50% of the cases, one of the arteries does not arise from the thyrocervical trunk.

⇨
GRANT'S 8.7, 8.8
ROHEN 175, 176
A.D.A.M. 7.48, 7.52
NETTER 27
CLEMENTE 704, 705
A.V.A. 4: 0.28.46

⇨
GRANT'S 8.8
ROHEN 176
A.D.A.M. 7.52
NETTER 27, 28
CLEMENTE 701, 702
A.V.A. 5: 1.26.00

⇦
GRANT'S 8.7
ROHEN 175, 176
A.D.A.M. 7.48
NETTER 22
CLEMENTE 699-701
A.V.A. 1: 0.17.34

⇦
GRANT'S 8.8
ROHEN 173
A.D.A.M. 7.44
NETTER 26
CLEMENTE 699
A.V.A. 5: 1.57.12

⇦
GRANT'S 8.8
ROHEN 178
A.D.A.M. 7.48
NETTER 27, 28
CLEMENTE 701-703
A.V.A. 5: 1.26.05

Structures Deep to Floor of Triangle

Remove the **fascial floor** (prevertebral fascia) of the posterior triangle. Expose the underlying muscles consisting of the **splenius capitis**, **levator scapulae**, and the **three scaleni**: scalenus posterior, scalenus medius, and scalenus anterior (Fig. 7.49).

Define the **scalenus anterior** and the **scalenus medius**. Clean these two muscles. Observe the following (Fig. 7.50):

- The two muscles are inserted into the first rib.
- An elongated triangular space is formed by the two muscles and rib 1. This is the **interscalene triangle**. Through this interval pass two important structures: the **subclavian artery** and the **brachial plexus**.
- The **subclavian vein** passes anterior to the scalenus anterior.

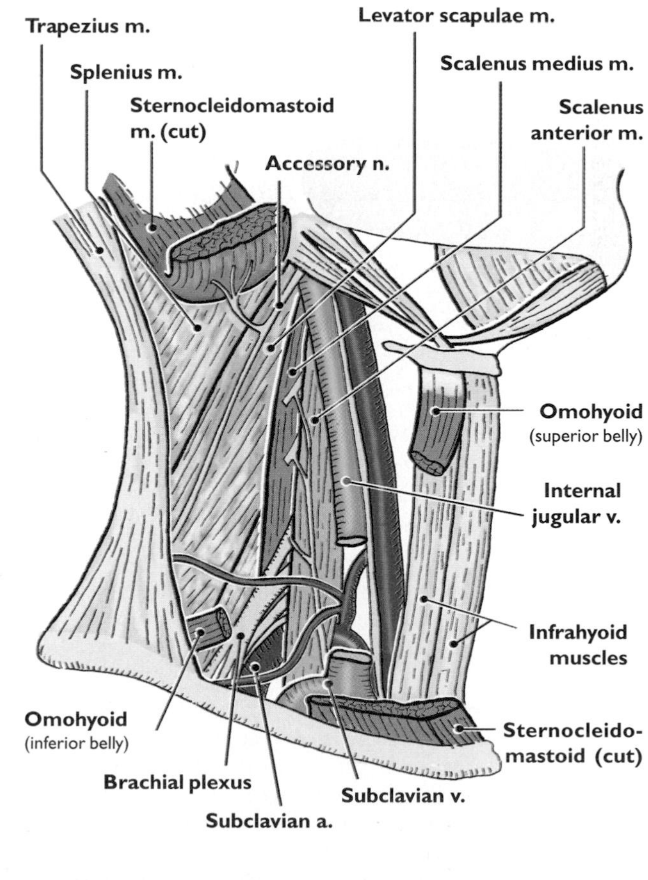

Figure 7.49. Following removal of the fascial floor (prevertebral fascia), the deep structures of the posterior triangle are exposed: muscles, nerves, and vessels.

- The transverse cervical artery and suprascapular artery commonly cross anterior to the scalenus anterior.
- The **phrenic nerve** (C3, C4, C5) descends vertically across the surface of the scalenus anterior toward the thorax. The nerve is intimately applied to the muscle; therefore, nerve and muscle are crossed anteriorly by the three vessels: transverse cervical artery, suprascapular artery, and subclavian vein.

GRANT'S 8.7-8.9
ROHEN 175, 180
A.D.A.M. 7.48
NETTER 27, 28
CLEMENTE 701-703
A.V.A. 5: 1.22.29

- The scalenus medius is pierced by motor nerves to the rhomboids (C5) and to the serratus anterior (C5, C6).

If not already done, clean the **axillary artery** and the **brachial plexus** at the level of the interscalene triangle. Review the brachial plexus, its rami, trunks, and divisions (*see* Chapter 6, pp. 196-197).

GRANT'S 8.9
ROHEN 178-181
A.D.A.M. 7.52
NETTER 28
CLEMENTE 701-703
A.V.A. 5: 1.26.35

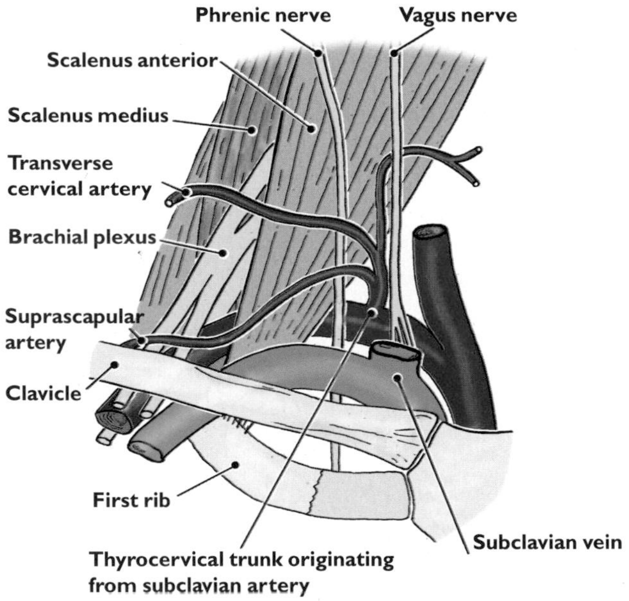

Figure 7.50. Relations of important nerves and vessels to the anterior and posterior scalenus muscles.

> ***Clinical Correlations:*** The **interscalene triangle** becomes clinically significant when it is too narrow and, therefore, compresses the structures passing through it. Anatomical variations, such as additional muscular slips, an accessory cervical rib, or exostosis on the 1st rib may narrow the available interval. As a result, the subclavian artery and/or the brachial plexus may be compressed. This compression may lead to ischemia and to disturbances in nerve function in the upper limb.

> The supraclavicular nerves and the phrenic nerve have essentially the same segmental origin, C3 and C4. This fact explains the phenomenon of "referred pain" in pleurisy. Irritation of the phrenic nerve in the diaphragmatic region may produce pain sensations in the cutaneous area supplied by the supraclavicular nerves (shoulder; clavicular region).

Anterior Triangle of Neck

General Remarks

GRANT'S 8.3, 8.12
ROHEN 153
NETTER 26
CLEMENTE 693

The boundaries of the **anterior triangle** of the neck are (Fig. 7.51A):

- Anteriorly, the median line of the neck;
- Posteriorly, the anterior border of the sternocleidomastoid;
- Superiorly, the inferior border of the mandible.
- The anterior triangle is further subdivided into smaller triangles: **muscular**, **carotid**, **submandibular**, and **submental**.

GRANT'S 8.3
ROHEN 153
CLEMENTE 693

Study a transverse section through the neck (Fig. 7.51B). The anterior part of the neck may be regarded as a "cervical cavity." It is bounded by walls:

- Posteriorly, by the cervical vertebrae;
- Posterolaterally, by the scaleni;
- Laterally, by the sternocleidomastoid;
- Anteriorly, by the strap-like infrahyoid muscles.

GRANT'S 8.2
ROHEN 150, 180
A.D.A.M. 7.29
NETTER 30
CLEMENTE 705, 714
A.V.A. 4: 2.21.38

The "cervical cavity" houses the cervical viscera, which lie in the median plane (Fig. 7.51B):

- The superior part of the digestive tract contains the pharynx and the esophagus;
- The superior part of the respiratory tract houses the larynx and the trachea;
- The thyroid gland lies anterior to the tube-like digestive and respiratory tracts.

Bony and Cartilaginous Landmarks

Study bony and cartilaginous landmarks that will be used as reference structures:

GRANT'S 8.4
ROHEN 154, 155
A.D.A.M. 7.24
NETTER 9, 71
CLEMENTE 712
A.V.A. 4: 1.39.09

- Hyoid bone, at the angle between floor of mouth and superior end of neck; palpate your own hyoid bone; distinguish body, greater horn, and lesser horn;
- Thyroid cartilage, the large cartilage of the larynx; in the midline, note and palpate the laryngeal prominence (Adam's apple);

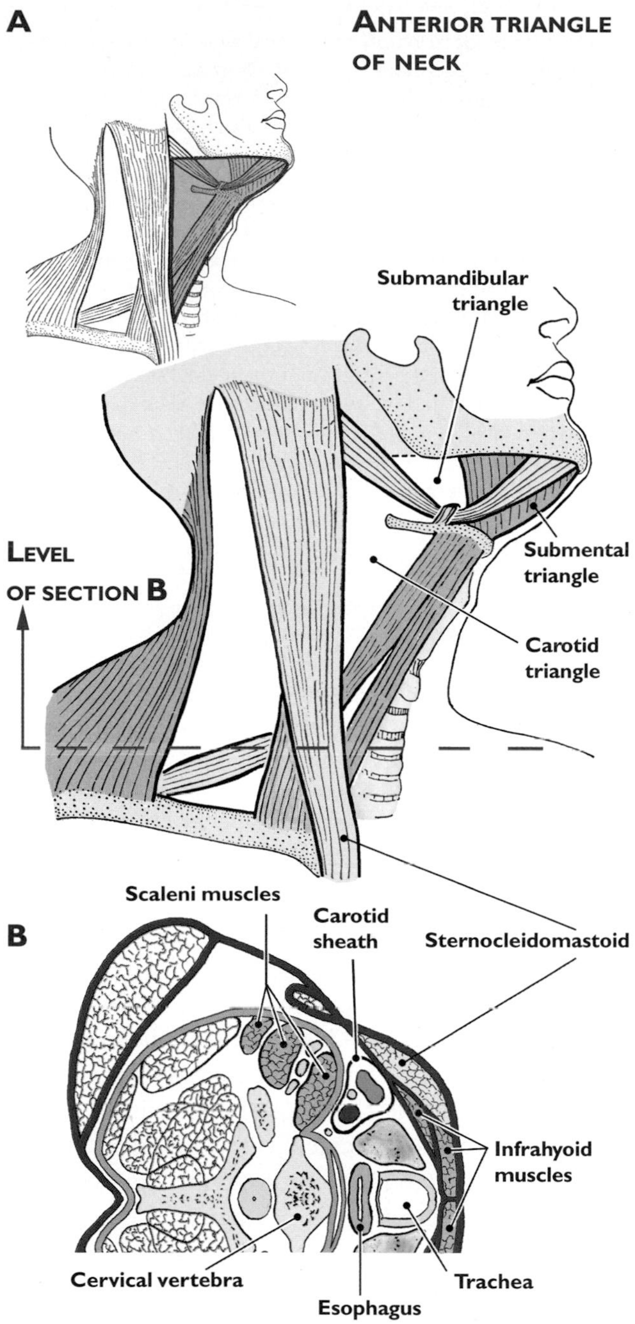

Figure 7.51. ***A***, Anterior triangle of neck and its subdivisions. ***B***, Transverse section through neck showing cervical viscera and surrounding boundaries.

- Thyrohyoid membrane, stretching between thyroid cartilage and hyoid bone;
- Cricoid cartilage, inferior to thyroid cartilage and superior to the 1st tracheal ring; it lies at the level of C6;
- Cricothyroid membrane, stretching between cricoid and thyroid cartilages; the cricothyroid muscles unite the two cartilages more laterally;
- Trachea; note its 1st, 2nd, and 3rd rings.

GRANT'S 8.4, 8.71
ROHEN 154, 155
A.D.A.M. 7.24
NETTER 71
CLEMENTE 712
A.V.A. 4: 2.09.31

Superficial Structures and Contents of Anterior Triangle

The big vessels and nerves lie to each side of the cervical viscera (Fig. 7.51B). Three major structures, **carotid artery**, **internal jugular vein**, and **vagus nerve**, are wrapped together in the fascial **carotid sheath** (Fig. 7.60B).

GRANT'S 8.13
ROHEN 167
A.D.A.M. 7.76
NETTER 27, 28

Arterial Supply

The **common carotid artery** bifurcates into the internal and external carotid arteries. The **external carotid artery** supplies almost all structures of the head and neck outside the cranial cavity. The **internal carotid artery** supplies the structures within the cranial and orbital cavities as well as the forehead. The **vertebral arteries**, which ascend in the neck through the foramina transversaria, enter the cranial cavity through the foramen magnum to contribute to the cerebral arterial circle (Fig. 7.62). A branch of the subclavian artery, the **thyrocervical trunk**, supplies the lower part of the neck.

GRANT'S 8.14A
ROHEN 164
A.D.A.M. 7.30, 7.31
NETTER 28
CLEMENTE 719, 721
A.V.A. 5: 1.27.07

Make a skin incision in the midline from the tip of the chin to the suprasternal notch. Remove entirely the skin from the anterior aspect of the neck.

Observe the fibers of the platysma. Reflect and remove it. Review the cutaneous nerve to the region of the anterior triangle, the transverse cervical nerve.

Superficial Veins (Fig. 7.46)

GRANT'S 8.11
ROHEN 166, 167
A.D.A.M. 7.32
NETTER 26, 64
CLEMENTE 709
A.V.A. 5: 1.57.09

Expect to find variations in the venous pattern. Review the course of the **external jugular vein**. Trace the **facial vein** along the lower border of the mandible to a point where it is joined by the anterior division of the **retromandibular vein**. The facial vein continues for a short distance and drains into the internal jugular vein deep to the sternocleidomastoid muscle. Follow the facial vein. If present, find the small **anterior jugular vein**. On occasion, this vein is connected to the facial vein by a communicating branch. Clean the deep fascia within the confines of the anterior triangle.

Muscular Triangle

The **muscular triangle** is separated from the carotid triangle by the superior belly of the omohyoid. On each side of the median line are four ribbon-like muscles that descend from the hyoid bone or the thyroid cartilage. These are the **infrahyoid muscles** (Fig. 7.52). Their names are descriptive of their attachments.

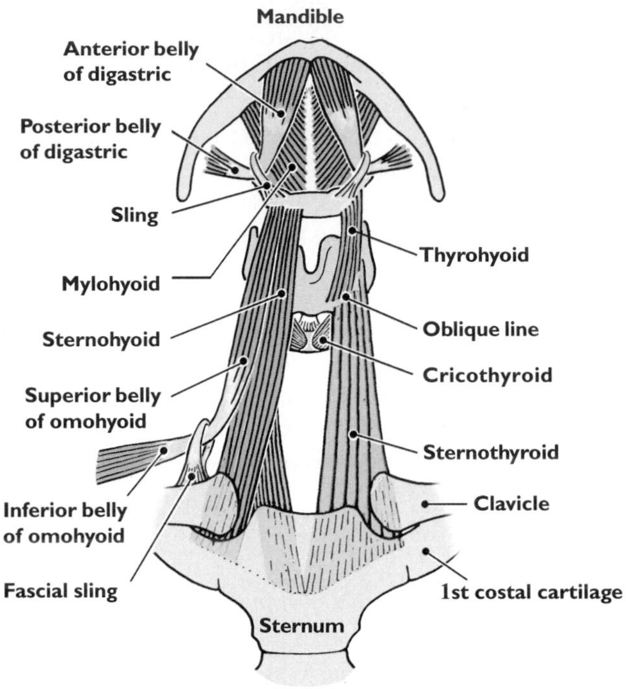

Figure 7.52. Muscles bounding the anterior median line of the neck. A diagram of the suprahyoid and infrahyoid muscles.

Infrahyoid Muscles

In a superficial plane, identify the **superior belly of the omohyoid** and the **sternohyoid**. Deep to these two muscles are the **sternothyroid** and the short **thyrohyoid**. The muscles are supplied by nerve branches from C1 to C3 via the **ansa cervicalis**. These nerves to the infrahyoid muscles will be identified later.

Widen the gap in the midline between the right and left infrahyoids by gently pulling the muscles laterally. Now, palpate and identify:

- **Laryngeal prominence**;
- **Cricoid cartilage**;
- **Cricothyroid membrane**;
- **1st tracheal ring**;
- **Isthmus of thyroid gland**.

Clinical Correlations: **Tracheotomy** (tracheostomy) is the formation of an opening into the trachea. As an emergency operation, it must be rapidly performed in cases with sudden obstruction of the vital airways (aspiration of foreign body; edema of larynx; paralysis of vocal cords). A superior (high) tracheotomy is performed superior to the level of the isthmus of the thyroid gland. An inferior (low) tracheotomy is done inferior to the isthmus.

The simplest and most rapid access to the airway inferior to the vocal cords may be created by opening the cricothyroid membrane, i.e., by performing a **cricothyrotomy**. This important, lifesaving procedure is often used prior to tracheotomy in certain emergency respiratory obstructions. Perform this essential procedure in the cadaver. Palpate the thyroid and cricoid cartilages and the membrane stretching between them. Then, incise the membrane transversely. Realize that only skin and some superficial fascia need to be traversed to reach the cricothyroid membrane. Once opened, an emergency airway can be maintained with almost any small hollow item (e.g., a piece of thin tubing or a straw).

Grant's 8.12, 8.24, 8.25
Rohen 176, 177
A.D.A.M. Table 7.5, 7.6
Netter 22, 24
A.V.A. 4: 2.36.46

Carotid Triangle

Grant's 8.13
Rohen 153
Netter 28
Clemente 693

The **carotid triangle** is bounded by the superior belly of the omohyoid, the posterior belly of the digastric, and the anterior border of the sternocleidomastoid. The common carotid artery ascends through the triangle. The pulse of the common carotid artery can be palpated and auscultated within the boundaries of this triangular space.

Nerves in the Carotid Triangle

Grant's 8.13, 8.16A
A.D.A.M. 8.22
Netter 27, 121
Clemente 701
A.V.A. 5: 1.18.12

Grant's 8.12B
Rohen 176, 177
A.D.A.M. 7.48
Netter 26, 27
Clemente 701, 702
A.V.A. 5: 1.20.20

Grant's 8.24, 8.25
Rohen 152, 153
A.D.A.M. Table 7.5
Netter 23
Clemente 706
A.V.A. 5: 2.36.22

The first objective is to find the **accessory nerve (XI)** as it enters the sternocleidomastoid muscle. Transect the sternocleidomastoid muscle about 5 cm superior to its insertion into sternum and clavicle. Free and clean the upper portion of the sternocleidomastoid from its surrounding fascia. Do not damage the nerves that radiate from the posterior border of the muscle into the posterior triangle. Notice the arterial branches that enter the muscle; then cut them. Find the accessory nerve where it enters the deep surface of the sternocleidomastoid: about 5 cm inferior to the tip of the mastoid process and about 2 cm posterior to the anterior border of the muscle (Fig. 7.49). Trace the accessory nerve superiorly as far as possible. The nerve may cross the internal jugular vein anteriorly or posteriorly. The nerve and the vein pass through the same opening, the jugular foramen.

To allow better access to deeper structures, cut the **facial vein** where it empties into the internal jugular vein.

The **tip of the greater horn of the hyoid bone** is an important reference point for many structures. The greater horn on one side is palpable only when the greater horn of the opposite side is steadied. Palpate the greater horn on the side of the dissection with one index finger while you press against the greater horn of the opposite side with your other index finger (Fig. 7.53).

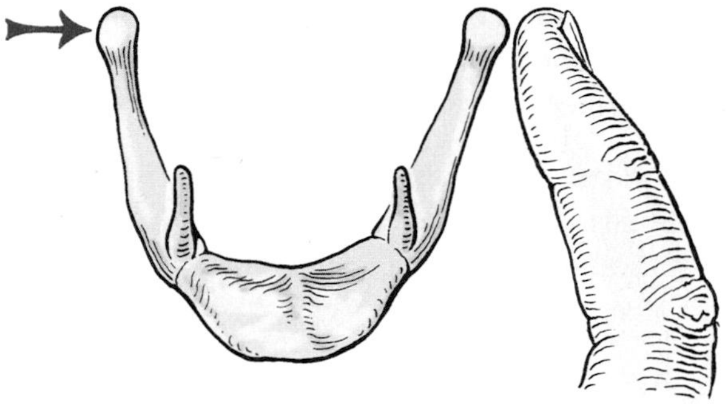

Figure 7.53. Steady the tip of one horn of the hyoid bone while palpating the other.

GRANT'S *8.16*
ROHEN 177
A.D.A.M. 8.23
CLEMENTE 724
A.V.A. 4: 1.39.20

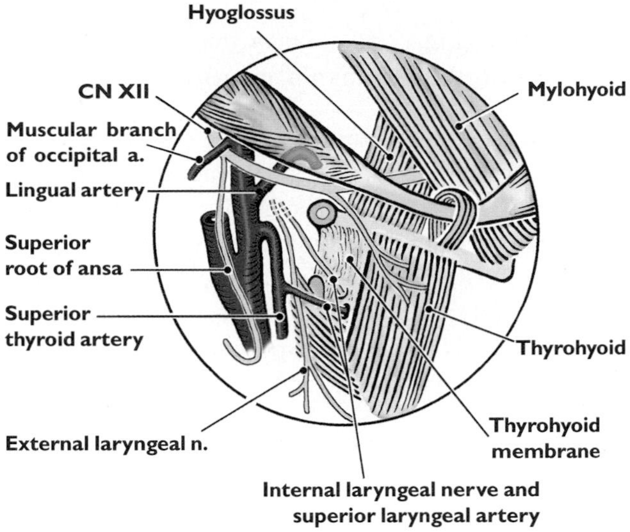

Figure 7.54. The tip of the greater horn of the hyoid bone (green bull's-eye) is the reference point for many structures: nerves, arteries, and muscles.

The next objective is to find the **hypoglossal nerve (XII)**. It is the motor nerve to the muscles of the tongue; therefore, it courses anteriorly. Palpate and locate the tip of the greater horn of the hyoid bone. Then, pick up the large, flat hypoglossal nerve just superior to the tip (Fig. 7.54). At this point, nerve fibers belonging to spinal cord segments C1 and C2 (mainly C1) and adhering to the hypoglossal nerve leave the nerve to supply the thyrohyoid muscle. Follow this slender branch across the tip of the greater horn to the lateral border of the **thyrohyoid muscle**.

GRANT'S *8.13, 8.16*
ROHEN 176, 177
A.D.A.M. 8.23
NETTER 27
CLEMENTE 701-703
A.V.A. 5: 1.19.06

Trace the **hypoglossal nerve** anteriorly and proximally. Verify that the posterior belly of the digastric muscle lies lateral to the nerve (Fig. 7.55). Retract the posterior belly of the digastric and demonstrate the course of the hypoglossal nerve. Proximally, study the relationship of the nerve to the occipital artery. Observe that a branch of the occipital artery, the muscular branch to the sternocleidomastoid, hooks over the nerve (Fig. 7.54).

GRANT'S *8.13, 8.16B*
ROHEN 176, 177
A.D.A.M. 8.23
NETTER 27
CLEMENTE 701-703
A.V.A. 5: 1.19.32

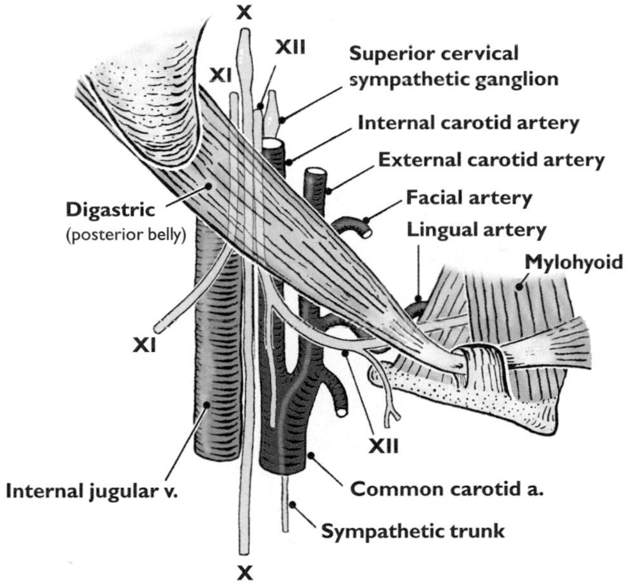

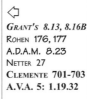

Figure 7.55. The posterior belly of the digastric muscle and structures deep to it.

Find the **superior root of the ansa cervicalis** that is closely adherent to nerve XII (Fig. 7.56). Study the components of the **ansa cervicalis**. The **superior root of the ansa** (descendens hypoglossi) is mainly composed of fibers from C1 that adhere to and run with the hypoglossal nerve. The **inferior root of the ansa** (descendens cervicalis; C2, C3) descends from the more superior neck region to join the superior root. Thus, a loop or ansa is formed. Dissect

GRANT'S *8.12B, 8.13*
ROHEN 176, 177
A.D.A.M. 7.48, 8.23
NETTER 27
CLEMENTE 701, 702
A.V.A. 5: 1.20.20

the ansa (Fig. 7.56). Trace nerve branches from it to the **infrahyoid muscles**.

The next objective is to find the **vagus nerve (X)** and one of its branches. The vagus lies in the carotid sheath, in the posterior angle between the internal jugular vein and the great arterial trunk. Pull the internal jugular vein and nerve XI laterally; pull the carotid arteries and nerve XII medially. This will expose the vagus (Fig. 7.55). Free the vagus and trace it inferiorly.

Find the **superior laryngeal nerve** and its major branch, the **internal laryngeal nerve** (Fig. 7.57). Proceed as follows:

- Relax the anatomical structures of the neck by flexing the head (bending it anteriorly).
- With scissors, sever the omohyoid and the sternohyoid close to the hyoid bone; reflect the muscles inferiorly.

⇦
GRANT'S 8.12B
A.D.A.M. 7.48, 8.23
NETTER 27
CLEMENTE 701, 702

⇦
GRANT'S 8.16
ROHEN 176-179
A.D.A.M. 7.76
NETTER 27, 65
CLEMENTE 703
A.V.A. 5: 1.14.02

⇦
GRANT'S 8.16
ROHEN 176-179
A.D.A.M. 8.17
NETTER 65
CLEMENTE 711
A.V.A. 5: 1.15.25

⇨
GRANT'S 8.27A, 9.14
ROHEN 176-179
A.D.A.M. 8.17
NETTER 65
A.V.A. 5: 1.15.46

- Next, carefully sever the exposed thyrohyoid muscle close to the hyoid bone; reflect it inferiorly.
- Now, the thyrohyoid membrane lies exposed (Fig. 7.54). Identify this membrane that extends between the thyroid cartilage and the hyoid bone. Palpate these two topographic landmarks.
- The **internal laryngeal nerve** pierces the thyrohyoid membrane just inferior to the greater horn of the hyoid bone to supply the superior portion of the larynx with sensory fibers (Figs. 7.54, 7.57).

Find the **external laryngeal nerve** that supplies the cricothyroid muscle and the adjacent part of the inferior constrictor (Fig. 7.57). Proceed as follows:

- Trace the internal laryngeal nerve proximally to a point where it is crossed by the internal carotid artery. Here, find the external laryngeal nerve.
- Trace the delicate nerve inferiorly.

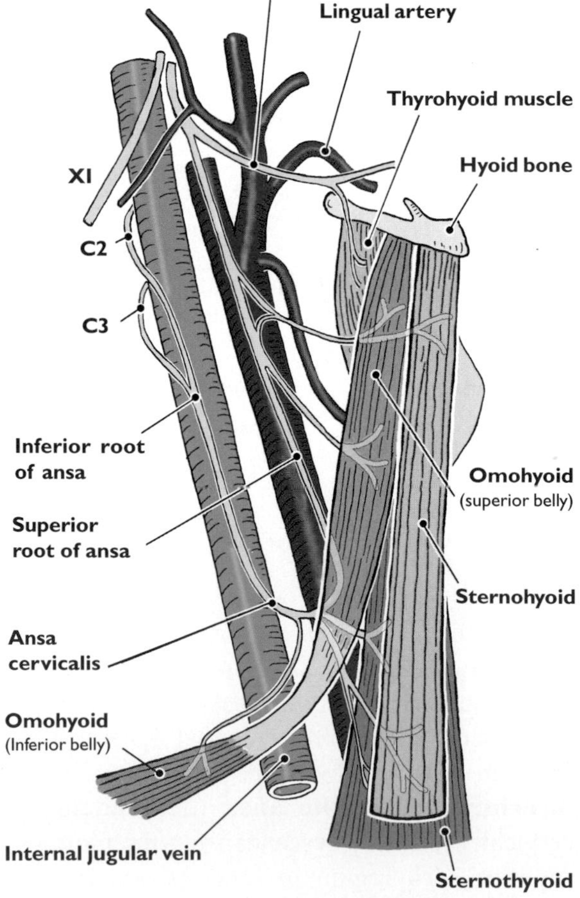

Figure 7.56. The ansa cervicalis.

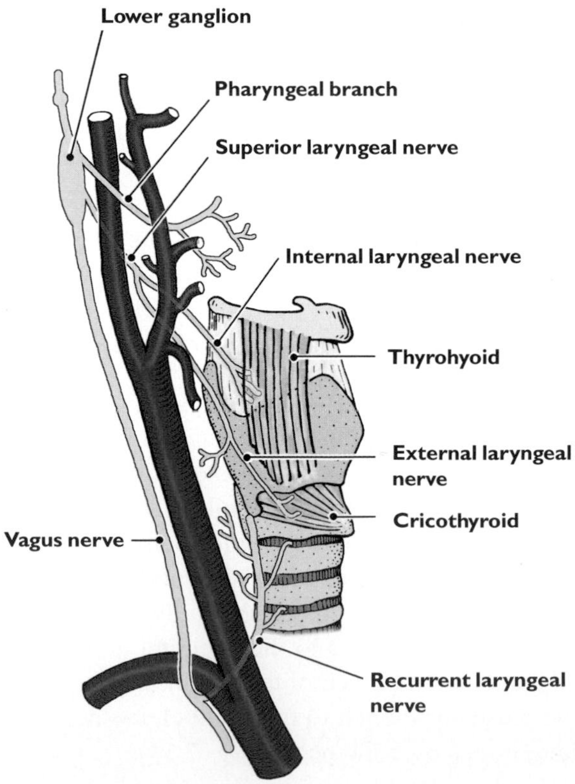

Figure 7.57. Laryngeal branches of the right vagus nerve (cranial nerve X)

- Carefully sever the sternothyroid muscle from the oblique line of the thyroid cartilage. Raise the muscle.
- Find the external laryngeal nerve deep to it.
- Trace the nerve to the **cricothyroid muscle**.

Arteries in the Carotid Triangle (Fig. 7.58). The arteries in this triangle are:

GRANT'S 8.13, 8.14
ROHEN 154, 178
A.D.A.M. 7.30
NETTER 29, 130
CLEMENTE 702
A.V.A. 5: 1.49.50

- Parts of the common, internal, and external carotid arteries; and
- The stems of most of the six collateral branches of the external carotid artery.

Remove the **carotid sheath**. Observe that the internal jugular vein lies in close lateral contact with the **common carotid artery** and the **internal carotid artery**. These two arteries have no collateral branches in the neck. The **external carotid artery**, which lies anteromedial to the internal carotid artery, gives off several branches before reaching the posterior belly of the digastric. Identify these branches (Fig. 7.58):

GRANT'S 8.13, 8.14A
ROHEN 164, 178
A.D.A.M. 7.76
CLEMENTE 702, 715
A.V.A. 5: 1.48.58

- **Superior thyroid artery**. Observe its origin just inferior and posterior to the tip of the greater horn of the hyoid bone (Fig. 7.54). The artery descends to the superior pole of the thyroid gland. Identify one of its branches, the superior laryngeal artery. This artery pierces the thyrohyoid membrane together with the internal laryngeal nerve (Fig. 7.54).

GRANT'S 8.14, 8.26A, 8.27A
ROHEN 179
A.D.A.M. 7.30
NETTER 28, 29
CLEMENTE 702
A.V.A. 5: 1.49.36

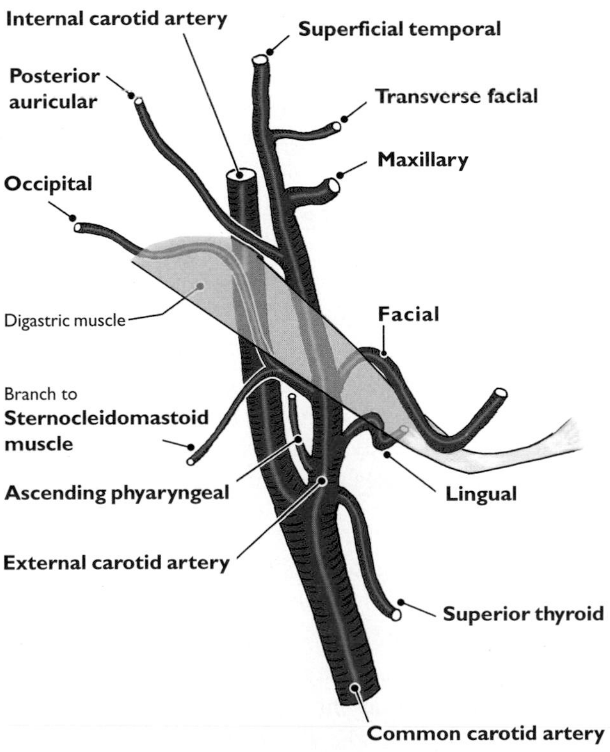

Figure 7.58. Arteries in the carotid triangle.

- **Lingual artery**. Identify its origin just posterior to the tip of the greater horn of the hyoid bone (Fig. 7.54). Expect to find variations.
- **Facial artery** (Fig. 7.58). It arises just superior to the lingual artery. In 20% of all cases, the lingual and facial arteries have a common stem. Expect to find variations.
- **Occipital artery**. It gives off a muscular branch to the sternocleidomastoid muscle.
- **Ascending pharyngeal artery**. Usually, it is the first branch to arise from the external carotid artery close to the carotid bifurcation. It is often difficult to find.

Clean the **bifurcation of the common carotid artery**. Notice the dilation of the superior end of the common carotid and the beginning of the internal carotid artery. Here, the walls of the artery are thinner, less muscular, and more elastic. This dilated region is the **carotid sinus**. The wall of this sinus contains pressoreceptors that respond to changes in blood pressure. Compare the gross anatomical features of the dissected vessels with a carotid arteriogram.

GRANT'S 9.13A - B
ROHEN 178
NETTER 29, 120
CLEMENTE 715
A.V.A. 5: 1.28.00

If time permits, look for the **carotid body**. It is a small mass of tissue, darker, and more firm than fat, located on the medial aspect in the crotch of the carotid bifurcation. The carotid body responds to changes in the chemical composition of the blood. The cranial nerve IX supplies the carotid body and sinus.

GRANT'S 9.14B
A.D.A.M. 8.16
NETTER 119
CLEMENTE 769

Veins in the Anterior Triangle

GRANT'S 8.11, 8.26A, 8.31
ROHEN 168, 169, 176
A.D.A.M. 7.32, 7.33
NETTER 26, 64
CLEMENTE 709, 710
A.V.A. 5: 1.35.54

Identify the following tributaries to the internal jugular vein:

- Common facial vein;
- Lingual vein;
- Superior thyroid vein, which accompanies the respective artery.

To clarify the dissection field, remove the tributaries of the internal jugular vein.

Submandibular Triangle

The **submandibular** or **digastric triangle** is bounded by the inferior border of mandible, anterior belly of digastric; and posterior belly of digastric.

GRANT'S 8.3, 8.17
ROHEN 153
A.D.A.M. TABLE 7.5
NETTER 24
CLEMENTE 693
A.V.A. 4: 2.04.29

Refer to a bony skull. Identify the following relevant bony landmarks of the **temporal bone**:

- **Mastoid process**;
- **Styloid process**; in many skulls, this long and sharp process is broken off due to rough handling of the bony specimen.

GRANT'S 7.2
ROHEN 25
NETTER 9-11
CLEMENTE 754
A.V.A. 4: 0.08.14

Examine the **inner aspect of the mandible** and identify the following:

GRANT'S 7.57B
ROHEN 36, 55
NETTER 10
CLEMENTE 869
A.V.A. 4: 1.28.40

- **Digastric fossa** for the attachment of the anterior belly of the digastric;
- **Mylohyoid line**, for the attachment of the mylohyoid muscle;
- **Submandibular fossa**, inferior to the mylohyoid line;
- **Mylohyoid groove**, in which course the nerves and vessels to the mylohyoid and the anterior belly of the digastric.

Part of the submandibular salivary gland and some lymph nodes fill the submandibular triangle. The **submandibular gland** is wrapped around the free posterior border of the mylohyoid like the letter U on its side.

Dissection

The deep part of the submandibular gland and its duct must not be disturbed. The superficial part of the gland, lying within the boundaries of the submandibular triangle, may be severed and removed. Proceed as follows:

- Clamp a hemostat or a forceps to the gland. Pull the gland medially.
- Free the superficial part of the gland from its surrounding fascia.
- Separate the facial artery and vein from the gland. Observe blood vessels supplying the glandular tissue.
- Cut through the gland at the posterior border of the mylohyoid and remove the superficial part of the gland.

Now, the **anterior and posterior bellies of the digastric** are in clear view and can be well defined. The two bellies are connected to each other by an **intermediate tendon** (Fig. 7.59). This tendon is held to the body and the greater horn of the hyoid bone by a **fibrous sling**. Observe that the intermediate tendon perforates a slender, round muscle, the **stylohyoid** (Fig. 7.59). Verify that the posterior belly of the digastric arises from the medial aspect of the mastoid process. The anterior belly arises from the digastric fossa of the mandible.

GRANT'S 8.17
NETTER 22-24
CLEMENTE 706, 724
A.V.A. 4: 1.42.59

Trace the **hypoglossal nerve (XII)** into the submandibular triangle. Observe that the nerve disappears under cover of the **mylohyoid muscle** (Fig. 7.55).

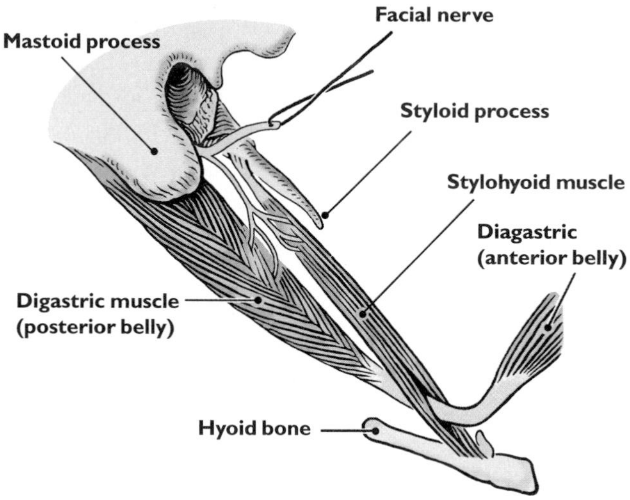

Figure 7.59. The stylohyoid muscle is perforated by the intermediate tendon of the digastric muscle.

Submental Triangle

GRANT'S 8.17
ROHEN 152, 153
A.D.A.M. TABLE 7.5
NETTER 23, 24
CLEMENTE 693, 725, 726

The **submental** (suprahyoid) **triangle** is bounded inferiorly by the body of the hyoid bone and laterally by the right and left anterior bellies of the **digastric muscles** (Fig. 7.52). The floor of the triangle is formed by the two **mylohyoid muscles**. These muscles arise from the mandible and are inserted into the body of the hyoid bone. The fibers of the right and left muscles meet in a median fibrous raphe.

Clean the anterior bellies of the digastric muscles. Occasionally, these anterior bellies are fused and, therefore, may hide the underlying mylohyoid muscle. If this is the case, separate the digastrics from each other and expose the floor of the submental triangle.

Pull the anterior belly of the digastric medially to expose the **mylohyoid nerve**, a branch of V_3. Observe that the nerve is sheltered by the lower border of the mandible. Its more distal portion is closely applied to the mylohyoid muscle. One of its nerve branches reaches the anterior belly of the digastric (the posterior belly of the digastric and the stylohyoid muscles are supplied by a branch of the facial nerve) (Fig. 7.59).

GRANT'S 8.17
A.D.A.M. 8.9
NETTER 41, 47
CLEMENTE 724
A.V.A. 5: 1.01.28

Cervical Viscera

The superior parts of the digestive tract (pharynx and esophagus) and the respiratory tract (larynx and trachea) will be dealt with in special assignments. The thyroid gland can be conveniently explored at this time.

Thyroid Gland (Fig. 7.60)

The infrahyoid and the sternocleidomastoid muscles have been reflected earlier. Therefore, the thyroid gland lies exposed. Verify that it extends between the carotid sheaths of the two sides. Identify the **right and left lobes**. The two lobes are connected by the isthmus, which usually covers the 2nd to 4th tracheal rings. In 50% of all cases, the gland has a **pyramidal lobe** that ascends from the **isthmus** superiorly, sometimes as high as the hyoid bone. Expect to find variations.

GRANT'S 8.26
ROHEN 170, 171, 178
NETTER 68, 69
CLEMENTE 712
A.V.A. 4: 2.36.20

GRANT'S 8.29C
NETTER 68
CLEMENTE 712, 715

Being an endocrine organ, the thyroid gland has a rich blood supply and drainage. Identify the **superior thyroid artery**. Demonstrate the **three paired veins** that drain the thyroid gland: **superior**, **middle**, and **inferior thyroid veins**. To find the **inferior thyroid artery**, on the respective side, pull the lobe of the thyroid gland anteriorly. Observe the origin of the artery from the thyrocervical trunk.

GRANT'S 8.26, 8.27, 8.31
ROHEN 164, 178
A.D.A.M. 7.30, 7.32, 7.52
NETTER 68
CLEMENTE 715
A.V.A. 5: 1.49.36

Cut the isthmus of the gland and turn the lobes laterally. Define and then sever the fascial band that attaches the capsule of the gland to the 1st tracheal ring (Fig. 7.60B). With a probe, display the **recurrent laryngeal nerve** that ascends just posterior to the gland on the side of the trachea.

GRANT'S 8.36B, 8.49
A.D.A.M. 7.43
NETTER 70
CLEMENTE 713
A.V.A. 4: 2.36.05

On the left side only, cut all blood vessels leading to or from the left lobe of the thyroid

GRANT'S 8.27, 8.31
NETTER 70
CLEMENTE 715
A.V.A. 5: 1.16.45

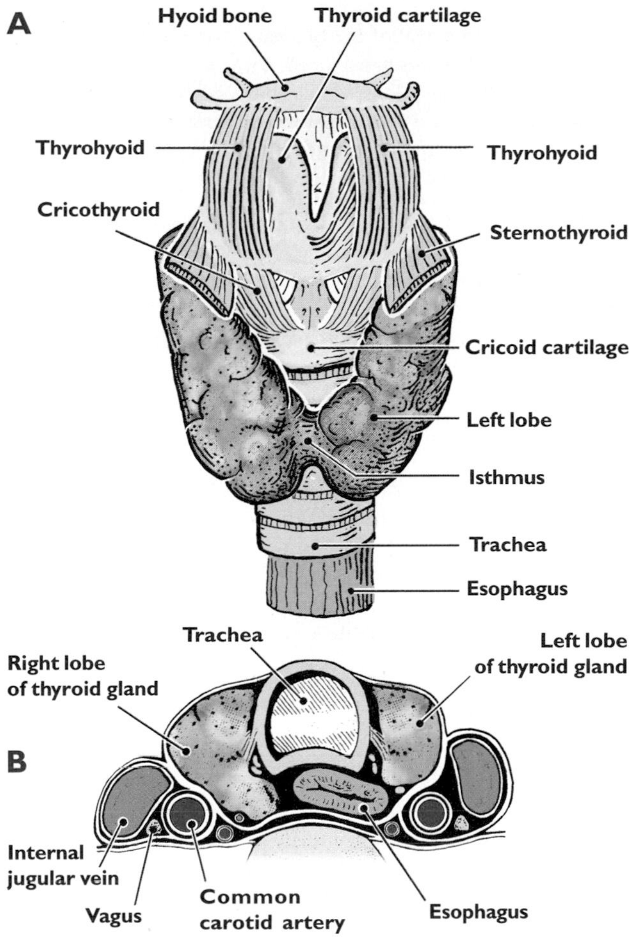

Figure 7.60. The thyroid gland and its relations in anterior view ***(A)*** and transverse section ***(B)***.

gland. Then, enucleate this lobe. Cut into the substance of the gland. Observe its characteristic colloid structure. Preserve the posterior aspect of the lobe, where the parathyroid glands may be found.

Parathyroid Glands

These small but vital glands lie along the posterior border of the thyroid gland between its capsule and its sheath. On the posterior aspect of the removed thyroid lobe, look for small brownish bodies, measuring about 5 mm in diameter. Usually, there are two parathyroid glands on each side. However, the total number may vary from 2 to 6.

Clinical Correlation: Physicians must be fully aware of the close relationship between thyroid gland, parathyroid glands, and the recurrent laryngeal nerves. If, during thyroidectomy (removal of thyroid gland), one or both recurrent laryngeal nerves are injured, paralysis of the laryngeal muscles will occur. Note how intimately the recurrent laryngeal nerve is related to the thyroid gland. Understand that a malignant tumor of the thyroid may easily lead to destruction of the recurrent laryngeal nerve or nerves.

The parathyroid glands play a vital role in the regulation of calcium and phosphorus metabolism. During thyroidectomy, these small endocrine glands are in danger of being damaged or of being removed. Appreciate this fact by studying the close relations between thyroid and parathyroid glands.

Root of the Neck

The root of the neck is also known as the thoracocervical region. It can be defined as the junction between the thorax and the neck. The boundaries of the root of the neck are:

GRANT'S 8.32, 8.33
ROHEN 181
A.D.A.M. 2.3
NETTER 24
CLEMENTE 711

- Anteriorly, the manubrium of the sternum;
- Laterally, the first ribs;
- Posteriorly, the body of the first thoracic vertebra.

The root of the neck is a vitally important area because it includes the **superior thoracic aperture**. Through this aperture pass all structures going from the head to the thorax and vice versa. During dissection of the root of the neck, some of these structures will be followed superiorly or inferiorly in reference to the superior thoracic aperture.

GRANT'S 8.32A
NETTER 24, 25
CLEMENTE 711
A.V.A. 5: 1.26.13

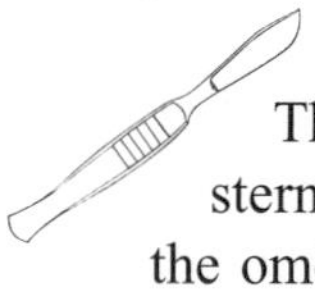

The sternocleidomastoid, sternohyoid, sternothyroid, and the superior belly of the omohyoid have been reflected earlier. If not already done, remove the fascia (loop) that binds the intermediate tendon of the omohyoid to the clavicle. Now, the root of the neck lies exposed, particularly on the left side, where the left lobe of the thyroid gland was resected.

To clarify the dissection field, cut the **common carotid artery** and the **internal jugular vein** (but not the vagus) about 2 cm superior to the clavicular level. Reflect the large vessels superiorly. Fix them in the reflected position with needles or a hemostat.

The next objective is to find the **thoracic duct** (Fig. 7.61). The duct opens at (or near) the angle between the **left subclavian vein** and the **left internal jugular vein**. The duct has approximately the same diameter as the superior thyroid vein. Usually, it is pale, collapsed, inconspicuous, and very easily torn.

GRANT'S 8.32
ROHEN 176
A.D.A.M. 7.42
NETTER 68, 227
CLEMENTE 715

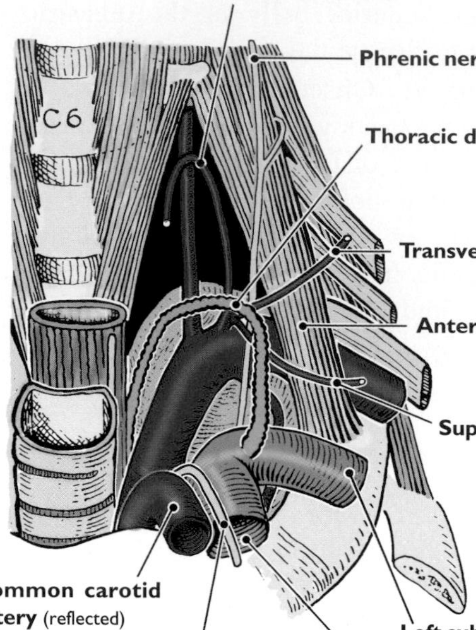

Figure 7.61. Root of the neck: drainage of the thoracic duct.

To find the thoracic duct, proceed as follows (Fig. 7.61):

- Pull the inferior portions of the severed common carotid artery and internal jugular vein anteriorly.
- Now, the duct lies exposed as it arches from the side of the esophagus laterally to the angle between internal jugular and subclavian veins.
- To clarify the dissection field, remove the vertebral vein. Usually, this vein descends posterior to the thoracic duct to empty dorsally into the brachiocephalic vein.
- Positively identify the thoracic duct.

GRANT'S 1.69
A.D.A.M. 7.42
CLEMENTE 716

The lymphatic drainage on the right side of the neck is different. Delicate lymphatic trunks empty into the right subclavian and jugular veins. You are not required to search for these lymph vessels.

Clean the **vagus nerve** and the **phrenic nerve.** Follow these structures into the thorax. Once again, verify that the phrenic nerve is intimately applied to the ventral surface of the scalenus anterior. The **transverse cervical** and **suprascapular arteries** pass directly anterior to the nerve and muscle. Trace these two arteries back to their origin from the **thyrocervical trunk**. This arterial trunk arises near the medial border of the scalenus anterior.

Identify a third branch of the thyrocervical trunk, the **inferior thyroid artery**. It passes posterior to the carotid sheath to enter the inferior pole of the thyroid gland. Expect to find variations. Often, the thyrocervical trunk does not give rise to all three arteries. On occasion, the arteries arise separately from the subclavian artery. Inferior to the origin of the thyrocervical trunk, observe the origin of the **internal thoracic artery** (Fig. 7.62).

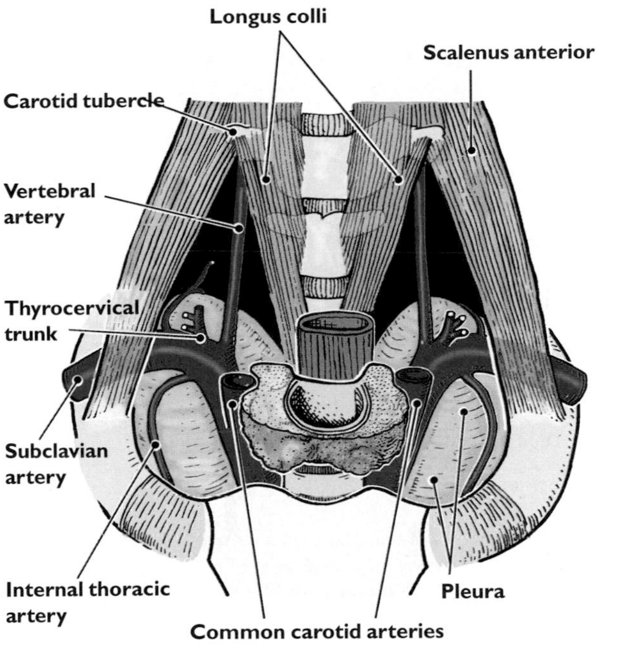

Figure 7.62. Triangle of the vertebral artery: branches of the subclavian artery.

The next objective is to find and partially trace the **vertebral artery**. It is the first and largest branch of the subclavian artery (Fig. 7.62). Identify this deeply running vessel in relation to two muscles, the scalenus anterior and the longus colli. These muscles form the two sides of the "triangle of the vertebral artery." The apex of this triangle is the transverse process of C6. The anterior tubercle of this transverse process is an important landmark. The common carotid artery passes anterior to the tubercle and may be compressed against it (hence the term "carotid tubercle"; Fig. 7.62). Trace the vertebral artery to the apex of the triangle where it enters the transverse foramen of C6. Review the course of the vertebral artery.

The **sympathetic trunk** and its ganglia may be examined now. However, these structures can be more conveniently studied in the prevertebral region after removal of the head.

GRANT'S 8.30, 8.33
ROHEN 164
NETTER 28
CLEMENTE 703
A.V.A. 5: 1.38.40

GRANT'S 8.30
ROHEN 164, 165
A.D.A.M. 7.30
NETTER 28
CLEMENTE 715
A.V.A. 5: 1.48.38

GRANT'S 8.33
ROHEN 164, 165
A.D.A.M. 7.31
NETTER 28
CLEMENTE 721
A.V.A. 5: 1.26.06

GRANT'S 8.14A, 8.33
ROHEN 164
A.D.A.M. 7.30, 7.31
NETTER 28
CLEMENTE 719, 721
A.V.A. 5: 1.31.28

Parotid Region

General Remarks

GRANT'S 7.9, 7.10
ROHEN 25
A.D.A.M. 7.9
NETTER 19
CLEMENTE 754
A.V.A. 4: 2.01.12

The parotid region is a restricted space occupied by the parotid gland and certain soft structures associated with it. Refer to a skull and define the bony space that forms the boundaries for the parotid bed (Fig. 7.63A):

- Posteriorly, the mastoid process;
- Anteriorly, the ramus of mandible;
- Superiorly, the floor of external acoustic meatus;
- Medially, the styloid process.

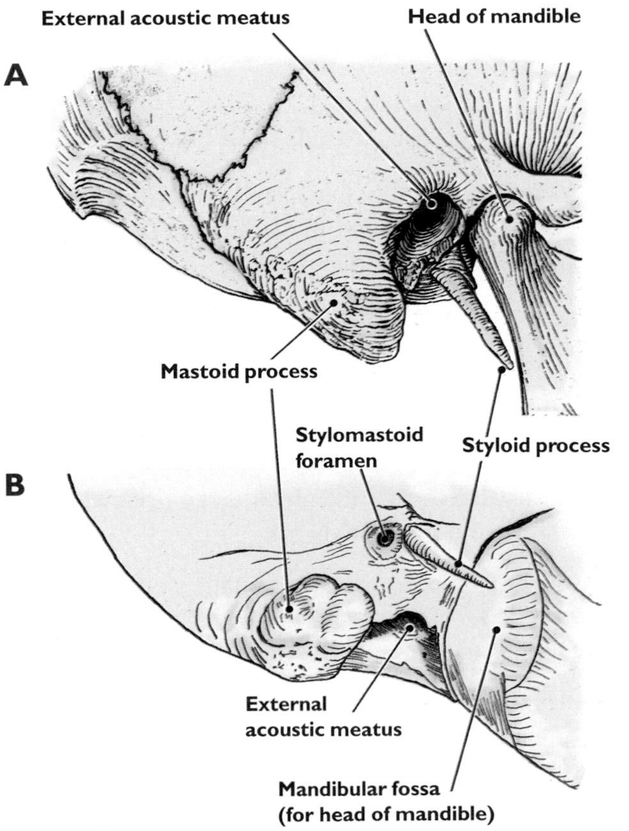

Figure 7.63. Pertinent bony landmarks of the parotid region. ***A***, Lateral view. ***B***, Inferior view at base of skull.

The posterior wall of the parotid region extends between the mastoid and styloid processes. Therefore, the muscles attached to these processes (sternocleidomastoid; posterior belly of digastric; stylohyoid) are closely related to the gland. The anterior wall of the parotid region is formed by the ramus of the mandible and the two muscles applied to it, the masseter and the medial pterygoid.

The parotid gland is traversed by branches of the facial nerve, arteries, and veins. This fact must be appreciated during dissection and during surgery.

GRANT'S 7.9, 7.10
ROHEN 25
A.D.A.M. 7.9
NETTER 19
CLEMENTE 754
A.V.A. 4: 2.02.33

Bony Landmarks

Refer to a bony skull and study the following pertinent landmarks (Fig. 7.63):

- On the **temporal bone**, identify the **styloid process**, the **mastoid process**, the **external acoustic meatus**, and the **mandibular fossa** for the head of the mandible.
- On the **mandible**, identify the **head**, the **neck**, and the posterior border of the **ramus**.
- On the exterior of the **base of the skull**, identify the **stylomastoid foramen**, located between the base of the **styloid process** and the **mastoid process** (Fig. 7.63B); the important facial nerve (cranial nerve VII) passes through this foramen.

GRANT'S 7.2
ROHEN 50
A.D.A.M. 7.9
NETTER 9
CLEMENTE 752
A.V.A. 4: 0.08.08

Structures of Parotid Region

Dissection

Observe the superficial extent of the parotid gland and the structures radiating from its anterior margin (Fig. 7.64A):

- **Parotid duct**;
- **Transverse facial artery**;
- Branches of the **facial nerve**. These structures have already been cleaned.
- Verify that the parotid gland is enclosed within fascia, the **parotid sheath**.

GRANT'S 7.10
ROHEN 76
A.D.A.M. 7.44
NETTER 19
CLEMENTE 735, 736
A.V.A. 4: 2.03.22

The first objective is to find the **stem of the facial nerve** (VII) as it emerges from the stylomastoid foramen. Proceed as follows:

- Make sure that the sternocleidomastoid is well cleaned where it attaches to the mastoid process. Reflect the muscle.
- With the handle of the scalpel, ease the parotid sheath and the parotid gland anteriorly. Hold it in this position with a hemostat.

GRANT'S 7.56, 9.11A
ROHEN 77
A.D.A.M. 8.11
NETTER 19
CLEMENTE 836
A.V.A. 4: 2.02.06

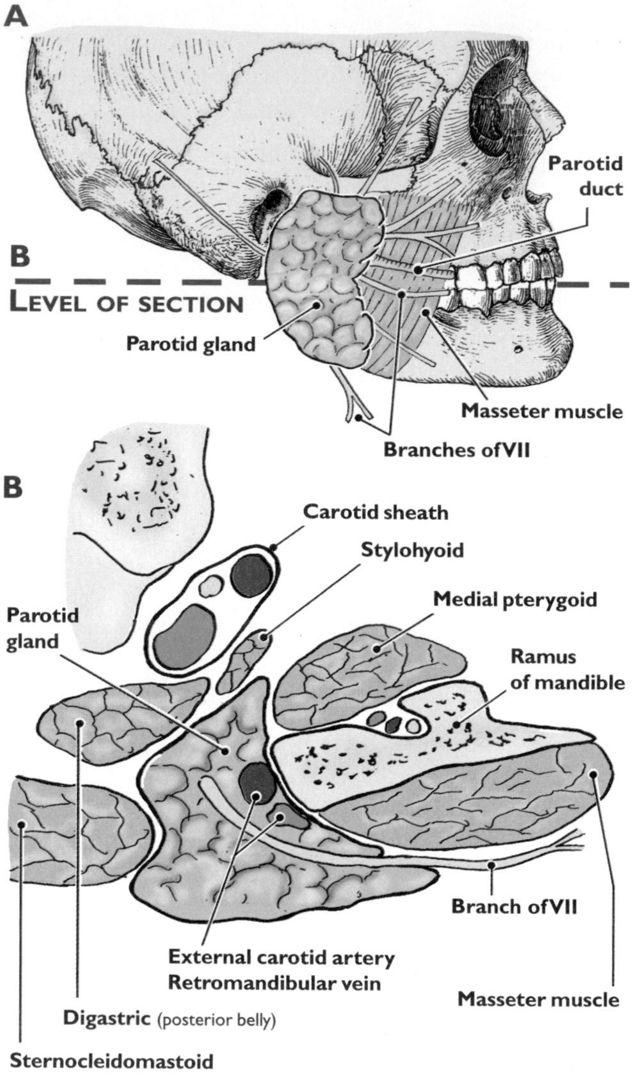

Figure 7.64. The parotid gland and its topographic relations. ***A***, Orientation in lateral view and level of section for the lower part of the illustration. ***B***, Transverse section demonstrates the relations of the gland to surrounding and traversing structures.

- Briefly, refer to a skull (Fig. 7.63B) and determine how you must aim the handle of the knife in order to reach the stylomastoid foramen.
- In the cadaver, push the handle in the same direction until it catches between the mastoid and styloid processes.
- Now, use a probe and search in the interval between the two processes. Reveal the facial nerve as it leaves the stylomastoid foramen to enter the parotid sheath.

Follow the **temporal branches of the facial nerve** superiorly. Trace them through the glandular tissue. You may find two communications with the **auriculotempo-**

GRANT'S 9.13D
A.D.A.M. 8.15
NETTER 19
CLEMENTE 735, 736
A.V.A. 4: 2.02.58

ral nerve (a branch of V_3) that carry secretory fibers to the parotid gland. Using blunt dissection, shell the gland out of its fascial bed. Follow the facial nerve branches deep through the substance of the gland (Fig. 7.65). Trace the auriculotemporal nerve toward the neck of the mandible. The nerve runs medial and deep to the parotid gland.

GRANT'S 7.55, 7.56
A.D.A.M. 8.15
NETTER 117, 128
CLEMENTE 749, 835
A.V.A. 4: 2.01.48

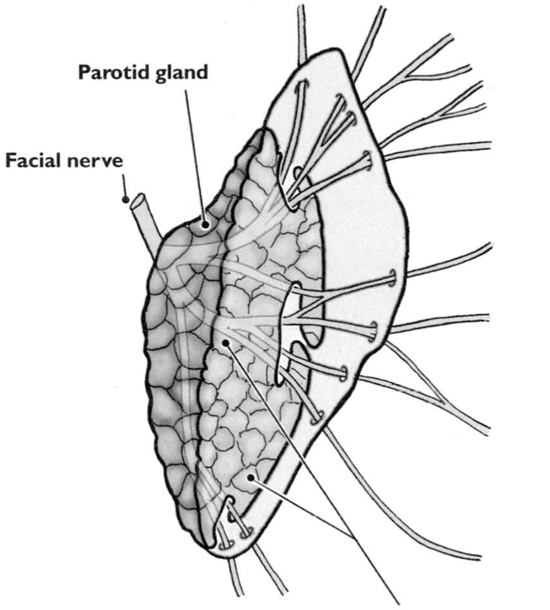

Figure 7.65. The facial nerve (VII) traverses the substance of the parotid gland.

The next objective is to identify the vessels that traverse the tissue of the parotid gland. Use scissors to spread the glandular tissue apart. Establish the course of the **retromandibular vein** (Fig. 7.64B). Next, trace the **external carotid artery** through the gland. The artery is deeply placed and sheltered by the ramus of the mandible (Fig. 7.64B). Posterior to the neck of the mandible, the external carotid artery divides into its two terminal branches, the **maxillary artery** and the **superficial temporal artery** (Fig. 7.58). Verify this.

GRANT'S 7.54
ROHEN 76
A.D.A.M. 7.44
NETTER 54, 55
CLEMENTE 735, 748
A.V.A. 5: 1.49.11

Cut the parotid duct close to the gland. Pull the gland posteriorly and inferiorly. Sever the facial nerve about 2 to 3 cm distal to the stylomastoid foramen, leaving the stump for future reference. Remove the parotid gland.

Now, examine the **parotid bed**. Identify the **posterior belly of the digastric** and the **stylohyoid**. Palpate the styloid process. Clean the **auriculotemporal nerve** posterior to the temporomandibular joint. Once more, examine the **facial nerve** as it leaves its canal in the temporal bone and exits through the stylomastoid foramen (Fig. 7.66). Mark the severed facial nerve by tying a piece of thread to it.

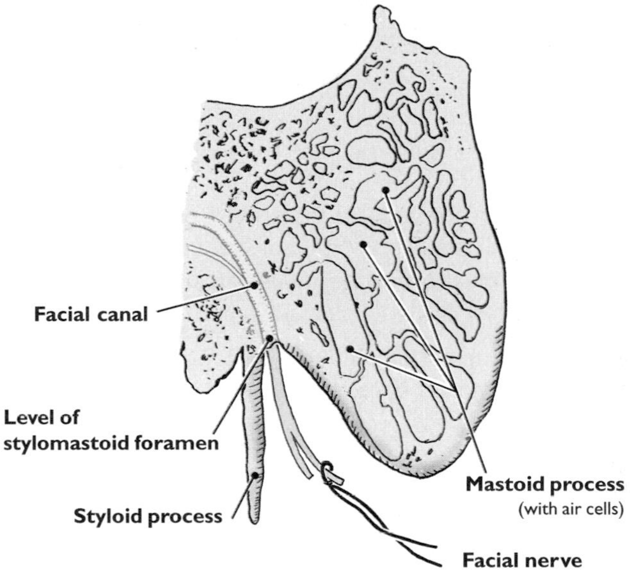

Figure 7.66. The section through the mastoid process and styloid process reveals the bony facial canal. The facial nerve is shown as it leaves the canal through the stylomastoid foramen.

Clinical Correlation: Appreciate the close relationship between the external ear canal and parotid gland (Gr., para, near; otos, = ear). A painful swelling of the parotid gland (e.g., as in mumps) characteristically pushes the ear lobe superiorly and laterally.

During parotidectomy (surgical excision of parotid gland), the facial nerve is in constant danger of being injured. In cases of benign parotid tumors, the stem of the facial nerve may be isolated at the stylomastoid foramen and the facial nerve branches may remain intact during removal of lobules of diseased parotid tissue. In malignant tumors, the facial nerve must be sacrificed. What will happen if the orbicularis oculi becomes nonfunctional as a result of facial nerve paralysis?

Temporal Region

General Remarks

GRANT'S 7.60, 7.61
ROHEN 25
A.D.A.M. 7.9
NETTER 48
CLEMENTE 748, 749
A.V.A. 4: 0.36.21

The **temporal region** consists of two fossae, the temporal fossa and the infratemporal fossa. The **temporal fossa** is located superior to the zygomatic arch. Its floor, consisting of portions of four bones, gives rise to the fan-shaped temporalis muscle, which is an important masticatory muscle. The **infratemporal fossa** is situated inferior and deep to the zygomatic arch. It contains two muscles of mastication, the mandibular nerve (V_3), and the maxillary vessels. The fossa lies deep; its lateral wall is the ramus of the mandible. The infratemporal and temporal fossae are in communication with each other through the interval between zygomatic arch and the cranial vault. The prominent masseter muscle is attached to the zygomatic arch.

GRANT'S 7.60, 7.61
ROHEN 25
A.D.A.M. 7.9
NETTER 48
CLEMENTE 748, 749
A.V.A. 4: 0.36.42

Bony Landmarks

GRANT'S 7.2, 7.60
ROHEN 25
NETTER 2, 9
CLEMENTE 754, 755
A.V.A. 4: 0.36.25

Refer to a bony skull and study the following pertinent landmarks:

- **Temporal lines**, curving backward from the frontal process of the zygomatic bone and indicating the margin of origin of the temporalis muscle; the temporal lines surround the **temporal fossa**; this fossa is formed by components of four different cranial bones: parietal bone, frontal bone, squamous part of temporal bone, and greater wing of sphenoid bone;
- **Zygomatic arch**, composed of the *zygomatic process* of the temporal bone and the *temporal process* of the zygomatic bone.

Refer to a **mandible**. On its *external surface* identify (Fig. 7.67A):

GRANT'S 7.57
ROHEN 55
A.D.A.M. 7.10
NETTER 10, 11
CLEMENTE 867-870
A.V.A. 4: 1.27.16

- **Ramus** and **angle**;
- **Mandibular notch** that is located between the **head of mandible** and **coronoid process**.

On the *inner aspect* of the mandible identify (Fig. 7.67B):

- **Lingula** for the attachment of the sphenomandibular ligament;
- **Mandibular foramen** for the transmission of the inferior alveolar nerves and vessels;
- **Mylohyoid groove** for the nerve and vessels to the mylohyoid and anterior belly of the digastric.

Remove the mandible from the bony skull, thus gaining access to the bony landmarks of the infratemporal fossa. View this area inferolaterally or from the base of the skull. Identify:

GRANT'S 7.61
ROHEN 25
NETTER 2
CLEMENTE 755
A.V.A. 4: 0.46.30

- **Lateral pterygoid plate** of the sphenoid bone;
- **Infratemporal** (posterior) **surface** of the maxilla;
- **Pterygopalatine fossa**, a wedge-shaped cleft that transmits blood vessels;
- **Greater wing of the sphenoid**, with two important foramina: **foramen ovale** and **foramen spinosum**.

Reposition the mandible on the bony skull and identify the **walls of the infratemporal fossa**:

- Laterally, the ramus of the mandible;
- Anteriorly, the posterior aspect of the maxilla; superiorly, it is limited by the inferior orbital fissure; medially, by the pterygopalatine fossa;
- The medial wall is the lateral plate of the pterygoid process.
- The roof of the infratemporal fossa is flat and formed by the greater wing of the sphenoid. The large foramen ovale transmits the mandibular nerve (V_3). The foramen spinosum is traversed by the middle meningeal vessels. The sphenomandibular ligament is attached near the spine of the sphenoid.

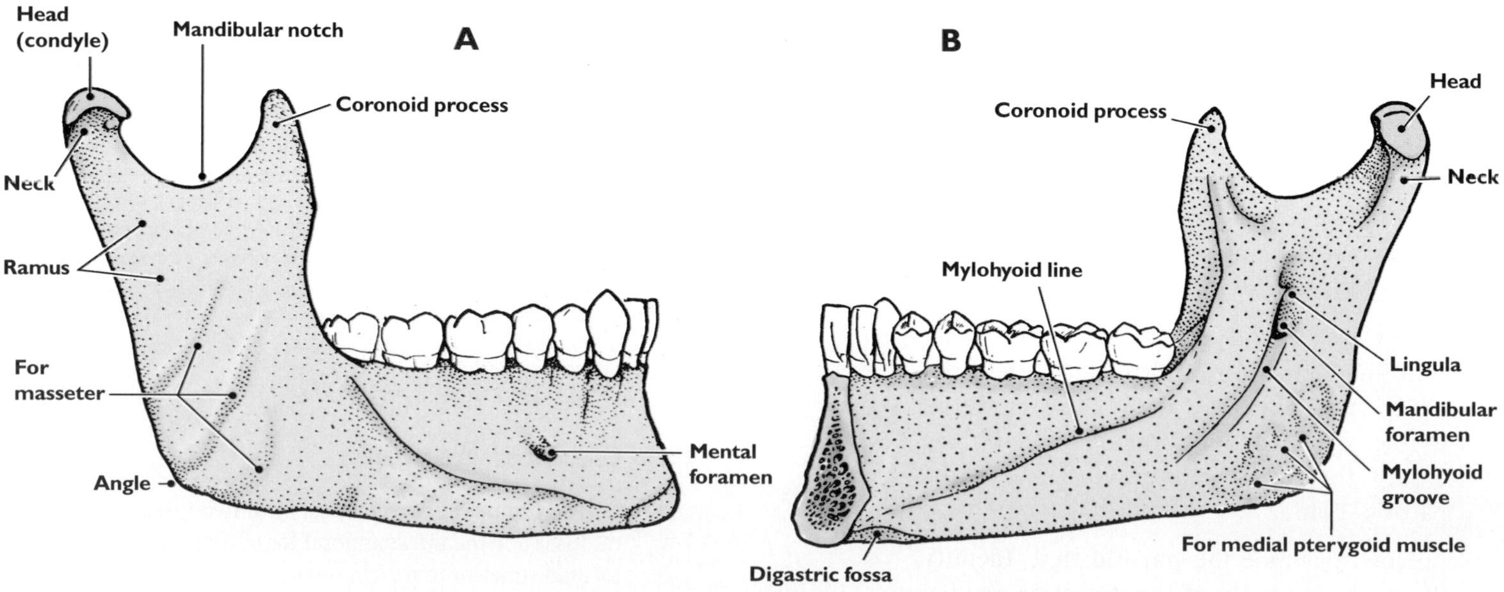

Figure 7.67. ***A***, External surface of mandible. ***B***, Internal aspect of mandible.

Structures of Temporal Region

Dissection

GRANT'S 7.8, 7.9
ROHEN 58
A.D.A.M. 7.23
NETTER 48
CLEMENTE 731, 733
A.V.A. 5: 0.53.23

Remove the remains of the masseteric fascia and clean the **masseter muscle** (Fig. 7.64). Detach the posterior third of the muscle from the zygomatic arch. Turn the detached portion of the masseter anteriorly to display the **masseteric nerve and vessels** passing through the mandibular notch.

GRANT'S 7.9
ROHEN 58
NETTER 48
CLEMENTE 731
A.V.A. 4: 1.36.41

Next, the masseter must be reflected inferiorly together with its bone of origin. Proceed as follows (Fig. 7.68):

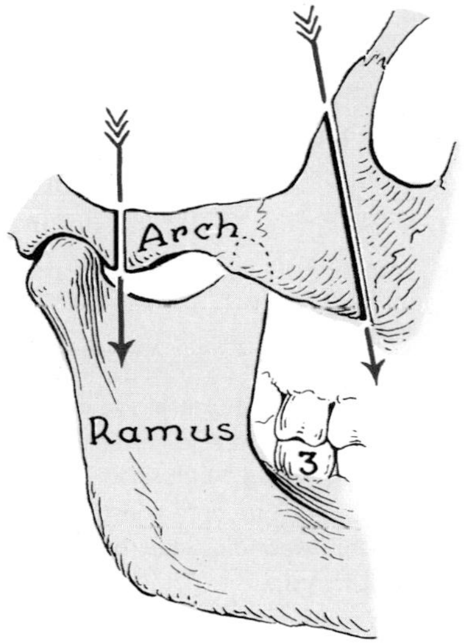

Figure 7.68. Two saw cuts *(arrows)* through the zygomatic arch.

- Pass a probe or closed forceps deep to the zygomatic arch to protect the underlying soft structures.
- Saw obliquely through the zygomatic bone as far anteriorly as possible.
- Next, saw through the zygoma as far posteriorly as possible.
- Reflect inferiorly the section of the zygomatic arch together with the attached masseter muscle. During this process, the nerve and vessels to the masseter will be torn.
- With the handle of a scalpel, detach the muscle fibers of the deep portion of the masseter from the superior portion of the ramus and from the lateral surface of the coronoid process.
- Detach the superficial portion of the muscle from the ramus of the mandible.
- Leave the masseter attached to the lower margin of the mandible.

Now, the **temporal fascia** is fully exposed. Review its attachment to the temporal line (it cannot be fully traced where the calvaria has been removed). Make a deep vertical cut through the fascia and evert it. Observe:

- The muscle fibers of the temporalis partly arise from the fascia.
- The temporalis inserts into the coronoid process of the mandible.
- The anterior portion of the temporalis is thick. Its fibers take a vertical direction (important for closure of the jaw). The fibers of the smaller posterior portion take a posterior sweep from the coronoid process.

The temporal fascia splits to enclose a small fat-pad between the temporalis and the lateral wall of the orbit. Notice that this fatty tissue is continuous with the buccal fat-pad on the buccinator. Remove the fat. Realize that in the emaciated person, the loss of the continuous fat-pads is responsible for the sunken cheeks and temples.

Infratemporal Fossa

GRANT'S 7.62
ROHEN 25, 58
A.D.A.M. 7.76
NETTER 48, 49
CLEMENTE 748
A.V.A. 5: 0.53.30

The infratemporal fossa contains two muscles of mastication, the mandibular nerve (V3), and the maxillary vessels. The fossa lies deep; its lateral wall is the ramus of the mandible. Therefore, access to the infratemporal fossa will necessitate partial removal of the ramus by means of three saw cuts.

Removal of Ramus of Mandible

GRANT'S 7.55
ROHEN 58
A.D.A.M. 7.52, 7.76
NETTER 48
CLEMENTE 733
A.V.A. 5: 0.53.34

First Saw Cut. To detach the coronoid process, proceed as follows (Fig. 7.69):

- Pass a probe or the blade of a forceps (*arrow* in Fig. 7.69) through the mandibular notch.
- Push the instrument obliquely inferiorly and anteriorly, in close contact with the mandible.

Now, the soft structures deep to the coronoid process are protected from the saw blade.

• Cut obliquely through the coronoid process. Reflect it together with the insertion of the temporalis muscle.

Raise the anterior and posterior borders of the temporalis until the nerves to the muscle are seen lying on the bone. These nerves are accompanied by deep temporal arteries. Study the muscle. Subsequently, remove the temporalis muscle entirely and discard it.

GRANT'S 7.62, 7.63
NETTER 65
CLEMENTE 749-751
A.V.A. 5: 0.53.40

Second Saw Cut

The objective of this procedure is to remove the superior part of the ramus of the mandible. However, the nerves and vessels just medial to the mandibular ramus must not be damaged. Proceed as follows (Fig. 7.69):

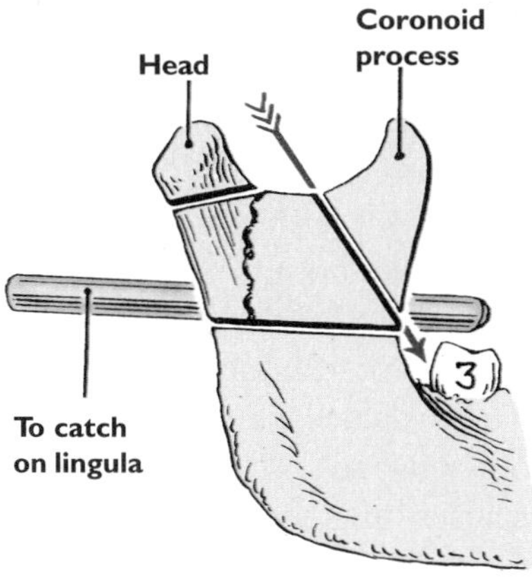

Figure 7.69. Three saw cuts through the mandible.

• With a pencil, mark the approximate position of the lingula (center of ramus) on the lateral surface of the ramus. Inferior to this pencil mark, the inferior alveolar nerve and vessels enter the mandible on its medial aspect.

• The inferior alveolar structures must be protected; therefore, the saw cut across the mandible must be made superior to the pencil mark. Pass the blade of an open forceps medial to the neck of the mandible. Keep in close contact with the bone. Work the instrument inferiorly until it is arrested by the lingula.

• Carefully make the prescribed saw cut and remove the bone fragment.

• Remaining bone, rough edges, or sharp spikes should be nibbled away with bone pliers. Guard your eyes against flying bone fragments.

Third Saw Cut (Fig. 7.69)

Cut through the neck of the mandible, just inferior to the temporomandibular joint. During the sawing procedure, protect the underlying soft structures with a probe or forceps.

GRANT'S 7.62
ROHEN 80-82
A.D.A.M. 7.76
NETTER 65
CLEMENTE 750, 751
A.V.A. 5: 1.00.32

Now, the **contents of the infratemporal fossa** lie exposed. Identify the **inferior alveolar nerve and artery** (the structures may be obscured by the mandibular periosteum inadvertently left behind during bone removal). Trace the nerve inferiorly; it enters the mandibular foramen. Trace the nerve proximally (superiorly); it leads to the inferior border of the lateral pterygoid muscle.

GRANT'S 7.62
ROHEN 80-82
A.D.A.M. 7.80
NETTER 65
CLEMENTE 750
A.V.A. 5: 1.00.50

Follow the **inferior alveolar nerve and vessels** into the (bony) mandibular canal. With small bone pliers (or with a dental drill), open the canal. Note branches of the nerve and arteries to the teeth. Finally, follow the distal portion of the inferior alveolar nerve through the mental foramen into the region of the chin and lower lip.

> ***Clinical Correlation:*** A mandibular block is produced by local anesthesia applied to the inferior alveolar nerve at the level of the mandibular foramen. Understand from your dissection that this block will not only anesthetize the mandibular teeth on the corresponding side, but also the lower lip and the chin inferior to it.

GRANT'S 7.62, 7.63, 7.65
ROHEN 80-82
A.D.A.M. 7.80
NETTER 65
CLEMENTE 750, 751
A.V.A. 5: 1.02.41

Pick up the **lingual nerve**, which is closely applied to the ramus of the mandible. This large nerve runs anterior to the inferior alveolar nerve. Trace it to the inferior border of the lateral pterygoid where it emerges. Posterior to the inferior alveolar nerve identify the delicate **mylohyoid nerve**.

Maxillary Artery (Fig. 7.70A)

GRANT'S 7.62, 7.63
ROHEN 65, 80
A.D.A.M. 7.76
NETTER 63, 65
CLEMENTE 750
A.V.A. 5: 1.52.36

Trace the artery through the infratemporal region. In most cases, it crosses superficial to the lateral pterygoid. However, in approximately one-third of all cases, it passes deep to the muscle.

To obtain a complete and extensive view of the infratemporal region, the **lateral pterygoid muscle** must be removed. Notice that the muscle has two heads: one arises from the roof of the fossa, the other from the lateral

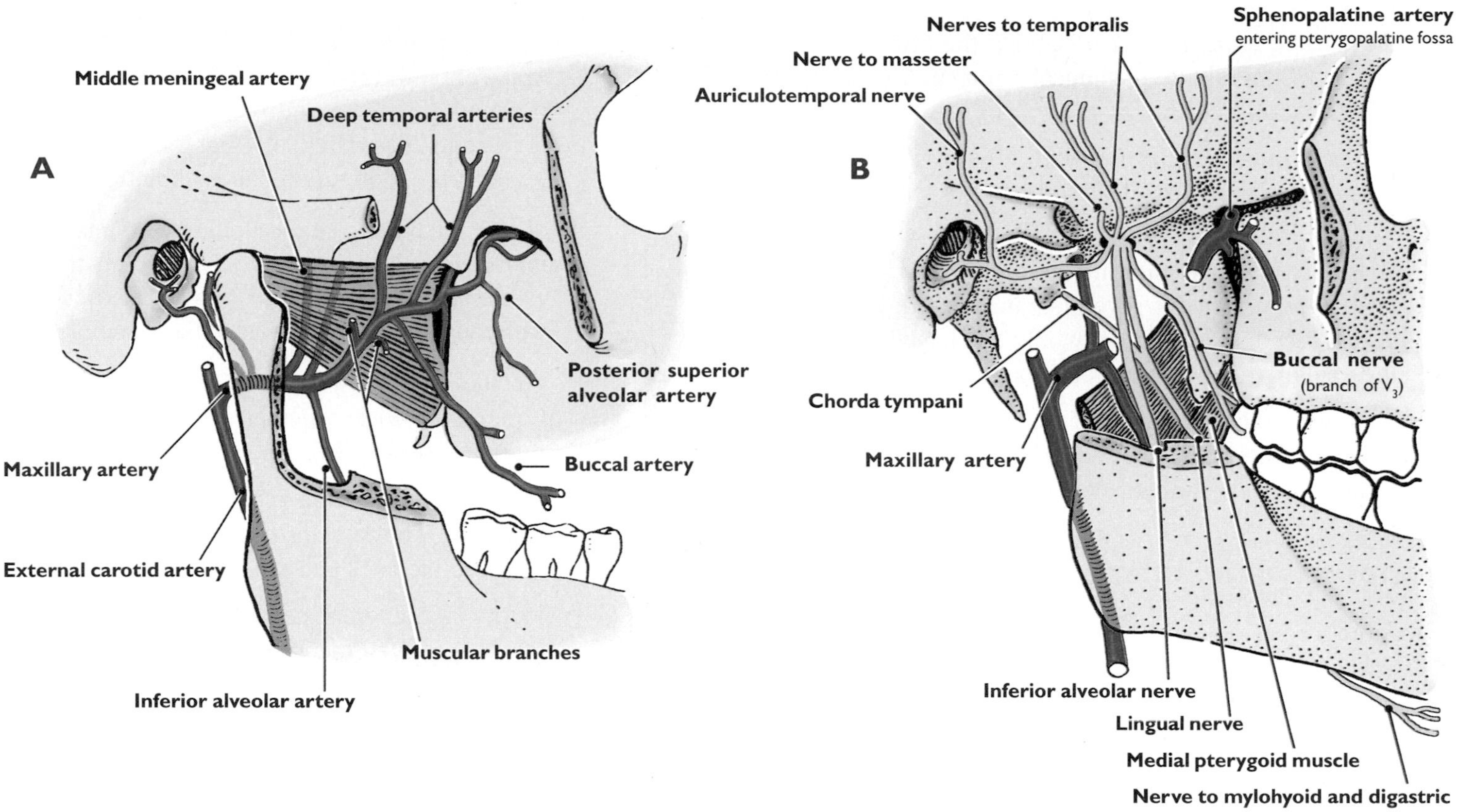

Figure 7.70. Arteries and nerves of the infratemporal fossa. ***A***, The maxillary artery and its branches. ***B***, The mandibular nerve (V_3) and its branches.

pterygoid plate. With the handle of the scalpel, free the superior border of the lateral pterygoid from the roof.

Next, define the inferior border of the muscle by inserting the handle into the interval between lateral and medial pterygoids. This interval is marked by the emergence of the **lingual nerve** and the **inferior alveolar nerve**. Work the handle anteriorly and superiorly and free the muscle from the lateral pterygoid plate.

Finally, sever the muscle close to its pointed insertion into the neck of the mandible and into the articular disc. Remove the muscle completely in a piecemeal fashion to preserve superficially positioned nerves and vessels.

Now, the nerves in the infratemporal fossa can be examined in detail (Fig. 7.70B):

- Identify the delicate **chorda tympani**. It joins the lingual nerve and it can be seen just posterior to the lingual nerve.

GRANT'S 7.62
ROHEN 81
A.D.A.M. 7.80
CLEMENTE 750
A.V.A. 5: 0.53.46

GRANT'S 7.63, 7.65
ROHEN 65, 80
NETTER 63, 65
CLEMENTE 750, 751
A.V.A. 5: 1.52.50

GRANT'S 7.63, 9.10A
ROHEN 81
A.D.A.M. 7.80
NETTER 65
CLEMENTE 751
A.V.A. 5: 1.02.52

- Follow the **inferior alveolar nerve** and the **lingual nerve** to the foramen ovale in the roof of the infratemporal fossa.
- Push a thin probe through the **foramen ovale**. Locate and palpate the tip of the probe in the middle cranial fossa. Estabish the continuity of nerve V_3 with the trigeminal ganglion.
- Identify and clean the **buccal nerve**. Its branches pierce the buccinator to supply the buccal mucosa with sensory fibers.
- Identify the auriculotemporal nerve. Follow it to the foramen ovale.

Clean the **maxillary artery**. Identify several branches (Fig. 7.70A):

- The **inferior alveolar artery**; follow it to the mandibular foramen; realize that it runs within the bony mandible to supply the mandibular teeth;
- The **middle meningeal artery**; follow it to the **foramen spinosum**. Stick a needle through the foramen spinosum. Find the needle tip in

the middle cranial fossa. Establish the continuity of the middle meningeal artery in the middle cranial fossa.

- Observe **muscular branches** to the muscles of mastication. Most of these branches have been torn or cut during dissection.
- Within the **pterygopalatine fossa**, the maxillary artery gives off several branches (Fig. 7.70A). At this time, identify only one banch: the **posterior superior alveolar artery**.

GRANT'S 7.63, 7.65
ROHEN 65, 80
A.D.A.M. 7.76
NETTER 63, 65
CLEMENTE 750, 751
A.V.A. 5: 1.53.28

Review the distribution of the mandibular division of the trigeminal nerve. Understand the importance of the delicate chorda tympani.

Temporomandibular Joint

Refer to a bony skull and examine the following landmarks (Fig. 7.71):

- On the temporal bone, identify the mandibular fossa and the articular tubercle.
- On the mandible, identify the neck and the head with its articular condyle.

GRANT'S 7.58, 7.59
ROHEN 56, 57
A.D.A.M. 7.23
NETTER 11
CLEMENTE 740-745
A.V.A. 4: 1.30.50

Dissection.

Although the superior portion of the mandibular ramus has been removed, the head and neck of the mandible are still intact. The capsule of the temporomandibular joint is lax. It is thickened laterally to form the temporomandibular ligament. Manipulate the head of the mandible to verify the movements permitted at this joint: hinge movements, protraction, and retraction.

Enter the point of the scalpel into the mandibular fossa close to the bone. Open freely the *superior cavity* of the joint. Remove the articular disc together with the head of the mandible.

GRANT'S 7.59
ROHEN 56, 57
A.D.A.M. 7.23
NETTER 11
CLEMENTE 742, 744
A.V.A. 5: 1.31.21

In the isolated specimen (head and neck of mandible with articular disc), study the following (Fig. 7.71):

- Observe the insertion of the severed lateral pterygoid. The remains of the muscle are attached to the neck and articular disc.
- Cut the disc anteroposteriorly and so open the *inferior cavity* of the joint. Observe the shape and varying thickness of the disc.

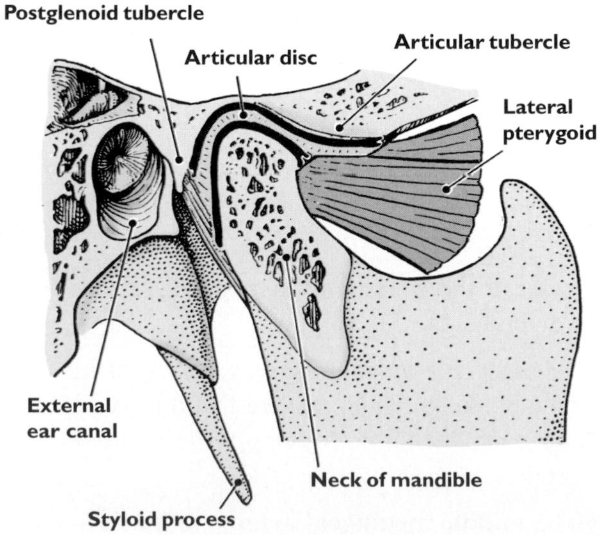

Figure 7.71. The temporomandibular joint (on parasagittal section)

Clinical Correlation: The presence of an articular disc implies two types of movements, one on each side of the disc. In the *lower cavity*, simple hinge movements between head and disc occur. In the *upper cavity*, the disc and head together glide on the articular tubercle during protraction of the mandible.

Place the little finger in the cartilaginous portion of your own external ear canal. Perform simple hinge movements of the mandible. Then protract and retract your lower jaw. By finger palpation, study the movements of the head of your own mandible.

Craniovertebral Joints and Removal of Head

General Remarks and Orientation

The head with the cervical viscera and the major nerves and vessels must be detached from the vertebral column and its associated musculature. This procedure will allow a posterior approach to the cervical viscera. Do not carry out any dissection at this time.

Study a midsagittal section of the head and neck region. Understand the following (Fig. 7.72):

GRANT'S 8.2A, 8.28
ROHEN 150, 170
NETTER 30
CLEMENTE 705, 714

- The logical plane for separation is the **retropharyngeal (retrovisceral) space** that is located between the visceral compartment (outlined in *red* in Figure 7.72) and the prevertebral fascia. This space contains loose fibrous tissue that is easily broken down. On a vertical plane, the retropharyngeal space extends from the base of the skull inferiorly into the superior part of the thorax.

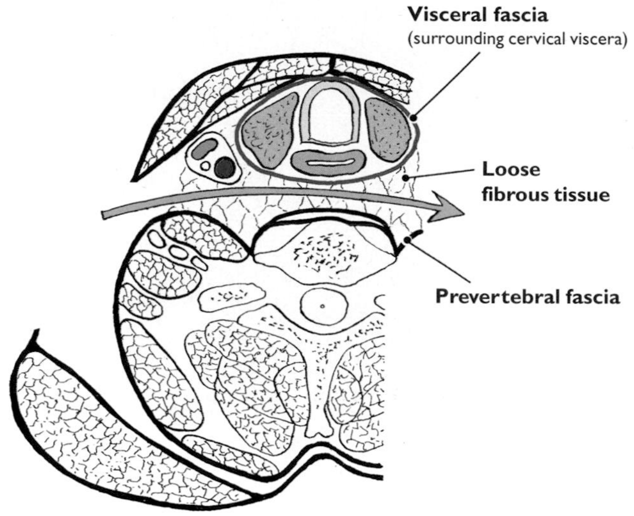

Figure 7.72. Transverse section of the neck. The arrow passes through the retropharyngeal or retrovisceral space, i.e., between visceral compartment and prevertebral fascia.

- The joints between cranium and vertebrae (craniovertebral joints) are the logical sites for separation between head and vertebral column. All ligaments holding these joints together must be severed in order to achieve separation.
- In addition, the muscles connecting the vertebrae with the base of the skull must be severed.
- Study a transverse section of the neck (Fig. 7.72). Identify the retropharyngeal (retrovisceral) space.

Dissection

GRANT'S 8.28
ROHEN 150, 170
NETTER 30
CLEMENTE 705, 714

Reflect the two sternocleidomastoid muscles. On both sides at once, insert the fingers of your right and left hands posterior to the carotid sheaths (*arrow* in Fig. 7.72). Push your fingers medially until they meet posterior to the cervical viscera. Your fingers are now in the **retropharyngeal (retrovisceral) space**. Work your fingers superiorly as high as the base of the skull; here is the superior limit of the retropharyngeal space. Work your fingers inferiorly toward the thorax; here, the space ends at the level of T3 where part of the prevertebral fascia fuses with the buccopharyngeal (visceral) fascia.

Before the head together with the cervical viscera can be removed, the **craniovertebral joints** must be studied and, subsequently, disarticulated. Knowledge of pertinent bony reference points is essential.

Bony Landmarks

GRANT'S 4.38-4.40
NETTER 15
CLEMENTE 639-642
A.V.A. 4: 0.10.19

Refer to a skeleton (or skull and cervical vertebral column) and identify the following pertinent landmarks (Fig. 7.73):

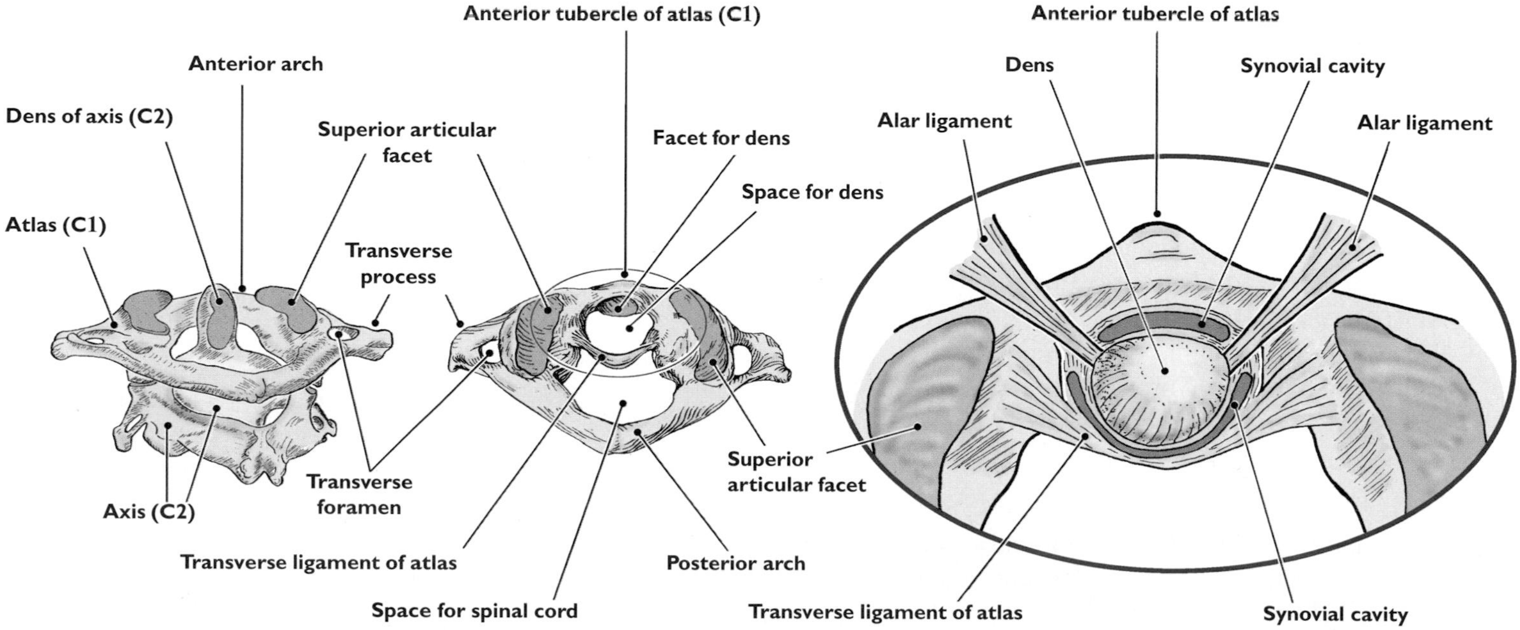

Figure 7.73. Essential bony landmarks and ligaments of the atlanto-axial joint. The enlarged inset shows a superior view of the middle atlanto-axial joint, i.e., the synovial joint between the dens of axis and anterior arch of atlas.

- **Axis**, C2. Note its **dens or odontoid process**, which is in apposition with the anterior arch of the atlas.
- **Atlas**, C1. Identify: **posterior arch**; **anterior arch** with facet for dens; transverse process; **superior articular facet**.
- Understand that the dens of the axis is held tight to the anterior arch by the **transverse ligament of the atlas**, which is bow-shaped and very strong.
- On the **occipital bone**, identify (Fig. 7.74): anterior and lateral margins of **foramen magnum**; right and left **occipital condyle**.
- The joint between the occipital condyle and the superior articular facet of the atlas is the **atlanto-occipital joint**.

GRANT'S 4.38-4.40
ROHEN 191
NETTER 15
CLEMENTE 639-642
A.V.A. 4: 0.13.00

GRANT'S 8.34
ROHEN 50, 51
NETTER 16
CLEMENTE 649
A.V.A. 4: 0.05.02

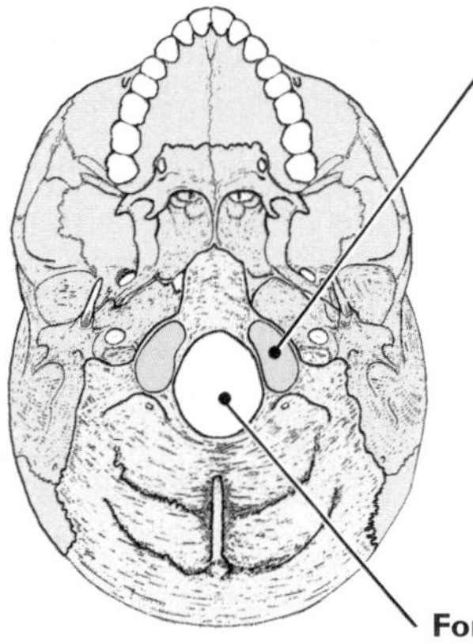

Figure 7.74. Occipital portion of skull (*yellow*): occipital condyle and foramen magnum.

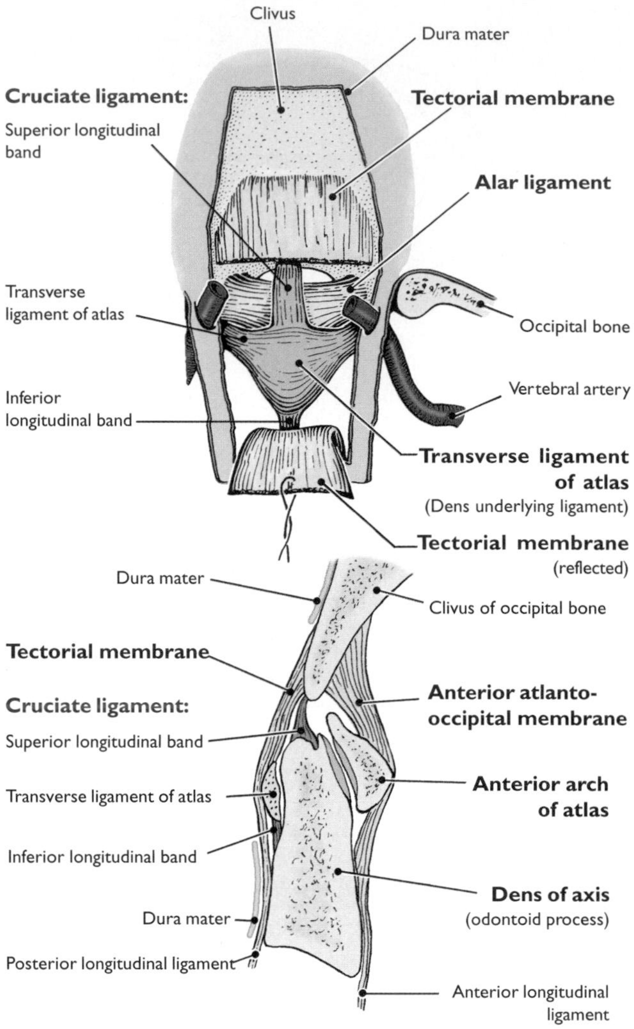

Figure 7.75. Craniovertebral joints in posterior view and sagittal section: tectorial membrane, cruciate ligament, and alar ligaments.

Craniovertebral Joints

Turn the cadaver into the prone position (face down). A large wedge-shaped portion of the occipital bone has been removed earlier. If not already done, resect the posterior arch of the atlas. Define the anterior border of the foramen magnum. Note the median knuckle-like eminence produced by the **dens of the axis**. Palpate the dens while rotating the head to the right and the left.

To expose the underlying ligaments, the **dura mater** and the **tectorial membrane** must be reflected. First, excise the dura mater in the following fashion (Fig. 7.75):

GRANT'S 4.40A
NETTER 15
CLEMENTE 649-653
A.V.A. 4: 0.20.35

- Make a transverse incision through the dura, about 3 cm inferior to the dorsum sellae.
- From each end of this incision, carry a cut inferiorly to the point where the vertebral artery pierces the dura. This is just medial to the points of exit of the hypoglossal nerves.
- With a probe, ease the dura from the underlying membrana tectoria. Turn inferiorly the flap of dura as far as possible (Fig. 7.75).

Next, examine the exposed **tectorial membrane**. Cut the membrane transversely superior to the anterior border of the foramen magnum. With the handle of a scalpel and a probe, raise the membrane and reflect it inferiorly as far as possible.

Now, the major ligaments of the craniovertebral region are exposed. Identify the following structures (Fig. 7.75):

- **Transverse ligament of atlas**; it holds the dens of the axis firmly to the anterior arch of the atlas.
- The transverse ligament and the vertically orientated **superior** and **inferior bands** are collectively known as the **cruciform ligament**.
- Next, identify the **alar ligaments** (check ligaments). They extend from the dens to the lateral margins of the foramen magnum. These strong paired ligaments are nearly as thick as a pencil. They check the lateral rotation and the side-to-side movements of the head. Observe the extent of rotation possible in the cadaver.
- Next, cut the alar ligaments close to the dens. Note that the rotation of the head is now very easy and extensive.

GRANT'S 4.39A, 4.40A
ROHEN 191
NETTER 15
CLEMENTE 650
A.V.A. 4: 0.21.42

GRANT'S 8.33
NETTER 25
CLEMENTE 717
A.V.A. 4: 0.28.15

GRANT'S 8.35
NETTER 62
CLEMENTE 888
A.V.A. 4: 2.22.30

Removal of Head

With a scalpel, cut along the anterior border of the foramen magnum, thereby severing a fine median strand extending from the tip of the dens to the anterior border of the foramen. Next, cut close to the lateral margins of the foramen magnum, thereby cutting the attachments of the alar ligaments. Carry cuts close to the medial and posterior aspects of the occipital condyles; this procedure will open the **atlanto-occipital joints**. Force a chisel into the atlanto-occipital joints and disarticulate the joints as much as possible.

At this point, it is advantageous to turn the cadaver into the supine position (face up). Once again, place your hands into the already defined **retropharyngeal (retrovisceral) space**. Pull the cervical viscera and the big vessels and nerves anteriorly. Thus, a convenient working space is created anterior to the prevertebral region. Now, proceed as follows:

GRANT'S 4.38
ROHEN 191
NETTER 15, 16
CLEMENTE 650, 651
A.V.A. 4: 0.23.28

GRANT'S 8.28
ROHEN 150, 170
A.D.A.M. 7.29
NETTER 30
CLEMENTE 705, 714

GRANT'S 8.33
NETTER 124
CLEMENTE 892
A.V.A. 5: 1.21.34

- Identify the **sympathetic trunk** and the large **superior cervical sympathetic ganglion**. Sever the sympathetic trunk on one side, just superior to the superior cervical ganglion, thus leaving it attached to the prevertebral region. On the other side, reflect the sympathetic trunk and its superior ganglion together with the cervical viscera (Fig. 7.79).
- Pull the cervical viscera anteriorly. Pass the knife between the transverse process of the atlas and the occipital bone. This procedure will sever the **rectus capitis lateralis** on each side (Fig. 7.76).
- Next, carry the cut more medially. Cut the **rectus capitis anterior** and the thick **longus capitis**.
- Carry the blade across the median plane just superior to the anterior arch of the atlas. This procedure will sever the **anterior atlanto-occipital membrane** (Fig. 7.75). Safeguard cranial nerves IX, X, XI, and XII.

Now, detach the head and the cervical viscera with relative ease. At this point, you have two options (consult with your instructor):

- Reflect the head and the attached cervical viscera inferiorly and anteriorly. This procedure will leave certain cervicothoracic relations intact. At the same time, it permits a posterior approach to the cervical viscera.
- Or, isolate the head and the cervical viscera. In that case, mobilize the trachea and the esophagus. If not already done, cut the esophagus in the thorax. Sever the contents of the carotid sheaths. Remove the head together with the attached cervical viscera.

Keep the cadaver moist at all times to make dissection possible.

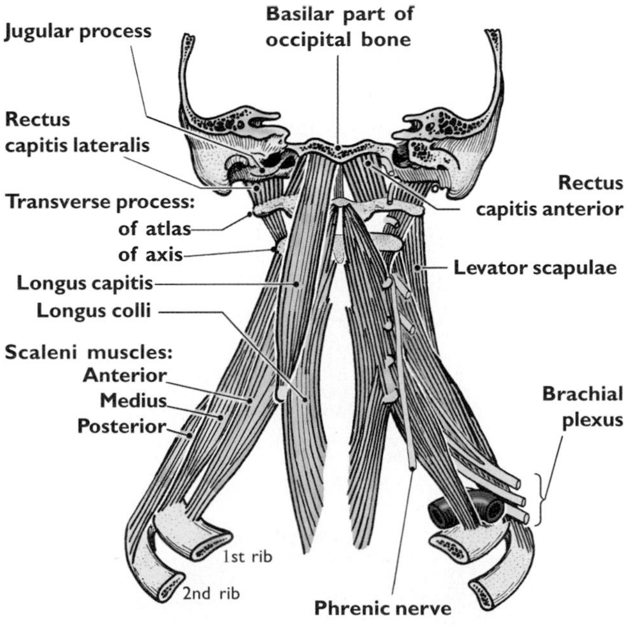

Figure 7.76. Prevertebral muscles and related nerves.

Prevertebral and Lateral Vertebral Regions

The head has been detached at the atlanto-occipital joint. During this procedure, the muscles between transverse processes of atlas and occipital bone were cut and the most superior portion of the longus capitis was severed.

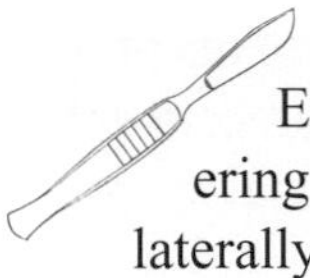

Examine the deep investing fascia covering the prevertebral muscles and more laterally positioned lateral vertebral muscles (scaleni). The fascia anterior to the vertebral column and extending between the transverse processes of the vertebrae is the prevertebral fascia (Fig. 7.77). It actually consists of two layers that are separated by loose connective tissue. With a forceps, pick up a fine fold of the more anterior layer, the alar fascia. Insert a probe into the interval between the alar fascia and the posterior layer of the prevertebral fascia. You are now in a space that has been termed by clinicians as the "danger space" (Fig. 7.77) because it constitutes a passageway for infections from the neck region all the way inferior into the posterior mediastinum.

On one side of the cadaver, the cervical part of the sympathetic trunk was left in place on the prevertebral muscles. Locate it. Identify the superior, middle, and inferior cervical sympathetic ganglia. The inferior cervical ganglion is positioned close to the anterior aspect of the head of rib 1. Frequently, the ganglion is fused with the 1st thoracic ganglion to form the cervicothoracic or stellate ganglion. Observe the rami communicantes that connect the sympathetic ganglia with the cervical spinal nerves.

Identify the longus colli, longus capitis, and scalenus anterior (Fig. 7.76). Remove these muscles from the anterior tubercles of the transverse processes of C3 through C6. Now, the cervical spinal nerves are exposed. Trace a ventral ramus to the gutter-like end of the corresponding transverse process on which it rests. Review the contributions of ventral rami C5 to C8 to the brachial plexus.

Follow the vertebral artery to the transverse foramen of C6. Be aware of possible variations.

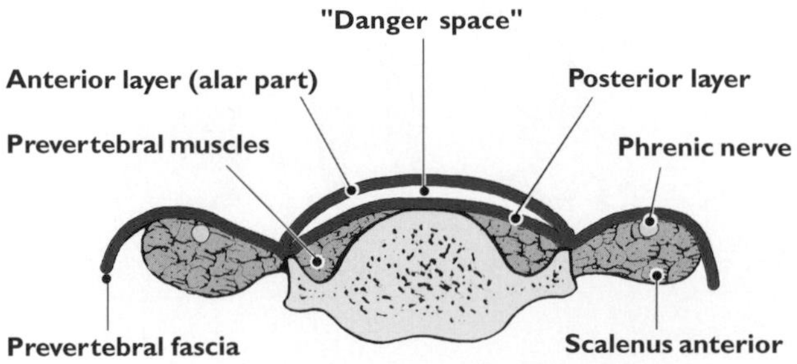

Figure 7.77. Prevertebral fascia and danger space.

⇦
GRANT'S 8.33
A.D.A.M. 7.27
NETTER 25
CLEMENTE 717
A.V.A. 4: 0.28.15

⇦
GRANT'S 8.14A
ROHEN 164
NETTER 28
CLEMENTE 719, 721
A.V.A. 5: 1.38.04

⇦
GRANT'S 8.2A, 8.28
ROHEN 150, 170
A.D.A.M. 7.29
NETTER 30
CLEMENTE 714, 718

⇨
GRANT'S 8.34
ROHEN 31, 160
A.D.A.M. 7.11
NETTER 5
CLEMENTE 781, 782

⇦
GRANT'S 8.33
ROHEN 161
NETTER 65
CLEMENTE 892
A.V.A. 5: 1.21.34

Exterior of Base of Skull

Bony Landmarks

Refer to a bony skull and study pertinent features.

Anterior Transverse Line (Fig. 7.78)

Pass a pencil or the handle of a probe through both mandibular notches across the base of the skull. The instru-

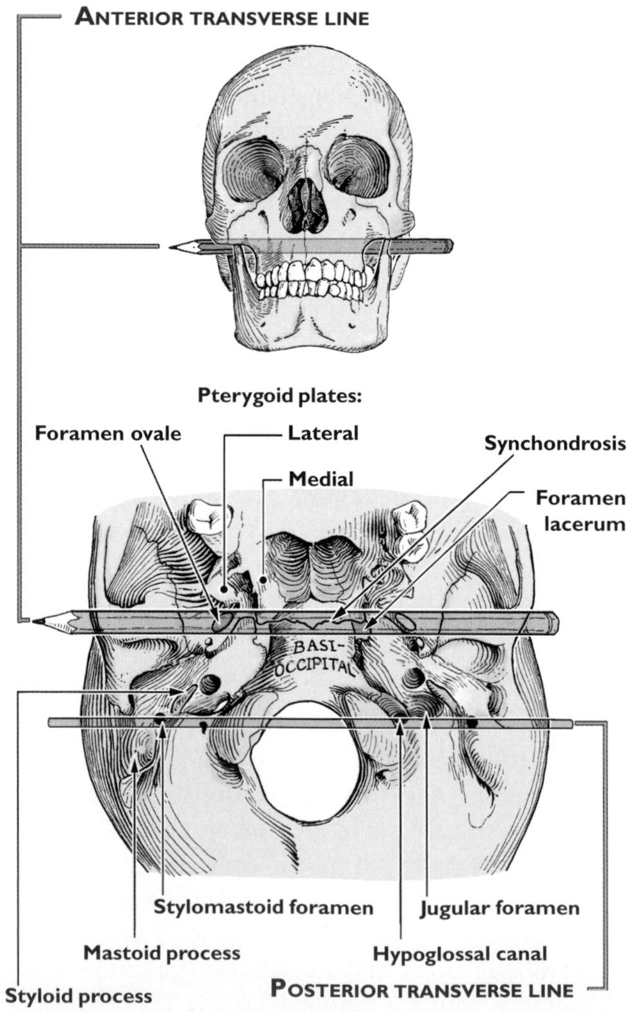

Figure 7.78. The anterior transverse line is marked by a pencil through both mandibular notches across the base of the skull. The posterior transverse line crosses both stylomastoid foramina.

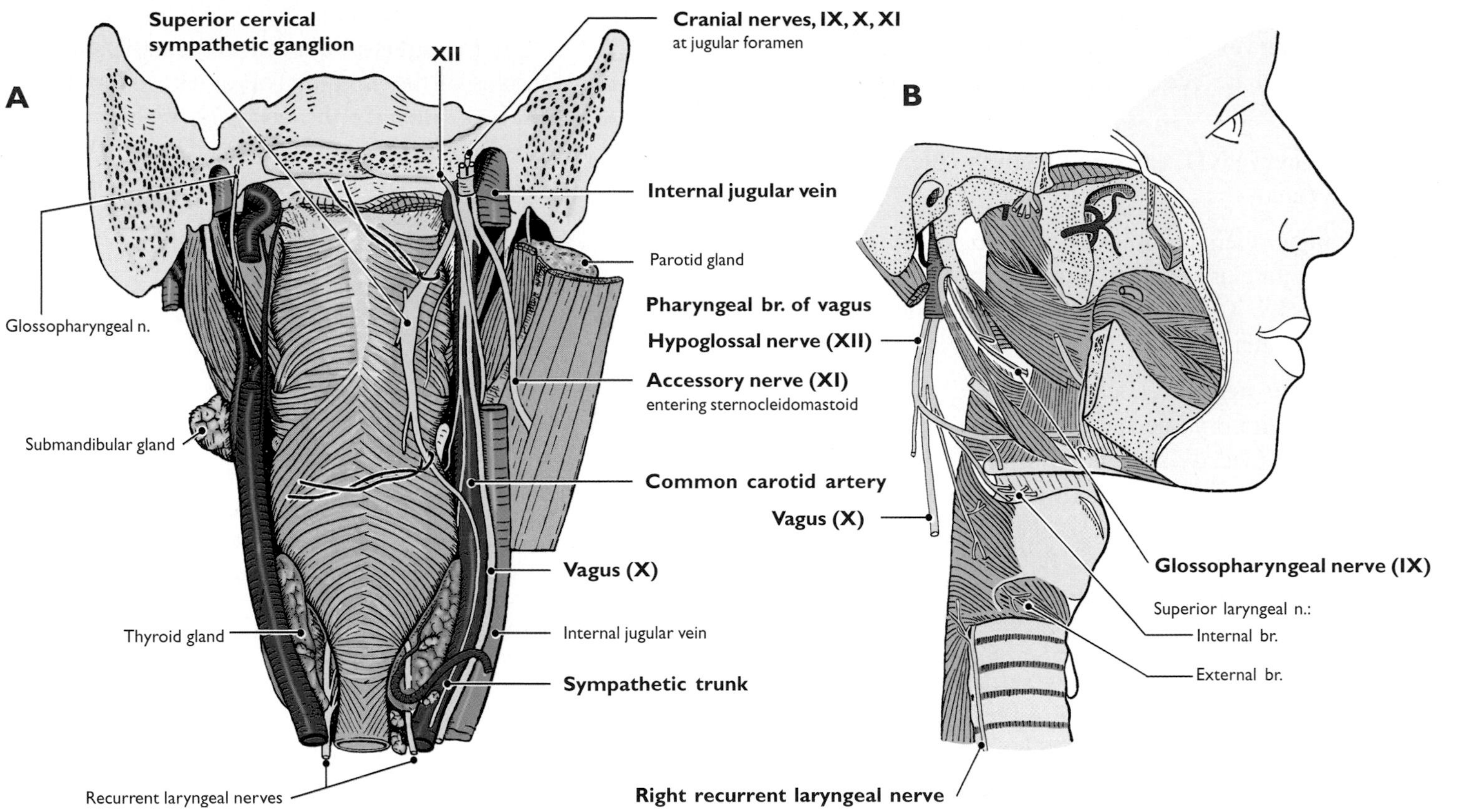

Figure 7.79. Nerves and vessels related to the pharyngeal wall. ***A*,** Posterior aspect. ***B*,** Lateral view.

ment marks a line that passes across the **foramen ovale** on each side.

Posterior Transverse Line (Fig. 7.78)

This line stretches across the base of the skull between the mastoid and styloid processes of the two sides. Observe that the line crosses the following landmarks:

- **Stylomastoid foramen**;
- **Jugular foramen**;
- **Hypoglossal canal**;
- **Occipital condyles**;
- **Foramen magnum**.

Examine the **jugular foramen** more closely, and observe that **three compartments** may be distinguished:

- **Anterior compartment**; it transmits the inferior petrosal sinus;
- **Intermediate compartment**, for the transmission of cranial nerves IX, X, and XI;
- **Posterior compartment**; it is the largest of the three compartments; it transmits mainly the sigmoid dural sinus, which here becomes the internal jugular vein.

GRANT'S 8.36
NETTER 65
CLEMENTE 892
A.V.A. 5: 1.28.52

GRANT'S 8.34
ROHEN 31, 160
A.D.A.M. 7.11
NETTER 5
CLEMENTE 781
A.V.A. 4: 0.08.15

GRANT'S 8.34, 8.36
ROHEN 31, 160, 161
A.D.A.M. 7.11, 8.1
NETTER 65
CLEMENTE 892

Structures at Base of Skull

Examine the nerves and vessels at the exterior of the base of the skull (Fig. 7.79). Pick up the cut end of the **common carotid artery**. Trace the **sympathetic trunk** (which lies posterior to the common and internal carotid arteries) superiorly to the carotid canal. Observe the long fusiform ganglion, the **superior cervical sympathetic ganglion**. The pharynx hangs from the pharyngeal tubercle, well anterior to the foramen magnum. The great vessels and nerves lie posterolateral to the posterior wall of the pharynx.

Identify the soft structures that traverse the foramina marked by the **posterior transverse line** (Figs. 7.78, 7.79):

- **Facial nerve**, emerging from the stylomastoid foramen;
- **Internal jugular vein**, beginning at the posterior compartment of the jugular foramen, where it is continuous with the sigmoid sinus and the inferior petrosal sinus;

- **Cranial nerves IX, X, and XI**, traversing the intermediate compartment of the jugular foramen;
- **Cranial nerve XII**, emerging from the hypoglossal canal.

Use bone pliers to remove the bone posterior to the jugular foramen. Now, follow cranial nerves IX, X, and XI from the neck into the posterior cranial fossa.

The **vagus nerve (X)** belongs to the digestive and respiratory tracts; therefore, it is logical that it proceeds straight inferiorly (Fig. 7.79). Trace the nerve between internal jugular vein and internal carotid artery. Just inferior to the jugular foramen, observe a 2-cm long swelling, the **inferior ganglion of the vagus** (nodose ganglion).

Grant's 8.36, 9.14
Rohen 161
A.D.A.M. 8.1, 8.17
Netter 65, 120, 124, 125
Clemente 892
A.V.A. 5: 1.14.02

The **superior laryngeal nerve** arises from the vagus about 2.5 cm inferior to the base of the skull. Trace this nerve to the larynx (Fig. 7.79).

The **pharyngeal branch of the vagus** nerve arises at a high level. Follow the branch between the internal and external carotid arteries to the pharyngeal wall (Fig. 7.79). Here it joins the pharyngeal plexus. Review the vagus nerve and its essential branches.

Grant's 8.36, 9.15
Rohen 161
A.D.A.M. 8.1, 8.22
Netter 65, 121, 124, 125
Clemente 892
A.V.A. 5: 1.18.10

The **accessory nerve (XI)** supplies the sternocleidomastoid and the trapezius muscles. At the base of the skull, it lies immediately lateral to the vagus nerve. Follow nerve XI through the interval between internal jugular vein and internal carotid artery toward the substance of the sternocleidomastoid (Fig. 7.79A). The accessory nerve crosses anterior to the internal jugular vein in 70%, and posterior to it in about 30% of all cases. Review nerve XI.

Grant's 9.13
A.D.A.M. 8.16
A.V.A. 5: 1.12.46

The **glossopharyngeal nerve (IX)** is destined for the pharynx and the back of the tongue; therefore, it must swing anteriorly (Fig. 7.79). In doing so, it passes between the internal and external carotid arteries. Separate the two carotid arteries. Observe a lumbrical-like muscle descending from the styloid process between the two arteries. This is the **stylopharyngeus**. The glossopharyngeal nerve is closely applied to its lateral side. Review nerve IX.

Grant's 9.16
Rohen 161
A.D.A.M. 8.23
Netter 122
A.V.A. 5: 1.19.05

The **hypoglossal nerve (XII)** supplies the muscles of the tongue. The quickest way to positively identify the nerve is to follow it proximally from the digastric triangle (Fig. 7.79B). At the base of the skull, the hypoglossal nerve is closely adherent to the inferior ganglion of the vagus. Review nerve XII.

Pharynx

General Remarks

The pharynx is the superior end of the respiratory and digestive tubes. It extends from the base of the skull to the inferior border of cricoid cartilage (vertebra C6). The **pharyngeal wall** consists of **five layers** or coats:

- **Areolar coat or layer**; it is continuous with the areolar layer of the buccinator; therefore, it is called the **buccopharyngeal fascia**; this layer facilitates movements of the pharynx; it also contains the pharyngeal plexus of veins and nerves;
- **Muscular layer**; it is composed of an *outer circular part* and an *inner longitudinal part*;
- **Fibrous layer or pharyngobasilar fascia**; it is especially strong where it anchors the pharynx to the base of the skull;
- Submucous layer, the **submucosa**;
- Mucous layer, the **mucous membrane**.

Muscular Layers

The outer circular part of the muscular layer consists of **three constrictors: superior, middle, and inferior** (Fig. 7.80). Each constrictor is fan-shaped. The narrow ends of the fans are fixed anteriorly. Posteriorly, the fans of the opposite sides meet in a median raphe. Laterally, there are gaps between the constrictors. Through these spaces pass vessels, nerves, and muscles. The constrictors overlap each other to some degree.

External Aspect of Pharynx

Grant's 8.35, 8.36
Rohen 162, 163
A.D.A.M. 7.57, 7.59
Netter 61
Clemente 891
A.V.A. 4: 2.14.06

Inspect and clean the posterior aspect of the pharyngeal constrictors. It is easiest to identify the **middle constrictor** first. Its fibers arise from the greater horn of the hyoid bone and from the inferior portion of the stylohyoid ligament (Fig. 7.80C). Palpate the greater horn of the hyoid bone. Positively identify the middle constrictor.

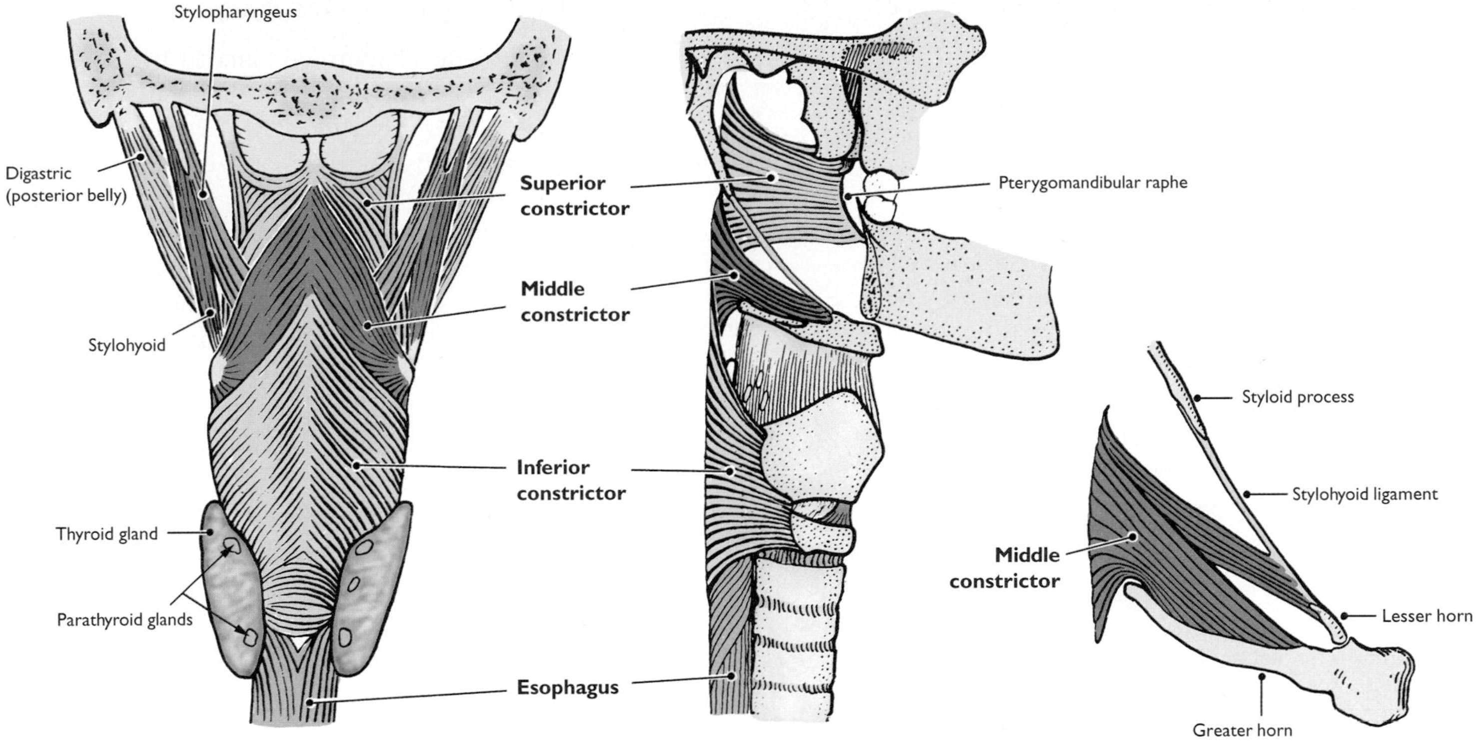

Figure 7.80. Muscles of the pharynx. ***A***, Posterior view. ***B***, Lateral view. ***C***, Origin of the middle constrictor from the hyoid bone and the stylohyoid ligament.

The muscle fibers *superior* to the middle constrictor belong to the **superior constrictor**. This muscle arises from the pterygomandibular raphe or ligament and from the bone at either end of it (Fig. 7.80B).

The muscle fibers *inferior* to the middle constrictor belong to the **inferior constrictor**. Observe the continuous origin of this muscle from the thyroid and cricoid cartilages (Fig. 7.80B). Demonstrate that the inferior constrictor overlaps the middle constrictor. Display the interval between the two muscles. Here, the **internal laryngeal nerve** and the superior laryngeal vessels pierce the thyrohyoid membrane.Examine the free inferior border of the inferior constrictor. Here, the **recurrent laryngeal nerve** enters the pharyngeal wall. Note that the most inferior fibers of the inferior constrictor are continuous with the circular fibers of the esophagus.

Demonstrate the interval between the middle and superior constrictors. The stylopharyngeus and the glossopharyngeal nerve (IX) pass through this gap. Verify this fact.

GRANT'S 8.35. 8.36
ROHEN 162, 163
NETTER 61
CLEMENTE 891
A.V.A. 4: 2.13.24

GRANT'S 8.35, 8.36
ROHEN 162, 163
NETTER 61
CLEMENTE 891
A.V.A. 4: 2.14.38

GRANT'S 8.37
ROHEN 159
A.D.A.M. 7.28, 7.59
NETTER 57, 60
CLEMENTE 890, 893
A.V.A. 4: 0.56.35

Internal Aspect of Pharynx

Incision

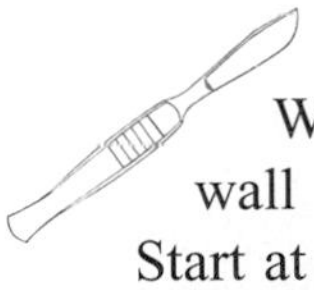

With scissors, slit open the posterior wall of the esophagus and the pharynx. Start at the level of the cricoid cartilage and carry the median section all the way superiorly to the base of the skull. With hooks or other instruments, reflect both sides of the opened pharyngeal wall laterally.

The interior of the pharynx communicates anteriorly with three cavities: nose, mouth, and larynx (Fig. 7.81). Accordingly, the **pharynx** is divided into **three parts: nasal pharynx, oral pharynx, and laryngeal pharynx**. The soft palate, ending in the uvula, separates the nasopharynx superiorly from the oral pharynx inferiorly.

Nasal Pharynx or Nasopharynx (Fig. 7.81)

It lies superior to the soft palate. Verify that it is a posterior extension of the nasal cavities. Refer to a skull and identify the two posterior nasal apertures or **choanae**, which are separated by the bony nasal septum. Look through the choanae. Identify scroll-like bones projecting from the lateral wall of each nasal cavity. These are the **middle concha** and the **inferior concha**. Turn to the cadaver. Identify the nasal septum, choanae, and conchae.

GRANT'S 8.37, 8.39
ROHEN 159
A.D.A.M. 7.28
NETTER 60
CLEMENTE 893
A.V.A. 4: 1.19.46

On each side of the nasopharynx, 1 to 1.5 cm posterior to the inferior concha, is the **pharyngeal orifice of the auditory tube**. Place a probe into the opening. Posterior to it, identify the **torus tubarius**, which is produced by the underlying cartilage of the auditory tube. Posterior to the torus, explore the **pharyngeal recess**, which extends laterally and posteriorly almost to the carotid canal.

> ***Clinical Correlation:*** The curved, bony roof of the nasopharynx is formed by the sphenoid and occipital bones. The mucous membrane on the roof and posterior wall contains a mass of lymphoid tissue, the pharyngeal tonsil or nasopharyngeal tonsil (Fig. 7.81). Enlarged pharyngeal tonsils are known as adenoids. Understand that large adenoids will obstruct the air passages from the nose through the nasopharynx, making mouth breathing necessary.
>
> Examine the close relation of the nasopharyngeal tonsil to the orifice of the auditory tube. Understand that enlarged adenoids will obstruct the ostium, thus interfering with the air exchange between the nasopharynx and the middle ear cavity.

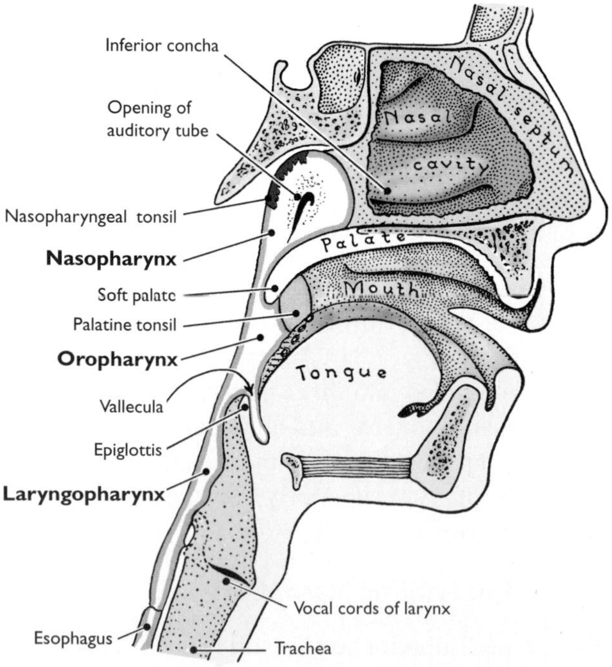

Figure 7.81. Pharynx and related structures (schematic sagittal section).

Oral Pharynx or Oropharynx

GRANT'S 8.37, 8.39
ROHEN 159
A.D.A.M. 7.28
NETTER 60
CLEMENTE 893
A.V.A. 4: 1.54.47

The oral pharynx is bounded by the soft palate superiorly and the epiglottis of the larynx inferiorly (Fig. 7.81). Push your finger anteriorly into the oral cavity. Palpate the posterior 1/3 of the tongue. Notice two folds of mucous membrane that descend from the soft palate. The anterior fold, the **palatoglossal arch**, descends to the junction of the anterior 2/3 and the posterior 1/3 of the tongue. The palatoglossal arch forms a dividing line between the oral cavity and the oral pharynx. The posterior fold, the **palatopharyngeal arch**, descends along the lateral wall of the pharynx. Between the two arches lies the **palatine tonsil**. Examine the arches and the tonsil on a transverse section through the head. Identify the right and left palatine arches in the cadaver.

> ***Clinical Correlation:*** Examine the palatine arches in your fellow students. Notice the two prominent folds in subjects who have undergone tonsillectomy and observe the empty tonsillar beds. Study the palatine tonsil in several subjects. Note that the tonsils vary in size from person to person.

Laryngeal Pharynx or Laryngopharynx

GRANT'S 8.37
ROHEN 159
A.D.A.M. 7.28, 7.59
NETTER 60
CLEMENTE 893
A.V.A. 4: 2.23.17

This portion of the pharynx extends from the epiglottis to the lower border of the cricoid cartilage (Fig. 7.81). Identify the epiglottis and the inlet (aditus) of the larynx. Palpate the cricoid cartilage through the mucous membrane. Place a probe into the right and left **piriform recesses**. Define the borders of the piriform recess (fossa): medially, the larynx; laterally, the thyroid cartilage and the thyrohyoid membrane; posteriorly, the inferior constrictor.

ROHEN 159
NETTER 61
CLEMENTE 893, 895

Carefully remove the mucosa of the piriform recess. Two nerves, which are submucous, are readily exposed. These are the **internal laryngeal nerve** and the **recurrent laryngeal nerve**. Identify the nerves. They will be studied more thoroughly during the dissection of the larynx.

> ***Clinical Correlation:*** The right and left piriform recesses are of clinical importance because foreign bodies (food particles; chicken or fish bones; accidentally swallowed

safety pins or coins) may become trapped here. These foreign materials cause irritation of the underlying musca. Since the muscosa is innervated by sensory fibers from the internal laryngeal and the recurrent laryngeal nerves, the trapped substances induce a choking sensation and severe coughing.

If the objects are sharp (e.g., fish bones), they may pierce the underlying mucosa and produce an infection and/or injury to the underlying nerves. Similarly, the nerves may be injured when the physician, in his/her effort to remove a foreign body, accidentally pierces the mucosa of the piriform recess.

Bisection of Head

General Remarks and Bony Landmarks

The nasal and oral cavities are not readily accessible in the undivided head. Therefore, the head must be bisected, close to the median plane. For practical purposes, it is best to carry the section just lateral to the nasal septum. Thus, one half of the head will have the nasal septum; the other half will have its nasal cavity fully opened.

GRANT'S *7.93*
NETTER 38
A.V.A. 4: 0.59.12

Usually, the **nasal septum** deviates somewhat to one side. Thus, the nasal cavity is slightly wider on one side, slightly narrower on the side of septal deviation. Refer to one or several skulls and verify this fact. Logically, the section should be made on the less obstructed side, just lateral to the nasal septum.

Orientation and Preparation

Examine a skull and study the bones through which you must saw:

- The saw cut must pass through the nasal bone and the remains of the frontal bone.
- Subsequently, you must saw just lateral to the crista galli through one of the cribriform plates of the ethmoid bone. Then, the cut must be carried midsagittally through the body of the sphenoid bone and part of the occipital bone to the anterior margin of the foramen magnum.
- You must saw through the hard palate that forms the floor of the nasal cavities and the roof of the oral cavity.

GRANT'S *8.60*
ROHEN 88, 141
A.D.A.M. 7.28
NETTER 57
CLEMENTE 890
A.V.A. 4: 1.00.10

Bisection Procedure

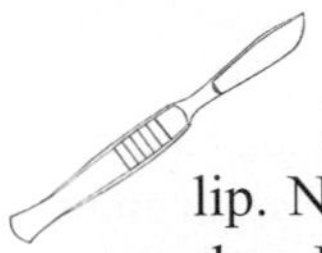

In the midline, cut through the upper lip. Next, explore each nasal cavity with a probe. Decide on which side of the nasal septum the bisection should be carried out. On the chosen side, carry out the following procedures:

- Divide the uvula and the soft palate in the midsagittal plane.
- Slit open the naris. Cut through the lateral portion of the septal cartilage all the way to the nasal bone.

ROHEN 159
NETTER 60, 61
CLEMENTE 893, 895

- If your instructors wish to use an electrical bandsaw for bisection, follow specific directions to be issued. Otherwise, insert a small saw into the nasal cavity. Keep the blade close to the septum. Cut superiorly through the nasal and frontal bones. Subsequently, saw through the cribriform plate, body of sphenoid, dorsum sellae, and basioccipital bone, until you reach the foramen magnum.
- Saw in an inferior direction through the floor of the nasal cavity. Divide the hard palate close to the midsagittal plane.
- Now, the two superior halves of the head will fall apart from each other. The tongue lies exposed.

GRANT'S *7.68B, 7.71*
ROHEN 145
A.D.A.M. 7.4
NETTER 52
CLEMENTE 860
A.V.A. 4: 1.45.49

Inspect the tongue. Verify the following statements (Fig. 7.82):

- The anterior 2/3 of the tongue lies horizontally in the mouth. This is the **oral part**.
- The posterior 1/3 of the tongue takes a curved vertical position and forms the ante-

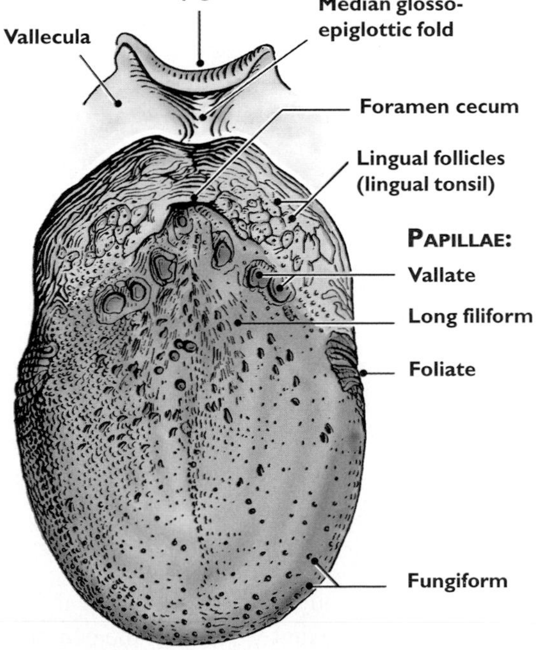

Figure 7.82. Dorsum of tongue.

rior wall of the oral pharynx. This is the **pharyngeal part** of the tongue.

- The boundary between the two parts is marked by the **sulcus terminalis**. This line has the shape of an inverted V. On each side, it runs from the palatoglossal arch posteriorly to a median pit, the **foramen cecum**.
- Large and conspicuous **vallate papillae**, 7 to 12 in number, occupy a V-shaped row just anterior to the sulcus terminalis. These papillae contain numerous taste buds (Fig. 7.82).
- The anterior 2/3 of the tongue is covered with **long filiform papillae**. Near the dorsum and margins of the tongue are the **fungiform papillae**. The lateral aspect of the tongue shows **foliate papillae**. These papillae also contain taste buds.
- A median fold of mucous membrane, the **median glossoepiglottic fold**, runs from the dorsum of the tongue to the **epiglottis**. On each side of this fold are the **valleculae**.
- The surface of the pharyngeal or posterior 1/3 of the tongue is conspicuously different from the oral part. It has no papillae. Its surface is uneven due to the presence of numerous lymphoid or **lingual follicles**. These encapsuled follicles are collectively known as the **lingual tonsil**.
- Be aware of the fact that the tongue is supplied by five different cranial nerves (V, VII, IX, X, XII).

Bisection of Mandible and Floor of Mouth

The next objective is to bisect the mandible together with the floor of the mouth and the tongue. Proceed as follows:

- Turn to the submental triangle between the anterior bellies of the digastric muscles.
- Split the thin median raphe of the mylohyoids and separate the muscles.
- Identify the underlying paired geniohyoids. With probe and scissors, separate these muscles from each other. Clean their pointed mandibular origins.
- Next, saw through the mandible in the midsagittal plane, exactly between the geniohyoid muscles.

◁
GRANT'S 7.68B, 7.71
ROHEN 145
A.D.A.M. 7.4
NETTER 52
CLEMENTE 860
A.V.A. 4: 1.46.09

◁
A.D.A.M. 7.4
NETTER 52
CLEMENTE 860
A.V.A. 4: 2.23.25

- Finally, bisect the tongue in the midsagittal plane from the tip to the hyoid bone and to the epiglottis. Take care not to destroy the epiglottis. Do not bisect the hyoid bone and the larynx at this time.

Nasal Cavities

Bony Landmarks

Refer to a skull and, in addition, to a bisected skull. Study and verify the following:

- The floor of the nasal cavity (which is also the roof of the oral cavity) is formed by the **bony palate**. Study its *inferior* surface.
- The anterior two-thirds of the bony palate consists of the **palatine processes of the maxilla**.
- The posterior one-third consists of the **horizontal plates of the palatine bones**.
- In the midline, immediately posterior to the incisor teeth, find the right and left **incisive foramina**.
- Medial to the 3rd molar tooth, locate the **greater palatine foramen**. Gently push a thin, flexible wire through the greater palatine foramen into the **greater palatine canal**.

▷
GRANT'S 7.83B
ROHEN 140
NETTER 3
CLEMENTE 827, 828
A.V.A. 4: 0.49.21

Examine the vertical part or **perpendicular plate of the palatine bone** that forms part of the lateral wall of the nasal cavity. The vertical plate has a **notch** on its superior border. This notch is in contact with the sphenoid bone; thus, the **important sphenopalatine (pterygopalatine) foramen** is formed. Identify the foramen in the bisected skull.

Next, coming from the lateral aspect of the skull, look through the **pterygopalatine fossa**. Detect the sphenopalatine foramen in the depth of the fossa. Understand that the foramen is a passageway for vessels and nerves from the pterygopalatine fossa to the nasal cavity.

▷
GRANT'S 7.87A
ROHEN 140, 141
NETTER 3
CLEMENTE 828
A.V.A. 4: 1.04.00

▷
GRANT'S 7.90A
A.D.A.M. 7.14
NETTER 39

▷
GRANT'S 9.11B
A.D.A.M. 7.11
NETTER 39
CLEMENTE 836

In the bisected bony skull, examine the **body of the sphenoid bone**. Locate the large **sphenoidal sinus**. Usually, the right and left sinuses differ in size. They are completely divided by a bony septum. Attempt to find the **posterior opening of the pterygoid canal**. This canal runs posteroanteriorly through the body of the sphenoid. Frequently, the canal causes a ridge on the floor of the sphenoid sinus. Pass a thin, flexible wire through the pterygoid canal. Note that the wire connects two foramina: **foramen lacerum** and **sphenopalatine foramen**. These relations are of importance. The greater petrosal nerve, carrying parasympathetic fibers, traverses the foramen lacerum and then the pterygoid canal to reach the pterygopalatine (sphenopalatine) ganglion.

Preferably in the bisected bony skull, examine the **lateral wall of the nasal cavity**. Identify the following:

- **Frontal process of maxilla**;
- **Vertical plate of palatine bone**;
- **Inferior concha** (turbinate);
- **Middle and superior conchae**; these structures are part of the ethmoid bone; they contain many small air cells; note the openings of some of these cells.

GRANT'S 7.85A
ROHEN 46
A.D.A.M. 7.15
NETTER 3
CLEMENTE 827, 828
A.V.A. 4: 1.01.15

Just superior to the inferior concha, find an opening that leads to the large **maxillary sinus**. Pass a wire through the **nasolacrimal canal**, and observe that the wire enters the nasal cavity under shelter of and lateral to the inferior concha. Pass a flexible wire from the **frontal sinus** into the nasal cavity.

GRANT'S 7.83A
ROHEN 46
A.D.A.M. 7.80
NETTER 3
CLEMENTE 828
A.V.A. 4: 1.07.04

Study the **bony roof of the nasal cavity**. Observe: nasal bone; small part of frontal bone; cribriform plate of ethmoid bone; body of sphenoid.

Examine the **bony nasal septum**. Identify the unpaired **vomer**. It articulates with the sphenoid and the bony palate. Identify the unpaired **perpendicular plate of the ethmoid**. Of course, the large septal cartilage is absent in the bony skull. Examine the two **choanae**, the posterior nasal apertures, and review their boundaries. Review the complex **ethmoid bone** and its relations to the nasal cavity.

Nasal Septum

Turn to the cadaver. Examine the half of the head that contains the **nasal septum**. Strip the mucoperiosteum completely off and identify the three main components of the septum: the **perpendicular plate of ethmoid**, the **vomer**, and the **septal cartilage** (Fig. 7.83).

GRANT'S 7.86A
ROHEN 139
A.D.A.M. 8.2, 8.8
NETTER 34
CLEMENTE 829, 830
A.V.A. 4: 1.14.45

Next, carefully remove the bony and cartilaginous parts of the septum. However, leave intact the mucoperiosteum lateral to it. Now, the vessels and nerves running along the nasal septum can be examined in the remaining mucoperiosteal membrane. The vessels are difficult to trace, unless they are injected. You are not required to dissect these structures. However, note that they exist.

The arteries form a network that receives its blood supply from various sources.

The **nerves to the nasal septum** are thin and run on either side of the bony and cartilagious septum. Observe the following (Fig. 7.84):

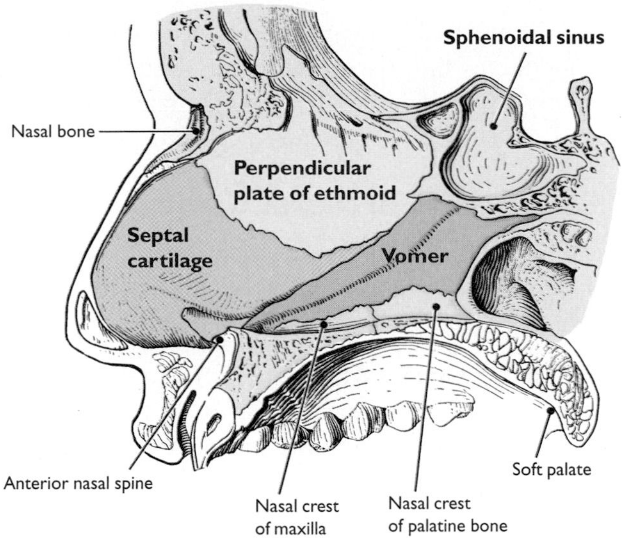

Figure 7.83. The septum of the nose is composed of three major components: septal cartilage, perpendicular plate of ethmoid, and vomer. The vomerine groove (*shaded*) is for the nasopalatine nerve and vessels.

GRANT'S 7.86C
ROHEN 143
NETTER 38
CLEMENTE 830
A.V.A. 5: 0.58.17

- The **nasopalatine nerve** is a branch of V_2 via the pterygopalatine ganglion. From the palatine side, pierce and mark the incisive canal with a needle. Now, you have a reference point. Using a probe and forceps, trace the thin nasopalatine nerve anteriorly toward the incisive canal.
- **Anterior ethmoidal nerve**; do not dissect this fine branch of V_1.
- Close to the cribriform plate is the **olfactory area** that contains olfactory nerve fibers.

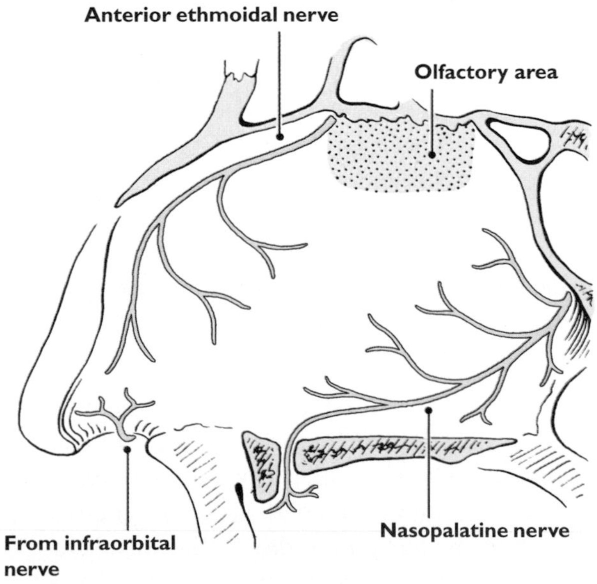

Figure 7.84. Diagram of nerve supply of nasal septum.

Remove all remains of the nasal septum, including the mucoperiosteum. Expose the lateral wall of the nasal cavity. The lateral wall of the other side is already exposed.

Lateral Wall of Nasal Cavity

In the cadaver, inspect the **lateral wall of the nasal cavity** (Fig. 7.85). Identify:

- **Inferior concha**. The space lateral to and inferior to it is the **inferior meatus**. Note that the free edge of the inferior concha is horizontal. About 1.5 cm posterior to the posterior limit of the inferior concha, identify the **pharyngeal orifice of the auditory tube**.
- **Middle concha**. The space lateral to and inferior to it is the **middle meatus**. Anteriorly, the free edge of the middle concha turns superiorly.
- **Superior concha**. This small structure extends from the roof to the front of the sphenoid. Lateral to and inferior to it is the **superior meatus**. The space posterosuperior to the superior concha is the **sphenoethmoidal recess**.
- **Nasal crest** or **agger**; an elevation in front of the middle concha covering the base of the ethmoidal crest.
- **Atrium**. It is located superior to the vestibule and anterior to the middle meatus.
- **Vestibule**; located superior to the nostril and anterior to the inferior meatus (*blue arrow* in Fig. 7.85). Note the presence of hairs on the mobile part.

Grant's 7.82
Rohen 140
Netter 32
Clemente 831
A.V.A. 4: 1.16.57

With scissors, cut away the **inferior concha**. Pass a stiff wire from the orbital cavity inferiorly through the **nasolacrimal duct** to the **inferior meatus**. Remove the mucoperiosteum from the lateral wall of the inferior meatus. Observe the **opening of the bony nasolacrimal canal**, which contains the nasolacrimal duct (Fig. 7.86B).

With scissors, cut away the **middle concha**. Identify a curved slit, the **hiatus semilunaris**. This hiatus has a sharp, inferior edge. Its more rounded superior edge is formed by the **ethmoidal bulla**, an elevation of the ethmoidal labyrinth.

Grant's 7.83A
Rohen 141
Netter 32
Clemente 832
A.V.A. 4: 1.17.30

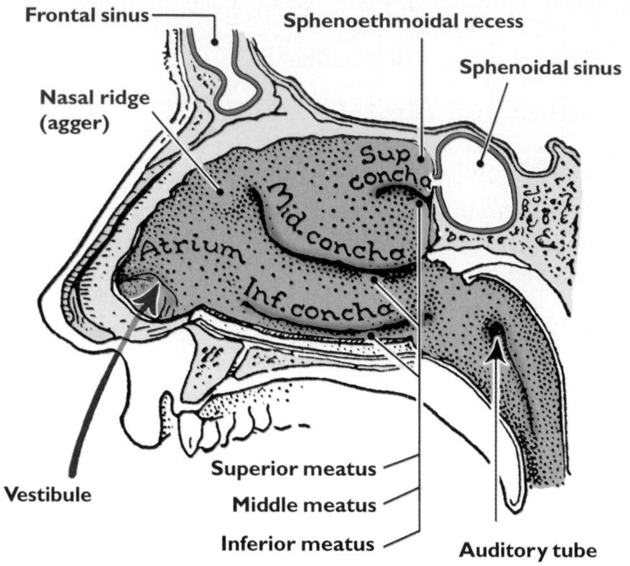

Figure 7.85. The lateral wall of the nasal cavity.

Identify the opened **frontal sinus** (Figs. 7.85, 7.86C). Pass a wire inferoposteriorly from the frontal sinus through the **frontonasal duct**. Usually, this duct opens into the upper portion of the **infundibulum**. The infundibulum is a narrow passage anterosuperior to the hiatus semilunaris.

> ***Clinical Correlation:*** In frontal sinus infections, irrigation of the sinus may be necessary. This is done with a specially curved cannula that is passed through the infundibulum and through the frontonasal duct. Study these important relations in the cadaver.

Grant's 7.84A, 7.87A
Rohen 140, 144
Netter 32, 33, 42, 43
Clemente 837-841
A.V.A. 4: 1.08.33

Observe that the **ethmoidal cells** (or sinuses) are located lateral to the middle and superior conchae (Fig. 7.86). Stay above (superior to) the hiatus semilunaris, and break into the **middle ethmoidal cells** of the ethmoidal bulla. Anteriorly, identify the **anterior ethmoidal cells**. Remove the superior concha to display one or more of the **posterior ethmoidal cells**. Pick away the partitions between the ethmoidal cells until you reach the thin **orbital plate** (lamina papyracea) of the ethmoid bone (Fig. 7.86). If you break through this plate, you will enter the orbital cavity.

Explore the **semilunar hiatus**. In it is the **ostium for the maxillary sinus** (Fig. 7.86A). Pass a probe into the maxillary sinus.

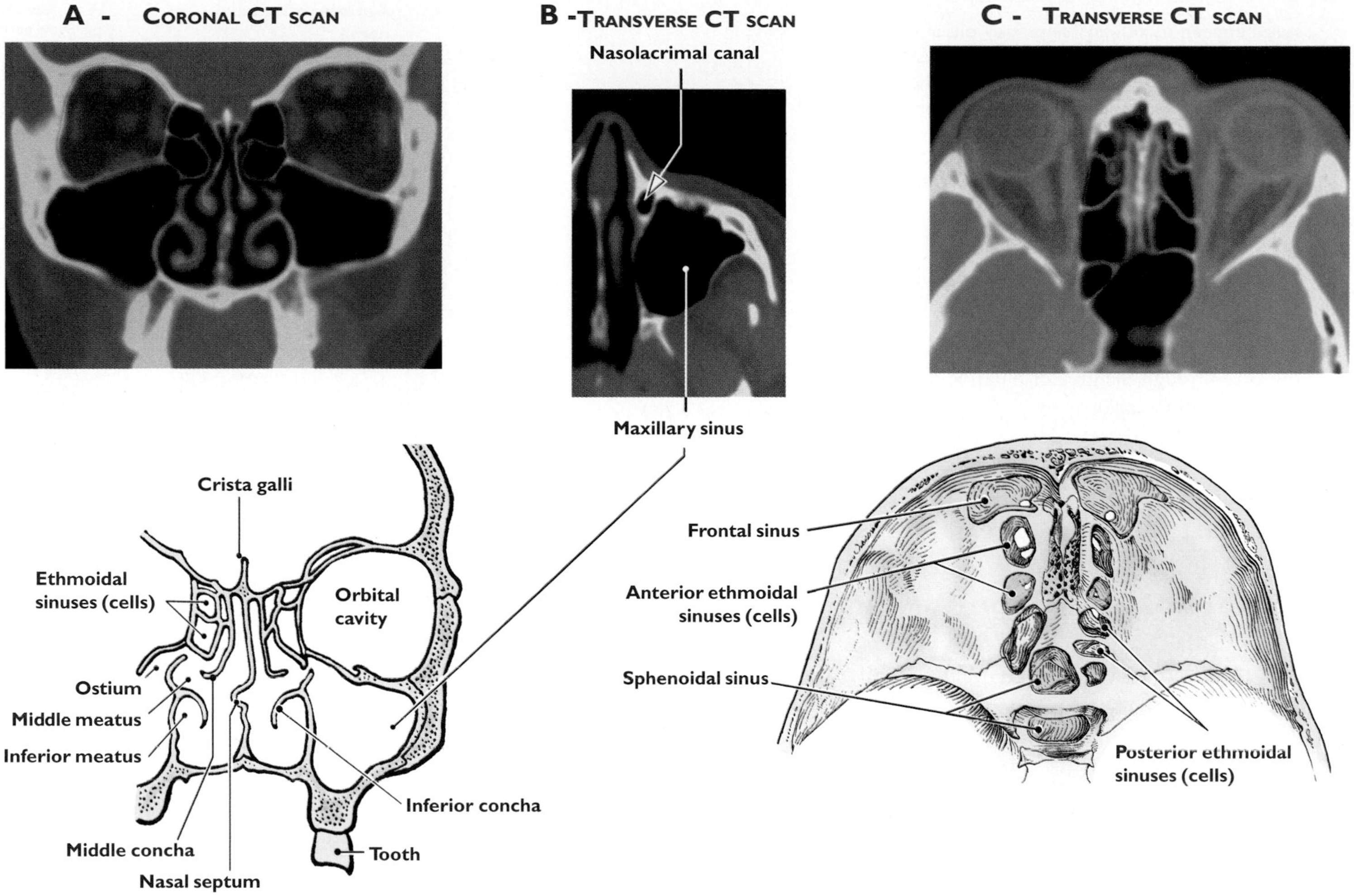

Figure 7.86. Correlations of anatomical sections and CT scans.

Clinical Correlation: Explore the **sphenoidal sinuses** or cells (Fig. 7.86). Find the orifice or ostium, which opens into the sphenoethmoidal recess. The size of the ostium may vary from 0.5 to 4.0 mm. Irrigation of an infected sphenoid sinus can be accomplished by inserting a special curved cannula through the ostium. Examine the orifice. Understand that it may not be accessible when the middle concha is too large or the septum is deviated. In that case, a trocar must be pushed directly through the anterior wall of the sphenoid into the sinus. Study these relations.

The **ostium of the maxillary sinus** can often be seen on a coronal CT scan of a sinus series (Fig. 7.86A). An infected maxillary sinus may be irrigated through its ostium. However, if difficulties are encountered, an artificial route of drainage is chosen. A curved trocar is pushed through the lateral wall of the inferior meatus into the maxillary sinus, close to its floor. With a probe, break through the thin lateral wall of the inferior meatus and create an artificial opening.

Now, with the aid of bone forceps, remove the medial wall of the **maxillary sinus**. Notice that it is a three-sided hollow pyramid.

⇨
GRANT'S 7.87, 7.88C
NETTER 43
CLEMENTE 788, 790
A.V.A. 4: 1.03.08

The average adult capacity is approximately 15 ml. Verify that the superior wall separates the sinus from the orbital cavity.

With forceps, remove the mucoperiosteum lining the maxillary sinus. Note a ridge on the orbital and anterior surfaces. This ridge is caused by the infraorbital canal. With a probe, break into the canal, open it along its length, and identify its contents: infraorbital nerve and accompanying vessels.

⇦
GRANT'S 7.84A, B
ROHEN 141
NETTER 32
CLEMENTE 832
A.V.A. 4: 1.18.05

Examine the floor of the maxillary sinus. Look for the roots of teeth that may project into the sinus.

Clinical Correlation: The roots of upper teeth, particularly of the molar teeth, may project into the adjacent maxillary sinus. Sometimes the roots are covered only with mucoperiosteum. Understand that an infection from a decaying tooth may readily spread into the sinus. During extraction of a molar or premolar tooth, the membrane superior to the projecting root may be torn. As a result, a fistula between mouth and sinus may occur. Under these conditions, a person cannot blow his or her cheeks; instead, the air from the oral cavity escapes though the fistula into the maxillary sinus and from there into the nose.

Sphenopalatine Foramen and Pterygopalatine Fossa

In the bony skull, identify the sphenopalatine foramen and the pterygopalatine fossa. Proceed as follows:

- Coming from the bony palate, gently push a thin, flexible wire through the greater palatine foramen into the greater palatine canal.
- Observe the wire as it emerges in the pterygopalatine fossa close to the sphenopalatine foramen.
- Identify the pterygoid canal and mark its course with a thin, flexible wire.
- Review the course of the maxillary nerve V2.

GRANT'S 7.61, 7.66, 9.11B
ROHEN 46
NETTER 2, 3, 33
CLEMENTE 835
A.V.A. 4: 1.09.26

The conchae and the medial wall of the maxillary sinus were removed earlier. The perpendicular plate of the palatine bone and the closely related greater palatine canal are still intact. Now, strip the mucoperiosteum from the perpendicular plate of the palatine bone. You will encounter the **posterior lateral nasal artery**. This artery is a branch of the **sphenopalatine artery**. After traversing the sphenopalatine foramen, the sphenopalatine artery divides into a **posterior septal branch** (for the septum) and the posterior lateral nasal branch. Most of its small branches have been cut during removal of the conchae. Do not dissect the arterial network of the lateral nasal wall. However, note that it exists.

GRANT'S 7.75B, 7.85C
ROHEN 139, 143
NETTER 37-39
CLEMENTE 834-836
A.V.A. 5: 0.57.37

GRANT'S 7.85B, 7.86B
ROHEN 142
NETTER 35, 36
CLEMENTE 830, 834

Sphenopalatine Foramen and Contents

The greater palatine canal leads to the **sphenopalatine foramen**. Make use of this fact. Insert a needle (about 30 mm or 1¼ inches long) into the greater palatine foramen, just medial to the 3rd molar tooth. Probe until you find the opening. Then, push the needle all the way through the greater palatine canal. The tip of the needle will be located anterior to the sphenoid bone and just lateral to the sphenopalatine foramen. Leave the needle in place. Now, use a probe and break down the medial wall

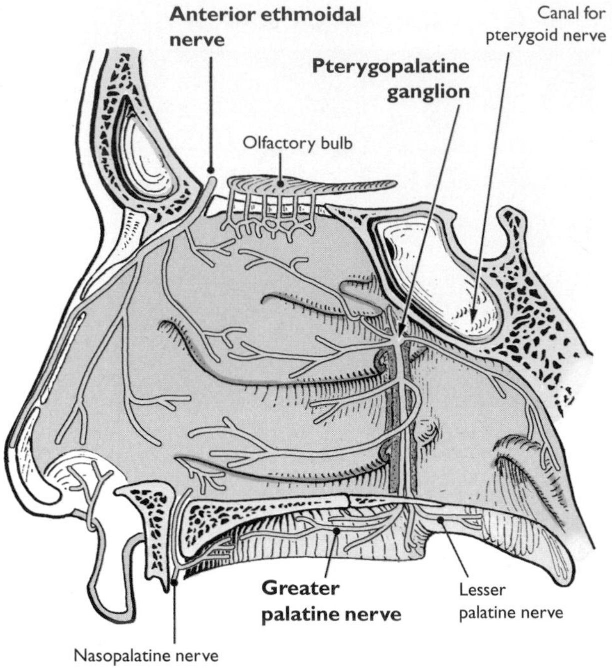

Figure 7.87. Diagram of nerve supply of lateral wall of nose.

of the greater palatine canal. This procedure will expose the contents of the canal: the **greater palatine nerve** (Fig. 7.87) and the greater palatine artery, a terminal branch of the maxillary artery.

Follow the greater palatine nerve superiorly to the sphenopalatine foramen. Here, find the small but important **pterygopalatine (sphenopalatine) ganglion** (Fig. 7.87).

GRANT'S 9.11B
ROHEN 143
A.D.A.M. 8.12
NETTER 39
CLEMENTE 836

If time permits, find the **nerve of the pterygoid canal**. Proceed as follows:

- Remove the mucoperiosteum from the sphenoid sinus.
- Find the ridge produced by the pterygoid canal (Fig. 7.87).
- With a probe, open the canal. Identify the thin nerve of the pterygoid canal.
- Follow the delicate nerve toward the pterygopalatine ganglion. The nerve of the pterygoid canal (Vidian nerve) consists of preganglionic parasympathetic fibers from the greater petrosal nerve, and postganglionic sympathetic fibers from the deep petrosal nerve.

GRANT'S 7.66, 7.67E
NETTER 35
CLEMENTE 751, 834
A.V.A. 5: 0.55.03

Next, turn the specimen over and approach it from its lateral aspect. Deep in the **pterygopalatine fossa**, identify the following pertinent structures:

- **Maxillary artery**, giving off the **greater palatine artery** and the **sphenopalatine artery**; the sphenopalatine artery is the one passing through the sphenopalatine foramen;
- **Maxillary nerve V_2**, coursing from the foramen rotundum posteriorly to the inferior orbital fissure anteriorly;
- **Pterygopalatine (sphenopalatine) ganglion**; it is attached to the maxillary nerve by two short stout medially running nerve branches.

If you cannot satisfactorily see the ganglion in relation to nerve V_2, remove the floor of the orbital cavity. Follow the infraorbital nerve posteriorly. Now, you have a clearer view of the pterygopalatine ganglion.

Palate, Tonsil, and Pharyngeal Wall

Hard Palate and Soft Palate

The palate consists of two portions (Fig. 7.88):

- The **hard palate,** comprising the anterior 2/3;
- The mobile **soft palate,** constituting the posterior 1/3 of the palate.

Small mucous glands, the **palatine glands,** are abundant over the palate. The pinpoint orifices of their ducts are evident.

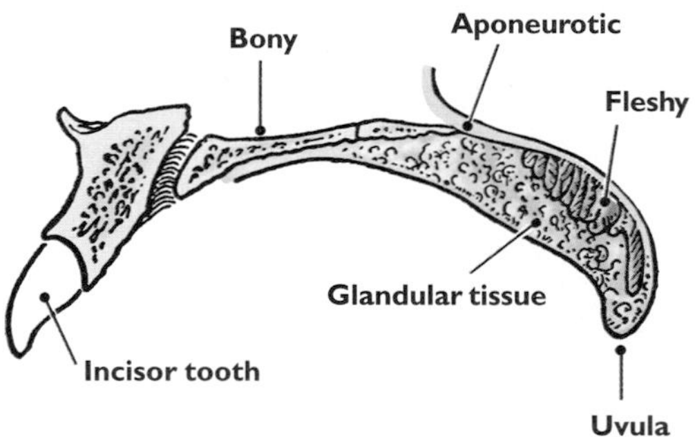

Figure 7.88. Hard palate and soft palate on sagittal section.

Mark the greater palatine fora men with a needle, as described earlier. The **greater palatine nerve and vessels** emerge from this foramen to be distributed to the hard palate. To demonstrate nerve and vessels, proceed as follows (Fig. 7.89):

GRANT'S 7.75
NETTER 46
CLEMENTE 845
A.V.A. 5: 0.57.37

GRANT'S 7.74
ROHEN 45, 56
NETTER 46, 57
CLEMENTE 871, 872
A.V.A. 4: 0.56.42

GRANT'S 8.39, 8.45
ROHEN 143, 145
A.D.A.M. 7.4
NETTER 58
CLEMENTE 843, 845, 860
A.V.A. 4: 1.55.19

GRANT'S 7.75
NETTER 46
CLEMENTE 845
A.V.A. 5: 0.57.18

- About 5 mm posterior to the marked greater palatine foramen, make a transverse cut through the thickness of the mucoperiosteum of the hard palate.
- With the rounded handle of the knife, ease the mucoperiosteum off the bony palate.
- Free the greater palatine nerve and vessels.
- Cut the reflected tissue close to the alveolar processes of the teeth.
- Identify the **greater palatine nerve** and follow it anteriorly to the mucosa of the hard palate.
- Identify the **lesser palatine nerve** and follow it posteriorly into the soft palalate.

Examine the soft palate, which had been cut earlier in the midsagittal plane. Observe (Fig. 7.88):

- The thickness of the soft palate is due mainly to glands;
- The strength of the soft palate depends on its aponeurosis situated in its anterior 1/3;
- Its mobility is due to muscles situated in its posterior 2/3. These muscles will be studied later.

Palatine Tonsil

The right and left **palatine tonsils** lie on each side of the oropharynx. The tonsil is called "palatine" because its superior 1/3 extends into the soft palate, a matter of clinical importance. Each tonsil is located in the triangular interval between the **palatoglossal arch** and the **palatopharyngeal arch** (Figs. 7.89, 7.90). In older individuals, the palatine tonsil may be inconspicuous.

Dissection

If the cadaver has no tonsils, remove the mucosa between the palatoglossal and palatopharyngeal arches and study the tonsillar bed.

If the tonsil is present, enucleate it (shell it out) as follows:

- As the first step, incise the mucous membrane along the palatoglossal arch (Fig. 7.90).
- As the second step, using blunt dissection, free the anterior border and the superior part

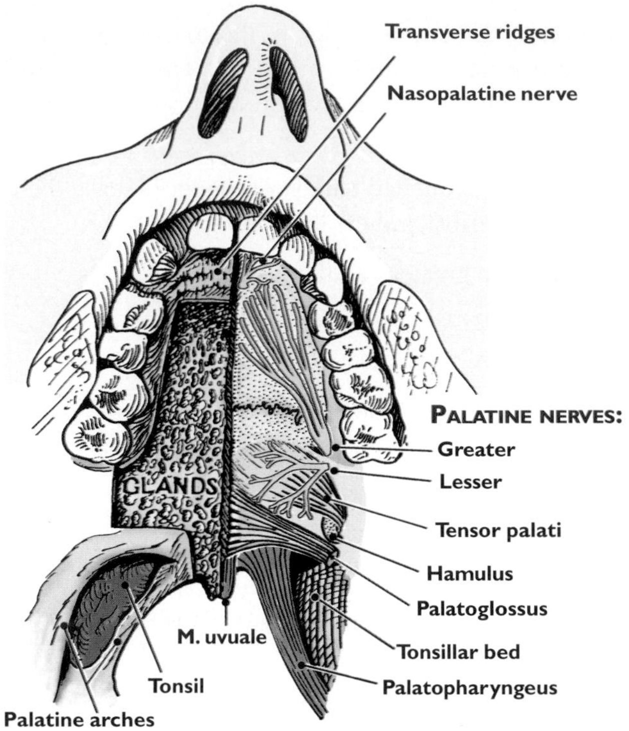

Figure 7.89. Structures related to the hard and soft palate.

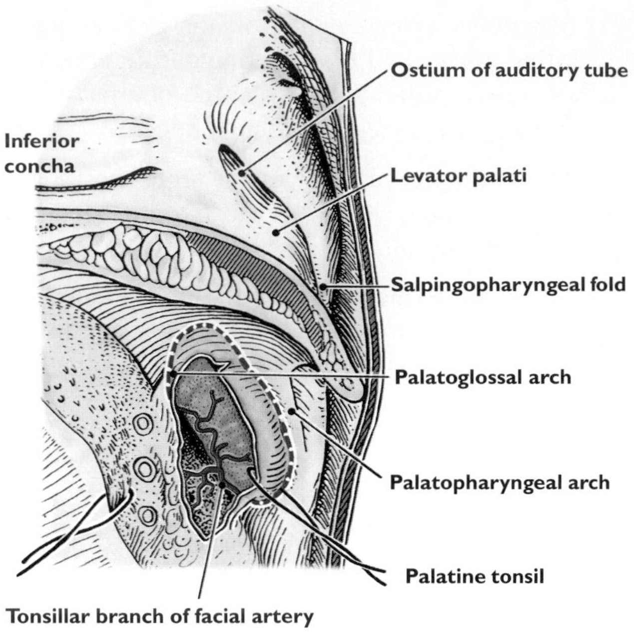

Figure 7.90. First step in removal of the palatine tonsil: incise the mucous membrane along the palatoglossal arch (*dotted blue line*).

of the tonsil (Fig. 7.91). This is easily done because the rounded lateral aspect of the tonsil has a fibrous capsule. This capsule is separated from the pharyngeal wall by a layer of loose areolar tissue. Work in the areolar space.

- Free the posterior part of the tonsil.
- Finally, detach the inferior part where the tonsil is most adherent. Note that the inferior pole of the palatine tonsil is continuous with the lymphoid tissue of the tongue, the **lingual tonsil**.

Examine the enucleated palatine tonsil. Section it. Observe the **crypts** that extend from the free surface of the tonsil to almost the level of the capsule.

⇦ *GRANT'S 8.44*

Examine the **bed of the palatine tonsil** (Fig. 7.92). The thin fibrous sheet covering the bed of the tonsil is part of the **pharyngobasilar fascia.** Remove it, and expose two muscles: **palatopharyngeus** and **superior constrictor.** These muscles are part of the muscular coat of the pharynx. The superior constrictor has a delicate, free, arched inferior border, which does not reach the inferior third of the tonsillar bed. If engorged, you may see the **paratonsillar vein.** This vein is often responsible for hemorrhage following tonsillectomy.

⇦ *GRANT'S 8.42*
A.D.A.M. 7.24
NETTER 58
A.V.A. 4: 2.17.38

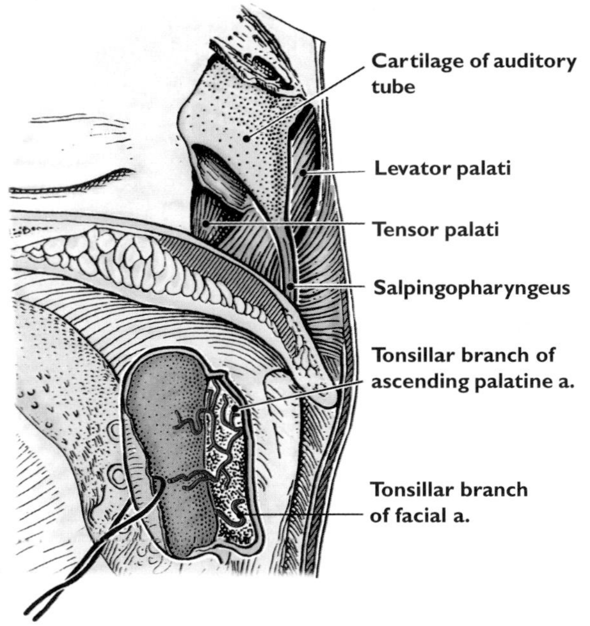

Figure 7.91. Second step in removal of the palatine tonsil: free the anterior and superior borders by blunt dissection; separate the inferior pole from the lymphoid tissue of the tongue.

Push a probe inferior to the free inferior border of the superior constrictor. Using the probe as a protective guide, carefully remove a small part of the superior constrictor just anterior to the palatopharyngeus (Fig. 7.92).

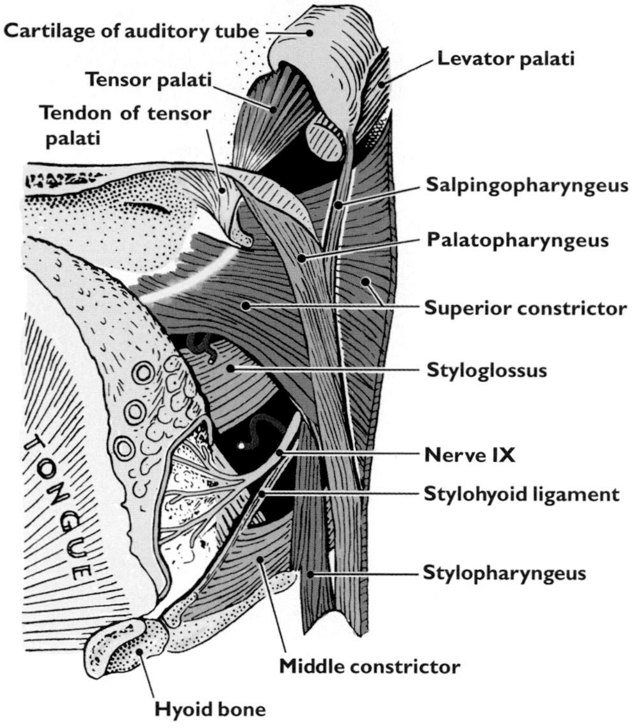

Figure 7.92. Bed of palatine tonsil; dissection of nasopharynx.

Now, the styloglossus and the glossopharyngeal nerve are exposed. Identify the **styloglossus.** It is a thick muscular band that passes from the tip of the styloid process to the lateral aspect of the tongue. Find the **glossopharyngeal nerve (IX)** that is also sensory to the area of the palatine tonsil. The nerve passes through the gap between the superior and the middle constrictors just lateral to the stylopharyngeus. It spreads out to the mucosa of the posterior 1/3 of the tongue. Follow the nerve proximally to the base of the skull. Review the distribution and functions of nerve IX.

Pharyngeal Wall

Carefully remove the mucous membrane from both surfaces of the soft palate, from the lateral pharyngeal wall, and from the nasopharynx. When removing the mucosa from the palatoglossal arch, the **palatoglossus** is displayed. After removal of the mucosa from the palatopharyngeal arch, the **palatopharyngeus** is exposed. The palatopharyngeus, salpingopharyngeus, and stylopharyngeus form the longitudinal musculature of the pharynx (Fig. 7.92).

GRANT'S 8.41
ROHEN 163
NETTER 59, 62
CLEMENTE 888
A.V.A. 4: 1.56.03

GRANT'S 8.40
NETTER 58
CLEMENTE 895
A.V.A. 4: 2.18.33

GRANT'S 8.40
ROHEN 64
NETTER 58, 59, 61
CLEMENTE 830
A.V.A. 4: 1.23.15

GRANT'S 8.39, 8.40
A.D.A.M. 7.24
NETTER 58, 59
CLEMENTE 895
A.V.A. 4: 2.17.38

Dissection Note: You may or may not be required to dissect the inferior part of the thin **palatopharyngeus muscle** as it descends, attaches itself to the posterior border of the thyroid cartilage, and blends with the lateral pharynx and the esophagus. Similarly, the muscle fibers of the **salpingopharyngeus** are difficult to dissect. It descends from the inferior part of the auditory tube (salpinx) and blends with the palatopharyngeus (Fig. 7.92).

The next objective is to display the **origin of the superior constrictor** from the **pterygomandibular raphe.** This raphe or ligament connects two bony landmarks: the **hamulus of the medial pterygoid plate**, and an area of the **mandible** just posterior to the 3rd molar tooth. Observe these bony landmarks in the skull. Then, palpate the hamulus in the cadaver. Now, you can positively identify the fibrous pterygomandibular raphe. Verify that two muscles meet at the raphe: **superior constrictor** and **buccinator.** In addition, examine these relations from the lateral aspect of the head.

Examine the free superior border of the superior constrictor. The gap between this border and the base of the skull is closed by the pharyngobasilar fascia. Passing through this gap are (Fig. 7.93): the **auditory tube,** the **levator palati,** and the **ascending pharyngeal artery.**

Auditory Tube (pharyngotympanic tube; Eustachian tube). It connects the nasopharynx with the tympanic cavity. It is about 36 mm long and consists of a cartilaginous

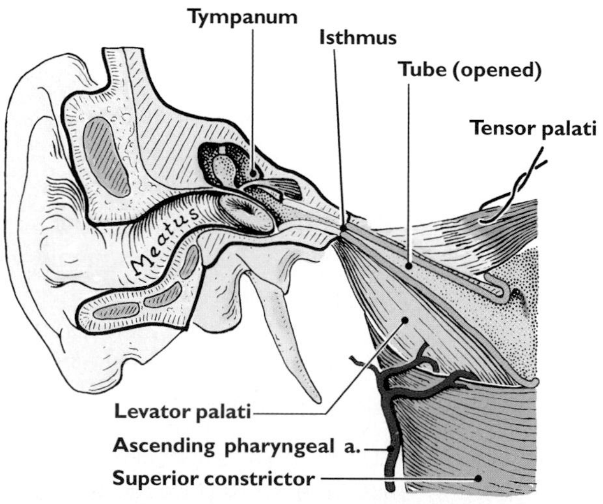

Figure 7.93. Auditory tube, levator palati, and ascending pharyngeal artery cross the superior border of the superior constrictor muscle.

and a bony portion. Refer to the base of a bony skull and look for the opening of the **osseous portion of the auditory tube**. Pass a thin, flexible wire through the canal. Now, look into the external ear canal. You will see the wire in the middle ear cavity (in the cadaver, the external ear canal and the middle ear cavity are separated by the tympanic membrane).

Grant's 8.40
Rohen 64
Netter 58, 59, 61
Clemente 830
A.V.A. 4: 0.52.50

The anterior 2/3 of the auditory tube is cartilaginous. Observe that the cartilage forms only the superior and medial walls of the tube. The inferior and lateral walls are membranous. The bony and the **cartilaginous portions of the auditory tube** meet at the **isthmus.** Here, the lumen of the tube is very narrow (Fig. 7.93).

Levator Veli Palatini or Levator Palati

Grant's 8.40, 8.45
Rohen 64
A.D.A.M. 7.24
Netter 46, 59, 61
Clemente 830
A.V.A. 4: 1.21.32

At the base of the skull, this muscle arises from the petrous bone and the medial portion of the cartilage of the auditory tube (Fig. 7.92). The **levator palati** elevates and retracts the soft palate (Fig. 7.94). Identify the muscle, which is slightly thicker than a pencil. Pass the handle of a scalpel between the levator and the floor of the auditory tube. Separate the two structures from each other. Cut the levator close to the base of the skull and reflect it.

Grant's 7.70, 7.72
Netter 65
Clemente 769

Free the **auditory tube** from the medial pterygoid plate. Cut it and remove its anterior portion. Observe the collapsed, slit-like lumen of the tube (Figs. 7.91, 7.93). Note the cartilaginous and membranous walls.

Grant's 7.75A, 8.40
Rohen 64
A.D.A.M. 7.24
Netter 46
Clemente 830
A.V.A. 4: 1.22.12

Now, the **tensor veli palatini (tensor palati)** lies exposed (Fig. 7.92). The muscle arises from the **scaphoid fossa.** Identify this bony landmark on the skull. Find the fossa at the superior end of the posterior border of the medial pterygoid plate. Once again, identify the **hamulus** of the medial pterygoid plate, which serves as a pulley for the tensor palati (Figs.7.89, 7.92). To render the soft palate "tense," the right and left tensors must pull it laterally. The thin, ribbon-like muscle ends in a tendon, which winds around the hamulus. In the cadaver, palpate the hamulus. Find the tendon of the tensor palati as it passes medially to its insertion into the palatine aponeurosis (Fig. 7.89).

Grant's 7.68
A.D.A.M. 7.4
Netter 45
Clemente 843
A.V.A. 4: 1.53.20

Continue with the dissection of the specimen from its medial side. Retract the tensor palati superiorly, or remove its superoposterior portion. This procedure will

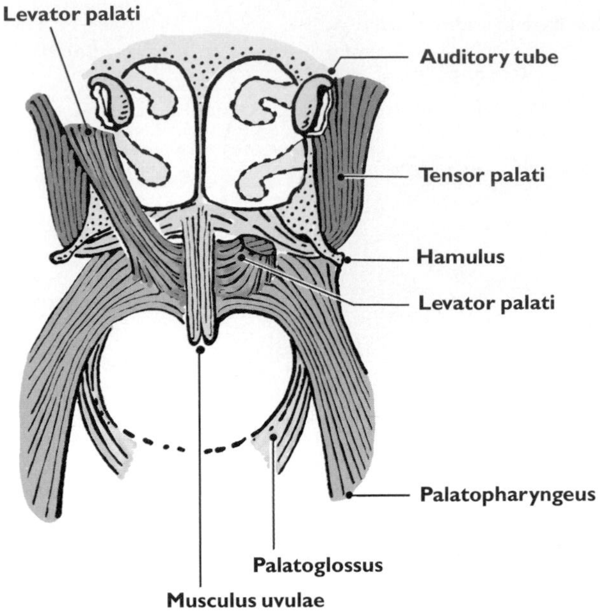

Figure 7.94. Schematic posterior view of nasopharynx and oropharynx. Five pairs of muscles of the soft palate.

expose the **mandibular nerve** (V_3) as it emerges from the **foramen ovale.** Coming from the medial side, carefully pass the tip of a probe through the foramen. Immediately inferior to the foramen and on the medial aspect of V_3 lies the small **otic ganglion**. The ganglion is difficult to find. Be aware of its functional importance.

Mouth and Tongue

Inspection and Palpation

Vestibule of the Mouth

The vestibule of the mouth is the U-shaped space bounded externally by the lips and cheeks and, internally, by the teeth and gums. The teeth and gums separate the vestibule from the oral cavity proper. With a clean or gloved index or middle finger, explore the vestibule of your own mouth. Have a skull on hand for reference. Palpate the following structures:

- **Mentalis,** passing from the incisive fossa of the mandible to the skin of the chin;
- Inferior border of **zygomatic arch**;
- **Maxilla,** its anterior (facial) and infratemporal surfaces;
- **Ramus** and **coronoid process of mandible; tendon of temporalis,** attached to the coronoid process;
- **Masseter,** easily palpated when the teeth are clenched;
- Posterior to the last molar tooth, the communication between vestibule and oral cavity proper;

- **Frenulum** of upper lip and frenulum of lower lip; the two frenula (L. *frenum*, bridle) are folds of mucosa attaching the lips to the gums in the median plane;
- **Orifice of the parotid duct;** a slightly elevated, whitish, constricted opening opposite the 2nd superior molar tooth; usually, this papilla can be readily palpated with the tip of the tongue; examine the right and left orifices.

GRANT'S 7.68
A.D.A.M. 7.4
NETTER 45
CLEMENTE 843

Oral Cavity Proper

Define its **borders:** laterally and anteriorly the teeth and gums; superiorly, the hard palate; inferiorly, the tongue; posteriorly and laterally, the palatoglossal arch, marking the border between oral cavity and oropharynx. In the living, inspect or palpate the following **structures of the oral cavity proper:**

GRANT'S 7.68
A.D.A.M. 7.4
NETTER 45
CLEMENTE 843
A.V.A. 4: 1.52.55

- **Sublingual region;** this region is located inferior to the mobile portions of the tongue;
- **Frenulum linguae;** connecting the tongue to the floor of the mouth; raise the tip of the tongue to see this median fold;
- **Deep lingual veins,** easily seen on each side of the frenulum;
- **Opening of submandibular duct;** observe it on each side of the root of the frenulum;
- **Plica sublingualis**, overlying the superior border of the sublingual salivary gland; several small sublingual ducts open onto this plica;
- **Hamulus of medial pterygoid plate**.

Sublingual Region

Refer to a bony mandible. Examine its medial aspect and identify two important bony landmarks:

GRANT'S 7.57
ROHEN 147
A.D.A.M. 7.18
NETTER 54, 55
CLEMENTE 769
A.V.A. 4: 1.28.44

- **Mylohyoid line,** for attachment of mylohyoid muscle;
- **Sublingual fossa,** for the sublingual gland and associated soft structures superior to the level of the mylohyoid muscle.

Turn to the bisected head of the cadaver. Examine the muscles of the floor of the mouth and of the tongue as they can be seen on median section: **mylohyoid, geniohyoid,** and the large, fan-shaped **genioglossus.**

GRANT'S 7.69
ROHEN 146
A.D.A.M. 7.28
NETTER 57
CLEMENTE 763-765
A.V.A. 4: 1.45.49

The next objective is to expose the sublingual gland. Before dissecting, it is important that you understand the following:

- Dissection of the lateral aspect of the gland is relatively simple, since no important structures intervene between gland and sublingual fossa of mandible.
- Dissection medial to the gland will require great care. Important structures (nerve, duct, vessels) will be found in the space between gland and genioglossus muscle of the tongue.
- The sublingual gland rests on the mylohyoid muscle.

GRANT'S 7.70
ROHEN 147
NETTER 54, 55
CLEMENTE 856-858
A.V.A. 4: 2.06.49

With these facts in mind, proceed as follows:

- Incise the mucous membrane between plica sublingualis and mandible. Start at the frenulum of the tongue. Carry the incision posteriorly, but not beyond the 2nd molar tooth.
- With a probe and handle of a scalpel, displace the **sublingual gland** medially.
- Identify the sublingual fossa of the mandible. Inferior to it, observe the origin of the mylohyoid.

Next, carefully incise the mucous membrane along the furrow between the **plica sublingualis** and the **tongue.** With a blunt instrument (probe or handle of scalpel), displace the gland laterally and the tongue medially. Identify the following (Fig. 7.95):

GRANT'S 7.70, 8.18
ROHEN 148, 149
NETTER 54, 55
CLEMENTE 856-858
A.V.A. 4: 2.05.52

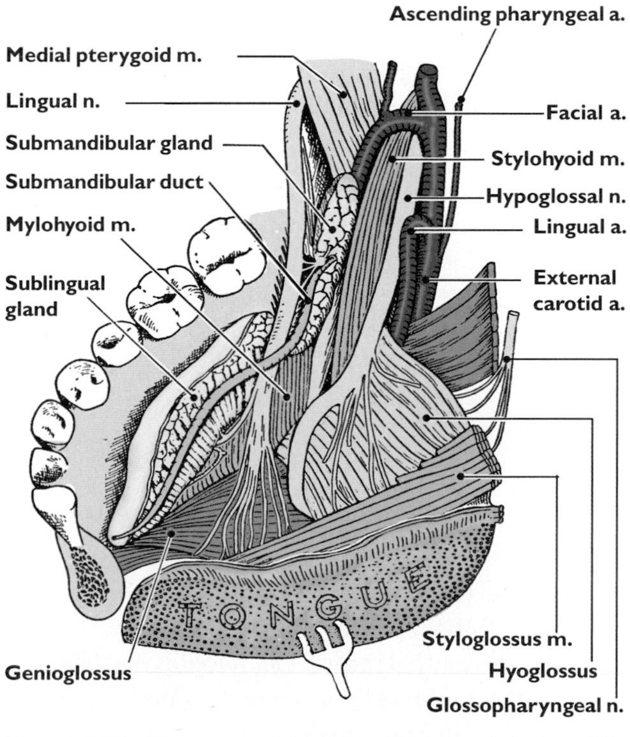

Figure 7.95. Dissection of the floor of the mouth (right side).

- **Sublingual salivary gland**; it is enveloped in a sheath of areolar tissue that fixes the gland to the floor of the mouth. Tease the tissue between superior border of sublingual gland and plica sublingualis and identify several very short and fine ducts. There are about 12 ducts that open on the summit of the plica.
- **Submandibular duct**; it runs diagonally across the medial aspect of the sublingual gland. Follow the duct anteriorly to its papilla just lateral to the frenulum linguae. Then, follow the duct posteriorly to the substance of the **submandibular salivary gland.**
- **Lingual nerve**; pick up the nerve posterior to the last molar tooth. Once again, verify that the nerve runs between ramus of mandible and medial pterygoid. Trace the lingual nerve anteriorly. The nerve describes a spiral around the submandibular duct. In successive order, the relations of the nerve to the duct are: lateral and superior to; inferior to; inferior and medial to; and finally superior and medial to the duct. Observe that the nerve divides into several branches to the tongue. These branches lie in the submucosa of the anterior 2/3 of the tongue (Fig. 7.95).
- **Submandibular ganglion**. Far posterior, in the vicinity of the 3rd molar tooth, look for the submandibular ganglion. This small ganglion is suspended from the lingual nerve by two or more short branches. Carefully tease the inferior surface of the lingual nerve to reveal the ganglion. Understand the functional importance of the ganglion.
- **Hypoglossal nerve (XII).** Pick up the nerve as it runs anteriorly between submandibular gland and hyoglossus, well inferior to the lingual nerve. Follow the nerve to the musculature of the tongue.

Tongue

Approach the bisected head from its lateral aspect. With a probe, define the attachment of the **mylohyoid** to the hyoid bone. Subsequently detach the muscle from the hyoid bone and reflect it superiorly. Now, the **hyoglossus** is fully exposed. Observe the two important nerves that cross the hyoglossus laterally: **hypoglossal nerve** and, more superiorly, the **lingual nerve.**

Grant's 7.70, 8.18
Rohen 148, 149
Netter 54, 55
Clemente 856-858
A.V.A. 4: 2.06.49

Grant's 8.18, 9.10B
Rohen 148, 149
Netter 53, 65
Clemente 856-858

Grant's 8.19-8.21
Rohen 62, 147
A.D.A.M. 7.24
Netter 53, 62
Clemente 863-865
A.V.A. 4: 2.15.50

Grant's 8.18-8.20
Rohen 146
A.D.A.M. 7.24
Netter 53, 54
Clemente 851, 863
A.V.A. 4: 1.49.24

With a probe, locate the origin of the **lingual artery** (Fig. 7.96). Understand that this artery runs medial to the hyoglossus. To expose the course of the artery, this muscle must be reflected. Proceed as follows: pass a probe deep to the attachment of the hyoglossus to the hyoid bone. Cut the muscle, and reflect it superiorly.

Now the course of the **lingual artery** is exposed. Follow its branches to the musculature of the tongue. Search for fine branches to the sublingual gland.

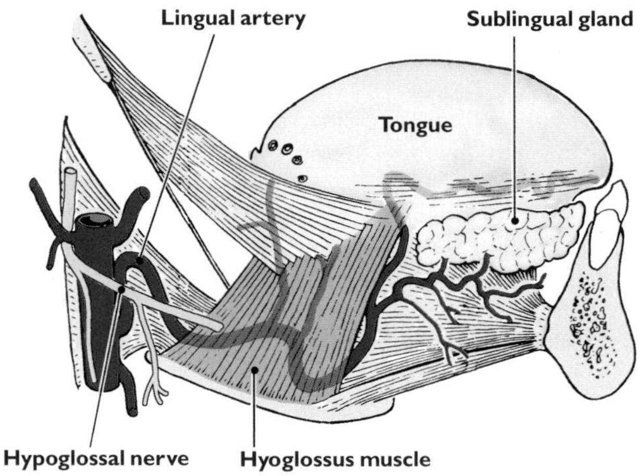

Figure 7.96. The hyoglossus muscle intervenes between the lingual artery and the hypoglossal nerve (XII).

Styloglossus (Fig. 7.97). Trace the muscle from the styloid process to the lateral aspect of the tongue. Note that its fibers interdigitate with those of the hyoglossus.

Genioglossus and Geniohyoid. Once again, examine these two muscles on median section. Separate the muscles with a probe. The geniohyoid is the one attached to the hyoid bone. Observe the large, fan-shaped genioglossus. With a probe, define its apical attachment to the genial tubercle of the mandible.

Next, cut the **genioglossus** close to the mandible. Observe that, as a result of this section, the tongue becomes quite mobile. Raise the tongue well posteriorly into the

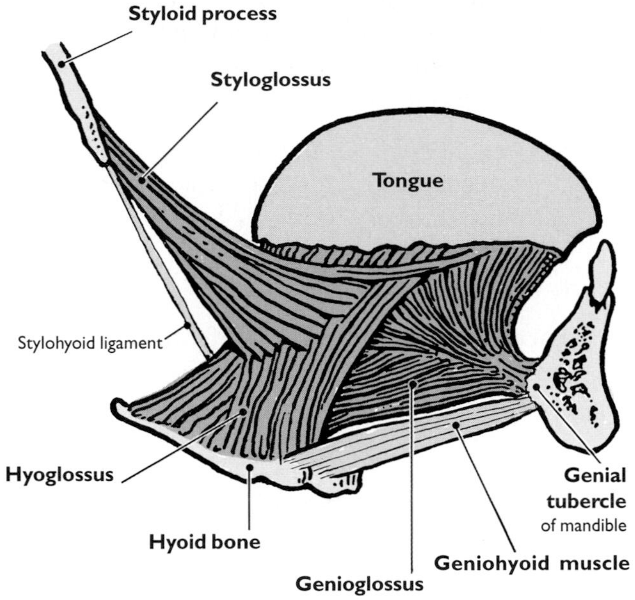

Figure 7.97. The three extrinsic muscles of the tongue and their three bony origins.

pharynx. Now, the underlying **geniohyoid** is exposed. Examine the attachments of this muscle to mandible and hyoid bone.

On one side of the bisected head only, make a **transverse section through the tongue.** Note the **intrinsic musculature of the tongue.** It consists of *vertical*, *transverse*, and *longitudinal fibers*. Review the hypoglossal nerve.

Clinical Correlation: The **genioglossus** is a paired muscle that is fused in the midline. Its function is to protrude the tongue (move it anteriorly; stretch it out). If one-half of the muscle does not function (hypoglossal paralysis on that side), the tongue cannot be protruded in a straight fashion; rather the intact side is protruded more, and the damaged side is protruded less or not at all. As a result, the stretched-out tongue deviates to the side of the lesion.

The genioglossus is of considerable clinical importance. If paralyzed (bilateral hypoglossal paralysis; deep general anesthesia), the tongue cannot be protruded and, due to its own weight, will relapse posteriorly against the posterior pharyngeal wall when the patient is in the supine position. As a result, the vital airway will be occluded with the attendant risk of suffocation.

Recent research has shown that the muscular tone of the genioglossus is greatly diminished during certain phases of sleep, thus enhancing the risk of intermittent airway occlusion during sleep. Obese patients with substantial fatty infiltration into the tongue are particularly vulnerable.

GRANT'S 8.48, 8.71
ROHEN 154, 155
A.D.A.M. 7.26, 7.54
NETTER 71
CLEMENTE 899-903
A.V.A. 4: 2.25.24

Larynx

General Remarks

The **skeleton of the larynx** is responsible for maintaining the shape of this organ. It consists of a series of articulating cartilages that are united by membranes (Fig. 7.98):

The **cricoid cartilage** (Gk., *krikos*, ring) is shaped like a signet ring; its large plate or lamina is positioned posteriorly, its arch anteriorly.

The inferior horns (or cornua) of the **thyroid cartilage** articulate with the cricoid cartilage at special facets. At these facets, the thyroid cartilage can be tilted anteriorly or posteriorly in a visor-like manner.

On the superior border of the lamina of the cricoid are the articular facets for the paired **arytenoid cartilages.** These small pyramidal cartilages are capable of various movements:

- Tilting anteriorly and posteriorly;
- Sliding toward or away from another;
- Rotary motion.

The posterior ends of the **vocal ligaments** are attached at the vocal processes of the arytenoid cartilages. The anterior ends of the vocal ligaments converge at the angle formed by the laminae of the thyroid cartilage.

NETTER 54
CLEMENTE 851

The **epiglottic cartilage** lies posterior to the tongue and hyoid bone (Fig. 7.98). The stalk of this cartilage is attached in the angle between the thyroid laminae, just superior to the vocal ligaments.

Laryngeal Muscles

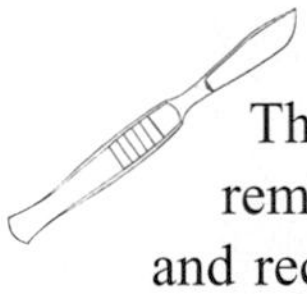

The mucosa of the piriform recess was removed earlier, and the internal laryngeal and recurrent laryngeal nerves were already partially exposed.

Now, strip the mucosa from the entire pharyngeal aspect of the larynx. This procedure will expose the following **intrinsic laryngeal muscles:**

GRANT'S 8.50
ROHEN 156
A.D.A.M. 7.26, 7.56
NETTER 72
CLEMENTE 905
A.V.A. 4: 2.32.20

- **Posterior cricoarytenoid muscles**. This pair of muscles arises from the posterior lamina of the cricoid and inserts into the muscular processes of the arytenoid cartilages.
- **Arytenoid muscle.** It unites the two arytenoid cartilages by *transverse fibers*. Some super-

ficial *oblique fibers* cross to the opposite side and toward the epiglottis. This part of the muscle is known as the *aryepiglotticus*.

Define the **cricothyroid joint**. Just posterior to the joint runs the recurrent laryngeal nerve. Cut through the ligamentous bands that hold the joint together. Disarticulate this synovial joint.

The next objective is to reflect a portion of the thyroid lamina in order to expose the remaining laryngeal muscles. Proceed as follows:

- Saw or cut the lamina of the thyroid cartilage about 8 mm to the left of the midline.
- Reflect the thyroid lamina, which is attached to the cricoid by the cricothyroid muscle.

Now, the following **laryngeal muscles** can be identified and studied (Fig. 7.98):

- **Cricothyroid,** stretching from the surface of the cricoid to the inferior border and inferior horn of the thyroid cartilage (Fig. 7.57 and 7.60A);

⇦
GRANT'S 8.50
ROHEN 156
A.D.A.M. 7.26, 7.56
NETTER 72
CLEMENTE 905
A.V.A. 4: 2.33.55

⇨
GRANT'S TABLE 8.5
ROHEN 157
A.D.A.M. TABLE 7.8
NETTER 72, 73
CLEMENTE 905, 906
A.V.A. 4: 2.27.55

⇦
GRANT'S 8.53
ROHEN 156
A.D.A.M. 7.26, 7.56, 7.57
NETTER 72
CLEMENTE 904-906
A.V.A. 4: 2.31.11

- **Lateral cricoarytenoid,** passing from the superior border of the cricoid and the cricothyroid ligament to the muscular process of the arytenoid cartilage;
- **Thyroarytenoid,** positioned superior to the lateral cricoarytenoid; it passes from the thyroid cartilage anteriorly to the arytenoid cartilage posteriorly; its superior and most medial fibers are the *vocalis*;
- **Vocalis,** applied lateral and inferior to the vocal ligament;
- **Thyroepiglotticus**, from thyroid cartilage to epiglottis.

Manipulate the arytenoid cartilages. Understand their movements in response to the actions of various laryngeal muscles. Only the **posterior cricoarytenoid** is capable of opening the **rima glottidis,** the interval between the true vocal cords. All other intrinsic laryngeal muscles close the rima glottidis. The cricothyroid muscle tilts the thyroid cartilage anteriorly and thus tenses the vocal cord (higher pitch of voice). Review the nerve supply to the laryngeal muscles.

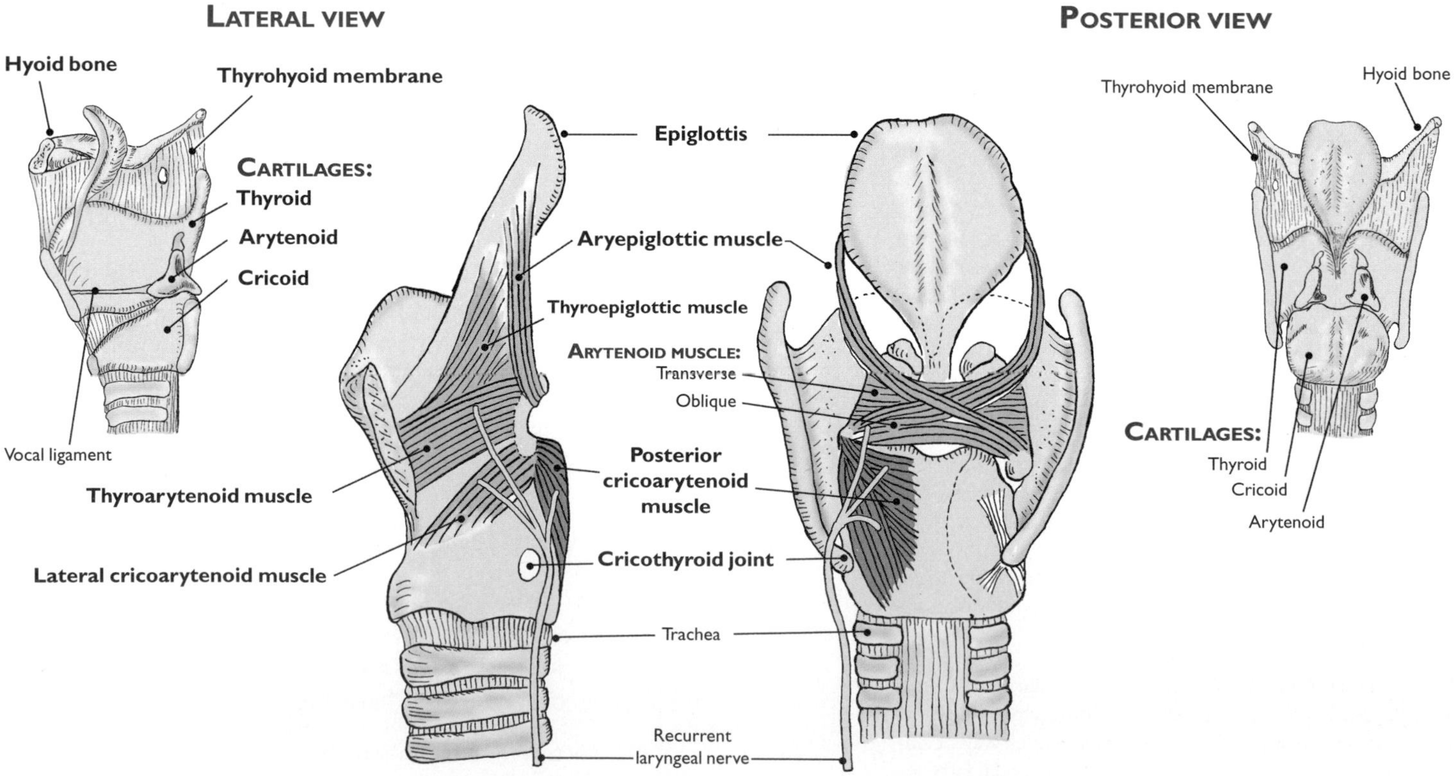

Figure 7.98. Cartilages and intrinsic muscles of larynx.

Clinical Correlation: Only the *posterior cricoarytenoid* is capable of opening the *rima glottidis*, the interval between the true vocal cords. Thus, this muscle is vital in maintaining the respiratory airway. **Laryngospasm** is a spasmodic closure of the glottic aperture. It is potentially life-threatening because breathing becomes impossible during the glottic closure. The spasm of the intrinsic laryngeal muscles that close the glottic aperture may be produced by irritating chemicals and sometimes as a dangerous side effect of certain medications.

The vocal cords can be readily visualized and inspected with the aid of a mirror (indirect laryngoscopy) or with a modern fiberoptic laryngoscope (direct laryngoscopy). Persistent hoarseness is always an indication for laryngoscopy. Persistent hoarseness may be caused by changes of the vocal cords; for example, by benign growths (polyps; warts) or by malignant tumors (cancer).

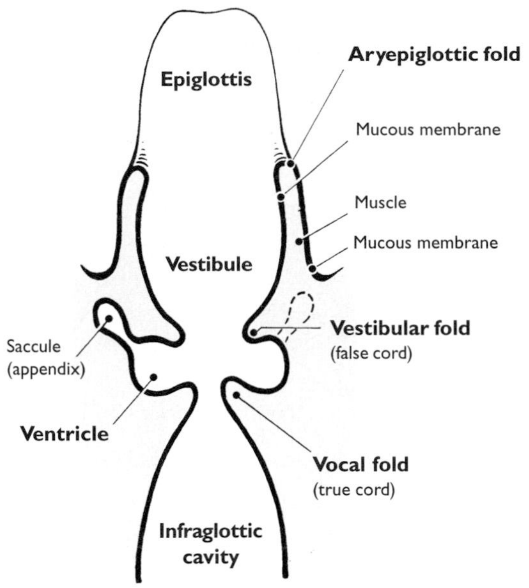

Figure 7.99. Subdivisions of the interior of the larynx.

Interior of Larynx

GRANT'S 8.54
ROHEN 157
A.D.A.M. 7.57
CLEMENTE 907-909
A.V.A. 4: 2.22.49

The **cavity of the larynx** has **three compartments** (Fig. 7.99):

- **Vestibule,** the compartment superior to the vestibular folds;
- **Ventricle,** the middle compartment between vestibular and vocal folds;
- **Infraglottic cavity,** inferior to the vocal folds and continuous with the trachea.

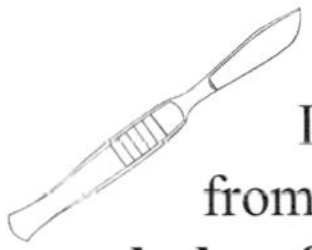

Inspect the interior of the larynx from its superior aspect. Observe the **vestibular folds** (ventricular folds; false cords) lying superolateral to the vocal cords (true cords).

GRANT'S 8.53
ROHEN 158
NETTER 74
CLEMENTE 898

The next objective is to expose the interior of the larynx. With heavy scissors, split the trachea, lamina of cricoid, and arytenoid muscle in the posterior median plane. In addition, cut the arch of the cricoid cartilage in the anterior median plane. Now, unfold the larynx.

GRANT'S 8.54-8.58
ROHEN 157
A.D.A.M. 7.57
CLEMENTE 907-909
A.V.A. 4: 2.23.53

Identify the **vestibular and vocal folds**. On each side, the depression between the two folds is the ventricle. The ventricle may extend into a recess, the saccule (Fig. 7.99). With a probe, explore ventricles and recesses.

Remove the mucous membrane from one half of the interior of the larynx. Start at the cricoid cartilage. Strip the mucosa from the triangular **cricothyroid ligament** (or conus elasticus). Observe that this membrane is attached inferiorly to the superior border of the cricoid ring. Superiorly, the free edge of the conus elasticus is thickened as the **vocal ligament.** The vocal ligament forms the basis for the vocal fold.

Next, remove the mucosa from the epiglottis and expose the epiglottic cartilage. Examine its attachment to the thyroid lamina.

Peel the mucosa from the area extending between the lateral border of epiglottic cartilage and arytenoid cartilage. The exposed membrane is the **quadrangular membrane.** Its free inferior border is the vestibular ligament, which supports the vestibular fold.

The laryngeal mucosa superior to the vocal cords is supplied with sensory fibers by the **internal laryngeal nerve**. Trace this nerve through the thyrohyoid membrane toward the interior of the larynx.

Middle Ear

General Remarks

GRANT'S 7.94C
ROHEN 118, 124
NETTER 87, 91
CLEMENTE 921, 922
A.V.A. 5: 2.31.34

The middle ear cavity or **tympanic cavity** is an air space contained within the temporal bone. Refer to schematic diagrams of the middle ear (Fig. 7.100), and study its boundaries:

- Laterally, the **tympanic membrane**; the small portion of tympanic cavity superior to the tympanic membrane is the **epitympanic recess**;

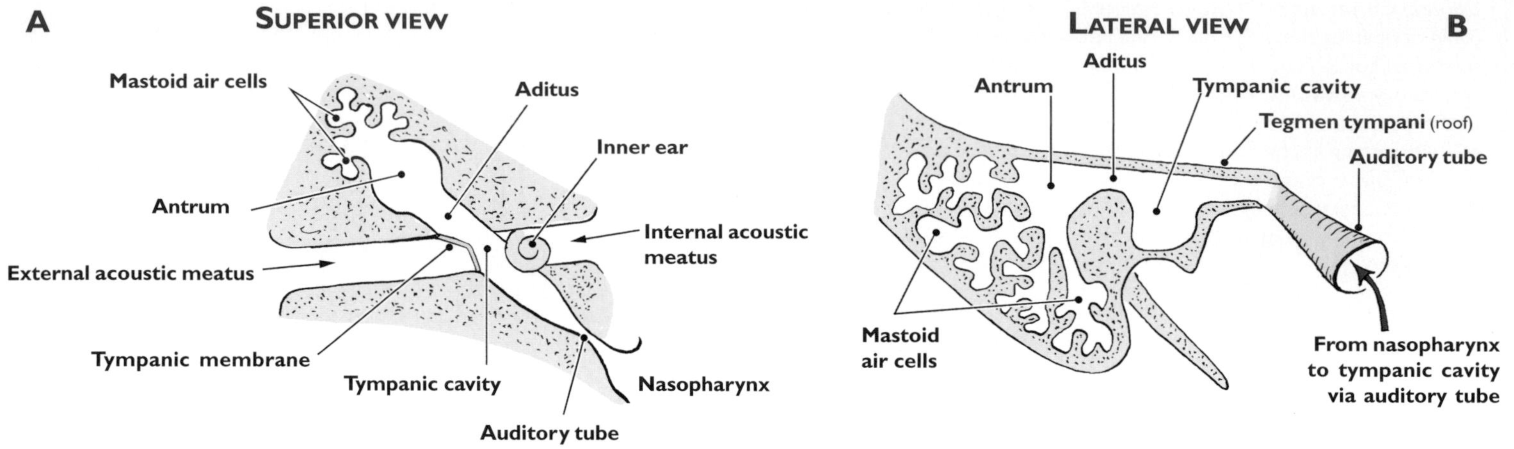

Figure 7.100. Schematic views of the middle ear and related structures. ***A***, Scheme of meatus and airway. ***B***, Diagram of tegmen tympani.

- Posteriorly, the mastoid wall; the superior portion of the wall is open; here, the **aditus** (L., *aditus,* inlet or access) leads to the **antrum** and **air cells of the mastoid process**;

Grant's 7.94C
Rohen 118, 124
Netter 87, 91
Clemente 921, 922
A.V.A. 5: 2.32.53

- Anteriorly, the **auditory tube** leads to the nasopharynx; just inferior to the auditory tube and anterior to the tympanic cavity is the carotid canal;
- Medially, the structures of the inner ear are contained within the temporal bone;
- Inferiorly, the floor of the tympanic cavity is closely related to the **jugular fossa** in which the superior jugular bulb is located;
- Superiorly, the roof or **tegmen tympani** is formed by a plate of the petrous portion of the temporal bone; the tegmen tympani separates the middle ear from the middle cranial fossa.

Each tympanic cavity contains a chain of **three auditory ossicles** that connect the tympanic membrane with the inner ear (Fig. 7.101). The middle ear cavity and its associated recesses and air cells are covered with mucous membrane.

Grant's 7.97A
Rohen 124
Netter 88, 89
Clemente 925, 926
A.V.A. 5: 2.36.12

The **facial nerve (VII)** traverses the temporal bone (Fig. 7.101). Its course is closely related to the inner and the middle ear. A branch of the facial nerve, the chorda tympani, passes between two of the auditory ossicles.

Grant's 7.100B, 9.11B
Rohen 123
A.D.A.M. 7.83
Netter 89
Clemente 931-936
A.V.A. 5: 2.32.20

Bony Landmarks

Refer to a skull and identify the following pertinent bony **landmarks:**

Grant's 7.4, 8.34
Rohen 31, 35, 121
A.D.A.M. 7.11, 7.12
Netter 5-7
Clemente 919, 9.20
A.V.A. 5: 2.27.10

- **Mastoid process**;
- **External acoustic meatus**;
- **Suprameatal spine,** just posterior to the superior part of the external acoustic meatus;

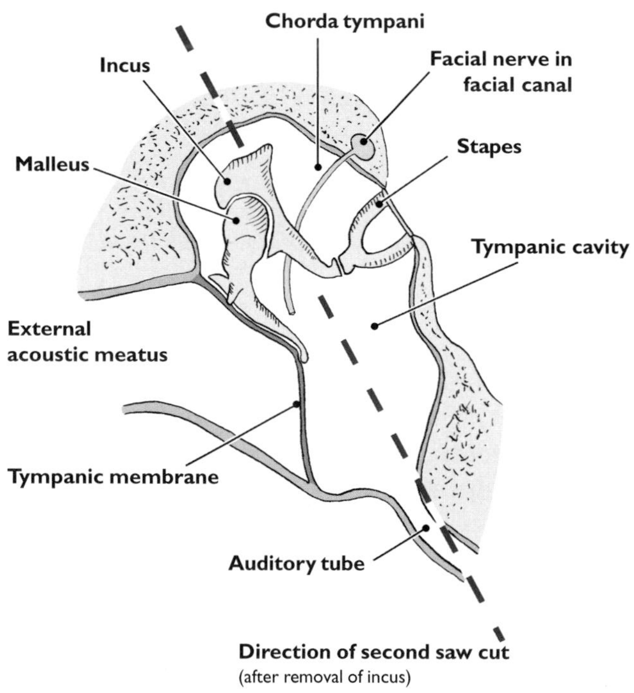

Figure 7.101. Ossicles of middle ear *in situ.*

- **Internal acoustic meatus**;
- **Hiatus** for greater petrosal nerve;
- **Tegmen tympani,** a plate of the petrous part of the temporal bone, located in the middle cranial fossa;
- **Jugular fossa** and jugular foramen;
- Bony portion of **auditory tube**;
- **Carotid canal**;
- **Stylomastoid foramen**.

Dissection of Middle Ear

If separate decalcified temporal bones are provided, make the cuts described with a very sharp scalpel or a single-edge razor blade. If only your cadaver specimen is available, the hard temporal bone must be sawed. Carry this dissection out on one side only. The objectives of this dissection are: to display the mastoid air cells; to expose the structures housed in the tympanic cavity; and to explore the walls of the tympanic cavity.

First Saw Cut. Saw coronally through the temporal bone. Start the saw cut just posterior to the suprameatal spine. Carry the cut into the cranial cavity, dividing the bone into two pieces. Now, examine the **mastoid cells.** Find the **antrum.** From the antrum pass a fine nylon thread through the **aditus** into the tympanic cavity.

⇦
GRANT'S 7.95, 7.99
NETTER 87, 118
CLEMENTE 935, 937
A.V.A. 5: 1.05.47

Identify certain soft structures that are relevant to this dissection. In the **middle cranial fossa,** remove the trigeminal ganglion and its three divisions. Define the **internal carotid artery** and the **middle meningeal artery** (or the foramen spinosum). In the **posterior cranial fossa,** identify the **facial nerve (VII)** and the **vestibulocochlear nerve (VIII)** as they pass through the internal acoustic meatus. Pass a probe into the meatus to gauge its length (approximately 19 mm). Remove the roof of the meatus. The bone is very hard. Use fine bone pliers. Protect your eyes against flying chips of bone. Observe the course of the **facial nerve**. Identify the **geniculate ganglion** and the **greater petrosal nerve.**

⇦
GRANT'S 7.100A
NETTER 89
CLEMENTE 937
A.V.A. 5: 2.34.38

Next, carefully remove the tegmen tympani. With sharp, pointed forceps, remove the incus. The incus is the strongest and the intermediate of the three auditory ossicles. Leave the malleus attached to the tympanic membrane.

⇦
GRANT'S 7.102
ROHEN 119, 120

Second Saw Cut. Stabilize the temporal bone as much as possible. Insert a fine saw into the gap created by the removal of the incus (Fig. 7.101). The saw cut is slightly oblique and parallel to the slope of the tympanic membrane. Anteriorly, the cut passes between the internal carotid artery and middle meningeal artery (foramen spinosum). Carefully split the bone into a medial and lateral piece. With skill, the auditory tube may be split longitudinally.

⇨
GRANT'S 7.100B
ROHEN 122
A.D.A.M. 7.82
NETTER 89
CLEMENTE 927
A.V.A. 5: 2.24.22

Remove the lateral piece. On it, examine the **lateral wall** of the tympanic cavity. Note the **tympanic membrane** with the attached handle of the **malleus.** The head of the malleus rises into the epitympanic recess. The **chorda tympani** is covered with mucous membrane. Identify it as it crosses the handle of the malleus medially. On the isolated piece, break down the anterior and inferior walls of the bony **external acoustic meatus**. Now, examine the lateral aspect of the tympanic membrane. Note that the membrane faces laterally, inferiorly, and anteriorly.

Anteriorly, the tympanic cavity leads to the **auditory tube.** Posteriorly, it leads to the **aditus ad antrum**. Verify these facts in the cadaver.

⇨
GRANT'S 7.101C
ROHEN 122
A.D.A.M. 7.83
NETTER 89
CLEMENTE 929-931
A.V.A. 5: 2.31.34

Examine the **medial wall** of the cavity. The features verge on the microscopic. Therefore, a magnifying lens is of great assistance. Observe at least the following features:

- **Promontory**, a gentle elevation on the medial wall, facing the tympanic membrane;
- **Stapes,** still in position in the **fenestra vestibuli** (oval window); you may be able to make out the delicate **stapedius tendon,** about 1 mm long, passing from the pyramid to the stapes;
- **Fenestra cochleae** (round window), at the bottom of a depression posteroinferior to the promontory;
- **Semicircular canals;** remove the mucosa from the medial wall of the tympanic cavity; with a probe, break into one of the three semicircular canals;
- **Tensor tympani**; it passes in a mucous fold from the medial wall to the superior part of the handle of the malleus (its tendon was divided by the saw cut);
- **Facial nerve** in the facial canal; follow the nerve proximally from the stylomastoid foramen; use a probe to force the canal open.

⇨
GRANT'S 7.104C
ROHEN 126
NETTER 91, 92
CLEMENTE 938

Dissection Note: If you wish to dissect the inner ear in detail, utilize a decalcified temporal bone. Refer to appropriate atlas illustrations. The details of the inner ear can be studied by carefully cutting, with a single-edge razor blade, thin slices of the temporal bone to expose the canals, chambers, and nerve pathways.

TEST 12

GAPP
GROSS ANATOMY PRACTICAL PRIMER

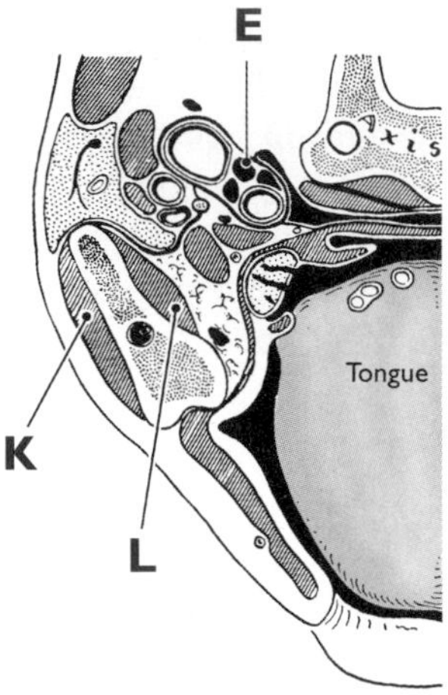

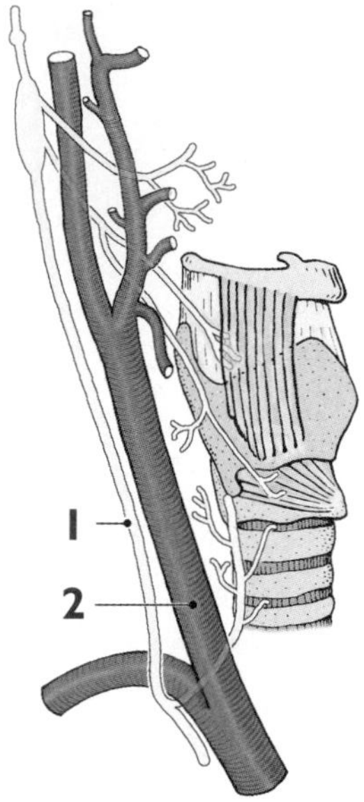

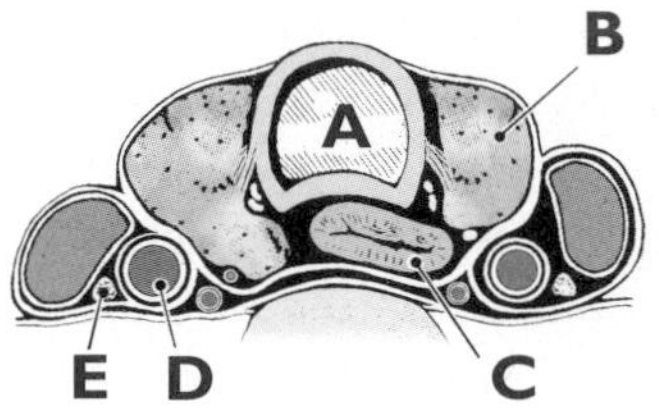

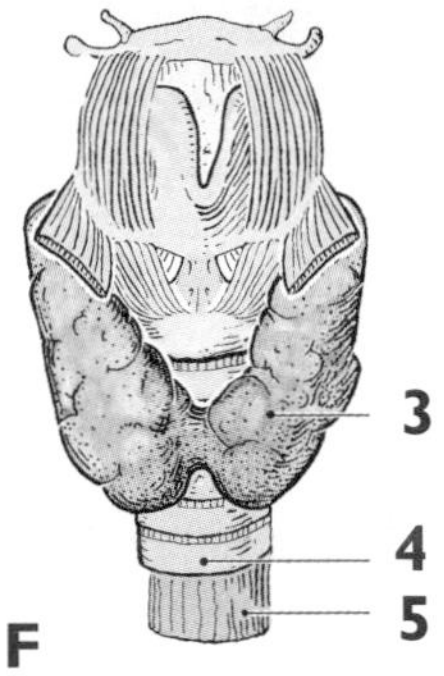

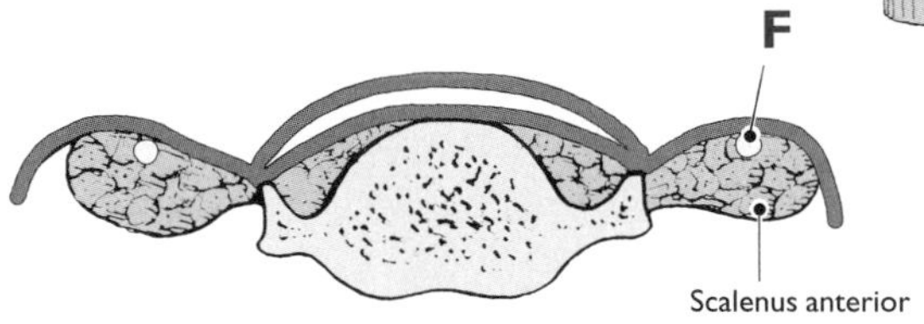

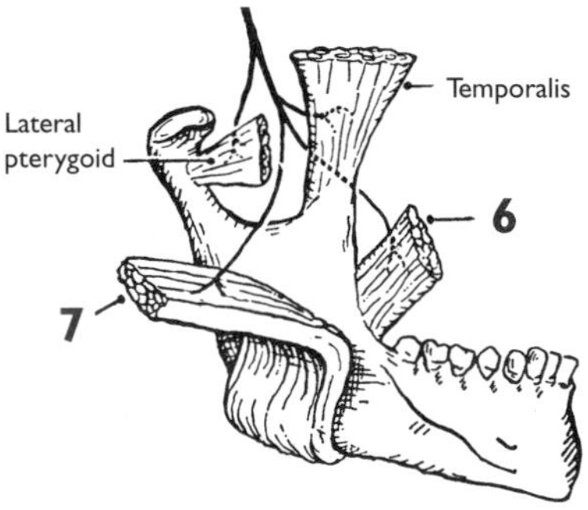

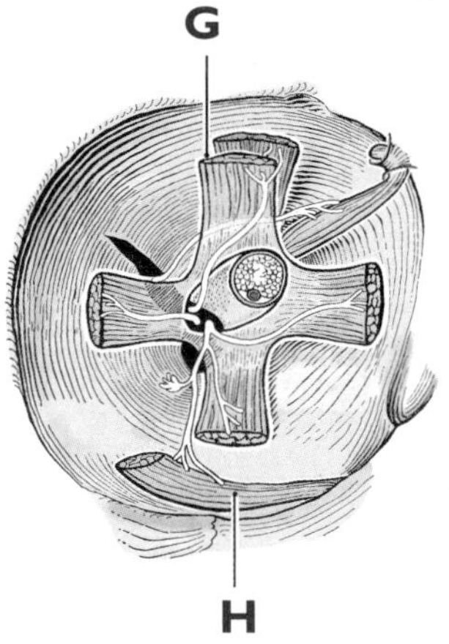

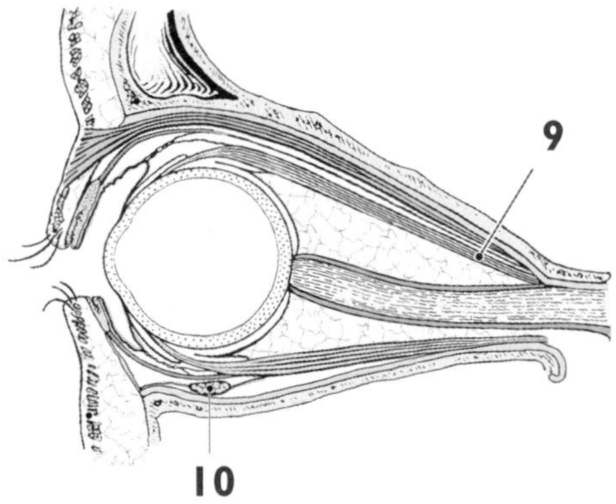

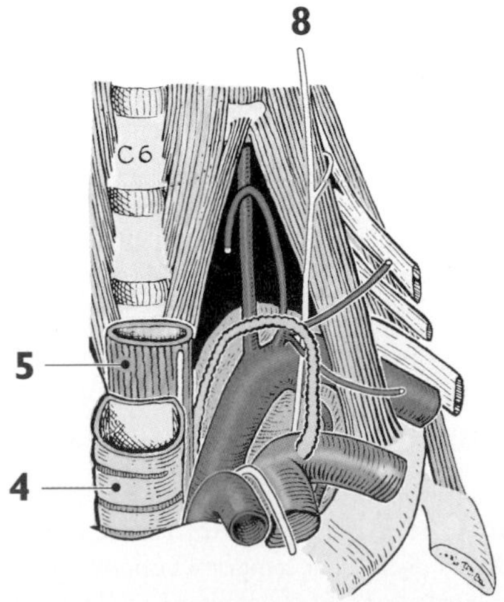

TEST YOUR 3-DIMENSIONAL CONCEPTUALIZATION.
MATCH THE NUMBERS WITH CORRESPONDING LETTERS:

1 ___	6 ___
2 ___	7 ___
3 ___	8 ___
4 ___	9 ___
5 ___	10 ___

GAPP TEST: IF YOU MADE AN ERROR, REVIEW AND GAIN A BETTER UNDERSTANDING OF THE CONCERNED 3-DIMENSIONAL ANATOMICAL CONCEPT. GAPP KEY: 1-E, 2-D, 3-B, 4-A, 5-C, 6-L, 7-K, 8-F, 9-G,10-H.

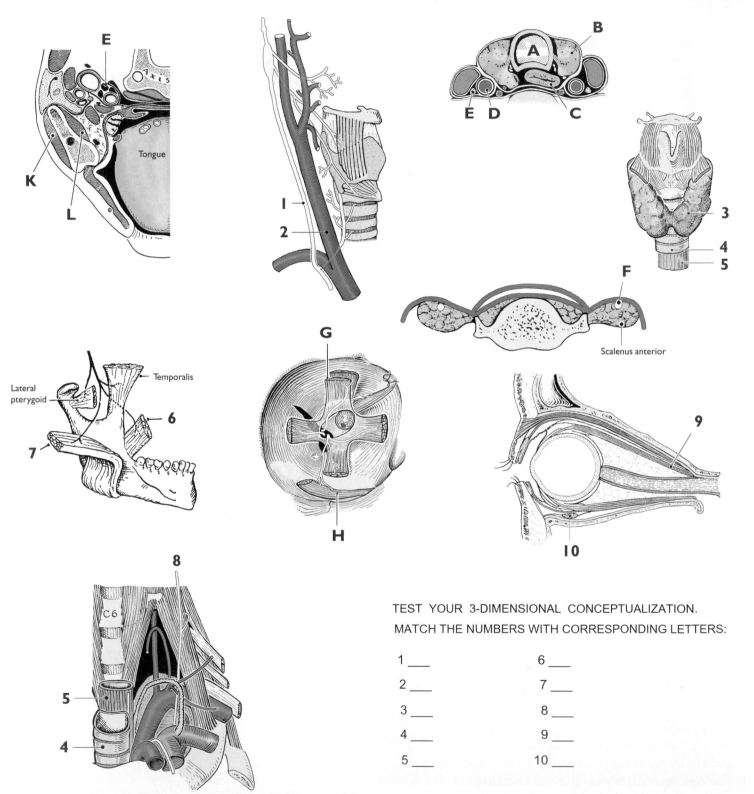

The Appendices

Appendix I - Lumbar Approach to the Kidney

General Remarks and Orientation

The **lumbar renal approach or retroperitoneal approach** to the kidney is an efficient surgical procedure. The lumbar approach does *not* involve the peritoneal cavity. Thus, contamination of the peritoneal cavity during surgery is avoided. The lumbar renal approach is indicated in a variety of renal disorders (inflammatory renal disease; renal cystic disease; tumors; calculi). On occasion, however, it is advantageous to reach the kidneys and their vessels via the transabdominal route (e.g., in kidney transplant procedures).

Level of Kidneys (Fig. A.1). In the recumbent position, the kidneys are at the level of vertebrae T12 to L3. Usually, the right kidney is slightly more inferior (1 cm) than the left one. The kidneys may move superiorly or inferiorly, depending on changes in posture and on respiratory movements. Also, there are individual variations in the precise positions of the kidneys.

Essential Posterior Relations (Fig. A.1). These relations must be understood before attempting the lumbar approach. The **superior pole of the right kidney** rises to the level of **rib 12.** The **superior pole of the left kidney** may be positioned as high as **rib 11.** The superior parts of the kidneys (with the attached suprarenal glands) are separated from the pleural cavities by the diaphragm. The medial aspect of the posterior surface of the kidney is in contact with the **quadratus lumborum.** The lateral aspect of the posterior surface is in contact with the **aponeurosis of the transversus abdominis.** The lumbar renal approach is greatly facilitated by the fact that the quadratus lumborum has an oblique lateral border. Appreciate this fact. (If the quadratus lumborum were square and if it were running from the iliac crest to the entire length of rib 12, this thick muscle would greatly impede the lumbar renal approach.)

Two nerves, which must not be cut during surgery, are in close relation to the posterior surface of the kidney (Fig. A.1): **subcostal nerve** (T12), just inferior to rib 12; and **iliohypogastric nerve** (L1), crossing obliquely the inferior pole of the kidney.

⇨ *Grant's 2.90* Netter 324 Clemente 373

⇨ Grant's 2.89 Netter 324 Clemente 435, 373

⇦ *Grant's 2.2F* Rohen 311 A.D.A.M. 3.31 Netter 311 Clemente 345

⇦ *Grant's 2.2F* Rohen 310-312 A.D.A.M. 3.31-3.33 Netter 312 Clemente 345-347 A.V.A. 3: 1.33.41

⇦ *Grant's 2.89, 2.91* Rohen 313 Netter 311, 312 Clemente 364 A.V.A. 3: 2.03.41

Important topographic knowledge can be gained by studying a transverse section through the kidneys (Fig. A.2). Again, note that the posterior surface of the kidney is related to the quadratus lumborum and the aponeurosis of the transversus abdominis. The psoas muscle lies medial to the kidney.

Review the tissues surrounding the kidney (Fig. A.2):

- **Fatty renal capsule** (adipose capsule; perinephric fatty tissue). This perirenal fat surrounds the kidney. It is thickest at the margins of the kidney. At the hilus, the renal vessels and the ureter are embedded in the fatty tissue.
- **Renal fascia** (of Gerota). It encloses both the kidney and its fatty capsule (Fig. A.2). Note the two parts of the renal fascia: **anterior layer** and **posterior layer**. It will be obvious that the renal fascia must be incised in order to gain access to the kidney. Dorsal to the renal fascia is the **paranephric fat** (pararenal fat).

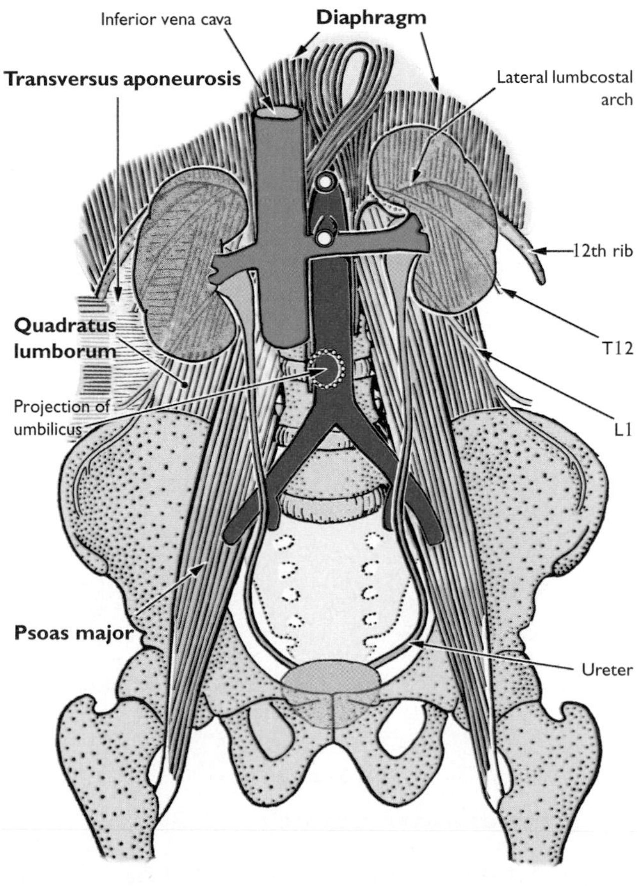

Figure A.1. Posterior relations of the kidneys.

Dissection

Place the cadaver into the prone or the lateral position. If not already done, remove the skin superior to the iliac crest. Identify the **lumbar fascia,** the **latissimus dorsi,** and the **external oblique** of the abdominal wall.

Incise the latissimus dorsi along the course of rib 12. Reflect the muscle. Palpate rib 12. Identify the thin **serratus posterior inferior.**

Next, incise the **external oblique** just inferior to the tip of rib 12, and turn it laterally. Make an incision through the **internal oblique** parallel to the free posterior border of the external oblique. Carry the cut all the way to the iliac crest. Reflect the internal oblique medially. Now, the **aponeurosis of the transversus abdominis** is exposed. Note that the aponeurosis is pierced by the **subcostal and iliohypogastric nerves.** These nerves must not be cut. Accordingly, the aponeurosis of the transversus must be incised between the two nerves.

Divide the aponeurosis of the transversus abdominis. Reflect the aponeurosis medially and expose the **quadratus lumborum.** Extend the incision superiorly. If necessary, detach the serratus posterior inferior from rib 12. Using blunt dissection, remove any fat you may encounter. This is the **paranephric fat** outside the renal fascia (Fig. A.2).

Expose the **renal fascia**. Incise it longitudinally. Palpate the kidney. Remove the **fatty renal capsule** posterior to the kidney. The structures of the hilus (renal artery, renal vein, renal pelvis, and ureter) lie just anterior to the quadratus lumborum. Gain access to these structures by retracting the quadratus lumborum medially and gently pulling the kidney laterally. Understand that the right kidney is less freely movable than the left one, since the right renal vein is much shorter than the left renal vein. Identify the **renal pelvis.** Obviously, the actual surgical approach must be more delicate than the gross anatomical exposure of the kidney.

GRANT'S 2.87
NETTER 312
A.V.A. 3: 1.33.06

GRANT'S 2.89
A.D.A.M. 3.33
NETTER 324, 325
CLEMENTE 372, 373

GRANT'S 2.88
NETTER 312
CLEMENTE 252, 360
A.V.A. 3: 1.44.32

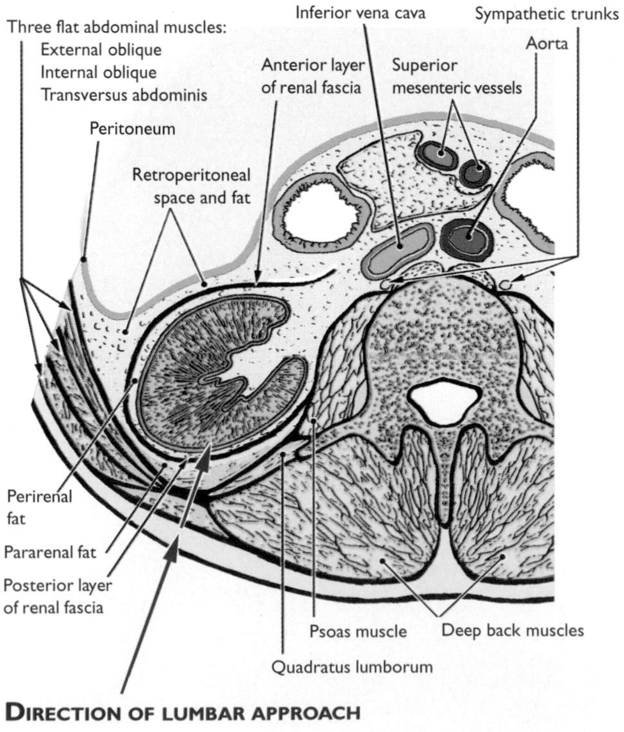

Figure A.2. Transverse section at the hilus of the right kidney. Direction of lumbar (surgical) approach to the kidney.

APPENDIX II - JOINTS

Joints of the Lower Limb

Sacroiliac Joint

GRANT'S 4.19A
ROHEN 421
A.D.A.M. 5.41
NETTER 330, 331
CLEMENTE 393
A.V.A. 3: 2.12.24

The synovial sacroiliac joint (articulation) is formed between the auricular surfaces of the **sacrum** and the **ilium**. Obtain an isolated hip bone (os coxae) and observe the **articular auricular surface of the ilium.** Identify the corresponding **auricular surface in the isolated sacrum.** Each bone has a **tuberosity** dorsal to its auricular surface. Procure an articulated pelvis and observe:

- The auricular surfaces are in apposition.
- The tuberosities are separated by a deep cleft.

Turn to the cadaver, which should be in the prone position (face down). Clean the following ligaments:

GRANT'S 4.22
NETTER 331
CLEMENTE 392
A.V.A. 3: 2.13.02

- **Sacrotuberous ligament** (Figs. A.4, A.5). Scrape the remainders of the gluteus maximus from it. Define the attachments of the ligament and clean its superior extension to the posterior iliac spines.
- **Sacrospinous ligament.** Define its attachments (Figs. A.4, A.5).

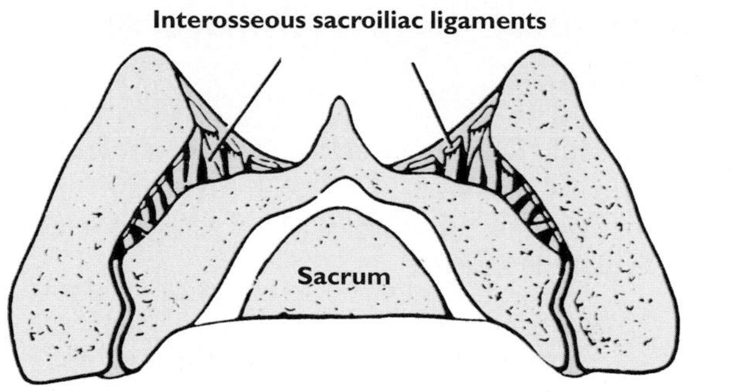

Figure A.3. Sacroiliac joint on transverse section. Note the interosseous sacroiliac ligaments anchoring the sacrum to the right ilium and left ilium.

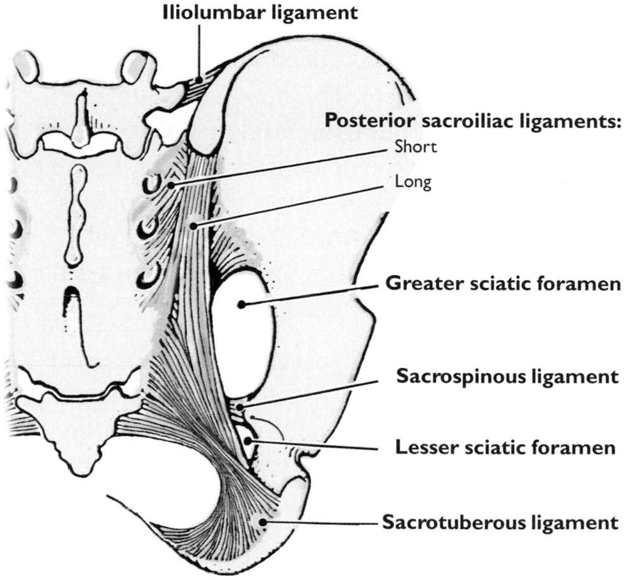

Figure A.4. Ligaments of the pelvis (posterior view).

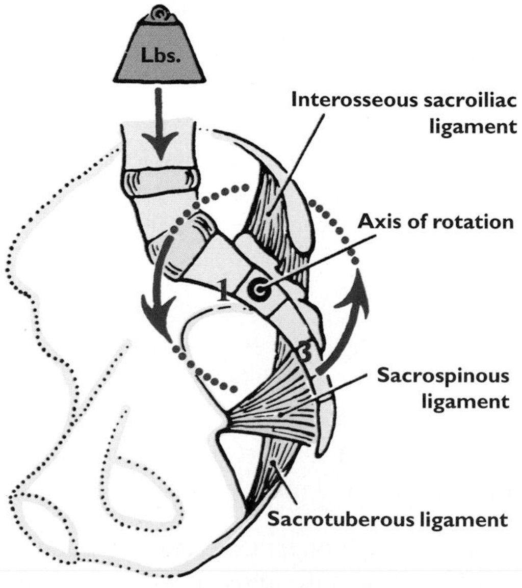

Figure A.5. Ligaments resisting rotation of the sacrum. The axis of rotation passes through S2.

GRANT'S 4.19B, 4.22
NETTER 331, 522
CLEMENTE 392

- **Posterior (dorsal) sacroiliac ligaments** (Fig. A.4). Observe long and short fasciculi that pass between the sacrum and the ilium in various directions.
- **Interosseous sacroiliac ligament** (Figs. A.3, A.5). It is exceedingly strong. It is the essential ligament of the joint. The interosseous sacroiliac ligament binds together the sacral and iliac tuberosities. This fact is best appreciated on transverse section (Fig. A.3) or on coronal section. To expose the ligament, you must remove the posterior (dorsal) sacroiliac ligaments.

GRANT'S 3.3A, 4.19A
NETTER 331, 521, 522
CLEMENTE 389, 393

Anteriorly, identify the thin **ventral sacroiliac ligament**. Cut through this ligament. It forms the ventral part of the joint capsule. Forcibly separate ilium and sacrum. Examine the cartilage-covered auricular surfaces of the joint.

Understand: Considerable weight is transmitted to the sacrum by the superimposed vertebral column. This force causes a tendency of the superior end of the sacrum to rotate anteriorly and of the inferior end of the sacrum to rotate posteriorly (Fig. A.5). The anterior rotation of the sacrum is mainly resisted by the interosseous sacroiliac ligaments and the posterior sacroiliac ligaments. The posterior rotation of the sacrum is resisted by the sacrospinous and sacrotuberous ligaments (Fig. A.5). On occasion, you will find synostosis (bony fusion) of the joint.

Hip Joint *(see Chapter 5)*

Knee Joint *(see Chapter 5)*

Ankle Joint *(see Chapter 5)*

Tibiofibular Joints

GRANT'S 5.64B
A.D.A.M. 5.5, 5.6
NETTER 479
CLEMENTE 589

Tibiofibular Joints (Fig. A.6). The fibula is moored to the tibia at its superior end, along its shaft, and at its inferior end at proximal, middle, and distal joints.

Examine an isolated fibula and a tibia. Observe a small, flat, round facet on the head of the fibula; a similar facet on the posterolateral aspect of the lateral condyle of the tibia.

GRANT'S 5.55
ROHEN 425
A.D.A.M. 5.3
NETTER 475, 476
CLEMENTE 575-577

In the cadaver, remove the popliteus tendon and the popliteus bursa posterior to the **proximal tibiofibular joint**. Verify

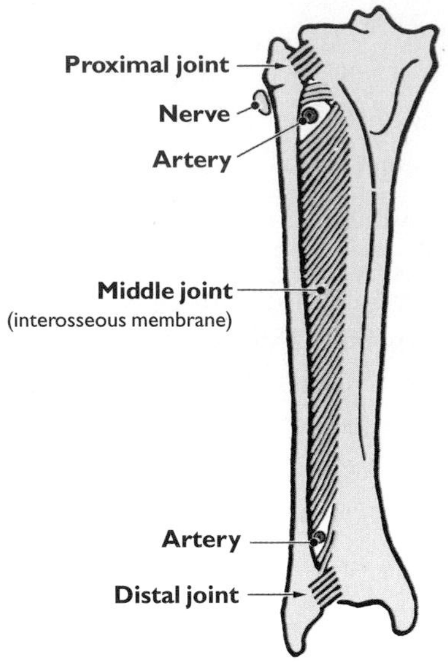

Figure A.6. Tibiofibular articulations. Note the unity of direction of the ligamentous fibers of the interosseous membrane.

that the joint capsule is strengthened by strong anterior and weak posterior fibers. Open the capsule and observe the small synovial cavity of this gliding joint.

Grant's 5.55
Rohen 425
A.D.A.M. 5.3
Netter 475, 476
Clemente 575-577

The *middle* and *distal tibiofibular joints* are *syndesmoses.* The **interosseous membrane** (middle joint) extends along the respective sides of tibia and fibula, producing a sharp line on each bone. Strip the muscles from the anterior and posterior aspect of the interosseous membrane. Observe the oval aperture between the proximal tibiofibular joint and the superior free margin of interosseous membrane. The *anterior tibial artery* passes through this opening (Fig. A.6). Observe the gap between the distal tibiofibular joint and the inferior free margin of interosseous membrane. The *perforating branch of the peroneal artery* passes through this opening (Fig. A.6).

Grant's 5.6, 5.64B
Netter 479
Clemente 589
A.V.A. 2: 1.16.31

Clean the anterior and posterior ligaments of the *distal tibiofibular joint* (Fig. A.6). These are the strong **anterior inferior** and **posterior inferior tibiofibular ligaments.** Grasp tibia and fibula well superior to the ankle, alternately squeezing the bones together and relaxing them. Note the yielding of the distal tibiofibular joint.

Grant's 5.86, 5.87
Rohen 425, 426
A.D.A.M. 5.5
Netter 479
Clemente 600-602
A.V.A. 2: 1.16.42

Joints of Inversion and Eversion
(see Chapter 5)

Joints Distal to the Transverse Tarsal Joint

Grant's 5.65C, 5.86A
Rohen 425-427
A.D.A.M. 2.55-2.56
Netter 488-492
Clemente 604-606
A.V.A. 2: 1.53.30

Intertarsal, Tarsometatarsal, and Intermetatarsal Joints. Review the bones of the foot. Frequently refer to an appropriate atlas illustration. Observe the **dorsal cuneonavicular ligaments.**

Grant's 5.86A
Netter 488-492
Clemente 604-606

Turn to the cadaver. Cut through the ligaments and open the **cuneonavicular joint** from the dorsum of the foot. Carry the incision to the **cubonavicular joint.** Explore the extent of the joint: anteriorly, it is continuous with the **intercuneiform and cuneocuboid joints.**

Grant's 5.86A, 5.94A
Netter 491, 492
Clemente 610, 611
A.V.A. 2: 1.53.34

Observe the bursa deep to the insertion of the tibialis anterior. This bursa communicates with the **first cuneometatarsal joint**. Open this joint from the dorsum of the foot. Leave the plantar ligaments intact to act as hinges. Open the joints between the tarsal and metatarsal bones. Identify the **intermetatarsal joints** (between metatarsal bones).

Grant's 5.81, 5.86A
Netter 491, 492
Clemente 610, 611
A.V.A. 2: 1.57.50

Metatarsophalangeal and Interphalangeal Joints. These are hinges, similar to the corresponding joints in the hand. Identify the **plantar ligaments** of the metatarsophalangeal joints. Observe the two sesamoid bones inferior to the head of the first metatarsal. Examine an **interphalangeal joint.** Observe that it possesses a plantar ligament and collateral ligaments.

Joints of the Upper Limb

Sternoclavicular Joint

Grant's 1.12B, 8.31
Rohen 356
A.D.A.M. 1.17, 5.71
Netter 171
Clemente 148
A.V.A. 1: 0.05.06

In the articulated skeleton, observe the relations between **sternum** and **clavicle**. Identify the **clavicular notch** of the manubrium sterni. This notch and the adjacent parts of the first costal cartilage articulate with the enlarged sternal (medial) end of the clavicle.

Turn to the cadaver. Anterior to the **sternoclavicular joint** is the tendon of the sternomastoid. Remove it. Dorsal to the joint are the broad, fleshy, strap-like sternohyoid and sternothyroid muscles.

Note the superolateral direction of the dense, parallel fibers of the anterior part of the **joint capsule.** This is the anterior sternoclavicular ligament. The costoclavicular ligament runs obliquely from the first costal cartilage to the inferior surface of the clavicle near its medial end. Clean the ligaments.

Cut through the anterior sternoclavicular ligament. In doing so, keep the blade of the scalpel close to the manubrium. Reflect the ligament. Now, the **articular disc** is exposed. It divides the articular cavity into two parts. Observe that the articular disc is attached in such a manner as to resist medial displacement of the clavicle. Inferiorly, it is attached to the first costal cartilage; superiorly, it is attached to the clavicle (Fig. A.7).

GRANT'S 8.31
ROHEN 356
A.D.A.M. 1.17
NETTER 171
CLEMENTE 148
A.V.A. 1: 0.42.38

On yourself, palpate the movements at the sternoclavicular joint. Move the scapula and, with it, the clavicle. Observe that the sternoclavicular joint allows a limited amount of movement in nearly every direction.

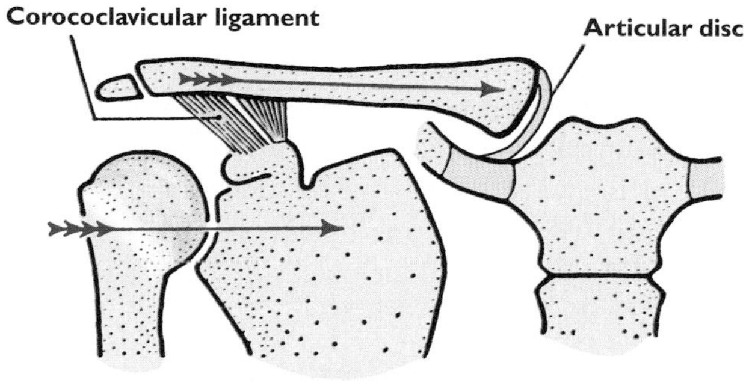

Figure A.7. Structures having unity of function: coracoclavicular ligament and articular disc of sternoclavicular joint.

Acromioclavicular Joint

Review the essential bony landmarks relevant to the acromioclavicular articulation and its associated ligaments: **acromion** and **coracoid process** of scapula; **lateral end of clavicle.**

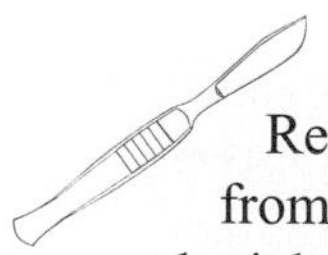

Remove the deltoid and the trapezius from the acromion and the lateral end of the clavicle. Thus, expose the **acromioclavicular joint**. The joint is subcutaneous; deep to it lies the subacromial bursa.

Identify the strong and important **coracoclavicular ligament** (Fig. A.7). Clean the two parts of the ligament, the **conoid ligament** and the **trapezoid ligament**.

Open the synovial acromioclavicular joint from its superior aspect. Remove the joint capsule completely; i.e., separate acromion from lateral end of clavicle.

Now, with the acromioclavicular joint disarticulated, the important functions of the coracoclavicular ligament can be studied. Realize that the ligament prevents the scapula from being driven medially (Fig. A.7).

On yourself, palpate the subcutaneous acromioclavicular joint. Observe that the joint enables the scapula to move vertically on the chest wall (as when shrugging the shoulders). The joint is essential to free elevation of the upper limb.

Shoulder Joint (see Chapter 6)

Elbow Joint (see Chapter 6)

Radioulnar Joints

GRANT'S 6.52, 6.53
A.D.A.M. 6.45
NETTER 409
CLEMENTE 118
A.V.A. 1: 0.04.55

The two bones of the forearm are united at the proximal, intermediate or middle, and distal radioulnar joints. The necessary rotary movements during supination and pronation take place in the proximal and distal radioulnar joints (Fig. A.8).

The **proximal radioulnar joint** (articulation) was considered with the elbow joint (see Chapter 6).

GRANT'S 6.23, 6.35A. 6.36A
ROHEN 356
A.D.A.M. 6.36
NETTER 396
CLEMENTE 72, 75

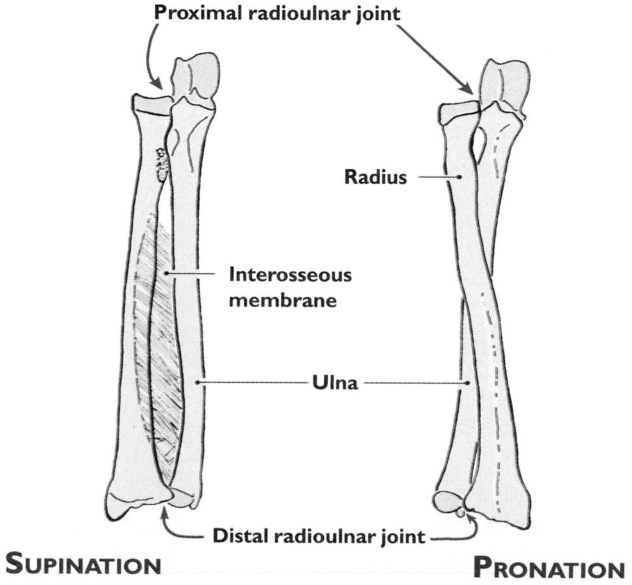

Figure A.8. Anterior view of right ulna and radius in supination and in pronation. Note proximal and distal radioulnar joints.

Intermediate (Middle) Radioulnar Joint (Fig. A.8). The shafts of the radius and ulna are united by the **interosseous membrane.** Remove or reflect all muscles from the anterior and posterior forearm, and expose the interosseous membrane. Note the direction of its fibers. The general direction of the fibers of the membrane is such that an upward thrust to the radius is transmitted to the ulna. Understand: During an upward thrust (fall on the hand), the forces are transmitted from hand via wrist joint to radius, from radius via interosseous membrane to ulna, from ulna (and radius) to humerus.

GRANT'S 6.53B
ROHEN 359
A.D.A.M. 6.45
NETTER 409
CLEMENTE 118
A.V.A. 1: 0.42.51

GRANT'S 6.87-6.89
ROHEN 359
NETTER 424. 425
CLEMENTE 126-128
A.V.A. 1: 0.49.22

Distal Radioulnar Joint (Fig. A.8). Cut through the anular ligament and release the head of the radius. Cut the interosseous membrane. Pass the blade of the scalpel through a sac-like recess, the **sacciform recess**. Now, enter the distal radioulnar joint. Do *not* injure the triangular **articular disc**.

GRANT'S 6.83-6.86
ROHEN 358, 359
A.D.A.M. 6.47
NETTER 409, 424, 425
A.V.A. 1: 0.47.52

Swing the radius laterally and view the **articular disc.** Observe:

- It is fibrocartilaginous. Its apex and its anterior and posterior margins are ligamentous.
- The apex is attached to the styloid process of the ulna.
- The base of the triangular disc is attached to the ulnar notch of the radius.
- The ligamentous borders of the disc spread far laterally on the radius.
- Commonly, the cartilaginous part of the disc is perforated (the disc is subjected to constant pressure and friction).

Wrist Joint (see *Chapter 6*)

Small Joints of the Hand

Review the bones of the hand. The osseofibrous **carpal tunnel** has already been opened (Chapter 6). Remove all contents from the carpal tunnel. Trace the tendon of the flexor carpi radialis through its special tunnel to the second metacarpal. Verify that the tubercle of the scaphoid acts as a pulley for the tendon. Observe that the lunate bulges conspicuously into the carpal tunnel.

Clean the **intercarpal, carpometacarpal, and intermetacarpal ligaments.** Open all joints from the palmar aspect. First, open the **midcarpal joint (transverse carpal joint)** by entering the scalpel between tubercle of scaphoid and tubercle of trapezium. Observe the sinuous surfaces of the opposed bones. Observe synovial folds that project into the joint.

Next, open the **carpometacarpal joints**. The carpometacarpal joint of the thumb (digit 1) has a loose capsule with parallel fibers. Manipulate the metacarpal bones. Observe the hinge movements at the bases of the 4th and 5th carpometacarpal joints. The flexion possible at these two joints allows the grip of the hand to be more secure.

Joints of the Digits

In the clefts between the fingers, the lumbrical muscles and the digital nerves and vessels pass anterior to the **deep transverse metacarpal ligaments.** The interossei pass dorsal to the ligaments. On each side, the deep transverse metacarpal ligaments are continuous with the palmar ligaments that form the proximal limit of the posterior wall of the fibrous digital flexor sheath.

GRANT'S 6.90
ROHEN 359
A.D.A.M. 6.59, 6.60
NETTER 427
CLEMENTE 128, 129
A.V.A. 1: 1.20.27

Metacarpophalangeal Joints. Cut one or more of the deep transverse metacarpal ligaments. Remove the interossei and the dorsal extensor expansion. Clean a pair of collateral ligaments. They are triangular and important. A *cord-like part* passes to the base of the adjacent phalanx; a *fan-like part* passes to the side of the palmar ligament. Verify: the strong, cord-like parts of the collateral ligaments are eccentrically attached to the flat metacarpal heads. The ligaments are slack during extension and taut during flexion. Therefore, the fingers cannot be spread (abducted) unless the hand is opened.

GRANT'S 6.83-6.86
A.D.A.M. 6.59, 6.60
NETTER 424, 430
CLEMENTE 126-128

Interphalangeal Joints. Study the collateral ligaments of the interphalangeal joints. These are hinge joints. Explore the synovial cavity of the joints. Inspect the articular surfaces that are covered with smooth cartilage.

APPENDIX III - EYEBALL OF BULL

General Remarks

The dissection of the *eyeball of the bull* is a convenient way to acquire a general knowledge of the gross anatomical features of the human eye.

The **eyeball** or **bulbus oculi** has **three concentric coats** (Fig. A.9):

- **External or fibrous coat:** *sclera* and *cornea;*
- **Middle or vascular coat:** *choroid, ciliary body* and *iris;*
- **Internal or retinal coat:** a). *Outer layer* of pigmented cells; b). *Inner layer*; the cells of this layer are nervous (visual) posterior to the ora serrata.

The **four refractive media** are (Fig. A.9):

- **Cornea;**
- **Aqueous humor;**
- **Lens;**
- **Vitreous body.**

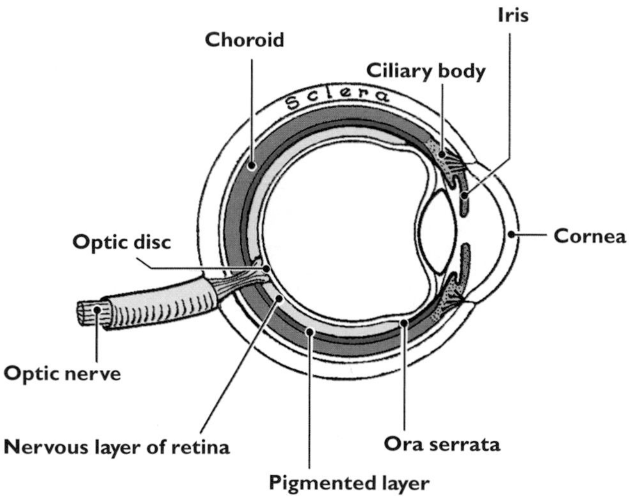

Figure A.9. Scheme of an eyebal (sagittal section).

Posterior and Anterior Halves of Eye

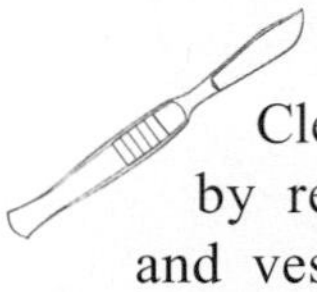

Clean the exterior of the eyeball or bulb by removing the adherent fat, muscles, and vessels. Leave the stump of the optic nerve intact. Anteriorly, sever the conjunctiva at the corneoscleral junction (margin) and remove it.

Divide the bulb into posterior and anterior halves by cutting with a sharp scalpel (new blade) around the equator. During this process, you will successively cut the sclera, choroid, retina, and the vitreous body.

GRANT'S 7.51
ROHEN 130
A.D.A.M. 7.71
NETTER 86
CLEMENTE 818, 821, 822

Examination of Posterior Half, Inner Aspect. The **retina** is dull and gray like an exposed photographic film and it is exceedingly friable. It is held in position and applied to the choroid by the vitreous body.

GRANT'S 7.51
ROHEN 129
A.D.A.M. 7.71
NETTER 82
CLEMENTE 819

Gently scoop out the jelly-like **vitreous body** with the handle of a scalpel. Now, the **retina** is no longer firmly applied to the choroid. As a result, it falls into folds, except at the optic disc. The **optic disc** is the site where the fibers of the optic nerve pierce the sclera, choroid, and outer retinal layer to spread out into the inner (optic) layer of the retina. The disc is a blind spot (compare with the human eye).

GRANT'S 7.51B
ROHEN 128, 129
NETTER 86
CLEMENTE 817

The **choroid** is the thin and pigmented vascular middle coat (Fig. A.10). Generally, it is easily detached as a whole from the sclera. At several spots, however, the choroid is bound to the sclera of the posterior half of the bulb:

- Where it is pierced by the optic nerve;
- Where the vorticose veins leave it near the equator to pierce the sclera (compare with the human eye).

There are certain differences between the human eye and the bull's eye: the pupil of the bull's eye is not round (compare the human eye, Fig. A.9, with the eyeball of a bull, Fig. A.10). There is no macula in the eye of the bull.

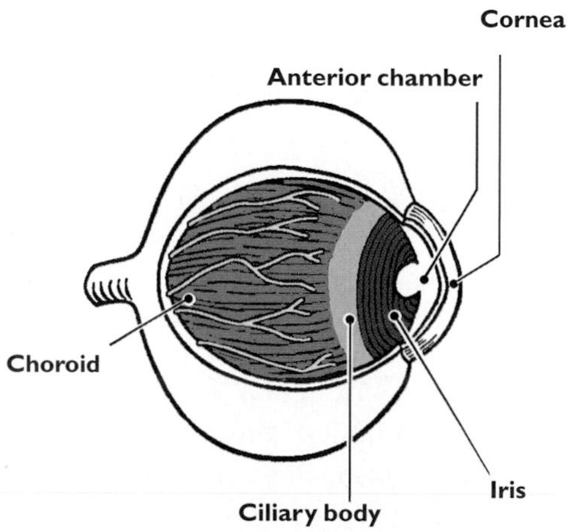

Figure A.10. Eyeball of a bull: the middle coat is exposed.

In the bull, but not in man, a wide triangular area of the choroid superior to the level of the optic disc has a greenish-blue metallic sheen. This is due to the presence of a fibrous sheet, the tapetum, between the layers of the choroid. In animals, this tapetum is responsible for the intense light reflections from the eyes at night.

Examination of Anterior Half, Inner Aspect. Observe the anterior part of the vitreous body. Gently remove it. The dull gray optic part of the retina ends well anterior to the equator in a slightly scalloped margin, the **ora serrata.**

Anterior to the ora serrata lies the ciliary zone. Here, about 70 black, finger-like ridges, the **ciliary processes,** converge on the equator of the **lens.** Note that the lens is suspended by numerous **zonular fibers** (compare with the human eye).

Grant's 7.51
Rohen 129
A.D.A.M. 7.71
Netter 83
Clemente 819, 820

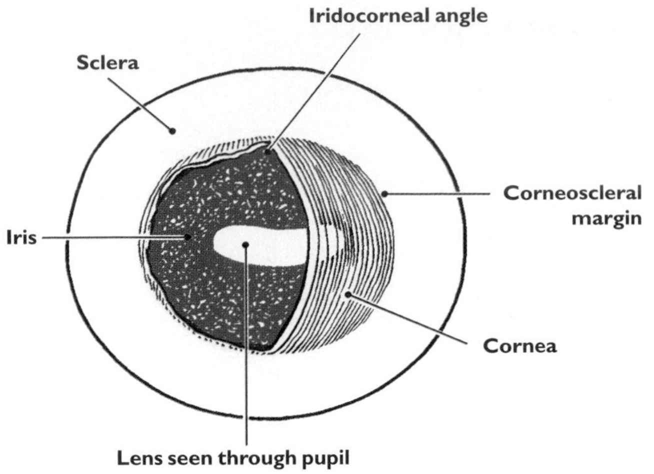

Figure A.11. Bull's eye: anterior approach - I.

Dissection (Anterior Approach)

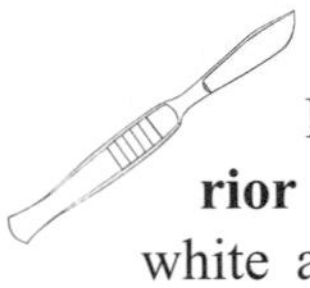

Dissection of the bull's eye; anterior approach (Fig. A.11). The sclera is white and tough. It is continuous with the transparent **cornea.** Through the cornea observe the dark **iris,** which surrounds the **pupil.** Posterior to the pupil is the lens. Proceed:

Grant's 7.51
Rohen 130
Netter 86
Clemente 820

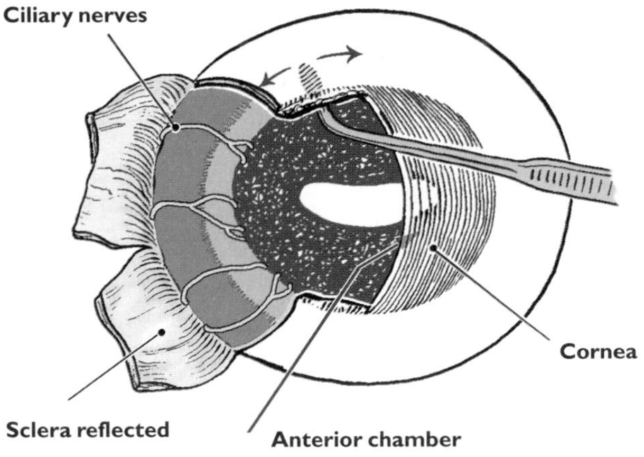

Figure A.12. Bull's eye: anterior approach - II.

- With a sharp scalpel, incise the cornea vertically.
- With scissors, cut horizontally along the corneoscleral junction. Leave the right quarter of the cornea intact. You have now opened the **anterior chamber** which, in the living, is filled with aqueous humor.
- Place a probe into the angle between iris and cornea, the **iridocorneal angle** (Fig. A.12).
- Pass the point of a probe through the pupil and into the space between the lens and the posterior surface of the iris. The probe is now in the **posterior chamber.**
- Remove a section of the iris (Fig. A.13).

Grant's 7.51
Rohen 129
A.D.A.M. 7.71
Netter 84
Clemente 819, 821, 823

Examine the exposed posterior chamber, which is triangular on transverse section. It is bounded anteriorly by the iris, posteriorly by the lens and zonular fibers, and laterally by the ends of the ciliary processes (compare with the human eye).

Grant's 7.51
Rohen 129
A.D.A.M. 7.71
Netter 85
Clemente 819, 821, 823

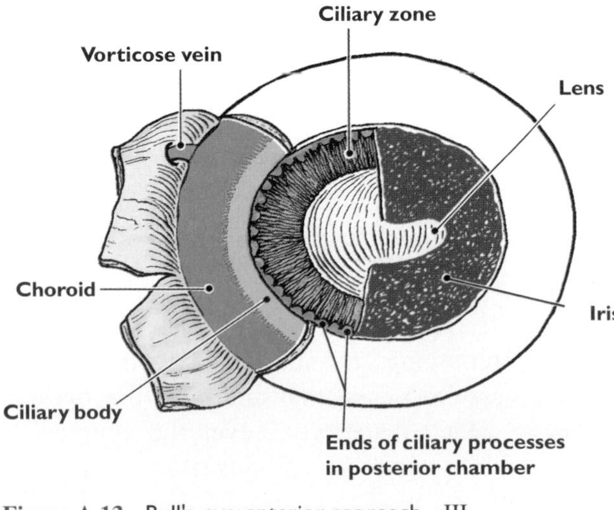

Figure A.13. Bull's eye: anterior approach - III.

Cut horizontally through the anterior portion of the capsule of the lens. The lens will pop out; if not, it can be easily extruded. Note that the anterior surface of the **lens** is less curved than the posterior surface. proceed:

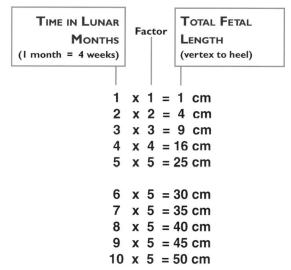

◁
GRANT'S 7.51
ROHEN 129
A.D.A.M. 7.71
NETTER 84
CLEMENTE 819, 821

- Place the point of a probe in the **iridocorneal angle** (Fig. A.13).
- Break through the firm attachment of the ciliary muscle to the anterior limit of the sclera.
- Detach the ciliary muscle widely.
- Press the probe against the sclera; this will avoid damage to the delicate choroidal coat.

With strong scissors, cut a sector of sclera and reflect it posteriorly. Observe the following (Figs. A.12 and A.13):

◁
GRANT'S 7.51
ROHEN 129
NETTER 83, 85
CLEMENTE 820

- A circular band, about 4 mm in width; this is the outer surface of the **ciliary body;** the ciliary body contains the ciliary muscle and the ciliary processes;
- Numerous white streaks; these are the **ciliary nerves;** they run toward the ciliary body and iris. Understand the function of these nerves.

APPENDIX IV FETUS AND PLACENTA

General Remarks

The dissection of a fetus will enhance any physician's understanding for pediatric problems, particularly regarding malformations. Frequently, a spontaneously aborted fetus is anatomically defective. In general, the student will be surprised how effortless and quickly the dissection of the fetus can be accomplished and how much general anatomical knowledge can be gleaned from such a dissection.

◁
ROHEN 271, 339
CLEMENTE 223, 433

The life of the growing fetus depends entirely on an intra-uterine organ, the placenta. The placenta is a most complex, temporary organ that performs several important functions:

- As an organ of respiration, it provides for the vital exchange of oxygen and carbon dioxide.
- As an organ of nutrition, it makes all essential nutrients available to the fetal blood.
- As and organ of excretion, it eliminates waste products by transporting them from the fetal blood into the maternal blood; subsequently, these waste products are eliminated by the mother.
- The placenta also functions as a powerful endocrine gland, regulating physiologic stability and economy of both fetus and mother.

Clinical Correlation: In view of the importance of the placenta, it is not surprising that placental dysfunctions or pathological changes of the placenta have grave consequences for the life of the fetus. Therefore, abnormal placental findings are often diagnostic of neonatal disease or death. At any rate, every physician should have a good understanding of the placenta. Its dissection is a most appropriate educational experience.

Determining the Age

Estimate the **age of the human fetus** available for dissection. The age of the fetus is often determined from its crown-rump length (sitting height). Estimation of age may also be based on the *total length* (vertex to heel). Utilize this simple and easily remembered formula to determine the approximate age of the fetus:

TIME IN LUNAR MONTHS (1 month = 4 weeks)		**Factor**		**TOTAL FETAL LENGTH** (vertex to heel)
1	x	1	=	1 cm
2	x	2	=	4 cm
3	x	3	=	9 cm
4	x	4	=	16 cm
5	x	5	=	25 cm
6	x	5	=	30 cm
7	x	5	=	35 cm
8	x	5	=	40 cm
9	x	5	=	45 cm
10	x	5	=	50 cm

Examples:

- After 3 lunar months or 12 weeks, the total length of the fetus is approximately $3^2 = 9$ cm long.
- A fetus measuring 20 cm in total length is approximately 4.5 lunar months or 18 weeks old.
- A premature baby born at 26 weeks (6.5 lunar months) of gestation is approximately 32 cm long.
- After 10 lunar months or 40 weeks, the mature newborn measures 50 cm from vertex to heel.

Note: The total length of a fetus may vary slightly from case to case, depending on genetic factors. Most full-term babies are between 46 to 55 cm (18 to 22 inches) long. The average is 50 cm or about 20 inches.

Exposure of Thoracic and Abdominal Viscera

Thoracic Incisions (Fig. A.14): Make two transverse incisions through the skin (A to B; C to D). Reflect the skin and the pectoral muscles. With scissors, cut through the soft, pliable rib cage from D to B and from C to A. Next, cut across the rib cage and sternum from A to B. Elevate the anterior chest wall. Cut across it from C to D, at the level of the diaphragm. Now, the thoracic viscera are exposed.

Abdominal Incisions (Fig. A.14): These incisions must be made in such a manner that the umbilical vein and the two umbilical arteries are not destroyed. Starting at point C, cut with scissors through the thin diaphragm and enter the abdominal cavity. Cut through all layers of the abdominal wall, and carry the incision to the midpoint of the inguinal region (E). Make an equivalent incision on the left side (D to F). Carefully lift up the right triangular flap of abdominal wall (D to C to E). Identify the umbilical ring at the inner surface of the abdominal wall. Here, several structures converge:

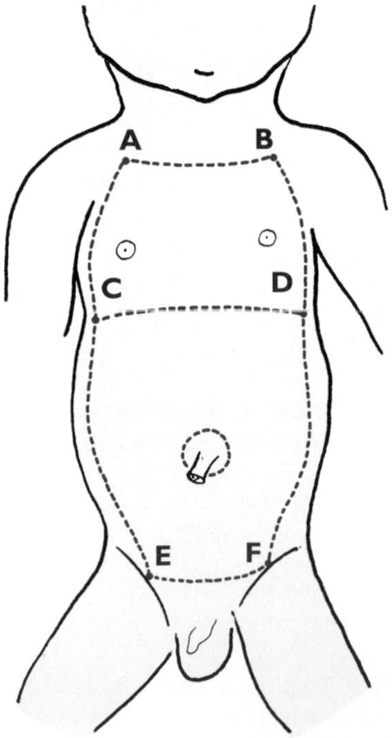

Figure A.14. Incisions to expose thoracic and abdominal viscera of fetus.

ROHEN 271
NETTER 217

- **Falciform ligament**; along its free margin identify the relatively thick **umbilical vein**;
- Right and left **umbilical arteries**;
- **Urachus**, contained in the median umbilical fold between the two umbilical arteries.

Using small scissors, dissect these structures from the abdominal wall, but leave them attached to the umbilical ring. Remove the entire abdominal wall, with the exception of a small circular region around the umbilicus. Now, the abdominal viscera are exposed. The umbilical region and the important structures converging upon it are still intact.

Cardiovascular and Respiratory Systems

Observe that the unexpanded **lungs** do not conceal the **pericardial sac**. The **thymus** is large and covers the upper part of the pericardial sac anteriorly.

ROHEN 271
NETTER 217
CLEMENTE 224

Identify the **umbilical vein**. In the living fetus, this vessel carries oxygenated blood from the placenta (Fig. A.15). Follow the vein along the free margin of the **falciform ligament** to the left **portal vein**. Most of the blood by-passes the liver via the **ductus venosus**, which connects the left portal vein with the inferior vena cava. The ductus venosus occupies a fissure at the posterior aspect of the liver. To expose this duct, dissect the liver away piece by piece. Demonstrate the continuity of the ductus venosus with the **inferior vena cava**.

To facilitate examination of the **heart**, remove the lungs, the thymus, and the brachiocephalic veins.

> **Clinical Correlation:** With scissors, cut off a piece of lung tissue and place it into a container with water. Does the tissue float or sink? Of forensic importance: The compact lungs of a still-born child are so dense that they sink. In contrast, previously aerated lungs float in water. Thus the pathologist can answer the question whether or not a newborn had ever breathed air.

ROHEN 270
NETTER 217
CLEMENTE 224

Incise the **pericardial sac**. Open the **right atrium**. Identify the large **foramen ovale**. Realize that, due to fluid dynamics, most of the oxygenated blood from the **inferior vena**

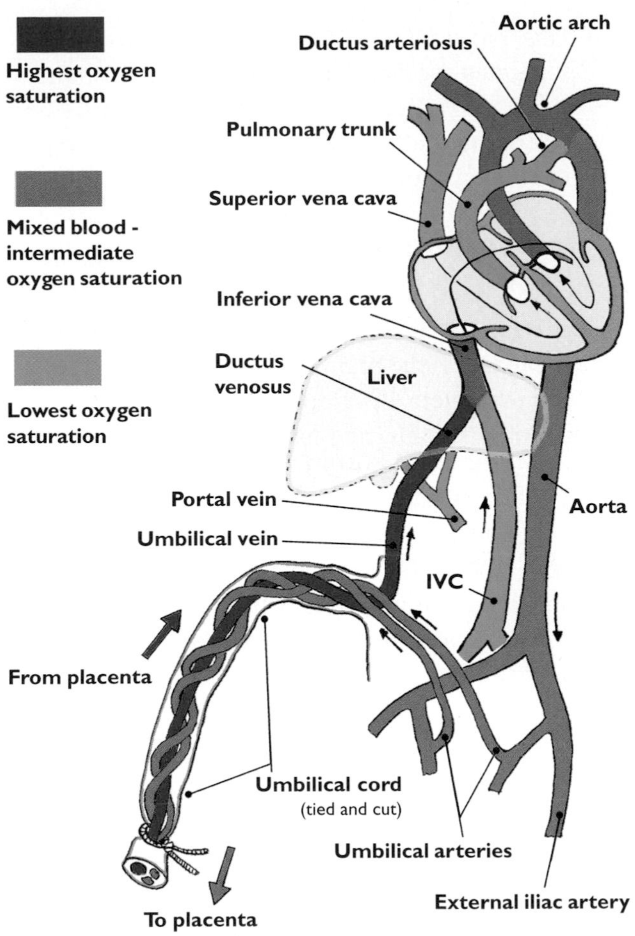

Figure A.15. Simplified diagram of fetal circulation.

cava passes through the foramen ovale into the **left atrium** (Fig. A.15). From there, the blood passes through the **left ventricle** to the **ascending aorta** and the **aortic arch**. Follow this path.

In contrast, and mainly due to fluid dynamics, the majority of deoxygenated blood from the **superior vena cava** passes through the right atrium into the **right ventricle** and on into the **pulmonary trunk** (Fig. A.15). From there, it passes through the large **ductus arteriosus** into the aorta. Follow this path. Verify that the ductus arteriosus reaches the aortic arch just inferior to the origin of the left subclavian artery.

Observe that the diameter of the pulmonary trunk is equal to that of the aorta. In the fetus, the wall of the right atrium is as thick as that of the left ventricle.

ROHEN 271
NETTER 217
CLEMENTE 223, 224

Follow the two **umbilical arteries** from the internal iliac arteries to the umbilical cord. Are there any sensory nerves in the umbilical cord? Is it painful for the newborn to have his or her umbilical cord tied and cut?

In the thoracic cavity, find the **right and left vagus nerve** and the bilateral **phrenic nerves**. Identify the **splanchnic nerves**. The **diaphragm** is only a thin, translucent membrane.

Gastrointestinal System

The **liver** is very large. Since there was no prior food intake, the **stomach** is empty. Identify the **cecum** with the attached appendix; it may not as yet have fully descended into its usual position. The cylindrical **rectum** almost fills the lesser pelvis. Identify the various parts of the **gastrointestinal tract**. The intestines are either empty or contain black meconium (consisting of epithelial cells, mucus, and bile). The **spleen** is conspicuous.

Remove the gastrointestinal tract, the liver, and the spleen. Find the **pancreas**.

Genito-Urinary System

Observe the large **suprarenal glands** covering the upper poles of the **kidneys**. Note the lobulated surface of the kidneys. Follow the sizeable **ureters** to the **urinary bladder**. Identify the **urachus**, which extends from the apex of the bladder to the umbilical ring.

GRANT'S 2.15B
NETTER 360
CLEMENTE 273, 448

If the fetus is a male, look for the **testes**. How far have they descended? During the 7th month, the testes are at the level of the inguinal canal. By the end of the 8th month, they are usually within the scrotal sac. Is the **processus vaginalis** open? Note that the scrotum of younger specimens is formed but empty.

ROHEN 270, 271
NETTER 217
CLEMENTE 224

If the fetus is a female, identify the **uterus**, **uterine tubes**, and **ovaries**.

Head and Neck

Cut away the auricle. Remove the scalp. Observe the following:

- There is no bony external acoustic meatus, but only a **tympanic ring**.
- The **tympanic membrane** is very close to the surface.
- There is no mastoid process. This leaves the **facial nerve** relatively unprotected (injuries to facial nerve after application of obstetrical forceps).
- The primary teeth have not yet erupted. Cut across the maxilla or the mandible and look for a **developing tooth**.
- There are no air sinuses. Therefore, the face is small.
- Identify the large **anterior fontanelle** and the smaller **posterior fontanelle** (Fig. A.16). These structures are of obstetrical and pediatric importance.
- Examine the thin and pliable bones of the calvaria.

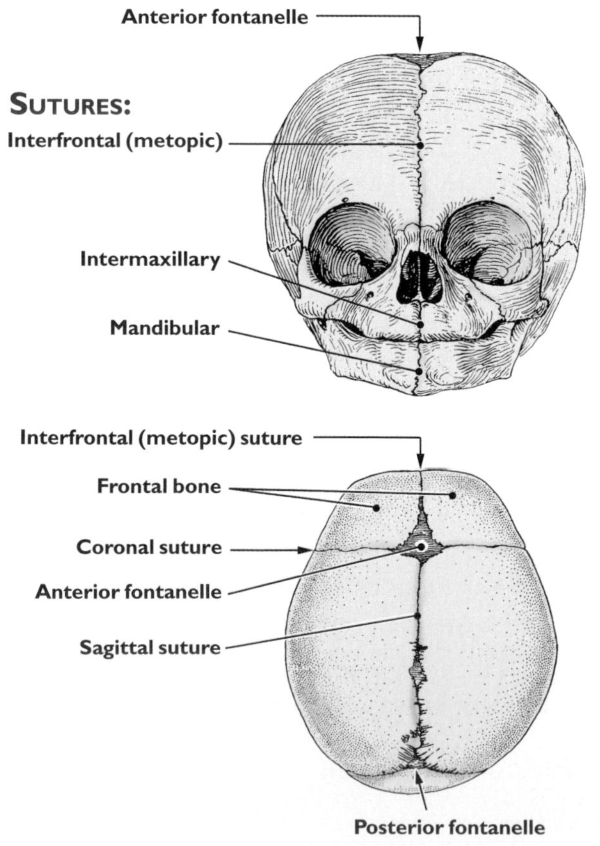

Figure A.16. Suture lines and fontanelles of skull of newborn.

NETTER 50
CLEMENTE 460

GRANT'S 7.6
CLEMENTE 760-763

ROHEN 271, 339
CLEMENTE 223, 433

- Observe the **frontal or metopic suture** that separates the two halves of the frontal bone (Fig. A.16). Remember: In the adult, this suture is normally closed and absent; however, in about 2% of all cases it persists.

Further Examination

Feel free to examine any structure of interest. If the brain is well preserved, note its incomplete development. Examine eyelids, digits, nails, and hair.

Make a longitudinal section through a long bone. It starts to ossify during the 2nd fetal month. Observe that the ends of the bone are cartilaginous. The skeletal age of children is commonly assessed by radiological examination.

Placenta

The **placenta** is an important organ which makes possible the metabolic interchange between mother and fetus. In smaller specimens, placenta and umbilical cord are often still attached to the fetus. By the fourth month of gestation (total fetal length 16 cm), the fetus and its placenta are approximately equal in weight. At that time, the placenta has developed its two components: the fetal portion and the maternal portion. The mature placenta at term averages 1/6 to 1/7 of the weight of the newborn. Examine a suitable specimen.

Placenta still attached to fetus via umbilical cord. Identify the rough **maternal aspect** of the placenta. By contrast, the **fetal aspect** is smooth; the **umbilical cord** is attached to its surface.

Expose the blood vessels within the umbilical cord. Under normal circumstances, you will find two **umbilical arteries** and a single **umbilical vein**. Follow these vessels to the umbilical region and establish their continuity within the fetus.

Mature Placenta (Fig. A.17). The organ may either be fresh or embalmed. Note its weight (approximately 450 to 600 grams) and its size (varying from 16 to 21 cm in diameter and 2.5 to 3.0 cm in thickness). Begin examination of the placenta by placing the rough maternal surface down on the table; the fetal surface points upward.

Fetal Membranes. Envision the fetus in the amniotic sac. Realize that this sac has ruptured to allow expulsion of the child. The so-called "water", the amniotic fluid, in which the child was suspended, has long been drained. Identify the torn fetal membranes (transparent amnion + slightly thicker chorion) adherent to the margins of the placenta and continuous with its smooth fetal aspect (Fig. A.17).

CLEMENTE 223

Examine the **umbilical cord** (Fig. A.17). It is approximately 50 to 55 cm long. It appears white, moist and coiled. Examine a cross section through the cord. Note that the diameter of the single **umbilical vein** is larger than that of the two **umbilical arteries**.

Dissect a portion of the cord and verify that the blood vessels are contained in a matrix of mucinous stroma (Wharton's jelly) and that they are coiled around each other. Follow the umbilical cord to the placenta. Usually, the cord is centrally attached. Marginal attachments are relatively rare.

Inspect the **fetal surface** (or inner surface) of the placenta. It is covered with smooth, shiny and transparent **amnion**. Subjacent to the amnion is the **chorionic plate** which has a mottled appearance. Note the fetal blood vessels radiating from the attachment of the umbilical cord (Fig. A.17).

CLEMENTE 223

Turn the placenta over and examine its **maternal surface** (Fig. A.17). It is granular and lobulated. There are between 15 to 20 lobes, termed **cotyledons**. The cotyledons are separated by grooves. These grooves correspond to incomplete **placental septa** or **decidual septa** which extend from the maternal surface toward the chorionic plate.

Clinical Correlation: In obstetrics, examination of the placenta is of great importance. An incomplete placenta (e.g., cotyledon left in the uterus) may result in serious *post-partum* complications, such as continued uterine bleeding and/or infections. In addition, abnormal placental findings are often diagnostic of neonatal disease or death.

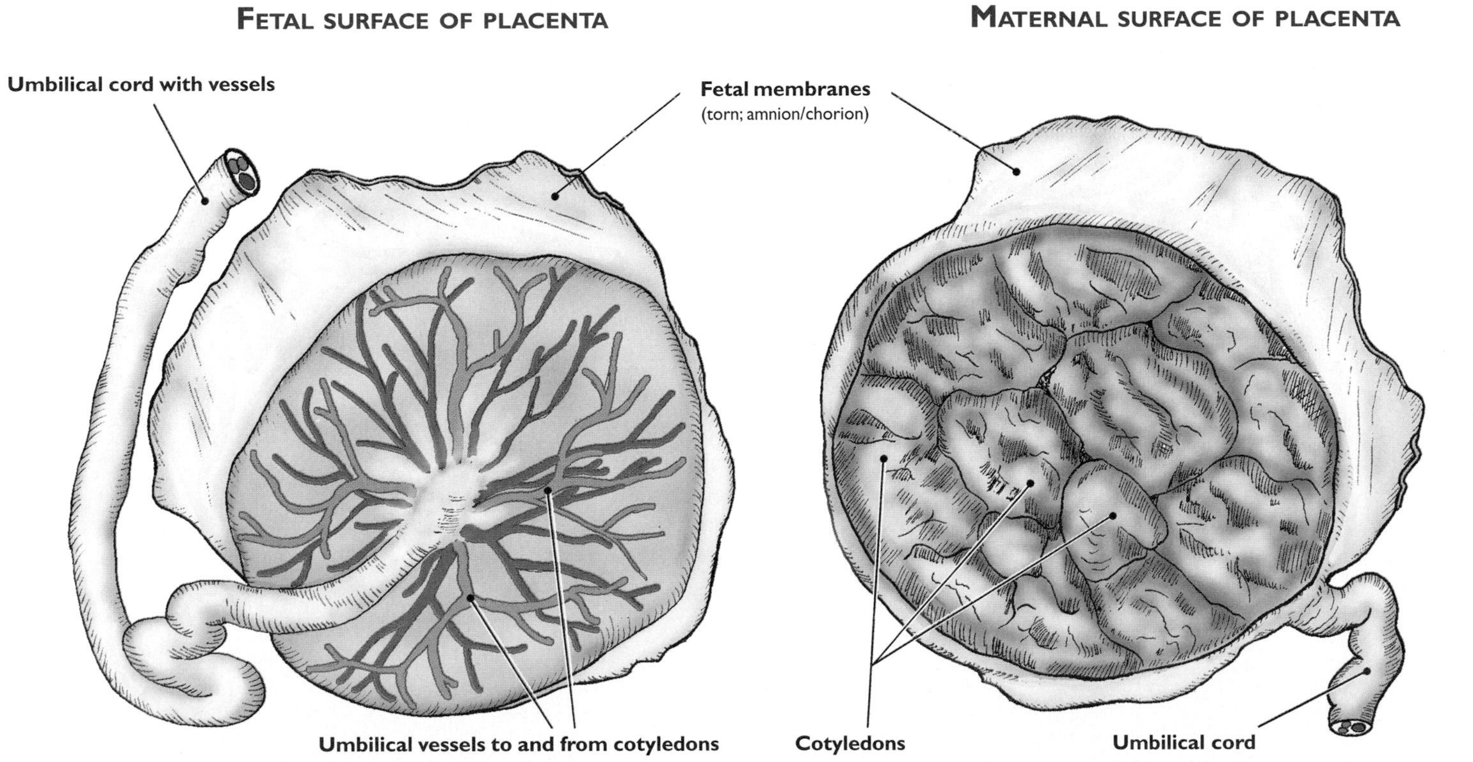

Figure A.17. Fetal and maternal aspects of the placenta at term (images are approximately 1/3 of actual size).

Notes

INDEX

B

C

D

E

F

G

H

M

N

O

P

Q

R

S

W

X

Z